Modeling Correlated Outcomes Using Extensions of Generalized Estimating Equations and Linear Mixed Modeling

George J. Knafl

Modeling Correlated Outcomes Using Extensions of Generalized Estimating Equations and Linear Mixed Modeling

Springer

George J. Knafl
School of Nursing
University of North Carolina at Chapel Hill
Chapel Hill, NC, USA

ISBN 978-3-031-41987-4 ISBN 978-3-031-41988-1 (eBook)
https://doi.org/10.1007/978-3-031-41988-1

Mathematics Subject Classification (2020): 62-04; 62-08; 62J02; 62P10

This Springer imprint is published by the registered company Springer Nature Switzerland AG
The registered company address is: Gewerbestrasse 11, 6330 Cham, Switzerland

Preface

Multiple outcome measurements taken as part of a research study for the same participant of that study are likely to be correlated. Examples include outcomes repeatedly measured over multiple times in longitudinal studies, under different treatments in crossover studies, and over multiple related measures in cross-sectional studies. Results of analyses that treat such outcome measurements as independent are questionable because possible outcome correlation has not been accounted for. When the outcome measurements are continuous and can be treated as multivariate normally distributed, they can be appropriately analyzed accounting for outcome correlation using linear mixed modeling (LMM). On the other hand, when the outcome measurements are categorical, calculation of likelihoods accounting for outcome correlation can pose computational problems. For this reason, generalized estimating equation (GEE) methods have been developed that specify equations to solve for estimation of mean parameters without specifying a likelihood while accounting for outcome correlation. GEE treats variances as specific functions of the means, possibly augmented with a constant dispersion parameter. GEE uses estimates of correlation parameters and of the dispersion parameter that are based on residuals.

Basing general variances/dispersions on multiple predictor variables can provide substantial benefits for modeling correlated outcomes. LMM supports possibly non-constant variances without modification. In that case, estimating equations for the variance parameters are generated using maximum likelihood. In contrast, GEE requires modification to provide estimating equations for variance/dispersion parameters. It can be demonstrated that the GEE estimating equations for the mean parameters can be generated by partially maximizing a likelihood function based on the multivariate normal density evaluated using the Pearson residuals. This likelihood function can be maximized in the variance/dispersion parameters to produce estimating equations for those parameters. Partially modified GEE combines these estimating equations for the variance/dispersion parameters with the standard GEE estimating equations for the mean parameters to obtain joint estimates for both types of parameters. Fully modified GEE maximizes the likelihood function in the mean and variance/dispersion parameters to generate joint estimating equations for both types of parameters. Partially and fully modified GEE use the standard GEE approach based on residuals to estimate the correlation parameters. Extended linear mixed modeling (ELMM) maximizes the likelihood function to generate joint estimating equations for the mean, variance/dispersion, and correlation parameters. LMM is the special case of ELMM with outcomes treated as normally distributed.

The likelihood function can also be used to compute model selection criteria for comparing alternative models for correlated outcomes. It can be combined with standard penalty functions to generate penalized likelihood criteria such as the Akaike information criterion and the Bayesian information criterion. It can also be used to compute likelihood cross-validation (LCV) scores with larger scores indicating better models. These model selection criteria can be used with existing adaptive regression methods to model nonlinear relationships for means and variances/dispersions of correlated outcomes in predictor variables. Consideration of nonlinearity in predictor variables can provide substantial benefits over standard models based on linearity in predictors for modeling of correlated outcomes.

This book provides formulations for standard GEE, partially modified GEE, fully modified GEE, and ELMM for modeling of correlated continuous, count/rate, dichotomous, polytomous, and discrete numeric outcomes including equations for computing associated gradient vectors and Hessian matrices. It provides a wide variety of example analyses of specific correlated outcomes of these types comparing results for standard GEE, partially modified GEE, fully modified GEE, and ELMM as well as demonstrating the benefits of considering non-constant variances/dispersions and nonlinearity of means and variances/dispersions. It also provides systematic strategies for conducting general adaptive analyses of correlated outcomes.

Supplementary materials are also available with each chapter. Download and unzip the folder Knafl.CorrOutcomesSM.zip to create the folder Knafl.CorrOutcomesSM. The file readme.txt in that folder provides a description of the other available files and subfolders. These include the genreg (for general regression) SAS macro used to generate GEE and ELMM models and their LCV scores, SAS code for loading in data and for analyzing those data as used in generating reported analyses, computational details for some of the more complex formulations not reported in the book for brevity, an Excel workbook for computing cutoffs for distinct percent decreases in LCV scores for comparing models, and the data files for conducting some reported analyses. URLs are also provided for obtaining data files from the Internet used in the other reported analyses.

Chapel Hill, NC, USA George J. Knafl

Acknowledgments

Thanks to Eva Hiripi of Springer for her support in the development of this book and to my wife Kathleen for all her encouragement on a daily basis. The development of the genreg macro used in reported analyses was partially supported by grants R01 AI57043 from the National Institute of Allergy and Infectious Diseases and R03 MH086132 from the National Institute of Mental Health.

About This Book

The book starts with an introduction in Chapter 1 followed by 15 more chapters organized into three parts. Part I addresses correlated sets of univariate outcomes of continuous, count/rate, and dichotomous types. Part II extends the material of Part I to address correlated sets of polytomous outcomes. Part III provides systematic strategies for conducting adaptive analyses of correlated outcomes as well as analyses demonstrating those strategies.

Part I has eight chapters. Chapters 2–5 provide formulations for standard GEE, partially modified GEE, fully modified GEE, and ELMM, respectively. Chapters 6–9 provide example analyses using standard GEE, partially modified GEE, fully modified GEE, and ELMM of specific correlated sets of univariate outcomes using, respectively, linear regression of continuous normally distributed outcomes, Poisson regression of Poisson distributed count/rate outcomes, logistic regression of Bernoulli distributed dichotomous outcomes, and exponential regression of positive continuous exponentially distributed outcomes.

Part II has five chapters. Chapter 10 provides formulations for multinomial regression of polytomous outcomes with nominal or ordinal values, Chapter 11 for ordinal regression of polytomous outcomes with ordinal values, and Chapter 12 for discrete regression of polytomous outcomes with discrete numeric values. Chapters 13–14 provide example analyses of a trichotomous correlated outcome using multinomial and ordinal regression in Chapter 13 and discrete regression in Chapter 14.

Part III has two chapters. Chapter 15 describes concise analyses for the data sets previously analyzed more extensively in Chapters 6–9 and 13–14, specifies systematic strategies for conducting concise adaptive analyses of correlated outcomes justified by the prior analyses reported in the chapter, provides an evaluation of the effectiveness of ELMM for analyzing theory-based models, and addresses future work needed for analyzing correlated outcomes. Chapter 16 uses the analysis strategies of Chapter 15 to conduct concise adaptive analyses of specific correlated outcomes not considered earlier and addressing contexts not considered earlier.

Contents

About the Author

George J. Knafl is Biostatistician and Professor Emeritus in the School of Nursing of the University of North Carolina at Chapel Hill where he taught statistics courses for doctoral nursing students, consulted with doctoral students and faculty on their research, and conducted his own research. He has over 45 years of experience in teaching, consulting, and research in statistics. He has continued to conduct research involving development of methods for searching through alternative models for different types of statistical data and application of those methods to the analysis of a variety of health science data sets. He is also Professor Emeritus in the College of Computing and Digital Media at DePaul University and has served on the faculties of the Schools of Nursing at Yale University and at the Oregon Health and Science University.

Abbreviations

AIC	Akaike information criterion
AR1	autoregressive order 1
BIC	Bayesian information criterion
DF	degrees of freedom
EC	exchangeable correlations
ELMM	extended linear mixed modeling
FaMM	Family Management Measure
GEE	generalized estimating equations
IND	independent
LCV	likelihood cross-validation
LMM	linear mixed modeling
QIC	quasi-likelihood information criterion
PD	percent decrease
TLC	Treatment of Lead-exposed Children
UN	unstructured

Chapter 1
Introduction

Abstract An overview is provided of the material covered in the book. Methods are formulated in the book for modifications/extensions of generalized estimating equations (GEE) and of linear mixed modeling (LMM) based on maximizing a likelihood function to generate estimating equations for parameter estimation. Example analyses are also provided in the book applying these methods to a variety of correlated sets of outcomes and using adaptive regression for modeling possible nonlinear relationships for those outcomes.

Keywords Adaptive regression modeling · Correlated outcomes · Extended linear mixed modeling · Generalized estimating equations

Introduction An overview is provided in the chapter of the material covered in the book. Section 1.1 provides background information, Sect. 1.2 an overview of Part I, Sect. 1.3 an overview of Part II, and Sect. 1.4 an overview of Part III.

1.1 Background

Computation of likelihoods for general correlated outcome (dependent, response, y) variables can be challenging except in limited cases due to their complexity. The GEE approach for modeling correlated outcomes was formulated by Liang and Zeger (1986) to circumvent this problem by addressing the marginal distribution rather than the full joint distribution. It extended generalized linear modeling (McCullagh, 1983; Wedderburn, 1974) to account for outcome correlation. GEE specifies estimating equations for mean parameters as would be generated by maximizing a likelihood, but without specifying a likelihood to avoid having to compute it. Estimates of correlation parameters and of a constant dispersion

Supplementary Information The online version contains supplementary material available at https://doi.org/10.1007/978-3-031-41988-1_1.

G. J. Knafl, *Modeling Correlated Outcomes Using Extensions of Generalized Estimating Equations and Linear Mixed Modeling*,
https://doi.org/10.1007/978-3-031-41988-1_1

parameter are then based on residuals. In the case of discrete outcomes, GEE implementations often only handle dichotomous outcomes with two outcome values, not general polytomous outcomes with more than two outcome values. Lipsitz et al. (1994) and Miller et al. (1993) provide extensions to handle correlated polytomous outcomes.

Knafl and Ding (2016) define a "likelihood" function L based on the multivariate normal density computed using the residuals and covariance matrices generated by the GEE approach. They note that the estimating equations for the mean parameters generated by maximizing L can be separated into the sum of two terms. The term corresponding to differentiating the residuals in the mean parameters while holding the covariances fixed in those parameters generates the standard GEE estimating equations. Thus, GEE modeling can be considered a "semi-maximum likelihood" or a "quasi-maximum likelihood" estimation method (see also Chaganty, 1997, who proposed an alternative "quasi-least squares" estimation method).

The availability of the function L allows for three related extensions of standard GEE modeling. First, it can be partially modified by maximizing L in variance/dispersion parameters to generate variance/dispersion estimating equations to combine with the standard GEE mean estimating equations (as initially addressed in Knafl & Ding, 2016). Second, a fully modified GEE approach can be defined by maximizing L jointly in parameters for the means as well as for the variances/dispersions. Both of these cases use the GEE approach for estimating correlations based on the residuals. The third possible modification maximizes L in all the model parameters including those for correlations as well as those for means and variances/dispersions. This third approach is extended linear mixed modeling (ELMM) in the sense that it involves fully maximizing the multivariate normal density function extended to general outcomes, not just normally distributed outcomes. It is standard linear mixed modeling (LMM) when the outcomes are treated as normally distributed.

The function L can be used to compute GEE model selection criteria. For example, it can be used to compute extensions of penalized likelihood criteria (Sclove, 1987) to address the GEE and ELMM contexts. It can also be used to compute likelihood cross-validation (LCV) scores for controlling the adaptive regression modeling process of Knafl and Ding (2016) to use in estimating nonlinear relationships for general correlated outcomes. In this book, standard GEE, partially modified GEE, fully modified GEE, and ELMM are formulated and their use in generating nonlinear relationships is demonstrated through example analyses. All example analyses are generated using SAS® Version 9.4 (SAS Institute, Inc., Cary, NC). A SAS macro and related SAS code have been implemented to support the methods and to generate example analyses.

Example analyses reported in the book are primarily adaptive, based on heuristic search through alternative models, i.e., sets of predictors, for the outcome variable. The search is controlled by LCV scores and tolerance parameters indicating how much of decrease (penalty) in the LCV score can be tolerated at given stages of the search process. This process generates an effective model for the data in the sense that the removal of any predictor from the final model generates a distinct decrease in that model's LCV score. In adaptive modeling, the choice of the model is data-driven, that is, based on its applicability to the data under analysis. Theory-based modeling is the more conventional approach used in the literature where a specific model is chosen based on a theoretical framework (also called a conceptual framework) and then assessed using hypothesis tests for zero parameter values. Adaptive modeling is more complicated than theory-based modeling. Furthermore, hypothesis tests for zero parameters of adaptive models are typically significant as a consequence of the adaptive modeling process and so are not appropriate to use for inferential purposes.

1.2 Overview of Part I

Part I addresses the analysis of correlated sets of univariate outcomes including continuous, count/rate, and dichotomous outcomes. This includes cases with the same univariate outcome repeatedly measured over multiple conditions such as times or patients of the same provider as well as cases with multiple related univariate outcomes such as multiple dimensions of quality of life. Chapter 2 provides an initial formulation for modeling of correlated sets of univariate outcomes as well as for standard GEE modeling of such outcomes. Chapters 3–5 cover extensions addressing partially modified GEE, fully modified GEE, and ELMM modeling, respectively, of correlated univariate outcomes.

Chapters 2–5 provide formulations for modeling of correlated continuous, count/rate, and dichotomous outcomes using linear, Poisson, logistic, and exponential regression methods. This includes generalized linear modeling of means with variances a specific function of the means and combined together with possibly non-constant dispersions into extended variances. Direct variance modeling is also considered with variances modeled only in terms of dispersions and not also treated as specific functions of the means. Correlation structures considered in these formulations include independent, exchangeable, spatial autoregressive order 1, and unstructured correlation structures.

Parameter estimation is based on solving estimating equations using a detailed multistep estimation process that extends Newton's method adjusted to account for possible estimation and convergence problems. For standard GEE, partially modified GEE, and fully modified GEE, this process is based on vectors and matrices treated as gradient vectors and Hessian matrices. For ELMM, parameter estimation is based on actual gradient vectors and Hessian matrices computed by differentiating the function L. Formulations are provided for all of these gradient vectors and Hessian matrices. For exchangeable and spatial autoregressive order 1 correlations, all ELMM computations can be computed without storing correlation matrices so that data with large numbers of correlated outcome measurements can be computed efficiently.

Chapters 6–9 provide example analyses of correlated univariate outcome data in the four contexts of linear, Poisson, logistic, and exponential regression, respectively. All four of these sets of analyses address cases with repeatedly measured univariate outcomes. The data analyzed in Chaps. 6–8 are equally spaced, while the data analyzed in Chap. 9 are unequally spaced. Analyses use adaptive methods (Knafl & Ding, 2016) to allow for possible nonlinear relationships. These methods are based on heuristic search through alternative models controlled by LCV scores for comparing those models.

Chapter 6 provides example analyses of dental measurements for girls and boys over ages 8, 10, 12, and 14 years. These analyses use linear regression methods based on the identity link function treating the dental measurements as normally distributed and correlated over ages for the same child. In this case, the function L is the multivariate normal density so that solving estimating equations based on derivatives for all model parameters is standard LMM. Means and variances of dental measurements are modeled as possibly nonlinear functions of child age, possibly changing with an additive effect to child gender, and/or possibly interacting with child gender.

Chapter 7 provides example analyses of seizure counts/rates for epilepsy patients in either a control or intervention group over periods prior to five clinic visits coded as 0–4. These analyses use Poisson regression methods based on the natural log link function treating the seizure counts as Poisson distributed and correlated over visits for the same patient. Models for the seizure counts are converted to models for seizure rates per week using an offset variable. Means and dispersions of seizure counts/rates are modeled as possibly nonlinear functions of visit, possibly changing with an additive effect to being in the intervention group, and/or possibly interacting with being in the intervention group.

Chapter 8 provides example analyses of dichotomous respiratory status levels of 0:poor or 1:good for patients with respiratory disorder on either placebo or active treatment over five clinic visits coded as 0–4. These analyses use logistic regression methods based on the logit link function treating the respiratory status levels as Bernoulli distributed and correlated over visits for the same patient. Treating 0:poor respiratory status level as the reference category, means, or equivalently probabilities for respiratory status 1:good, and dispersions are modeled as possibly nonlinear functions of visit, possibly changing with an additive effect to being on active treatment, and/or possibly interacting with being on active treatment.

Chapter 9 provides example analyses of blood lead levels for children taking either a placebo or the chelating agent succimer over 0, 1, 4, and 6 weeks. These analyses use exponential regression methods based on the log link function treating the blood lead levels as exponentially distributed and correlated over weeks for the same patient. Means and dispersions of blood lead levels are modeled as possibly nonlinear functions of week, possibly changing with an additive effect to being on succimer, and/or possibly interacting with being on succimer.

1.3 Overview of Part II

Part II addresses handling of correlated sets of polytomous outcomes with three or more possible outcome values. Chapters 10–12 cover methods for modeling such outcomes. Chapters 13 and 14 provide example analyses of such outcomes.

Chapter 10 addresses multinomial regression applied to polytomous outcomes having either nominal or ordinal values assigned to outcome categories. Chapter 11 covers ordinal regression applied to either individual or cumulative polytomous outcomes having ordinal values assigned to outcome categories. These alternatives apply to outcomes with $K + 1$ possible values corresponding to categories coded as 0, 1, $\cdots$, K, thereby generalizing logistic regression modeling of dichotomous outcomes with two possible values corresponding to categories coded as 0 and 1. They involve modeling correlated sets of multiple dichotomous outcomes determined by recoding each univariate polytomous outcome into a multivariate set of dichotomous indicators for that outcome taking on its possible values (except for one value treated as a reference category). Chapter 12 covers the related case of discrete outcomes with a finite number of possible numeric outcome values, including polytomous outcomes with ordinal categories, but as correlated sets of univariate outcomes rather than as correlated sets of multivariate outcomes. Three discrete regression alternatives are considered based on either multinomial, ordinal, or censored Poisson probabilities. Multinomial regression and multinomial probabilities are based on generalized logits for individual outcome values that depend on the same predictors but with different intercept and slope parameters. Ordinal regression and ordinal probabilities are based on cumulative logits for cumulative outcome values that depend on the same predictors with different intercept parameters and the same slope parameters. Censored Poisson probabilities are based on the same predictors with the same intercept and slope parameters.

Chapter 13 provides example analyses of multinomial and ordinal regression modeling of a polytomous outcome recoded as multiple dichotomous outcomes. Chapter 14 provides example analyses of discrete regression modeling of the same polytomous outcome without recoding it using multinomial, ordinal, and censored Poisson probabilities. The outcome for analyses in both chapters is trichotomous respiratory status, coded as 0:poor, 1:fair, or 2:good for patients with respiratory disorder on either placebo or active treatment over five clinic visits coded as 0–4. The dichotomous respiratory status outcome analyzed in Chap. 8 is obtained by recoding 1:fair and 2:good into the single value of 1:good.

Chapter 13 analyses use multinomial regression methods based on generalized logits applied to the trichotomous respiratory status levels correlated over visits for the same patient. Treating 0:poor respiratory status level as the reference category, probabilities of 1:fair and 2:good respiratory status levels at one time for one patient have 2×2 dimensional correlation matrices based on the multinomial distribution. Chapter 13 analyses also use ordinal regression methods based on cumulative logits applied to the trichotomous respiratory status levels treated as correlated over visits for the same patient. This generates cumulative probabilities for having respiratory status levels $\leq$0:poor, $\leq$1:fair, and $\leq$ 2:good, which are differenced to generate individual probabilities for having respiratory status levels 0:poor, 1:fair, and 2: good. Ordinal analyses are conducted using outcomes based on indicators either for the individual ordinal probabilities or for the cumulative ordinal probabilities. Treating 2:good respiratory status level as the reference category, indicators for individual ordinal probabilities of 0:poor and 1:fair respiratory status levels at one time for one patient have 2×2 dimensional correlation matrices based on the multinomial distribution. Treating $\leq$2:good respiratory status level as the reference category, indicators for cumulative ordinal probabilities of $\leq$0:poor and $\leq$1:fair respiratory status levels at one time for one patient have 2×2 dimensional correlation matrices similar to but not the same as those determined by the multinomial distribution. Combined correlation matrices have $5 \cdot 5 = 25$ component correlation matrices of dimension 2×2. Combined correlation structures considered include independent, exchangeable, spatial autoregressive order 1, and unstructured. Methods for efficiently computing exchangeable and spatial autoregressive order 1 without storing the correlation matrices do not extend to associated combined correlation matrices. The diagonal component matrices are functions of the probabilities and so can be different for different patients, complicating computation of parameter estimates. The multinomial, individual ordinal, and cumulative ordinal probabilities as well as the dispersions for trichotomous respiratory status are modeled as possibly nonlinear functions of visit, possibly changing with an additive effect to being on active treatment, and/or possibly interacting with being on active treatment.

Chapter 14 analyses use discrete regression methods applied to the trichotomous respiratory status levels correlated over visits for the same patient as also analyzed in Chap. 13. Correlation structures considered include independent, exchangeable, spatial autoregressive order 1, and unstructured correlations. Correlation matrices have dimension 5×5 and so are less complex than the correlation matrices used in analyses of Chap. 13. Computations for exchangeable and spatial autoregressive order 1 correlation can be conducted efficiently without storing correlation matrices. Three types of probabilities are considered. Multinomial and ordinal probabilities are computed in the same way as probabilities for multinomial and ordinal regression, respectively. Censored Poisson probabilities are computed for the first K outcome values using standard Poisson probabilities. The probability for the last outcome value is set so that the probabilities sum to 1 and so equals the standard Poisson probability for all values larger than or equal to K; hence these are censored Poisson probabilities. The multinomial, ordinal, and censored Poisson probabilities as well as the dispersions for trichotomous respiratory status treated as a discrete outcome are modeled as possibly nonlinear functions of visit, possibly changing with an additive effect to being on active treatment, and/or possibly interacting with being on active treatment.

1.4 Overview of Part III

Analyses reported in Chaps. 6–9 of Part I and Chaps. 13 and 14 of Part II are purposely more detailed than is typically required to adaptively analyze a data set with correlated outcomes. All of these data sets have repeatedly measured longitudinal outcomes with no missing outcome values. Part III demonstrates how to conduct concise analyses of these and other data sets. Chapter 15 provides concise analyses for the data sets analyzed in Chaps. 6–9 and 13 and 14 as covered in Sects. 15.1–15.6, respectively, and uses these results to specify in Sect. 15.8 analysis strategies for general adaptive analysis of correlated outcomes. Example analyses so far emphasize adaptive modeling issues. However, theory-based analyses also need to be conducted for correlated outcomes. For this reason, Sect. 15.9 provides an evaluation of the effectiveness of ELMM for analyzing theory-based models. Chapter 15 ends with Sect. 15.10 addressing future work needed for analyzing correlated outcomes.

Chapter 16 demonstrates the use of the analysis strategies specified in Chap. 15 using data not previously analyzed and of different kinds. Section 16.1 provides analyses of correlated cross-sectional outcomes corresponding to different scales of a survey instrument measuring problematic aspects of family management of childhood chronic conditions for single mothers. Sections 16.2–16.4 provide analyses of correlated dyadic data for partnered parents with some missing outcome measurements on conduct-disordered behaviors of children with chronic conditions including a continuous, count, and dichotomous outcome measure of the intensity, number of problems, and a high level of conduct-disordered behaviors, respectively.

References

Chaganty, N. R. (1997). An alternative approach to the analysis of longitudinal data via generalized estimating equations. *Journal of Statistical Planning and Inference, 63*, 39–54.

Knafl, G. J., & Ding, K. (2016). *Adaptive regression for modeling nonlinear relationships*. Springer.

Liang, K.-Y., & Zeger, S. L. (1986). Longitudinal data analysis using generalized linear models. *Biometrika, 73*, 13–22.

Lipsitz, S. R., Kim, K., & Zhao, L. (1994). Analysis of repeated categorical data using generalized estimating equations. *Statistics in Medicine, 13*, 1149–1163.

McCullagh, P. (1983). Quasi-likelihood functions. *Annals of Statistics, 11*, 59–67.

Miller, M. E., Davis, C. S., & Landis, J. R. (1993). The analysis of longitudinal polytomous data: Generalized estimating equations and connections with weighted least squares. *Biometrics, 49*, 1033–1044.

Sclove, S. L. (1987). Application of model-selection criteria to some problems in multivariate analysis. *Psychometrika, 52*, 333–343.

Wedderburn, R. W. M. (1974). Quasi-likelihood functions, generalized linear models, and the Gauss-Newton method. *Biometrika, 61*, 439–447.

Part I
Continuous, Count, and Dichotomous Outcomes

The chapters of Part I address modeling of correlated sets of univariate outcomes including continuous, count/rate, and dichotomous outcomes. Chapter 2 addresses standard GEE modeling with constant dispersions while providing an initial formulation for the modeling and analysis of correlated univariate outcomes. Chapter 3 extends the formulation to partially modified GEE modeling allowing for non-constant dispersions by augmenting standard GEE estimating equations for means with estimating equations for dispersions. Chapter 4 extends the formulation further to address fully modified GEE modeling with revised estimating equations for means along with the estimating equations for dispersions used in partially modified GEE modeling. Standard, partially modified, and fully modified GEE modeling use the GEE approach for estimating correlation parameters computed with residuals. Chapter 5 extends the formulation even further to address combined estimation of mean, dispersion, and correlation parameters by augmenting the estimating equations for means and dispersions of fully modified GEE to include estimating equations for correlation parameters. Chapters 6–9 provide example analyses of correlated univariate outcome data using partially modified GEE, fully modified GEE, and ELMM modeling. Chapter 6 addresses such analyses in the context of linear regression for real-valued continuous outcomes under the normal distribution with identity link function. Chapter 7 addresses such analyses in the context of Poisson regression for count/rate outcomes under the Poisson distribution with natural log link function. Chapter 8 addresses such analyses in the context of logistic regression for dichotomous outcomes under the Bernoulli distribution with logit link function. Chapter 9 addresses such analyses in the context of exponential regression for positive continuous outcomes under the exponential distribution with natural log link function.

Chapters 2–5 provide technical details for standard GEE, partially modified GEE, fully modified GEE, and extended linear mixed modeling, respectively. These chapters can be skipped by readers more interested in the data analyses reported in Chaps. 6–9.

Chapter 2
Standard GEE Modeling of Correlated Univariate Outcomes

Abstract Formulations are provided for correlated sets of univariate outcomes allowing for missing values, generalized linear modeling of means for such outcomes, correlation structures, and the standard generalized estimating equations (GEE) approach to modeling those outcomes. Four cases for generalized linear modeling of means are considered: linear regression with the identity link function for normally distributed continuous outcomes, Poisson regression with the natural log link function for Poisson distributed count outcomes and related rate outcomes, logistic regression with the logit link function for dichotomous 0/1-valued outcomes, and exponential regression with the natural log link function for exponentially distributed positive-valued continuous outcomes. Four correlation structures are considered: independent, exchangeable, spatial autoregressive order 1, and unstructured correlations. Formulations of a likelihood function for addressing standard GEE modeling and of likelihood cross-validation (LCV) scores for GEE model selection are provided. Two approaches for computing LCV scores are considered: matched-set-wise deletion and measurement-wise deletion. An overview of adaptive regression for modeling nonlinear relationships is provided as well as descriptions for the four data sets to be used in later adaptive analyses.

Keywords Adaptive regression modeling · Correlated outcomes · Generalized estimating equations · Likelihood cross-validation

Introduction In this chapter, formulations are provided for correlated univariate outcomes in Sect. 2.1, generalized linear modeling of means for such outcomes in Sect. 2.2, correlation structures in Sect. 2.3, and the standard GEE approach to modeling those outcomes in Sect. 2.4. Four cases for generalized linear modeling of means are considered: linear, Poisson, logistic, and exponential regression in Sects. 2.2.1–2.2.4, respectively. Four correlation structures are considered: independent, exchangeable, spatial autoregressive order 1, and unstructured correlations in Sects.

Supplementary Information The online version contains supplementary material available at https://doi.org/10.1007/978-3-031-41988-1_2.

G. J. Knafl, *Modeling Correlated Outcomes Using Extensions of Generalized Estimating Equations and Linear Mixed Modeling*,
https://doi.org/10.1007/978-3-031-41988-1_2

2.3.1–2.3.4, respectively. Formulations of a likelihood function for standard GEE modeling, of likelihood cross-validation scores for model selection, and an overview of adaptive regression for modeling nonlinear relationships are also provided in Sects. 2.5–2.7, respectively. Descriptions are provided in Sect. 2.8 for the four data sets to be used in the analyses of Chaps. 6–9.

2.1 Correlated Univariate Outcomes

Assume that univariate outcome values y_{sc} are measured over $m(s)$ conditions indexed by $c \in C(s)$, a subset of the full set of conditions $C = \{c : 1 \leq c \leq m\}$, for matched sets of outcomes with indexes $s \in S = \{s : 1 \leq s \leq n\}$. Let $SC = \{sc : c \in C(s), s \in S\}$ denote the full set of

$$m(SC) = \sum_{s \in S} m(s)$$

observed index pairs. Combine the $m(s)$ outcome values over $c \in C(s)$ into $m(s) \times 1$ vectors $\boldsymbol{y}_s$ for $s \in S$.

The matched sets are usually called subjects as is appropriate when the conditions are times at which, or treatments under which, each study subject/participant is measured. However, the matched sets can correspond to sets of study subjects/participants, for example, members of the same family or patients of the same provider, and then the conditions correspond to individual subjects/participants, not the matched sets.

2.2 Generalized Linear Modeling

Assume that predictor values $x_{sc,j}$ for $1 \leq j \leq r$ are measured for $sc \in SC$. For each $sc \in SC$, combine the r predictor values into $r \times 1$ vectors $\boldsymbol{x}_{sc}$ and, for $s \in S$, let $\boldsymbol{X}_s$ denote the $m(s) \times r$ predictor matrices with rows $\boldsymbol{x}_{sc}^{\mathrm{T}}$ (i.e., the transpose of $\boldsymbol{x}_{sc}$). Denote the mean or expected value of y_{sc} as $\mu_{sc} = \mathrm{E}y_{sc}$ for $sc \in SC$. For $s \in S$, combine the means μ_{sc} over $c \in C(s)$ into the $m(s) \times 1$ vectors $\boldsymbol{\mu}_s$. The residuals are $e_{sc} = y_{sc} - \mu_{sc}$. Combine these into the $m(s) \times 1$ residual vectors

$$\boldsymbol{e}_s = \boldsymbol{y}_s - \boldsymbol{\mu}_s.$$

Use a generalized linear model (McCullagh & Nelder, 1999) for the means satisfying

$$g(\mu_{sc}) = \mathbf{x}_{sc}^{\mathrm{T}} \cdot \boldsymbol{\beta}$$

for a $r \times 1$ vector $\boldsymbol{\beta}$ of coefficient parameters and for some link function g. Thus,

$$\frac{\partial g(\mu_{sc})}{\partial \beta_j} = \frac{dg(\mu_{sc})}{d\mu} \cdot \frac{\partial \mu_{sc}}{\partial \beta_j} = x_{sc,j}$$

giving

$$\frac{\partial \mu_{sc}}{\partial \beta_j} = \frac{x_{sc,j}}{\frac{dg(\mu_{sc})}{d\mu}}$$

for $sc \in SC$ and $1 \leq j \leq r$. When $x_{sc,1} = 1$ for $sc \in SC$, the first entry β_1 of $\boldsymbol{\beta}$ is an intercept parameter.

The variance function $V(\mu)$ indicates how the variances depend on the means (examples are provided in Sects. 2.2.1–2.2.4). Assuming constant dispersions for now based on the single dispersion parameter φ, define the extended variances for the outcomes y_{sc} as

$$\sigma_{sc}^2 = \varphi \cdot V(\mu_{sc}).$$

Let $\boldsymbol{\sigma}_s$ denote the $m(s) \times 1$ vector with entries

$$\sigma_{sc} = (\varphi \cdot V(\mu_{sc}))^{1/2}.$$

The standardized residuals are $stde_{sc} = e_{sc}/\sigma_{sc}$, and the Pearson residuals are

$$Pres_{sc} = \varphi^{1/2} \cdot stde_{sc} = \frac{e_{sc}}{V^{1/2}(\mu_{sc})}.$$

Combine the standardized residuals and Pearson residuals into their respective $m(s) \times 1$ vectors $\boldsymbol{stde}_s$ and $\boldsymbol{Pres}_s$ for $s \in S$. Four examples under different outcome distributions and link functions are presented next.

2.2.1 Linear Regression with Identity Link Function

Outcomes y_{sc} are continuous real-valued and are treated as normally distributed. The link function is the identity function $g(\mu) = \mu$ for $-\infty < \mu < \infty$ with derivative

$$\frac{dg(\mu)}{d\mu} = 1.$$

This is the canonical choice for the link function for the normal distribution. The variance function is $V(\mu) = 1$ so that the constant dispersion parameter is the same as the usual constant variance parameter. Formally, the extended variances are

$$\sigma_{sc}^2 = \varphi \cdot V(\mu_{sc}) = \varphi$$

(the same as the variances), the extended standard deviations are $\sigma_{sc} = \varphi^{1/2}$, and the standardized residuals are

$$stde_{sc} = \frac{y_{sc} - \mu_{sc}}{\varphi^{1/2}}.$$

The means satisfy $\mu_{sc} = \boldsymbol{x}_{sc}^{\mathrm{T}} \cdot \boldsymbol{\beta}$ with partial derivatives

$$\frac{\partial \mu_{sc}}{\partial \beta_j} = \frac{x_{sc,j}}{\frac{dg(\mu_{sc})}{d\mu}} = x_{sc,j}$$

for $sc \in SC$ and $1 \leq j \leq r$.

2.2.2 *Poisson Regression with Natural Log Link Function*

Outcomes y_{sc} are count-valued, that is, nonnegative integer-valued, and are treated as Poisson distributed. The link function is the natural log function $g(\mu) = \log \mu$ for $0 < \mu < \infty$ with derivative

$$\frac{dg(\mu)}{d\mu} = \frac{1}{\mu}.$$

This is the canonical choice for the link function for the Poisson distribution. The variance function is $V(\mu) = \mu$. The means satisfy $\mu_{sc} = \exp\left(\boldsymbol{x}_{sc}^{\mathrm{T}} \cdot \boldsymbol{\beta}\right)$ with partial derivatives

$$\frac{\partial \mu_{sc}}{\partial \beta_j} = \frac{x_{sc,j}}{\frac{dg(\mu_{sc})}{d\mu}} = x_{sc,j} \cdot \mu_{sc}$$

for $sc \in SC$ and $1 \leq j \leq r$. The extended variances are

$$\sigma_{sc}^2 = \varphi \cdot V(\mu_{sc}) = \varphi \cdot \mu_{sc},$$

the extended standard deviations are $\sigma_{sc} = (\varphi \cdot \mu_{sc})^{1/2}$, and the standardized residuals are

$$stde_{sc} = \frac{y_{sc} - \mu_{sc}}{\sigma_{sc}}$$

for $sc \in SC$.

Outcome counts y_{sc} often have associated totals $T_{sc} > 0$ and the model for the mean counts μ_{sc} is then converted to a model for the associated rates $y'_{sc} = y_{sc}/T_{sc}$ (or proportions when T_{sc} are also counts) by adding the offset variable $o_{sc} = \log T_{sc}$ to the log of the mean counts. Formally, replace $\boldsymbol{x}_{sc}^{\mathrm{T}} \cdot \boldsymbol{\beta}$ with $\boldsymbol{x}_{sc}^{\mathrm{T}} \cdot \boldsymbol{\beta} + o_{sc}$ so that the mean counts are

$$\mu_{sc} = \exp\left(\boldsymbol{x}_{sc}^{\mathrm{T}} \cdot \boldsymbol{\beta} + o_{sc}\right)$$

and then

$$\mu'_{sc} = Ey'_{sc} = \frac{\mu_{sc}}{T_{sc}} = \exp\left(\boldsymbol{x}_{sc}^{\mathrm{T}} \cdot \boldsymbol{\beta}\right)$$

are the mean rates. Combine the offsets o_{sc} into the $m(s) \times 1$ vectors $\boldsymbol{o}_s$.

2.2.3 Logistic Regression with Logit Link Function

Outcomes y_{sc} are dichotomous with two possible values 0 and 1 and are treated as Bernoulli distributed so that $\mu_{sc} = \mathrm{P}(y_{sc} = 1)$. The link function is the logit function

$$g(\mu) = \mathrm{logit}(\mu) = \log \frac{\mu}{1-\mu}$$

for $0 < \mu < 1$ with derivative

$$\frac{dg(\mu)}{d\mu} = \frac{1}{\mu \cdot (1-\mu)}.$$

This is the canonical choice for the link function for the Bernoulli distribution. The variance function is $V(\mu) = \mu \cdot (1 - \mu)$. The means satisfy

$$\mu_{sc} = \frac{\exp\left(\boldsymbol{x}_{sc}^{\mathrm{T}} \cdot \boldsymbol{\beta}\right)}{1 + \exp\left(\boldsymbol{x}_{sc}^{\mathrm{T}} \cdot \boldsymbol{\beta}\right)}$$

with partial derivatives

$$\frac{\partial \mu_{sc}}{\partial \beta_j} = \frac{x_{sc,j}}{\frac{dg(\mu_{sc})}{d\mu}} = x_{sc,j} \cdot \mu_{sc} \cdot (1 - \mu_{sc})$$

for $sc \in SC$ and $1 \leq j \leq r$. The extended variances are

$$\sigma_{sc}^2 = \varphi \cdot V(\mu_{sc}) = \varphi \cdot \mu_{sc} \cdot (1 - \mu_{sc}),$$

the extended standard deviations are

$$\sigma_{sc} = (\varphi \cdot \mu_{sc} \cdot (1 - \mu_{sc}))^{1/2},$$

and the standardized residuals are

$$stde_{sc} = \frac{y_{sc} - \mu_{sc}}{\sigma_{sc}}$$

for $sc \in SC$.

2.2.4 Exponential Regression with Natural Log Link Function

Outcomes y_{sc} are continuous positive-valued and are treated as exponentially distributed. The link function is the natural log function $g(\mu) = \log \mu$ for $0 < \mu < \infty$ with derivative

$$\frac{dg(\mu)}{d\mu} = \frac{1}{\mu}.$$

The variance function is $V(\mu) = \mu^2$. The means satisfy $\mu_{sc} = \exp\left(\boldsymbol{x}_{sc}^{\mathrm{T}} \cdot \boldsymbol{\beta}\right)$ with partial derivatives

$$\frac{\partial \mu_{sc}}{\partial \beta_j} = \frac{x_{sc,j}}{\frac{dg(\mu_{sc})}{d\mu}} = x_{sc,j} \cdot \mu_{sc}$$

for $sc \in SC$ and $1 \leq j \leq r$. The extended variances are

$$\sigma_{sc}^2 = \varphi \cdot V(\mu_{sc}) = \varphi \cdot \mu_{sc}^2,$$

the extended standard deviations are $\sigma_{sc} = \varphi^{1/2} \cdot \mu_{sc}$, and the standardized residuals are

$$stde_{sc} = \frac{y_{sc} - \mu_{sc}}{\sigma_{sc}}$$

for $sc \in SC$.

The natural log function is not the canonical choice for the link function for the exponential distribution. The canonical choice is the reciprocal function $g(\mu) = 1/\mu$ for $0 < \mu < \infty$, but that generates means $\mu_{sc} = 1/\left(\boldsymbol{x}_{sc}^{\mathrm{T}} \cdot \boldsymbol{\beta}\right)$ so that the estimation process needs adjustment to guarantee positive values for all $\boldsymbol{x}_{sc}^{\mathrm{T}} \cdot \boldsymbol{\beta}$. The natural log link function does not have this shortcoming.

The gamma distribution generalizes the exponential distribution and has an extra parameter ν with $\nu = 1$ corresponding to the exponential distribution. McCullagh and Nelder (1999) cover the more general gamma distribution and not the exponential distribution, but the variance function $V(\mu) = \mu^2$ is the same for both cases. Consequently, standard GEE formulations are the same for the gamma distribution as for the exponential distribution, as is also the case for partially modified GEE, fully modified GEE, and ELMM to be covered in Chaps. 3–5, respectively. For this reason, only the exponential case is considered.

2.3 Modeling Correlations

Denote the $m(s) \times m(s)$ covariance matrix for the outcome vector $\boldsymbol{y}_s$ as $\boldsymbol{\Sigma}_s$ for $s \in S$. Use the GEE approach (Liang & Zeger, 1986) to model $\boldsymbol{\Sigma}_s$ as

$$\boldsymbol{\Sigma}_s = \boldsymbol{DIAG}(\boldsymbol{\sigma}_s) \cdot \boldsymbol{R}_s(\boldsymbol{\rho}) \cdot \boldsymbol{DIAG}(\boldsymbol{\sigma}_s)$$

where $\boldsymbol{DIAG}(\boldsymbol{\sigma}_s)$ is the $m(s) \times m(s)$ diagonal matrix with diagonal entries σ_{sc} for $c \in C(s)$ and $\boldsymbol{R}_s(\boldsymbol{\rho})$ is a $m(s) \times m(s)$ correlation matrix determined by a $p \times 1$ vector $\boldsymbol{\rho}$ of correlation parameters, varying with the assumed correlation structure. The full $m \times m$ correlation matrix $\boldsymbol{R}(\boldsymbol{\rho})$ is called the working correlation matrix. Four useful correlation structures are described next.

2.3.1 Independent Correlations

Under independent (IND) correlations, the correlation matrices $\boldsymbol{R}_s(\boldsymbol{\rho}_{\text{IND}})$ have entries $r_{c,c'}(\boldsymbol{\rho}_{\text{IND}}) = 0$ for $c \neq c'$ with $c, c' \in C(s)$. In this case, $\boldsymbol{\rho}_{\text{IND}}$ is the constant scalar with value 0.

2.3.2 Exchangeable Correlations

Under exchangeable correlations (EC), the correlation matrices $\boldsymbol{R}_s(\boldsymbol{\rho}_{\text{EC}})$ have entries $r_{c,c'}(\boldsymbol{\rho}_{\text{EC}}) = \rho_{\text{EC}}$ for $c \neq c'$ with $c, c' \in C(s)$. In this case, $\boldsymbol{\rho}_{\text{EC}}$ is a scalar parameter denoted by ρ_{EC}. This is the correlation structure used in standard repeated measures modeling. IND correlations correspond to the special case $\rho_{\text{EC}} = 0$.

2.3.3 Autoregressive Order 1 Correlations

Under non-spatial autoregressive order 1 (AR1) correlations, the correlation matrices $\boldsymbol{R}_s(\boldsymbol{\rho}_{\text{AR1}})$ have entries

$$r_{c,c'}(\boldsymbol{\rho}_{\text{AR1}}) = \rho_{\text{AR1}}^{|c' - c|}$$

where $-1 < \rho_{\text{AR1}} < 1$, $c, c' \in C(s)$, and $|c - c'|$ denotes the absolute value of the difference $c - c'$. In the special case with $c - c' = 0$, $\rho_{\text{AR1}}^{|c' - c|}$ equals 1 even when $\rho_{\text{AR1}} = 0$. In this case, $\boldsymbol{\rho}_{\text{AR1}}$ is a scalar parameter denoted by ρ_{AR1} and called the autocorrelation. IND correlations correspond to the special case $\rho_{\text{AR1}} = 0$. The correlations are well defined for all cases because the differences $c - c'$ are all integers. This assumes that outcome measurements within matched sets are truly ordered, as when the conditions correspond to times or dosages, and not nominally indexed, for example, as when the conditions c correspond to nurses working on the same hospital unit. Moreover, this treats outcome measurements as equally spaced, even when that is not the case. Statistical software typically assumes AR1 correlations are non-spatial in the GEE context.

Spatial AR1 correlations are also possible for handling non-equally spaced outcomes measured at values $t(c)$ strictly increasing in the integer indexes $c \in C$ (e.g., increasing measurement times or dosages). For the special case of non-spatial AR1, $t(c) = c$ for $c \in C$. In the more general spatial AR1 case, assume that the autocorrelation is nonnegative, that is, $\rho_{\text{AR1}} \geq 0$, so that $\rho_{\text{AR1}}^{|t(c') - t(c)|}$ is well defined for all ρ_{AR1} in the interval [0, 1) and all $c, c' \in C(s)$. In the special case with $t(c') - t(c) = 0$, $\rho_{\text{AR1}}^{|t(c') - t(c)|}$ equals 0 even when $\rho_{\text{AR1}} = 0$. To justify the assumption of a nonnegative autocorrelation, consider the case with equally spaced data and all distances $t(c') -$

$t(c)$ equal to a constant $d > 1$ as for the dental measurement data defined later in Sect. 2.8.1 with $t(c) = 8$, 10, 12, and 14 years for $1 \le c \le 4$ so that $d = 2$ years. Although no dental measurements are recorded for intermediate years, the child would have such dental measurements and so, under the spatial AR1 correlation structure, the correlation between dental measurements 2 years apart would be the square of the correlation 1 year apart and so the former correlation is necessarily nonnegative. The correlation between dental measurements at any positive real-valued number d' of years apart would also be positive as it is the square of the correlation of dental measurements $d'^{1/2}$ years apart. Similar arguments hold for any data for which a spatial autoregression correlation structure is applicable with continuous values $t(c)$.

2.3.4 Unstructured Correlations

Under unstructured (UN) correlations, the correlation matrices $\boldsymbol{R}_s(\boldsymbol{\rho}_{\mathrm{UN}})$ have entries

$$r_{c,c'}(\boldsymbol{\rho}_{\mathrm{UN}}) = \rho_{\mathrm{UN},c,c'}$$

for $c < c'$ with $c, c' \in C(s)$. In this case, $\boldsymbol{\rho}_{\mathrm{UN}}$ is a $(m \cdot (m - 1)/2) \times 1$ vector. When $m = 2$, the EC, AR1, and UN correlation structures are all the same and are based on a single correlation parameter.

2.4 Standard GEE Modeling

Standard GEE modeling (Liang & Zeger, 1986) assumes constant dispersions based on a constant dispersion parameter φ so that $\boldsymbol{\Sigma}_s$

$$\boldsymbol{\Sigma}_s = \varphi \cdot \boldsymbol{DIAG}(\boldsymbol{V}(\boldsymbol{\mu}_s)) \cdot \boldsymbol{R}_s(\boldsymbol{\rho}) \cdot \boldsymbol{DIAG}(\boldsymbol{V}(\boldsymbol{\mu}_s)),$$

and only the matrices $\boldsymbol{DIAG}(\boldsymbol{V}(\boldsymbol{\mu}_s))$ and $\boldsymbol{R}_s(\boldsymbol{\rho})$ vary with $s \in S$ where $\boldsymbol{V}(\boldsymbol{\mu}_s)$ denotes the $m(s) \times 1$ vector with entries $V(\mu_{sc})$ for $c \in C(s)$. The generalized estimating equations are given by $\boldsymbol{E}(\boldsymbol{\beta}) = \boldsymbol{0}$ where $\boldsymbol{0}$ is the $r \times 1$ vector of entries equal to 0,

$$\boldsymbol{E}(\boldsymbol{\beta}) = \sum_{s \in S} \boldsymbol{E}_s(\boldsymbol{\beta}) = \sum_{s \in S} \boldsymbol{D}_s^{\mathrm{T}} \cdot \boldsymbol{\Sigma}_s^{-1} \cdot \boldsymbol{e}_s,$$

and the $m(s) \times r$ matrices

$$\boldsymbol{D}_s = \frac{\partial \boldsymbol{\mu}_s}{\partial \boldsymbol{\beta}}$$

for $s \in S$ with entries

$$D_{sc,j} = \frac{\partial \mu_{sc}}{\partial \beta_j}$$

for $c \in C(s)$ and $1 \le j \le r$. Let

$$\boldsymbol{E}'(\boldsymbol{\beta}) = -\sum_{s \in S} \boldsymbol{D}_s^{\mathrm{T}} \cdot \boldsymbol{\Sigma}_s^{-1} \cdot \boldsymbol{D}_s.$$

The standard GEE estimation process iteratively solves $\boldsymbol{E}(\boldsymbol{\beta}) = \boldsymbol{0}$ as follows. Given the current value $\boldsymbol{\beta}_i$ for $\boldsymbol{\beta}$, the next value is given by

$$\boldsymbol{\beta}_{i+1} = \boldsymbol{\beta}_i - \boldsymbol{E}'^{-1}(\boldsymbol{\beta}_i) \cdot \boldsymbol{E}(\boldsymbol{\beta}_i),$$

thereby adapting Newton's method with $\boldsymbol{E}(\boldsymbol{\beta})$ in the role of the gradient vector and $\boldsymbol{E}'(\boldsymbol{\beta})$ in the role of the Hessian matrix. $\boldsymbol{E}(\boldsymbol{\beta})$ is only a gradient-like vector and $\boldsymbol{E}'(\boldsymbol{\beta})$ a Hessian-like matrix, but these will be referred to in what follows as a gradient vector and a Hessian matrix for brevity.

The constant dispersion parameter φ is estimated using the Pearson residuals $Pres_{sc}(\boldsymbol{\beta})$ evaluated at a given value for the coefficient parameter vector $\boldsymbol{\beta}$. The bias-adjusted estimate $\varphi(\boldsymbol{\beta})$ of the dispersion parameter φ satisfies

$$\varphi(\boldsymbol{\beta}) = \frac{\sum_{s \in S} \boldsymbol{Pres}_s^{\mathrm{T}}(\boldsymbol{\beta}) \cdot \boldsymbol{Pres}_s(\boldsymbol{\beta})}{m(SC) - r}.$$

Bias-adjusted estimates like this one assume that the denominator is greater than 0, $m(SC) - r > 0$ in this case. One can use instead bias-unadjusted estimates dividing by the associated count, $m(SC)$ in this case. Next, the correlation parameter vector $\boldsymbol{\rho}(\boldsymbol{\beta})$ is estimated using standardized residuals $stde_{sc}(\boldsymbol{\beta})$ for $sc \in SC$, computed using $\varphi(\boldsymbol{\beta})$ along with the Pearson residuals $Pres_{sc}(\boldsymbol{\beta})$ (see Sect. 2.4.1 for details). For any correlation structure, once the GEE estimate $\boldsymbol{\beta}(SC)$ of the coefficient parameter vector $\boldsymbol{\beta}$ is computed using the observations indexed by SC, the GEE estimate of the dispersion parameter φ is $\varphi(SC) = \varphi(\boldsymbol{\beta}(SC))$ and the GEE estimate of the correlation parameter vector $\boldsymbol{\rho}$ is $\boldsymbol{\rho}(SC) = \boldsymbol{\rho}(\boldsymbol{\beta}(SC))$ (computed using $\boldsymbol{\beta}(SC)$ and $\varphi(SC)$).

2.4.1 Estimating the Correlation Structure

How $\boldsymbol{\rho}$ is estimated varies with the correlation structure as described next. Let

$$CC = \{cc' : c < c', c, c' \in C\}$$

denote the full set of $m(CC) = m \cdot (m - 1)/2$ possible distinct ordered index pairs. The IND structure assumes all correlations equal the constant value $\rho_{\text{IND}} = 0$ for all choices of the parameter vector $\boldsymbol{\beta}$, and so then there is no need for an estimate of $\boldsymbol{\rho}$.

For the EC structure, let

$$CC' = \{cc' : c < c'; c, c' \in C(s), s \in S\}$$

denote the subset of CC containing the $m(CC')$ observed distinct ordered index pairs. For a given value of the coefficient parameter vector $\boldsymbol{\beta}$, the bias-adjusted estimate of the EC correlation parameter ρ_{EC} is given by

$$\rho_{\text{EC}}(\boldsymbol{\beta}) = \frac{\sum\limits_{cc' \in CC'} stde_{sc}(\boldsymbol{\beta}) \cdot stde_{sc'}(\boldsymbol{\beta})}{m(CC') - r}$$

assuming $m(CC') - r > 0$.

For the AR1 structure, let

$$CC'(+1) = \{cc' : c' = c + 1; c, c' \in C(s), s \in S\}$$

denote the set containing the $m(CC'(+1))$ observed consecutive index pairs. In the non-spatial AR1 case, for a given value of the coefficient parameter vector $\boldsymbol{\beta}$, a bias-adjusted estimate of the autocorrelation parameter ρ_{AR1} is given by

$$\rho_{\text{AR1}}(\boldsymbol{\beta}) = \frac{\sum\limits_{cc' \in CC'(+1)} stde_{sc}(\boldsymbol{\beta}) \cdot stde_{sc'}(\boldsymbol{\beta})}{m(CC'(+1)) - r}$$

assuming $m(CC'(+1)) - r > 0$. For the spatial AR1 structure, let $d(i)$ $1 \leq i \leq n_d$ denote the n_d unique positive distances apart for $cc' \in CC'(+1)$ and let $CC'(+1, i)$ be the subset of $CC'(+1)$ satisfying

$$CC'(+1, i) = \{cc' : cc' \in CC(+1), |t(c') - t(c)| = d(i)\}$$

of size $m(CC'(+1, i))$. For a given value of the coefficient parameter vector $\boldsymbol{\beta}$, define the n_d bias-adjusted estimates $\rho_{\text{AR1}}(\boldsymbol{\beta}, i)$ of $\rho_{\text{AR1}}(\boldsymbol{\beta})$ as

$$\rho_{\mathrm{AR1}}(\boldsymbol{\beta}, i) = \left(\max\left(\frac{\sum\limits_{cc\prime \in CC\prime(+1,i)} stde_{sc}(\boldsymbol{\beta}) \cdot \mathrm{stde}_{sc\prime}(\boldsymbol{\beta})}{m(CC'(+1,i)) - r}, 0\right)\right)^{1/d(i)}$$

assuming $m(CC'(+1, i)) - r > 0$. When $m(CC'(+1, i)) - r \le 0$, use $m(CC'(+1, i))$ in its place. An estimate of the spatial autocorrelation ρ_{AR1} is given by the average of the n_d estimates $\rho_{\mathrm{AR1}}(\boldsymbol{\beta}, i)$, that is

$$\rho_{\mathrm{AR1}}(\boldsymbol{\beta}) = \frac{\sum\limits_{i=1}^{n_d} \rho_{\mathrm{AR1}}(\boldsymbol{\beta}, i)}{n_d}.$$

In the non-spatial case, $n_d = 1$ and the spatial estimate is equivalent to the non-spatial estimate and is the same when $d(1) = 1$.

For the UN structure, the correlation parameter vector $\boldsymbol{\rho}_{\mathrm{UN}}$ has $m \cdot (m - 1)/2$ entries $\rho_{\mathrm{UN},\,c,\,c'}$ for $cc' \in CC$. For $cc' \in CC$, let

$$S(cc') = \{s : c, c' \in C(s), s \in S\}$$

denote the set of $m(S(cc'))$ matched set indexes s with observed measurements in $C(s)$ for the ordered index pair cc'. For a given value of the coefficient parameter vector $\boldsymbol{\beta}$, the bias-adjusted estimate of the UN correlation parameter $\rho_{\mathrm{UN},\,cc'}$ is given by

$$\rho_{\mathrm{UN},c,c'}(\boldsymbol{\beta}) = \frac{\sum\limits_{s \in S(cc')} stde_{sc}(\boldsymbol{\beta}) \cdot stde_{sc'}(\boldsymbol{\beta})}{m(S(cc')) - r}$$

assuming $m(S(cc')) - r > 0$, for $cc' \in$ CC. The correlation parameter vector $\boldsymbol{\rho}_{\mathrm{UN}}$ is estimated by combining the estimates $\rho_{\mathrm{UN},\,c,\,c'}(\boldsymbol{\beta})$ of the UN correlation parameters over $cc' \in CC$ into the $(m \cdot (m - 1)/2) \times 1$ vector $\boldsymbol{\rho}_{\mathrm{UN}}(\boldsymbol{\beta})$.

2.4.2 *Estimating the Covariance Matrix for Mean Parameter Estimates*

Two estimates of the covariance matrix for the estimated parameter vector $\boldsymbol{\beta}(SC)$ can be computed. The model-based estimate treats the assumed model as the true model for the data, while the robust empirical estimate allows the true model for the data to differ from that of the assumed model. The model-based estimate is

$$\Sigma_{\mathrm{MB}}(\boldsymbol{\beta}(SC)) = -\boldsymbol{E}'^{-1}(\boldsymbol{\beta}(SC)).$$

The robust empirical estimate (Claeskens & Hjort, 2008) is

$$\Sigma_{\mathrm{RE}}(\boldsymbol{\beta}(SC)) = \boldsymbol{E}'^{-1}(\boldsymbol{\beta}(SC)) \cdot \boldsymbol{G}(\boldsymbol{\beta}(SC)) \cdot \boldsymbol{G}^{\mathrm{T}}(\boldsymbol{\beta}(SC)) \cdot \boldsymbol{E}'^{-1}(\boldsymbol{\beta}(SC))$$

where $\boldsymbol{G}(\boldsymbol{\beta}(SC))$ is the $r \times m(SC)$ matrix with $r \times m(s)$ component matrices $\boldsymbol{G}_s(\boldsymbol{\beta}(SC))$ for $s \in S$ satisfying

$$\boldsymbol{G}_s(\boldsymbol{\beta}(SC)) = (\boldsymbol{D}_s^{\mathrm{T}} \cdot \Sigma_s^{-1}) \circ \boldsymbol{e}_s^{\mathrm{T}}$$

where $\circ$ denotes elementwise multiplication of the entries of each row of the matrix $\boldsymbol{D}_s^{\mathrm{T}} \cdot \boldsymbol{\Sigma}_s^{-1}$ by the associated entries of the row vector $\boldsymbol{e}_s^{\mathrm{T}}$. Note that $\boldsymbol{E}(\boldsymbol{\beta}(SC))$ equals the $r \times 1$ vector generated by summing the rows of $\boldsymbol{G}(\boldsymbol{\beta}(SC))$. The diagonal entries of $\boldsymbol{\Sigma}_{\mathrm{MB}}(\boldsymbol{\beta}(SC))$ and $\boldsymbol{\Sigma}_{\mathrm{RE}}(\boldsymbol{\beta}(SC))$ are estimates of variances for the parameter estimates given by the entries of $\boldsymbol{\beta}(SC)$. These can be used to generate z tests of zero coefficient parameter values.

2.4.3 *Parameter Estimation Problems*

The standard GEE modeling process can have estimation problems. First, correlation estimates might not generate valid correlation matrices. This is more likely to happen for UN correlation structures but can also happen for EC and AR1 correlation structures when the associated correlation parameter estimates fall outside appropriate bounds. Also, the estimation process might not converge in the sense that the maximum $\max(|\boldsymbol{E}(\boldsymbol{\beta})|)$ of the absolute values of the entries of the gradient vector $\boldsymbol{E}(\boldsymbol{\beta})$ does not converge to 0. This happens more often for models for the means with zero intercepts. Furthermore, the GEE estimation process can converge slowly. Adjustments are possible to limit these problems, but details on these adjustments are provided later in Sect. 3.6. Details on the full estimation process are presented later in Sect. 3.7.

2.5 The Likelihood Function

Denote the observations for the matched set $s \in S$ by $O_s = \{\boldsymbol{y}_s, \boldsymbol{X}_s\}$ (also add in the offset vector $\boldsymbol{o}_s$ when used in the Poisson regression case). Let

$$\boldsymbol{\theta} = \begin{pmatrix} \boldsymbol{\beta} \\ \varphi \end{pmatrix}$$

be the $(r + 1) \times 1$ vector of the mean and dispersion parameters. The correlation parameter vector $\boldsymbol{\rho}$ has not been included in $\boldsymbol{\theta}$ because it is a function of $\boldsymbol{\beta}$ and φ. Using the multivariate normal likelihood, define the likelihood function $L(SC;\boldsymbol{\theta})$ as the product of the terms $L(O_s;\boldsymbol{\theta})$ satisfying

$$\ell(O_s;\boldsymbol{\theta}) = \log L(O_s;\boldsymbol{\theta}) = -\boldsymbol{e}_s^{\mathrm{T}} \cdot \boldsymbol{\Sigma}_s^{-1} \cdot \boldsymbol{e}_s/2 - (\log|\boldsymbol{\Sigma}_s|)/2 - (m(s) \cdot \log(2 \cdot \pi))/2$$

for $s \in S$, where $|\boldsymbol{\Sigma}_s|$ is the determinant of the covariance matrix $\boldsymbol{\Sigma}_s$ and π is the usual constant. Similarly define $L(SC';\boldsymbol{\theta})$ for any subset SC' of SC with $L(SC';\boldsymbol{\theta}) = 1$ when SC' is the empty set. In general, $L(SC;\boldsymbol{\theta})$ is only a likelihood-like or extended likelihood function serving the same purpose as a likelihood while not necessarily integrating to 1, but that distinction is ignored for brevity. For normally distributed y_{sc}, $L(SC;\boldsymbol{\theta})$ is the actual likelihood determined by the multivariate normal distribution. Knafl and Ding (2016, Sect. 10.7.1) note that the vector $\frac{\partial \ell(SC;\boldsymbol{\theta})}{\partial \boldsymbol{\beta}}$ of partial derivatives of $\ell(SC;\boldsymbol{\theta})$ can be separated into the sum of two terms. The first term, corresponding to differentiating the $\boldsymbol{e}_s$ part of each $\ell(O_s;\boldsymbol{\theta})$ with respect to $\boldsymbol{\beta}$ while holding $\boldsymbol{\Sigma}_s$ fixed in $\boldsymbol{\beta}$, equals the gradient quantity $\boldsymbol{E}(\boldsymbol{\beta})$ used in standard GEE modeling. Chaganty (1997) recognized this relationship between the standard GEE estimating equations and the partial derivatives, but his quasi-least squares approach utilizes only the least squares part $\sum_{s=1}^{n} \boldsymbol{e}_s^{\mathrm{T}} \cdot \Sigma_s^{-1} \cdot \boldsymbol{e}_s$ of the log-likelihood $\ell(SC;\boldsymbol{\theta})$ to generate estimating equations rather than the full log-likelihood.

The standard GEE modeling process technically only requires that $\boldsymbol{\Sigma}_s$ be invertible for $s \in S$ or, equivalently, that $\boldsymbol{R}_s(\boldsymbol{\rho})$ be invertible for $s \in S$. Consideration of the likelihood function $L(O_s;\boldsymbol{\theta})$ imposes the stronger restriction that $\boldsymbol{\Sigma}_s$ be positive definite for $s \in S$ so that $\boldsymbol{e}_s^{\mathrm{T}} \cdot \boldsymbol{\Sigma}_s^{-1} \cdot \boldsymbol{e}_s > \mathbf{0}$ for all non-zero residual vectors $\boldsymbol{e}_s \neq \mathbf{0}$ and so that the determinants $|\boldsymbol{\Sigma}_s| > 0$ and then associated $\log|\boldsymbol{\Sigma}_s|$ terms are well defined. This holds if the working correlation matrix $\boldsymbol{R}(\boldsymbol{\rho})$ for the full set C of m conditions is positive definite.

Given that the likelihood function L is only an extended likelihood and not a true likelihood, the robust estimate of the covariance matrix for standard GEE mean parameter estimates (see Sect. 2.4.2) seems more appropriate to use for conducting z tests for zero model parameters than the model-based estimate since it allows for the true model to be different from the assumed model. An even better way to allow for indeterminant models would be to use bootstrapping to generate confidence intervals for testing for zero model parameters.

An advantage of having the likelihood function L for GEE modeling is that it can be used to compute model selection criterion. For example, penalized likelihood criteria (Sclove, 1987) like the Akaike information criterion (AIC) and the Bayesian information criterion (BIC) can be readily generalized to handle GEE models using associated penalty factors (Sect. 2.6.3). A likelihood cross-validation score can also be defined (Sect. 2.6) for evaluating and comparing GEE models, and then these scores can be used to adaptively search through alternative GEE models for a given set of measurements (Sect. 2.7). A penalized model selection criterion related to the AIC called the quasi-likelihood information criterion (QIC) has been formulated (Pan, 2001) for GEE model selection, but the QIC score does not fully account for the correlation structure. Model selection criteria based on the likelihood function L fully account for the correlation structure in contrast to the QIC score.

2.6 Likelihood Cross-Validation

In k-fold cross-validation, the measurements are partitioned into k disjoint subsets called folds (Burman, 1989), and the fold measurements are predicted using parameter estimates computed using the remaining measurements. In k-fold likelihood cross-validation (LCV), these deleted fold predictions are scored using the associated likelihood function such as the function L defined in Sect. 2.5.

One possibility for the partitioning of the data into folds is matched-set-wise deletion with all measurements within the same matched set allocated to the same fold. Randomly partition the index set S into k disjoint folds $F(h)$ for $1 \leq h \leq k$ with all $C(s)$ measurements for a matched set s assigned to the same fold $F(h(s))$ where $h(s) = \text{int}(k \cdot u_s) + 1$ for independent, uniform random values u_s in $(0, 1)$ and int $(k \cdot u_s)$ denotes the integer part of $k \cdot u_s$. The LCV score for a standard GEE model (or any of its extensions to be addressed in Chaps. 3–5) based on the coefficient parameter vector $\boldsymbol{\theta}$ satisfies

$$\text{LCV} = \prod_{h=1}^{k} \prod_{s \in F(h)} L^{1/m(SC)}(O_s; \boldsymbol{\theta}(S \backslash F(h)))$$

where $\boldsymbol{\theta}(S\backslash F(h))$ denotes the estimate of $\boldsymbol{\theta}$ using the data for matched sets with indexes s in the complement $S\backslash F(h)$ of the fold $F(h)$. The LCV score is normalized by the total number $m(SC)$ of observed measurements over all matched sets $s \in S$ rather than by the total number n of matched sets.

Another possibility is to use measurement-wise deletion. Randomly partition the index set SC into k disjoint folds $F(h)$ for $1 \leq h \leq k$. For $sc \in SC$, the measurement index sc is assigned to the fold $F(h(sc))$ where $h(sc) = \text{int}(k \cdot u_{sc}) + 1$ for independent, uniform random values u_{sc} in $(0, 1)$. Let $U(h)$ for $1 \leq h \leq k$ denote the union of all folds $F(h')$ for $1 \leq h' \leq h$ and $U(0)$ the empty fold. For a subset SC' of SC and a fixed $s \in S$, let

$$SC(s, SC') = \{s'\text{c} : s'\text{c} \in SC', s' = s\},$$

that is, the index pairs sc in SC' for a fixed $s \in S$. Define the LCV score to satisfy

$$\mathrm{LCV} = \prod_{h=1}^{k} \prod_{s \in S} \mathrm{LCV}_{s,h}^{1/m(SC)}$$

where

$$\mathrm{LCV}_{s,h} = L(SC(s, F(h)) | U(h-1); \boldsymbol{\theta}(S \backslash F(h))) = \frac{L(SC(s, U(h)); \boldsymbol{\theta}(S \backslash F(h)))}{L(SC(s, U(h-1)); \boldsymbol{\theta}(S \backslash F(h)))}.$$

Informally, $\mathrm{LCV}_{s,h}$ for $s \in S$ and $1 \leq h \leq k$ are the conditional likelihood terms for the set $SC(s, F(h))$ of measurements sc of the matched set s in fold $F(h)$ conditioned on the measurements sc of the matched set s in the union $U(h - 1)$ of the prior folds using the deleted estimate $\boldsymbol{\theta}(S \backslash F(h))$ of the parameter vector $\boldsymbol{\theta}$.

Use the same initial seed to generate folds for all models of the same set of measurements so that their LCV scores are comparable. Also, the order of the measurements needs to stay the same because measurements can get assigned to different folds when the order changes.

Measurement-wise deletion seems important to use with data having missing outcome measurements for some matched sets (i.e., with $m(s) < m$ for some $s \in S$) or with data having only one matched set (i.e., $n = 1$) or only a small number of matched sets. On the other hand, matched-set-wise deletion seems reasonable to use with data sets containing the full set of m outcome measurements for each of n matched sets (i.e., $m(s) = m$ for all $s \in S$ so that $m(SC) = m \cdot n$) with n not too small, as for the example data sets described in Sect. 2.8.

Since fold assignment is random, as the number k of folds increases, the chance of one or more empty folds increases. Empty folds out of k randomly assigned folds are ignored when computing associated LCV scores, but these scores are based on a smaller number of folds than k and so are not actually k-fold LCV scores. This seems an indication that k is set too large relative to the number n of matched sets for matched-set-wise deletion and too large relative to the number $m(SC)$ of measurements for measurement-wise deletion. In such cases, only smaller values for the number of folds seem appropriate to use in setting the number of folds for analyzing the data. For matched-set-wise deletion, a smaller number n of matched sets increases the chance of empty folds even for relatively small numbers of folds. Similarly, for measurement-wise deletion, a smaller number $m(SC)$ of measurements increases the chance of empty folds. For cases with such small numbers, it may be better to use what is called leave-one-out LCV with each matched set in its own fold for matched-set-wise deletion and with each measurement in its own fold for measurement-wise deletion. An example is provided in Chap. 12 of Knafl and Ding (2016).

2.6.1 Choosing the Number of Folds

An appropriate choice is needed for the number k of folds to use in analyses; this can change with the data. A recommended approach for making this choice is provided by Knafl and Ding (2016, Sect. 2,8). Briefly, select an important benchmark adaptive analysis for a data set and vary the value of k starting at five folds over multiples of five folds until a local maximum in the LCV score occurs for this analysis. Use that first local maximum k^* in k for all subsequent analyses of the data set. In the case where the LCV score decreases from the first value at $k = 5$ to the second one at $k = 10$, $k^* = 5$ may not necessarily be an appropriate choice. In that case, also consider values of k larger than 10. If the LCV score is also smaller for $k = 15$, use $k^* = 5$ in subsequent analyses. Otherwise, continue searching and use the next local maximum instead. Examples of choosing k are given in Chaps. 6–9 and 13–16. For data sets with a large number of measurements, a small number of folds such as $k = 5$ can be used to reduce computation times (as for the analyses of Chap. 13) with the understanding that generated models might not be competitive alternatives to models that would be generated using larger numbers of folds.

It is important that models generated using k^* folds be consistent with models generated using other choices for the number of folds. This can be assessed by computing k^*-fold LCV scores for models generated using other number of folds. If these models generate competitive k^*-fold LCV scores, any number of folds could be used. A smaller number of folds than k^* generating a model with a competitive k^*-fold LCV score may be preferable to use instead of k^* in order to reduce computation times, especially when UN correlations are preferable over simpler correlation structures.

2.6.2 LCV Ratio Tests

A larger LCV score of either kind indicates a better model but not necessarily a distinctly (or substantially or significantly) better model. LCV ratio tests, computed using the χ^2 distribution as for standard likelihood ratio tests, can be used to assess this issue. LCV ratio tests are expressed in terms of a cutoff for a distinct (or substantial or significant) percent decrease (PD) in the LCV score.

Let M_1 and M_2 be two models for the same data with LCV scores satisfying

$$\mathrm{LCV}(M_1) < \mathrm{LCV}(M_2).$$

The associated quantities $\mathrm{LCV}^{m(SC)}(M_1)$ and $\mathrm{LCV}^{m(SC)}(M_2)$ serve in the role of likelihoods so that

$$\delta = 2 \cdot \log \mathrm{LCV}^{m(SC)}(M_1) - 2 \cdot \log \mathrm{LCV}^{m(SC)}(M_2)$$

is treated as $\chi^2(\mathrm{DF})$ distributed using an appropriate choice for the degrees of freedom DF. The percent decrease PD satisfies

$$\frac{\mathrm{PD}}{100} = \frac{\mathrm{LCV}(M_2) - \mathrm{LCV}(M_1)}{\mathrm{LCV}(M_2)} = 1 - \exp\left(-\frac{\delta}{2 \cdot m(SC)}\right)$$

and so is significant at level α when

$$\frac{\mathrm{PD}}{100} > 1 - \exp\left(-\frac{\Delta(1-\alpha, \mathrm{DF})}{2 \cdot m(SC)}\right)$$

where the $\Delta(1 - \alpha, \mathrm{DF})$ is the $(1 - \alpha) \cdot 100^{\mathrm{th}}$ percentile of the $\chi^2(\mathrm{DF})$ distribution. The cutoff is therefore set to

$$1 - \exp\left(-\frac{\Delta(1-\alpha, \mathrm{DF})}{2 \cdot m(SC)}\right),$$

which decreases with increased numbers $m(SC)$ of measurements. If the PD is greater than the cutoff, then model M_2 with the larger LCV score provides a distinct (or substantial or significant) improvement over model M_1 with the smaller LCV score. Otherwise, model M_1 is a competitive alternative to model M_2. If model M_1 is also simpler than model M_2 (e.g., with fewer parameters or based on only main effects rather than including interaction effects), then model M_1 is preferable as a parsimonious, competitive alternative to model M_2.

LCV ratio tests are usually conducted using DF = 1 because, in most cases, the removal of a single predictor from the model generates a model with one less parameter. One exception is multinomial regression with a categorical outcome having $K + 1$ possible values (as covered in Chap. 10), in which case removal of one predictor for the means results in the removal of K parameters. Consequently, two multinomial regression models for the means are usually compared using LCV ratio tests based on DF = K. LCV ratio tests can be applied to non-nested models. These are usually conducted conservatively using the smallest possible non-zero DF = 1. In cases when the model M_1 with the smaller LCV score has more than one less parameter than the model M_2 with the larger LCV score, the cutoff based on DF = 1 may not be an appropriate choice and a more nuanced assessment can be needed. See Sects. 8.6 and 9.6 for examples.

A common example of the use of an LCV ratio test is in assessing nonlinearity of the means for a continuous outcome variable in a continuous predictor x. This involves comparing the LCV score for the adaptive model for the means accounting for possible nonlinearity in x (as described in Sect. 2.7) to the LCV score for the standard linear polynomial model with the means depending on an intercept and untransformed x. The means are reasonably treated as linear in x if the LCV score for the linear polynomial model is larger than the LCV score for the adaptive model or if the PD in the LCV scores for the linear polynomial model compared to the adaptive model is not distinct (i.e., less than or equal to the associated cutoff). Otherwise, the means are distinctly nonlinear in x.

The comparison of models based on different correlation structures needs special handling. Consider two models with the same number of mean and variance/ dispersion parameters. When one model has IND correlations and the other either spatial AR1 or EC correlations, a cutoff based on DF $= 1$ is appropriate for comparing these models because they differ by one correlation parameter. This is also the case when one model has spatial AR1 correlations and the other EC correlations since these two correlation structures are both based on a single correlation parameter. However, when one model has UN correlations and the other has either spatial AR1 or EC correlations, a cutoff based on

$$\mathrm{DF} = \frac{m \cdot (m-1)}{2} - 1$$

seems a more appropriate choice. Further adjustments of DF can be appropriate when the two models have different numbers of mean and variance/dispersion parameters as well as different correlation structures.

LCV ratio tests are most appropriately conducted between two models generated by the same modeling approach applied to the same data set using the same number of folds. LCV scores are not comparable for models generated using different data sets including two different subsets of the same data set. Models generated by the same modeling approach applied to the same data set but computed using different numbers of folds are compared in reported analyses to assess which number of folds to use in subsequent analyses. A larger score can indicate a better choice of the number of folds to use in subsequent analyses, but a smaller number of folds generating a smaller LCV score may be a reasonable alternative to reduce computation times if the smaller number of folds generates a consistent model. In any case, these LCV scores are not assessed using LCV ratio tests.

Models generated by two different modeling approaches (e.g., partially modified GEE and fully modified GEE) applied to the same data set using the same number k of folds can be compared as follows. Let M_1 and M_2 denote the models generated by the first and second modeling approaches, respectively. Compute the k-fold LCV score for model M_2 using the modeling approach used to generate model M_1 and compare this k-fold LCV score using an LCV ratio test to the k-fold LCV score for model M_1. Examples are provided in reported analyses. The modeling approach to use to compute common LCV scores is determined in example analyses as follows. When comparing models generated by fully modified GEE and partially modified GEE, use fully modified GEE to compute common LCV scores since it more fully utilizes the likelihood function L used in computing LCV scores. When comparing models generated by ELMM and either fully modified GEE or partially modified GEE, use ELMM to compute common LCV scores since it fully utilizes the likelihood function L.

2.6.3 Penalized Likelihood Criteria

The likelihood function L of Sect. 2.5 can be combined with standard penalty factors to compute penalized likelihood criteria (Sclove, 1987) for model selection as alternatives to using LCV. These are usually expressed as scores with smaller values indicating better models. They can be used in adaptive modeling (as described in Sect. 2.7) in place of LCV scores but need to be adjusted so that larger values indicate better models. For example, the Akaike information criterion (AIC) bases the penalty factor on the number of parameters dim($\boldsymbol{\theta}$) and satisfies

$$\mathrm{AIC} = -2 \cdot L(SC;\boldsymbol{\theta}) + 2 \cdot \dim(\boldsymbol{\theta}).$$

To use AIC in adaptive modeling, adjust it to

$$\mathrm{AIC}' = \exp\left(-\frac{\mathrm{AIC}}{2 \cdot m(SC)}\right).$$

As a second example, the Bayesian information criterion (BIC) score bases the penalty factor on both the number of parameters dim($\boldsymbol{\theta}$) and the number of measurements $m(SC)$. It satisfies

$$\mathrm{BIC} = -2 \cdot L(SC;\boldsymbol{\theta}) + 2 \cdot (\log(m(SC))) \cdot \dim(\boldsymbol{\theta}).$$

To use BIC in adaptive modeling, adjust it to

$$\mathrm{BIC}' = \exp\left(-\frac{\mathrm{BIC}}{2 \cdot m(SC)}\right).$$

AIC and BIC are the most commonly used penalized likelihood criteria. AIC/BIC ratio tests analogous to LCV ratio tests can be conducted using adjusted AIC and BIC scores.

Adjusted AIC or adjusted BIC scores can be used in place of LCV scores in adaptive modeling to reduce computation times, especially for data sets with large numbers of measurements, but generated models might not be competitive alternatives to models that would be generated using LCV scores. However, for very large numbers of measurements, Adjusted AIC scores approximate LCV scores (Claeskens & Hjort, 2008). Knafl et al. (2018) provide an example using a data set with a singleton univariate outcome (i.e., all matched sets consist of $m = 1$ measurement) and $m(SC) = 37{,}781$.

2.7 Adaptive Regression Modeling of Means

Knafl and Ding (2016) provide a thorough formulation of adaptive regression modeling allowing for nonlinear relationships in general regression contexts (see their Chap. 20 for details). An overview is presented here assuming standard GEE modeling for now. Positive predictor values $x_{sc,j} > 0$ for modeling means can be power transformed using arbitrary real-valued powers. These can be generalized to arbitrary power transforms of general real-valued (i.e., possibly negative, zero, or positive) predictor values $x_{sc,j}$ (see Knafl & Ding, 2016, Sect. 4.6). Power-transformed predictors are called fractional polynomials (Royston & Altman, 1994). The modeling process is controlled by tolerance parameters indicating how much of a change in the LCV score can currently be tolerated at given stages of the process.

Adaptive modeling first expands (or grows) the model for the means in one or more power transforms of a set of primary predictors. For each primary predictor currently under consideration for inclusion in the model, the best power for that transform is the power that generates the largest LCV score with that transform added to the currently expanded model. The primary predictors can include indicator (dummy) predictors requiring no transformation. A primary predictor can be dropped from consideration for inclusion if its best transform generates too small of an LCV score (as determined by a tolerance parameter). The transform generating the best LCV score among all primary predictors currently under consideration for inclusion is the one added next to the model. The expansion stops when this best LCV score is too small (as determined by a tolerance parameter). A heuristic used in reported analyses that is not considered in Knafl and Ding (2016) is that the expansion is restricted to add only a maximum of five transforms to the model for the means in order to reduce computation times.

Adaptive modeling then contracts (or prunes) the expanded model. Transforms in the current model are removed one at a time and the powers for the remaining transforms are adjusted to improve the LCV score. The next transform to be removed is the one generating the best LCV score with its removal. Transforms can be dropped from consideration for removal if the LCV score generated by their removal at some step in the contraction is too small (as determined by a tolerance parameter). The contraction stops when the removal of the next transform decreases the LCV score by too much (as determined by a tolerance parameter with value set using an LCV ratio test). If no transforms are removed from the expanded model, the powers of the transforms of that model are adjusted to improve the LCV score. The final adaptively generated model is an effective choice in the sense that the removal of each of its transforms generates a distinct (or substantial or significant) PD in the LCV score.

The adaptive process can optionally consider geometric combinations of predictors, that is, products of power transforms of primary predictors, generalizing standard interactions, and power transforms of these products. This provides for a nonlinear assessment of the issue called moderation (Baron & Kenny, 1986). By default, the process considers models for the means with zero intercepts, but can be restricted to consider only non-zero intercept models. Multiple transforms of the same primary predictor but with different powers are considered by default, but the process can be restricted to consider at most one transform per primary predictor. Unit dispersions GEE models (i.e., with $\varphi = 1$) can also be optionally considered rather than only constant dispersions GEE models (i.e., with the value of φ estimated). Models based on specific sets of power transforms can be adaptively retransformed by adjusting their powers to improve the model's LCV score.

Model-based and robust empirical tests for zero parameters (Sect. 2.4.2) can be conducted for adaptively generated models. However, these tests are usually significant as a consequence of the model selection process, and so should either not be considered or should only be reported for descriptive rather than for inferential purposes. For this reason, results for such tests are not reported in example analyses.

2.8 Example Data Sets

Example data analyses are provided in Chaps. 6–9 for the four cases of linear, Poisson, logistic, and exponential regression of Sects. 2.2.1–2.2.4. The associated four data sets are described next and involve correlated univariate outcomes with all matched sets having no missing outcome measurements.

2.8.1 The Dental Measurement Data

Data on dental measurements for $n = 27$ children, including 16 boys and 11 girls, over the four ages of 8, 10, 12,and 14 years old are reported and analyzed by Potthoff and Roy (1964) in their growth curve modeling paper. The outcome variable for this data set is called dentmeas and contains values for dental measurements of the distance in mm from the center of the pituitary to the pterygomaxillary fissure. The possible predictor variables are age and the indicator male for the child being a boy. There are $m(SC) = 108$ outcome measurements with four measurements available for each child, and so none missing, and the four measurements are equally spaced 2 years apart. The cutoff using DF $= 1$ for a distinct percent decrease in LCV scores (Sect. 2.6.2) for these data with 108 measurements is 1.76%. Chapters 4 and 5 of Knafl and Ding (2016) provide a variety of example analyses of these data as well as code for conducting such analyses. Results are reported in Chap. 6 for analyses of these data, which may differ somewhat from those reported in Knafl and Ding (2016) because a different estimation process is used (as described in Sects. 3.7 and 4.3).

2.8.2 The Epilepsy Seizure Rate Data

Data on seizure counts over a baseline period and over intervals between four post-baseline clinic visits, coded as 0–4, for $n = 59$ patients with epilepsy are analyzed and published by Thall and Vail (1990). The outcome variable is called count and contains numbers of seizures. The possible predictor variables are visit and the indicator int for the patient being in the intervention group given the antiepileptic drug progabide as opposed to being in the control group given a placebo with 31 patients in the intervention group and 28 patients in the control group. The associated numbers of weeks over which seizure counts were counted are loaded into the variable called dltatime; the baseline period is 8 weeks long, while all four post-baseline periods are 2 weeks long. The offset variable computed as log (dltatime) is used to convert Poisson regression models for seizure counts into models for seizure rates per week. There is a total of $m(SC) = 295$ outcome measurements with five measurements available for each patient, and so none missing. The measurements are treated as equally spaced due to coding visits as 0–4. The cutoff using DF = 1 for a distinct percent decrease in LCV scores (Sect. 2.6.2) for these data with 295 measurements is 0.65%. Chapters 14 and 15 of Knafl and Ding (2016) provide a variety of example analyses of the post-baseline data as well as code for conducting such analyses. The full set of data, including baseline and post-baseline outcome measurements, are analyzed in Chap. 7.

2.8.3 The Dichotomous Respiratory Status Data

Data on respiratory status levels at baseline and at four post-baseline clinic visits, coded as 0–4, for $n = 111$ patients with respiratory disorder are analyzed and are published in Koch et al. (1989). The dichotomous outcome variable for this data set is called status0_1 with values 0:poor and 1:good and is analyzed by Stokes et al. (2012). The possible predictor variables are visit and the indicator active for the patient being on an active as opposed to a placebo treatment. There is a total of $m(SC) = 555$ outcome measurements with five measurements available for each of 111 patients, 54 on active treatment and 57 on a placebo, and so none missing. The measurements are treated as equally spaced due to coding visits as 0–4. The cutoff using DF = 1 for a distinct percent decrease in LCV scores (Sect. 2.6.2) for these data with 555 measurements is 0.35%. Chapters 10 and 11 of Knafl and Ding (2016) provide a variety of example analyses of the post-baseline data as well as code for conducting such analyses. The full set of data, including baseline and post-baseline outcome measurements, are analyzed in Chap. 8.

2.8.4 The Blood Lead Level Data

Data on blood lead levels for $n = 100$ children over 0, 1, 4, and 6 weeks are available (Treatment of Lead-exposed Children (TLC) Trial Group, 2000). Blood lead levels range from 2.8 to 63.9 μg/dL. The outcome variable for this data set is called lead and contains the blood lead levels. The possible predictor variables are week and the indicator succimer for the child being treated with the chelating agent succimer versus being on a placebo. There are $m(SC) = 400$ outcome measurements with four measurements available for each patient, 50 taking succimer and 50 taking a placebo, and so none missing. The measurements are not equally spaced. The cutoff using DF $= 1$ for a distinct percent decrease in LCV scores (Sect. 2.6.2) for these data with 400 measurements is 0.48%. These data are analyzed in Chap. 9.

References

Baron, R. M., & Kenny, D. A. (1986). The moderator-mediator variable distinction in social psychology research: Conceptual, strategic, and statistical considerations. *Journal of Personality and Social Psychology, 51*, 1173–1182.

Burman, P. (1989). A comparative study of ordinary cross-validation, ν-fold cross-validation and the repeated learning-testing methods. *Biometrika, 76*, 503–514.

Chaganty, N. R. (1997). An alternative approach to the analysis of longitudinal data via generalized estimating equations. *Journal of Statistical Planning and Inference, 63*, 39–54.

Claeskens, G., & Hjort, N. L. (2008). *Model selection and model averaging*. Cambridge University Press.

Knafl, G. J., & Ding, K. (2016). *Adaptive regression for modeling nonlinear relationships*. Springer.

Knafl, G. J., Toles, M., Beeber, A. S., & Jones, C. B. (2018). Adaptive classification methods for predicting transitions in the nursing workforce. *Open Journal of Statistics, 8*, 497–512. https://doi.org/10.4236/ojs.2018.83032. https://www.scirp.org/Journal/PaperInformation.aspx?PaperID=85246

Koch, G. G., Carr, C. F., Amara, I. A., Stokes, M. E., & Uryniak, T. J. (1989). Categorical data analysis. In D. A. Berry (Ed.), *Statistical methodology in the pharmaceutical sciences* (pp. 391–475). Marcel Dekker.

Liang, K.-Y., & Zeger, S. L. (1986). Longitudinal data analysis using generalized linear models. *Biometrika, 73*, 13–22.

McCullagh, P., & Nelder, J. A. (1999). *Generalized linear models* (2nd ed.). Chapman & Hall/CRC.

Pan, W. (2001). Akaike's information criterion in generalized estimating equations. *Biometrics, 57*, 120–125.

Potthoff, R. F., & Roy, S. N. (1964). A generalized multivariate analysis of variance model useful especially for growth curve problems. *Biometrika, 51*, 313–326.

Royston, P., & Altman, D. G. (1994). Regression using fractional polynomials of continuous covariates: Parsimonious parametric modeling. *Applied Statistics, 43*, 429–467.

Sclove, S. L. (1987). Application of model-selection criteria to some problems in multivariate analysis. *Psychometrika, 52*, 333–343.

Stokes, M. E., Davis, C. S., & Koch, G. G. (2012). *Categorical data analysis using the SAS system* (3rd ed.). SAS Institute.

Thall, P. F., & Vail, S. C. (1990). Some covariance models for longitudinal count data with overdispersion. *Biometrics, 46*, 657–671.

Treatment of Lead-exposed Children (TLC) Trial Group. (2000). Safety and efficacy of succimer in toddlers with blood lead levels of 20–44 μg/dL. *Pediatric Research, 48*, 593–599.

Chapter 3
Partially Modified GEE Modeling of Correlated Univariate Outcomes

Abstract Formulations are provided for a partially modified approach to standard generalized estimating equations (GEE) methods for modeling correlated sets of univariate outcomes. This approach allows for non-constant dispersions by combining extra estimating equations for dispersion parameters with standard GEE estimating equations for mean parameters. The extra estimating equations are generated by maximizing an appropriate likelihood function in the dispersion parameters. Generalizations of standard GEE estimates of correlation parameters are provided accounting for non-constant dispersions along with tests for significant mean and dispersion parameter estimates. The special case with constant dispersions is formulated and compared to standard GEE. Possible degeneracy in correlation estimates is addressed. A detailed estimation process is described that limits the impact of estimation problems through extensions of Newton's method. The issue of variation in measurement conditions is addressed as well.

Keywords Correlated outcomes · Generalized estimating equations · Newton's method · Non-constant dispersions

Introduction This chapter provides formulations for non-constant dispersions in Sect. 3.1, estimating equations for dispersion parameters in Sect. 3.2, estimates of correlation parameters in Sect. 3.3, and tests for significant mean and dispersion parameter estimates in Sect. 3.4. An example with constant dispersions is presented in Sect. 3.5, possible degeneracy in correlation estimates is addressed in Sect. 3.6, and a detailed estimation process is described in Sect. 3.7 that limits the impact of estimation problems (as initially addressed in Sect. 2.4.3). The issue of variation in measurement conditions is addressed in Sect. 3.8.

Supplementary Information The online version contains supplementary material available at https://doi.org/10.1007/978-3-031-41988-1_3.

G. J. Knafl, *Modeling Correlated Outcomes Using Extensions of Generalized Estimating Equations and Linear Mixed Modeling*,
https://doi.org/10.1007/978-3-031-41988-1_3

3.1 Including Non-constant Dispersions

Using the notation of Sects. 2.1 and 2.2 and the extended quasi-likelihood approach (McCullagh & Nelder, 1999; Nelder & Pregibon, 1987), define the extended variances for the outcomes y_{sc} as $\sigma_{sc}^2 = \varphi_{sc} \cdot V(\mu_{sc})$ where φ_{sc} are possibly non-constant dispersions and examples of the variance function $V(\mu_{sc})$ depending on the means μ_{sc} are provided in Sects. 2.2.1–2.2.4. For $s \in S$, let $\boldsymbol{\sigma}_s$ denote the $m(s) \times 1$ vector with entries

$$\sigma_{sc} = (\varphi_{sc} \cdot V(\mu_{sc}))^{½}$$

for $c \in C(s)$. The residuals are $e_{sc} = y_{sc} - \mu_{sc}$, standardized residuals are $stde_{sc} = e_{sc}/\sigma_{sc}$, and the Pearson residuals are

$$Pres_{sc} = \varphi_{sc}^{½} \cdot stde_{sc} = \frac{e_{sc}}{V^{½}(\mu_{sc})}.$$

Combine the residuals, standardized residuals, and Pearson residuals over $c \in C(s)$ into their respective $m(s) \times 1$ vectors $\mathbf{e}_s$, $\boldsymbol{stde}_s$, and $\boldsymbol{Pres}_s$ for $s \in S$.

Assume that predictor values $v_{sc,j}$ for $1 \le j \le q$ are measured for $sc \in SC$. For $sc \in SC$, combine the q predictor values into the $q \times 1$ vector $\mathbf{v}_{sc}$ and, for $s \in S$, let $\mathbf{V}_s$ denote the $m(s) \times q$ predictor matrices with rows $\mathbf{v}_{sc}^{\mathrm{T}}$ for $c \in C(s)$. For $sc \in SC$, model the natural log of the dispersions in terms of these predictors, that is,

$$\log \varphi_{sc} = \mathbf{v}_{sc}^{\mathrm{T}} \cdot \boldsymbol{\gamma}$$

where $\boldsymbol{\gamma}$ is a $q \times 1$ vector of coefficient parameters. When $v_{sc,1} = 1$ for $sc \in SC$, the first entry γ_1 of $\boldsymbol{\gamma}$ is an intercept parameter. Similar notation for predictor values $x_{sc,j}$ and associated parameter vector $\boldsymbol{\beta}$ for the means is defined in Sect. 2.2.

For the linear regression case of Sect. 2.2.1, the variance function is $V(\mu) = 1$. Hence, the extended variances $\sigma_{sc}^2 = \varphi_{sc}$ are the same as the dispersions and the above formulation for dispersion modeling is actually variance modeling.

For the Poisson regression case of Sect. 2.2.2 with an offset variable $o_{sc} = \log T_{sc}$ included to convert the model for the counts y_{sc} to one for rates $y'_{sc} = y_{sc}/T_{sc}$, it can be added to the dispersions as well as to the means. Let the dispersions satisfy

$$\log \varphi_{sc} = \mathbf{v}_{sc}^{\mathrm{T}} \cdot \boldsymbol{\gamma} + o_{sc}$$

so that the extended variances for the counts y_{sc} satisfy

$$\sigma_{sc}^2 = \varphi_{sc} \cdot V(\mu_{sc}) = \varphi_{sc} \cdot \mu_{sc}$$

$$= \exp\left(\boldsymbol{v}_{sc}^{\mathrm{T}} \cdot \gamma\right) \cdot \exp\left(\boldsymbol{x}_{sc}^{\mathrm{T}} \cdot \boldsymbol{\beta}\right) \cdot \exp^2(o_{sc})$$
$$= \exp\left(\boldsymbol{v}_{sc}^{\mathrm{T}} \cdot \gamma\right) \cdot \exp\left(\boldsymbol{x}_{sc}^{\mathrm{T}} \cdot \boldsymbol{\beta}\right) \cdot T_{sc}^2$$

and then the variances for the rates y'_{sc} satisfy

$$\sigma'^2_{sc} = \frac{\sigma_{sc}^2}{T_{sc}^2} = \varphi'_{sc} \cdot \mu'_{sc}$$

where $\mu'_{sc} = \exp\left(\boldsymbol{x}_{sc}^{\mathrm{T}} \cdot \boldsymbol{\beta}\right)$ and $\varphi'_{sc} = \exp\left(\boldsymbol{v}_{sc}^{\mathrm{T}} \cdot \boldsymbol{\beta}\right)$. The standardized residuals for the counts satisfy

$$stde_{sc} = \frac{y_{sc} - \mu_{sc}}{\sigma_{sc}} = \frac{y_{sc} - \mu'_{sc} \cdot T_{sc}}{\sigma'_{sc} \cdot T_{sc}}$$

and so are the same as the standardized residuals for the rates

$$stde'_{sc} = \frac{y'_{sc} - \mu'_{sc}}{\sigma'_{sc}}.$$

Standard GEE modeling in the Poisson regression case can also be adjusted to consider offsets for constant dispersions although this is not usually an option for implementations of standard GEE modeling even when offsets for the means are included.

3.2 Adding Estimating Equations for the Dispersions Based on the Likelihood

GEE modeling can be partially modified to handle non-constant dispersions (Knafl & Ding, 2016). As in Sect. 2.5, define the likelihood function $L(SC;\boldsymbol{\theta})$ as the product of the terms $L(O_s;\boldsymbol{\theta})$ satisfying

$$\ell(O_s;\boldsymbol{\theta}) = \log L(O_s;\boldsymbol{\theta}) = -\boldsymbol{e}_s^{\mathrm{T}} \cdot \boldsymbol{\Sigma}_s^{-1} \cdot \boldsymbol{e}_s/2 - (\log|\boldsymbol{\Sigma}_s|)/2 - (m(s) \cdot \log(2 \cdot \pi))/2$$

for $s \in S$, where $O_s = \{\boldsymbol{y}_s, \boldsymbol{X}_s, \boldsymbol{V}_s\}$ (also add in the offset vector $\boldsymbol{o}_s$ when used in the Poisson regression case of Sect. 2.2.2) denotes an observation, $\boldsymbol{\Sigma}_s$ is the $m(s) \times m(s)$ covariance matrix satisfying

$$\boldsymbol{\Sigma}_s = \boldsymbol{DIAG}(\boldsymbol{\sigma}_s) \cdot \boldsymbol{R}_s(\rho) \cdot \boldsymbol{DIAG}(\boldsymbol{\sigma}_s),$$

$|\boldsymbol{\Sigma}_s|$ is the determinant of $\boldsymbol{\Sigma}_s$, and π is the usual constant. Let

$$\boldsymbol{\theta} = \begin{pmatrix} \boldsymbol{\beta} \\ \boldsymbol{\gamma} \end{pmatrix}$$

be the $(r + q) \times 1$ vector composed of the mean and dispersion parameter vectors $\boldsymbol{\beta}$ and $\boldsymbol{\gamma}$ with r and q entries, respectively. The correlation parameter vector $\boldsymbol{\rho}$ (as defined in Sect. 2.3) has not been included in $\boldsymbol{\theta}$ because it is a function of $\boldsymbol{\beta}$ and $\boldsymbol{\gamma}$ (see Sect. 3.3). Differentiate the log-likelihood $\ell(SC;\boldsymbol{\theta})$ with respect to the vector $\boldsymbol{\gamma}$ of coefficient parameters while holding the correlation vector $\boldsymbol{\rho}$ fixed in the current parameter vector $\boldsymbol{\gamma}$ to provide the q estimating equations

$$\boldsymbol{E}(\boldsymbol{\gamma}) = \sum_{s\in S} \boldsymbol{E}_s(\boldsymbol{\gamma}) = \sum_{s\in S} \frac{\partial_0 \ell(O_s;\boldsymbol{\theta})}{\partial_0 \boldsymbol{\gamma}} = \frac{\partial_0 \ell(SC;\boldsymbol{\theta})}{\partial_0 \boldsymbol{\gamma}} = \mathbf{0}$$

where the operator notation $\frac{\partial_0}{\partial_0 \gamma}$ is used to indicate that this is not a full partial derivative in γ due to not accounting for the effect of γ on $\boldsymbol{\rho}$. Now, combine these with the r standard GEE mean estimating equations $\boldsymbol{E}(\boldsymbol{\beta}) = \mathbf{0}$ as defined in Sect. 2.4 to solve for joint estimates of $\boldsymbol{\beta}$ and $\boldsymbol{\gamma}$. Then, iteratively solve for

$$\boldsymbol{E}(\boldsymbol{\theta}) = \begin{pmatrix} \boldsymbol{E}(\boldsymbol{\beta}) \\ \boldsymbol{E}(\boldsymbol{\gamma}) \end{pmatrix} = \mathbf{0}$$

with $\boldsymbol{E}(\boldsymbol{\theta})$ in the role of the gradient vector and the $(r + q) \times (r + q)$ matrix $\boldsymbol{E}'(\boldsymbol{\theta})$ in the role of the Hessian matrix. $\boldsymbol{E}'(\boldsymbol{\theta})$ has four component matrices: the $r \times r$ matrix $\boldsymbol{E}'(\boldsymbol{\beta})$ for the mean coefficients as used in standard GEE modeling, the $q \times q$ matrix

$$\boldsymbol{E}'(\boldsymbol{\gamma}) = \frac{\partial_0 \boldsymbol{E}(\boldsymbol{\gamma})}{\partial_0 \boldsymbol{\gamma}}$$

for the q dispersion coefficients, the $r \times q$ matrix

$$\boldsymbol{E}'(\boldsymbol{\beta},\boldsymbol{\gamma}) = \frac{\partial_0 \boldsymbol{E}(\boldsymbol{\beta})}{\partial_0 \boldsymbol{\gamma}},$$

and its transpose $\boldsymbol{E}'(\boldsymbol{\gamma},\boldsymbol{\beta}) = \boldsymbol{E}'^{\mathrm{T}}(\boldsymbol{\beta},\boldsymbol{\gamma})$.

Note that

$$\log|\boldsymbol{\Sigma}_s| = \log|\boldsymbol{R}_s(\boldsymbol{\rho})| + \sum_{c\in C(s)} \boldsymbol{v}_{sc}^{\mathrm{T}} \cdot \boldsymbol{\gamma} + \sum_{c\in C(s)} \log V(\mu_{sc}),$$

$$\varphi_{sc} = \exp\left(\boldsymbol{v}_{sc}^{\mathrm{T}} \cdot \boldsymbol{\gamma}\right), \text{ and}$$

$$\boldsymbol{e}_s^{\mathrm{T}} \cdot \boldsymbol{\Sigma}_s^{-1} \cdot \boldsymbol{e}_s = \boldsymbol{stde}_s^{\mathrm{T}} \cdot \boldsymbol{R}_s^{-1}(\boldsymbol{\rho}) \cdot \boldsymbol{stde}_s.$$

Consequently, $\boldsymbol{E}(\boldsymbol{\gamma})$ is the sum over $s \in S$ of $\boldsymbol{E}_s(\boldsymbol{\gamma})$ with entries

$$E_{s,j}(\gamma) = \boldsymbol{vstde}_{s,j}^{\mathrm{T}} \cdot \boldsymbol{R}_s^{-1}(\rho) \cdot \boldsymbol{stde}_s - \sum_{c \in C(s)} v_{sc,j}/2$$

where $\boldsymbol{vstde}_{s,j}$ is the $m(s) \times 1$ vector with entries

$$vstde_{sc,j} = v_{sc,j} \cdot stde_{sc}/2$$

for $sc \in SC$ and $1 \leq j \leq q$. $\boldsymbol{E}'(\gamma)$ is the sum over $s \in S$ of $\boldsymbol{E}'_s(\gamma)$ with entries

$$E'_{s,j,j'}(\gamma) = -\boldsymbol{vvstde}_{s,j,j'}^{\mathrm{T}} \cdot \boldsymbol{R}_s^{-1}(\rho) \cdot \boldsymbol{stde}_s - \boldsymbol{vstde}_{s,j}^{\mathrm{T}} \cdot \boldsymbol{R}_s^{-1}(\rho) \cdot \boldsymbol{vstde}_{s,j'}$$

where $\boldsymbol{vvstde}_{s,j,j'}$ is the $m(s) \times 1$ vector with entries

$$vvstde_{sc,j,j'} = v_{sc,j} \cdot v_{sc,j'} \cdot stde_{sc}/4$$

for $sc \in SC$ and $1 \leq j, j' \leq q$. $\boldsymbol{E}'(\boldsymbol{\beta}, \boldsymbol{\gamma})$ is the sum over $s \in S$ of $\boldsymbol{E}'_s(\boldsymbol{\beta}, \boldsymbol{\gamma})$ with q $r \times 1$ column vectors

$$\begin{aligned} \boldsymbol{E}'_{s,j}(\boldsymbol{\beta}, \boldsymbol{\gamma}) = & -\boldsymbol{D}_s^{\mathrm{T}} \cdot \boldsymbol{DIAG}(\boldsymbol{v\sigma inv}_{s,j}) \cdot \boldsymbol{R}_s^{-1}(\rho) \cdot \boldsymbol{stde}_s \\ & -\boldsymbol{D}_s^{\mathrm{T}} \cdot \boldsymbol{DIAG}(\mathbf{1}/\boldsymbol{\sigma}_s) \cdot \boldsymbol{R}_s^{-1}(\rho) \cdot \boldsymbol{vstde}_{s,j} \end{aligned}$$

where $\boldsymbol{v\sigma inv}_{s,j}$ is the $m(s) \times 1$ vector with entries

$$v\sigma inv_{sc,j} = \frac{v_{sc,j}}{2 \cdot \sigma_{sc}}$$

for $sc \in SC$ and $1 \leq j \leq q$. When offsets are included, they are just carried along without any other effect on the computations.

The formulations for LCV scores given in Sect. 2.5 and LCV ratio tests of Sect. 2.6 readily generalize to handle this more general context. The adaptive regression modeling process of Sect. 2.7 also generalizes. Primary predictors are considered for dispersions as well as for means, possibly different ones. Transforms of predictors for means and for dispersions are considered for adding to the model in the expansion and for removal in the contraction phase. It is also possible to apply the adaptive modeling process to just the means holding the dispersions fixed or to just the dispersions holding the means fixed. The only heuristic used in reported analyses that is not considered in Knafl and Ding (2016) is that the expansion is restricted to add only a maximum of five transforms to the model for the dispersions together with a maximum of five transforms to the model for the means in order to reduce computation times.

3.3 Estimating the Correlation Structure

Given a value for the vector $\boldsymbol{\theta}$ of all coefficient parameters, an estimate of the correlation parameter vector $\boldsymbol{\rho}$ can be based on the associated standardized residuals $stde_{sc}(\boldsymbol{\theta})$ determined by non-constant dispersions $\varphi_{sc}(\gamma)$ computed with the current value for γ. Calculate the revised correlation estimates for the correlation structures of Sect. 2.3 using the formulas of Sect. 2.4.1 evaluated with these revised standardized residuals $stde_{sc}(\boldsymbol{\theta})$.

3.4 Estimating the Covariance Matrix for Coefficient Parameter Estimates

Let

$$\boldsymbol{\theta}(SC) = \begin{pmatrix} \boldsymbol{\beta}(SC) \\ \boldsymbol{\gamma}(SC) \end{pmatrix}$$

denote the estimate of the coefficient vector $\boldsymbol{\theta}$ obtained by solving the partially modified GEE equations $\boldsymbol{E}(\boldsymbol{\theta}) = \mathbf{0}$ using the observations with indexes in SC. As in Sect. 2.4.2 for standard GEE, two estimates of the covariance matrix for the estimated parameter vector $\boldsymbol{\theta}(SC)$ can be computed: the model-based and robust empirical estimates. The model-based estimate is

$$\Sigma_{\mathrm{MB}}(\boldsymbol{\theta}(SC)) = -\boldsymbol{E}'^{-1}(\boldsymbol{\theta}(SC)).$$

The robust empirical estimate is

$$\Sigma_{\mathrm{RE}}(\boldsymbol{\theta}(SC)) = \boldsymbol{E}'^{-1}(\boldsymbol{\theta}(SC)) \cdot \boldsymbol{G}(\boldsymbol{\theta}(SC)) \cdot \boldsymbol{G}^{\mathrm{T}}(\boldsymbol{\theta}(SC)) \cdot \boldsymbol{E}'^{-1}(\boldsymbol{\theta}(SC))$$

where $\boldsymbol{G}(\boldsymbol{\theta}(SC))$ is the $(r + q) \times m(SC)$ matrix with $(r + q) \times m(s)$ component matrices $\boldsymbol{G}_s(\boldsymbol{\theta}(SC))$ for $s \in S$ satisfying

$$\boldsymbol{G}_s(\boldsymbol{\theta}(SC)) = \begin{pmatrix} \boldsymbol{G}_s(\boldsymbol{\beta}(SC)) \\ \boldsymbol{G}_s(\boldsymbol{\gamma}(SC)) \end{pmatrix}.$$

$\boldsymbol{G}_s(\boldsymbol{\beta}(SC))$ has the same formulation as in Sect. 2.4.2. $\boldsymbol{G}_s(\boldsymbol{\gamma}(SC))$ is the $q \times m(s)$ matrix with rows $\boldsymbol{G}_{s,j}(\boldsymbol{\gamma}(SC))$ for $1 \leq j \leq q$ satisfying

$$\boldsymbol{G}_{s,j}(\boldsymbol{\gamma}(SC)) = (\boldsymbol{vstde}_{s,j}^{\mathrm{T}} \cdot \boldsymbol{R}_s^{-1}(\boldsymbol{\rho})) \circ \boldsymbol{stde}_s^{\mathrm{T}} - \boldsymbol{v}_{s,j}^{\mathrm{T}}/2$$

where $\circ$ denotes elementwise multiplication and $\boldsymbol{v}_{s,j}$ is the $m(s) \times 1$ vector with entries $v_{sc,j}$ for $c \in C(s)$. Note that $\boldsymbol{E}(\boldsymbol{\theta}(\mathrm{SC}))$ equals the $(r + q) \times 1$ vector generated by summing the rows of $\boldsymbol{G}(\boldsymbol{\theta}(SC))$. The diagonal entries of $\boldsymbol{\Sigma}_{\text{MB}}(\boldsymbol{\theta}(SC))$ and $\boldsymbol{\Sigma}_{\text{RE}}(\boldsymbol{\theta}(SC))$ are estimates of variances for the parameter estimates given by the entries of $\boldsymbol{\theta}(SC)$. These can be used to generate z tests of zero coefficient parameter values. Results of such tests are not reported in example adaptive analyses because adaptively determined models have parameters that are usually significant as a consequence of the adaptive modeling process.

3.5 The Constant Dispersion Model

A simple partially modified GEE modeling example is the constant dispersion model with $q = 1$, $v_{sc,1} = 1$ for $sc \in SC$, and a single dispersion parameter γ. The estimating equation corresponding to γ is

$$E(\gamma) = \sum_{s \in S} \left(\exp(-\gamma) \cdot \boldsymbol{Pres}_s^{\text{T}}(\boldsymbol{\beta}) \cdot \boldsymbol{R}_s^{-1}(\rho) \cdot \boldsymbol{Pres}_s(\boldsymbol{\beta}) \right) / 2 - m(SC)/2 = 0$$

so that the associated constant dispersion estimate $\varphi(SC)$ satisfies

$$\varphi(SC) = \exp(\gamma(SC)) = \frac{\sum_{s \in S} \boldsymbol{Pres}_s^{\text{T}}(\boldsymbol{\beta}(SC)) \cdot \boldsymbol{R}_s^{-1}(\rho(SC)) \cdot \boldsymbol{Pres}_s(\boldsymbol{\beta}(SC))}{m(SC)}.$$

In contrast, the constant dispersion estimate $\varphi_{\text{GEE}}(SC)$ used in standard GEE modeling satisfies (Sect. 2.4)

$$\varphi_{\text{GEE}}(SC) = \frac{\sum_{s \in S} \boldsymbol{Pres}_s^{\text{T}}(\boldsymbol{\beta}(SC)) \cdot \boldsymbol{Pres}_s(\boldsymbol{\beta}(SC))}{m(SC) - r},$$

and so differs in having a bias-adjusted denominator and in not accounting for the correlation structure in the numerator. Standard GEE models can be generated from constant dispersions partially modified GEE models by multiplying the estimate $\varphi(SC)$ by $\varphi_{\text{GEE}}(SC)/\varphi(SC)$. This works because both types of models use the standard GEE estimating equations $\boldsymbol{E}(\boldsymbol{\beta}) = \boldsymbol{0}$ for $\boldsymbol{\beta}$. However, this involves computing two estimates $\varphi(SC)$ and $\varphi_{\text{GEE}}(SC)$. A more efficient approach is generated by assuming unit dispersions so that $\varphi(SC) = 1$ does not need to be computed and only $\varphi_{\text{GEE}}(SC)$ needs to be computed.

3.6 Degeneracy in Correlation Parameter Estimation

Correlation parameter estimates need to be bounded to avoid degeneracy. Since these parameters are correlations, they clearly need to lie within the open interval $(-1, 1)$. Also, as noted in Sect. 2.5, the working correlation matrix for the full set C of m conditions needs to be positive definite. Correlation parameter estimates generated for standard and partially modified GEE as defined in Sects. 2.4.1 and 3.3 can violate these boundedness and positive definiteness restrictions.

Positive definiteness holds for the EC structure if ρ_{EC} falls within $(-1/(m-1), 1)$ (see Sect. 5.3.2 for details) and for the AR1 structure if ρ_{AR1} falls within $[0, 1)$ (see Sect. 5.4.1 for details). Set $\rho_{\mathrm{Lo}} = -1/(m-1) + \delta_1$ for the EC structure and $\rho_{\mathrm{Lo}} = 0$ for the AR1 structure. Also set $\rho_{\mathrm{Hi}} = 1 - \delta_1$ for both these structures. Set δ_1 to some small positive number like 0.0001. Restricting correlation estimates to fall within the bounds given by the closed interval $[\rho_{\mathrm{Lo}}, \rho_{\mathrm{Hi}}]$, a subset of $(-1, 1)$, guarantees a positive definite estimated correlation matrix for these two correlation structures. Consequently, if an estimate falls outside the closed interval $[\rho_{\mathrm{Lo}}, \rho_{\mathrm{Hi}}]$, a straightforward adjustment would be to change it to the closer endpoint of this interval. This appears to be the adjustment used by PROC GENMOD of SAS Version 9.4 using $\delta_1 = 0.0001$ (an issue apparently not addressed in the SAS documentation) since correlation parameter estimates equal to 0.9999 are generated by PROC GENMOD in rare cases.

The problem is not that easily resolved for the UN correlation structure. First of all, the estimated correlation matrix may have one or more entries that lie outside of the interval $(-1, 1)$. This can be rectified as follows. If there are entries larger than $1 - \delta_1$, adjust the largest such value to be equal to $1 - \delta_1$ and the other such values to proportionally smaller values. If there are entries smaller than $-1 + \delta_1$, adjust the smallest such value to be equal to $-1 + \delta_1$ and the other such values to proportionally larger values. However, this does not guarantee that the adjusted correlation matrix is positive definite. To address this possibility, let $\boldsymbol{R}_0$ denote the standard or partially modified GEE estimate of the $m \times m$ UN working correlation matrix for the full set C of m conditions given in Sect. 2.4.1 possibly adjusted as above for out-of-range entries. $\boldsymbol{R}_0$ can be checked for positive definiteness using the decomposition

$$\boldsymbol{R}_0 = \boldsymbol{A} \cdot \boldsymbol{DIAG}(\boldsymbol{\lambda}) \cdot \boldsymbol{A}^{\mathrm{T}}$$

where $\boldsymbol{\lambda}$ is the vector of eigenvalues λ for $\boldsymbol{R}_0$. The dependence of $\boldsymbol{R}_0$, $\boldsymbol{A}$, and $\boldsymbol{\lambda}$ on $\boldsymbol{\theta}$ has been suppressed to simplify the notation. $\boldsymbol{R}_0$ is positive definite if the smallest entry $\min(\boldsymbol{\lambda})$ of $\boldsymbol{\lambda}$ is positive. Problems can occur when $\min(\boldsymbol{\lambda})$ is negative, zero, or too small a positive value. Let δ_2 be a small positive value like $\delta_2 = 0.005$. Adjust $\boldsymbol{R}_0$ if $\min(\boldsymbol{\lambda}) < \delta_2$ as follows. Let

$$0 < \eta = \frac{1 - \delta_2}{1 - \min(\boldsymbol{\lambda})} < 1$$

and $\boldsymbol{R}' = \eta \cdot \boldsymbol{R}_0 + (1 - \eta) \cdot \boldsymbol{I}$ where $\boldsymbol{I}$ is the associated identity matrix. $\boldsymbol{R}'$ is the correlation matrix with associated vector $\boldsymbol{\lambda}'$ of eigenvalues λ'. These eigenvalues satisfy

$$(\boldsymbol{R}' - \lambda' \cdot \boldsymbol{I}) \cdot \boldsymbol{x} = \boldsymbol{0}$$

or, equivalently,

$$\left(\boldsymbol{R}_0 - \frac{\lambda' - (1 - \eta)}{\eta} \cdot \boldsymbol{I}\right) \cdot \boldsymbol{x} = \boldsymbol{0}$$

so that the eigenvalues of $\boldsymbol{R}_0$ satisfy

$$\lambda = \frac{\lambda' - (1 - \eta)}{\eta}$$

and then the eigenvalues of $\boldsymbol{R}'$ satisfy $\lambda' = \lambda \cdot \eta + 1 - \eta$ or that the minimum eigenvalue $\min(\boldsymbol{\lambda}')$ of $\boldsymbol{R}'$ satisfies

$$\min(\boldsymbol{\lambda}') = \min(\boldsymbol{\lambda}) \cdot \eta + 1 - \eta = -\eta \cdot (1 - \min(\boldsymbol{\lambda})) + 1 = -(1 - \delta_2) + 1 = \delta_2.$$

In this way, a correlation matrix with a problematic minimum eigenvalue can be adjusted to have a positive minimum eigenvalue equal to δ_2, and so be positive definite. Consequently, when $\min(\boldsymbol{\lambda}) \geq \delta_2$, use the working correlation matrix $\boldsymbol{R} = \boldsymbol{R}_0$ to compute $\boldsymbol{E}(\boldsymbol{\theta})$ and $\boldsymbol{E}'(\boldsymbol{\theta})$; otherwise use $\boldsymbol{R} = \boldsymbol{R}'$.

3.7 The Estimation Process

Let $\boldsymbol{\theta}_i$ denote the current value for the coefficient vector $\boldsymbol{\theta}$ for the means and dispersions with $r + q$ entries. In the standard GEE case of Chap. 2, replace $\boldsymbol{\theta}$ by $\boldsymbol{\beta}$. Let $\boldsymbol{\rho}(\boldsymbol{\theta}_i)$ denote the correlation parameter vector estimate generated by $\boldsymbol{\theta}_i$, possibly adjusted as described in Sect. 3.6 to resolve any degeneracy problems. The vectors $\boldsymbol{\theta}_i$ and $\boldsymbol{\rho}(\boldsymbol{\theta}_i)$ generate the current values for the vector $\boldsymbol{E}(\boldsymbol{\theta}_i)$ and the matrix $\boldsymbol{E}'(\boldsymbol{\theta}_i)$ treated in what follows as the gradient vector and the associated Hessian matrix, respectively. The next parameter vector $\boldsymbol{\theta}_{i+1}$ can be determined using a series of steps as described next. Step 0 is to use Newton's method with

$$\boldsymbol{\theta}_{i+1,0} = \boldsymbol{\theta}_i - \boldsymbol{E}'^{-1}(\boldsymbol{\theta}_i) \cdot \boldsymbol{E}(\boldsymbol{\theta}_i).$$

Denote the entries of the gradient vector $\boldsymbol{E}(\boldsymbol{\theta})$ as $E_j(\boldsymbol{\theta})$ for $1 \leq j \leq r + q$ and the maximum of the absolute values of these entries as

$$\max(|\boldsymbol{E}(\boldsymbol{\theta})|) = \max\left\{|E_j(\boldsymbol{\theta})| : 1 \leq j \leq r + q\right\}.$$

Convergence to a solution to the estimating equations requires that $\max(|\boldsymbol{E}(\boldsymbol{\theta}_i)|)$ converges to 0. However, $\max(|\boldsymbol{E}(\boldsymbol{\theta}_{i+1,0})|)$ need not be smaller than $\max(|\boldsymbol{E}(\boldsymbol{\theta}_i)|)$. Even when it is smaller, it can often be improved with a Step 1 adjustment as described next and, in some cases, convergence does not occur unless a Step 1 adjustment is always included in the estimation process. So, to be conservative, this adjustment is always included in the estimation process.

3.7.1 Step 1 Adjustment

Let

$$\boldsymbol{\theta}_{i+1,1}(d) = \boldsymbol{\theta}_i - d \cdot \boldsymbol{E}'^{-1}(\boldsymbol{\theta}_i) \cdot \boldsymbol{E}(\boldsymbol{\theta}_i).$$

A search algorithm is needed to identify an effective choice d' for d in the sense that $\max(|\boldsymbol{E}(\boldsymbol{\theta}_{i+1,1}(d'))|)$ is close to the minimum value for $\max(|\boldsymbol{E}(\boldsymbol{\theta}_{i+1,1}(d))|)$ over possible values of d. This can require consideration of $d < 0$ or $d > 1$. An algorithm for doing this is presented next. If $\max(|\boldsymbol{E}(\boldsymbol{\theta}_{i+1,0})|) < \max(|\boldsymbol{E}(\boldsymbol{\theta}_i)|)$, set $d_0 = 0$; otherwise set $d_0 = 1$, thereby initially searching over $\boldsymbol{\theta}_{i+1,1}(d)$ around the choice of d_0 generating the better value of $\max(|\boldsymbol{E}(\boldsymbol{\theta}_{i+1,1}(d))|)$ for the two choices $d = 0$ and $d = 1$.

Iteration 1. Solve for a d within one decimal digit around $d = d_0$ as follows. Set $digits = 1$. Consider values for d of $d_0(t) = d_0 + t \cdot 10^{-digits}$ for t an integer between ± 10. Start with $t = 1$ so that $d_0(1) = d_0 + 0.1$. If

$$\max(|\boldsymbol{E}(\boldsymbol{\theta}_{i+1,1}(d_0(1)))|) < \max(|\boldsymbol{E}(\boldsymbol{\theta}_i)|),$$

continue searching over larger values of t until

$$\max(|\boldsymbol{E}(\boldsymbol{\theta}_{i+1,1}(d_0(t+1)))|) \geq \max(|\boldsymbol{E}(\boldsymbol{\theta}_{i+1,1}(d_0(t)))|),$$

and set $d_1 = d_0(t)$. Otherwise, start with $t = -1$ so that $d_0(1) = d_0 - 0.1$, and search over smaller values for t until

$$\max(|\boldsymbol{E}(\boldsymbol{\theta}_{i+1,1}(d_0(t+1)))|) \geq \max(|\boldsymbol{E}(\boldsymbol{\theta}_{i+1,i}(d_0(t)))|),$$

and set $d_1 = d_0(t)$. When $d_0 = 0$, the stopping condition for positive t may not hold for any t, in which case, $d_1 = d_0(+10) = 1$. Also, the stopping condition for positive t might hold for $t = 1$, in which case $d_1 = d_0(0) = 0$. The stopping condition for negative t may not hold for any t, in which case, $d_1 = d_0(-10) = -1$. Also, the stopping condition for negative t might hold for $t = -1$, in which case $d_1 = d_0(0) = 0$. Similar results hold when $d_0 = 1$.
Iteration 2. Solve for a d within two decimal digits around d_1 as follows. Set $digits = 2$. Consider values for d of $d_1(t) = d_1 + t \cdot 10^{-digits}$ for t an integer between ± 10. Search first through positive t and possibly through negative t as in the search for iteration 1, defining d_2.
Iteration j. Solve for a d within j decimal digits around d_{j-1} as follows. Set $digits = j$. Consider values for d of $d_{j-1}(t) = d_{j-1} + t \cdot 10^{-digits}$ for t an integer between ± 10. Search first through positive t and possibly through negative t as in the search for iteration 1, defining d_j.

To stop the step 1 adjustment search, set a maximum j^* for the number of digits; for example, a maximum of $j^* = 5$ digits would identify a $d' = d_5$ within ± 0.00001 of a local minimum in d for $\max(|\boldsymbol{E}(\boldsymbol{\theta}_{i+1,1}(d))|)$. However, it may be possible to stop the search earlier. For example, if the percent decrease for $\max(|\boldsymbol{E}(\boldsymbol{\theta}_{i+1,1}(d_j))|)$ compared to $\max(|\boldsymbol{E}(\boldsymbol{\theta}_{i+1,1}(d_{j-1}))|)$ for any $j < j^*$ is within a certain small tolerance, stop the search and use $d' = d_j$, rather than considering larger j. Formally, stop the search at j if

$$\max\left(\left|\boldsymbol{E}\left(\boldsymbol{\theta}_i\left(d_{j-1}\right)\right)\right|\right) > \max\left(\left|\boldsymbol{E}\left(\boldsymbol{\theta}_{i+1,1}\left(d_j\right)\right)\right|\right) \geq (1-\tau_1) \cdot \max\left(\left|\boldsymbol{E}\left(\boldsymbol{\theta}_i\left(d_{j-1}\right)\right)\right|\right)$$

for some tolerance τ_1. This indicates that further search should not change the results by much.

When $d_0 = 0$, in extreme conditions the first iteration will stop at $d_1 = -1$, the second iteration at $d_2 = -1.1$, the third iteration at $d_3 = -1.11$, and so on. In all cases, not just extreme ones, it will stop at a value less than or equal to 1. When $d_1 = 1$, in extreme conditions the first iteration will stop at $d_1 = 2$, the second iteration at $d_2 = 2.1$, the third iteration at $d_3 = 2.11$, and so on. In all cases, not just extreme ones, it will stop at a value greater than or equal to 0. Thus, the final choice will be in a bounded interval with bounds depending on the starting value of d_0 and on the maximum number of iterations j^*. In some cases, searches over a larger set of values d might generate a better result, but the next iteration is likely to do as well or better.

The parameter vector $\boldsymbol{\theta}_{i+1,1}(d')$ generated by the step 1 adjustment may not always be an effective alternative to $\boldsymbol{\theta}_{i+1,0}$. When $d' = 0$, $\boldsymbol{\theta}_{i+1,1}(d') = \boldsymbol{\theta}_{i+1,0}$. When $d' \neq 0$, $\max(|\boldsymbol{E}(\boldsymbol{\theta}_{i+1,1}(d))|)$ might not be too much smaller than $\max(|\boldsymbol{E}(\boldsymbol{\theta}_{i+1,0})|)$ and a step 2 adjustment may be needed (Sect. 3.7.2). Skip this step 2 adjustment and set $\boldsymbol{\theta}_{i+1} = \boldsymbol{\theta}_{i+1,1}(d')$ if $\boldsymbol{\theta}_{i+1,1}(d')$ provides at least a fixed percent decrease over $\max(|\boldsymbol{E}(\boldsymbol{\theta}_i)|)$, that is, if

$$\max(|\boldsymbol{E}(\boldsymbol{\theta}_{i+1,1}(d'))|) < (1-\tau_2)\cdot\max(|\boldsymbol{E}(\boldsymbol{\theta}_i)|)$$

for some tolerance τ_2. However, a step 2 adjustment can be time-consuming and so is best avoided if possible. Consequently, also skip the step 2 adjustment if $\max(|\boldsymbol{E}(\boldsymbol{\theta}_{i+1,1}(d'))|)$ is not too large, that is, if $\max(|\boldsymbol{E}(\boldsymbol{\theta}_{i+1,1}(d'))|) < \tau_3$. Otherwise, conduct the step 2 adjustment, that is, when $\max(|\boldsymbol{E}(\boldsymbol{\theta}_{i+1,1}(d'))|)$ does not provide much of an improvement over $\max(|\boldsymbol{E}(\boldsymbol{\theta}_i)|)$ and $\max(|\boldsymbol{E}(\boldsymbol{\theta}_{i+1,1}(d'))|)$ is also large.

3.7.2 Step 2 Adjustment

Let $\boldsymbol{\theta}'_i = \boldsymbol{\theta}_{i+1,1}(d')$ and $\boldsymbol{\theta}_{i+1,2}(\boldsymbol{\Delta}) = \boldsymbol{\theta}'_i - \boldsymbol{\Delta}$ for a $(r+q)\times 1$ vector $\boldsymbol{\Delta}$ with entries δ_j. A search algorithm is needed to identify an effective choice $\boldsymbol{\Delta}'$ for $\boldsymbol{\Delta}$ in the sense that $\max(|\boldsymbol{E}(\boldsymbol{\theta}_{i+1,2}(\boldsymbol{\Delta}'))|)$ is close to the overall minimum in $\boldsymbol{\Delta}$ for $\max(|\boldsymbol{E}(\boldsymbol{\theta}_{i+1,2}(\boldsymbol{\Delta}))|)$. The step 2 adjustment has two stages. Stage 1 identifies a choice for $\boldsymbol{\Delta}$ by systematically identifying entries δ_j. Stage 2 searches over choices $\boldsymbol{\Delta}' = d\cdot\boldsymbol{\Delta}$ using an approach similar to the step 1 adjustment. Let $\mathbf{1}_j$ denote the $(r+q)\times 1$ vector with value 1 in its jth entry and value 0 elsewhere.

Stage 1, Start with $\boldsymbol{\Delta}_0 = \mathbf{0}$.

Stage 1, iteration j. The prior iteration has identified $\boldsymbol{\Delta}_{j-1}$ having entries $\delta_{j-1,j'}$ for $1 \le j' \le r+q$ with $j-1$ of these entries set to a non-zero value and the other $r+q-j+1$ entries equaling 0.

Stage 1, iteration j, sub-iteration j'. If $\delta_{j-1,j'} \ne 0$, skip this sub-iteration. Otherwise, conduct a search in two sub-stages. For sub-stage 1, start with $power = 0$, $j'' = 0$, $\delta_{j-1,j',j''} = 1$, $sign = +1$, and

$$\boldsymbol{\Delta}_{j-1,j''} = \boldsymbol{\Delta}_{j-1} + sign\cdot\mathbf{1}_j\cdot\delta_{j-1,j',j''},$$

If

$$\max\left(\left|\boldsymbol{E}\left(\boldsymbol{\theta}_{i+1,2}\left(\boldsymbol{\Delta}_{j-1,j''}\right)\right)\right|\right) \ge \max(|\boldsymbol{E}(\boldsymbol{\theta}'_i)|),$$

reset $sign = -1$, recompute $\boldsymbol{\Delta}_{j-1,j''} = \boldsymbol{\Delta}_{j-1} \cdot + sign \cdot \mathbf{1}_j\cdot\delta_{j-1,j',j''}$, and if

$$\max\left(\left|\boldsymbol{E}\left(\boldsymbol{\theta}_{i+1,2}\left(\boldsymbol{\Delta}_{j-1,j''}\right)\right)\right|\right) \ge \max(|\boldsymbol{E}(\boldsymbol{\theta}'_i)|),$$

stop sub-iteration j'. Otherwise, increment j'' and continue the search with sign as set with $j'' = 0$. With $power = j'' > 0$, $\delta_{j-1,j',j''} = 10^{power}$, and

$$\boldsymbol{\Delta}_{j-1,j''} = \boldsymbol{\Delta}_{j-1} + sign\cdot\mathbf{1}_j\cdot\delta_{j-1,j',j''},$$

stop the search if

$$\max\left(\left|\boldsymbol{E}\left(\boldsymbol{\theta}_{i+1,2}\left(\boldsymbol{\Delta}_{j-1,j''}\right)\right)\right|\right) \geq \max(|\boldsymbol{E}(\boldsymbol{\theta}'_i)|).$$

Set a maximum value j''^* for j'', and stop the search when $j'' = j''^* + 1$ (without computing anything for this value of j''). If the final value $j''(end)$ of the search over j'' satisfies

$$j''(end) = j''^* + 1,$$

then

$$\max\left(\left|\boldsymbol{E}\left(\boldsymbol{\theta}_{i+1,2}\left(\boldsymbol{\Delta}_{j-1,j''^*}\right)\right)\right|\right) < \max(|\boldsymbol{E}(\boldsymbol{\theta}'_i)|),$$

so set $\boldsymbol{\Delta}_{j-1,j''} = \boldsymbol{\Delta}_{j-1} + sign \cdot \mathbf{1}_j \cdot \delta_{j-1,j',j''^*}$ and skip sub-stage 2. Otherwise, conduct sub-stage 2 searching on either side of $\delta_{j-1,j',j''\ (end)}$ over increasing numbers of decimal digits. Sub-stage 1 chooses $j''(end)$ in such a way that sub-stage 2 searches in the positive and negative directions will eventually result in an increase in the maximum absolute value of the associated gradient entries. The logic of the sub-stage 2 search is similar to the search conducted in the step 1 adjustment except that it is conducted over multiples of one entry of $\boldsymbol{\Delta}$ starting at a power of 10 rather than over a multiple of $\boldsymbol{E}'^{-1}(\boldsymbol{\theta}_i) \cdot \boldsymbol{E}(\boldsymbol{\theta}_i)$ starting at 0, and so the details are not presented. Sub-stage 2 uses the same maximum number of iterations j''^* as for sub-stage 1. It also uses a stopping tolerance τ_4 analogous to the tolerance τ_1 used to stop the step 1 adjustment. Iteration j generates $\boldsymbol{\Delta}_j$. Stage 1 stops after $r + q$ such iterations addressing all $r + q$ parameters have been conducted.

Stage 2. The full stage 1 search generates an initial $\boldsymbol{\Delta}$ built up one entry at a time. This $\boldsymbol{\Delta}$ now plays the role of the adjustment $\boldsymbol{E}'^{-1}(\boldsymbol{\theta}_i) \cdot \boldsymbol{E}(\boldsymbol{\theta}_i)$ used in Newton's method. Stage 2 determines an appropriate multiple $d \cdot \boldsymbol{\Delta}$ to use in place of $\boldsymbol{\Delta}$ similar to the step 1 adjustment of $\boldsymbol{E}'^{-1}(\theta_i) \cdot \boldsymbol{E}(\boldsymbol{\theta}_i)$. However, this has to be conducted in two sub-stages as in the stage 1 sub-iterations, first identifying in sub-stage 1 a power j of 10 for which sub-stage 2 searches on either side of 10^j over increasing numbers of decimal digits will eventually result in an increase in the maximum absolute value of the gradient entries. The logic of these two sub-stage searches is similar to prior searches and so the details are not presented. Stage 2 generates a final choice $\boldsymbol{\Delta}' = d' \cdot \boldsymbol{\Delta}$. It has a maximum number of iterations j'''^* and a stopping tolerance τ_5. Let $\boldsymbol{\theta}_{i+1} = \boldsymbol{\theta}_i - \boldsymbol{\Delta}'$.

3.7.3 *Stopping the Estimation Process*

To stop the overall estimation process, first set a maximum number i^* of iterations and stop the search if $i = i^*$ and use $\boldsymbol{\theta}_{i^*}$. This maximum would be set to allow for a relatively large number of iterations. Set a stopping tolerance τ_6 and stop the search if $\max(|\boldsymbol{E}(\boldsymbol{\theta}_i)|) < \tau_6$. For $i > 1$, the current proportional decrease in $\max(|\boldsymbol{E}(\boldsymbol{\theta})|)$ is

$$PD_i = \frac{\max(|\boldsymbol{E}(\boldsymbol{\theta}_{i-1})|) - \max(|\boldsymbol{E}(\boldsymbol{\theta}_i)|)}{\max(|\boldsymbol{E}(\boldsymbol{\theta}_{i-1})|)}.$$

For $i > 2$, let $I(PD_i < PD_{i-1})$ be the indicator for a decrease in consecutive proportional decreases where I denotes an indicator function for a logical condition equal to 1 when the logical condition holds and 0 otherwise. Also, let *stopcnt*(i) denote the number of decreases in the consecutive proportional decrease up to iteration i, that is,

$$stopcnt(i) = \sum_{i'=2}^{i} I(PD_{i'} < PD_{i'-1}).$$

Set a tolerance τ_7 for a small proportional decrease and a maximum number *maxPD* for decreases in the proportional decrease. Stop the search if $PD_{i+1} < \tau_7$ or if *stopcnt*(i) > *maxPD*. This adjusts for slowly converging cases. Altogether, the search stops if the maximum absolute gradient entry is small enough, its proportional decrease compared to the prior iteration is small enough, the number of decreases in consecutive proportional decreases occurs too many times, or the number of iterations gets too large.

3.7.4 Initial Estimates

An initial estimate $\boldsymbol{\beta}_0$ of $\boldsymbol{\beta}$ for standard GEE modeling can be the estimate generated by generalized linear modeling treating the *m*(*SC*) measurements as independent of each other even when they include multiple measurements within matched sets (see Sect. 4.4 for more on such singleton univariate outcomes). This is the default approach used by PROC GENMOD of SAS Version 9.4 (a fixed starting point can also be optionally specified). Knafl and Ding (2016) proposed an extension of generalized linear modeling of independent measurements to support non-constant dispersions (see Sect. 4.4). This can be used to generate an initial estimate $\boldsymbol{\theta}_0$ of $\boldsymbol{\theta}$ for partially modified GEE modeling. These initial estimates can be ineffective in the sense that the maximum absolute value of the gradient entries increases in the first few iterations; that is, $\max(|\boldsymbol{E}(\boldsymbol{\theta}_i)|)$ is much larger than $\max(|\boldsymbol{E}(\boldsymbol{\theta}_{i+1,0})|)$ for the first few iterations i. Resolution of this problem can be addressed by executing the step 2 adjustment. Formally, if

$$\max(|\boldsymbol{E}(\boldsymbol{\theta}_{i+1,0})|) > \max(|\boldsymbol{E}(\boldsymbol{\theta}_i)|) + \tau_8 \cdot \max(|\boldsymbol{E}(\boldsymbol{\theta}_i)|)$$

for some positive tolerance τ_8 starting with $i = 0$, then execute the step 2 adjustment even if the step 1 adjustment provides at least a fixed percent decrease as defined in

Sect. 3.7.1 using the tolerance τ_2. Stop considering this adjustment after the first iteration i for which

$$\max(|\boldsymbol{E}(\boldsymbol{\theta}_{i+1,0})|) \leq \max(|\boldsymbol{E}(\boldsymbol{\theta}_i)|) + \tau_8 \cdot \max(|\boldsymbol{E}(\boldsymbol{\theta}_i)|).$$

3.7.5 Other Computational Issues

When predictors are arbitrary power transforms of primary predictors, they can have extreme values that can cause convergence problems if left unadjusted. This can be ameliorated by bounding the predictor matrices. Let $\boldsymbol{X}$ be the $m(SC) \times r$ composite predictor matrix formed by combining the n predictor matrices $\boldsymbol{X}_s$ over $s \in S$ with r $m(SC) \times 1$ column vectors $\boldsymbol{x}_j$ and let $\boldsymbol{\beta}_0$ be the associated initial mean parameter vector with entries $\beta_{0,j}$. Let $xmax_j$ be the maximum of the absolute values of the entries of $\boldsymbol{x}_j$ or the value 1 if $\boldsymbol{x}_j$ is the zero vector and define the adjusted composite predictor matrix $\boldsymbol{X}'$ to have columns $\boldsymbol{x}_j/xmax_j$ and the adjusted initial estimate $\boldsymbol{\beta}'_0$ to have entries $\beta'_{0,j} = \beta_{0,j} \cdot xmax_j$ for $1 \leq j \leq r$. Adjust, in the same way, the composite predictor matrix $\boldsymbol{V}$ formed by combining the n predictor matrices $\boldsymbol{V}_s$ over $s \in S$ with column bounds $vmax_j$ for $1 \leq j \leq q$ into the adjusted $m(SC) \times q$ composite predictor matrix $\boldsymbol{V}'$ and the initial parameter vector $\boldsymbol{\gamma}_0$ into the adjusted dispersion parameter vector $\boldsymbol{\gamma}'_0$. Apply the estimation process to the adjusted composite predictor matrices $\boldsymbol{X}'$ and $\boldsymbol{V}'$ using the starting vector

$$\boldsymbol{\theta}'_0 = \begin{pmatrix} \boldsymbol{\beta}'_0 \\ \boldsymbol{\gamma}'_0 \end{pmatrix}.$$

This generates a solution

$$\boldsymbol{\theta}'(SC) = \begin{pmatrix} \boldsymbol{\beta}'(SC) \\ \boldsymbol{\gamma}'(SC) \end{pmatrix}$$

with entries $\beta'_j(SC)$ for $1 \leq j \leq r$ and $\gamma'_j(SC)$ for $1 \leq j \leq q$. The associated solution

$$\boldsymbol{\theta}(SC) = \begin{pmatrix} \boldsymbol{\beta}(SC) \\ \boldsymbol{\gamma}(SC) \end{pmatrix}$$

for the original composite predictor matrices $\boldsymbol{X}$ and $\boldsymbol{V}$ has entries $\beta_j(SC) = \beta'_j(SC)/xmax_j$ for $1 \leq j \leq r$ and $\gamma_j(SC) = \gamma'_j(SC)/vmax_j$ for $1 \leq j \leq q$.

Another problem is that the computation of the product $a \cdot b$ of two non-zero numbers a and b with signs sign(a) and sign(b) can cause floating point overflow. This can be avoided as follows. Let *logmax* be a large number for which its exponent exp(*logmax*) can be computed without overflow; the value $logmax = 700$ works for Windows systems. Define

$$logab = \min(\log|a| + \log|b|, logmax)$$

and set the product $a \cdot b$ of a and b to

$$a \cdot b = \text{sign}(a) \cdot \text{sign}(b) \cdot \exp(logab).$$

Similar adjustments can be made when the product involves vectors or matrices. In cases where the vector's entries are to be summed, the sum of terms each bounded by exp(*logmax*) may also generate floating point overflow. In such cases, use a smaller bound for each entry that guarantees that their sum is bounded by exp(*logmax*). Further adjustments for computational issues are provided by Knafl and Ding (2016, Sects. 20.4.10 and 20.4.11).

3.7.6 Recommended Tolerance Settings

Analyses reported in Chaps. 6–8 use the following recommended tolerance settings. For the step 1 adjustment, the maximum for the number of digits is set to $j^* = 5$ with stopping tolerance $\tau_1 = 0.0001$. The step 2 adjustment is skipped if it provides at least a fixed percent decrease over $\max(|\boldsymbol{E}(\boldsymbol{\theta}_i)|)$ of $\tau_2 = 10^{-7}$ or $\max(|\boldsymbol{E}(\boldsymbol{\theta}_i)|)$ is not too large, that is, if it is less than $\tau_3 = 5$. The latter tolerance is set relatively large because the step 2 adjustment can result in substantial increases in computation times. The step 2 adjustment is executed in the first few iterations if $\max(|\boldsymbol{E}(\boldsymbol{\theta}_{i+1,0})|)$ exceeds $\max(|\boldsymbol{E}(\boldsymbol{\theta}_i)|)$ by the multiple $\tau_8 = 2$ of $\max(|\boldsymbol{E}(\boldsymbol{\theta}_i)|)$. For sub-stage 1 of the step 2 adjustment, the maximum for the number of digits is set to $j''^* = 7$. For sub-stage 2 of the step 2 adjustment, the maximum for the number of digits is also set to $j''^* = 7$ and with stopping tolerance $\tau_4 = 0.01$. For stage 2 of the step 2 adjustment, the maximum for the number of digits is set to $j'''^* = 7$ with stopping tolerance $\tau_5 = 0.005$.

For stopping the estimation process, the maximum number of iterations is set to $i^* = 300$ (but this has little effect since the number of iterations is typically much smaller). The tolerance for a small proportional decrease is $\tau_7 = 10^{-7}$, for the maximum number of proportional decreases is $maxPD = 2$, and for a small maximum absolute gradient entry is $\tau_6 = 10^{-6}$.

3.8 Variation in Measurement Conditions

The formulation intentionally allows for measurements within matched sets over possibly different condition subsets *C*(*s*) of the maximal condition set *C*. The correlation estimates of Sect. 2.4.1 for standard GEE estimation and of Sect. 3.3

for partially modified GEE estimation take this variation in measurement into account as does the likelihood function $L(SC;\boldsymbol{\theta})$.

Allowing the condition sets $C(s)$ to change with the matched sets $s \in S$ supports varying numbers of outcome measurements within matched sets. Natural predictors $x_{sc,j}$ and $v_{sc,j}$ to consider for inclusion in such cases would be ones measuring condition set differences. For example, when the matched sets correspond to parents of a child with some kind of chronic illness (as considered in analyses reported in Chap. 16), single-parent families can have only one study participant, while partnered-parent families can have both parents participating, only the mother (i.e., the primary caregiver) participating, or only the father participating. The smaller number of participants for single-parent families is not a consequence of missing data, but a smaller number for partnered-parent families is. Possible condition set difference predictors in this case include indicator variables based on parent type (father or mother), family type (single or partnered), number of participating parents (1 or 2), and participation types (only mother participating or not; only father participating or not).

Allowing the condition sets $C(s)$ to change with the matched sets $s \in S$ also adjusts for missing outcome measurements within the matched sets. Natural predictors $x_{sc,j}$ and $v_{sc,j}$ to consider for inclusion in such cases would be ones measuring outcome missingness. For example, possible missingness predictors include the number $m(s)$ of non-missing outcome measurements (or, equivalently, the number $m - m(s)$ of missing outcome measurements) along with indicators for a given outcome measurement missing (y_{sc} missing or not for each c, $1 \leq c \leq m$). However, different sizes $m(s)$ for condition sets $C(s)$ is not always due to missing data, but because matched sets are not the same size. Examples of such matched sets include nurses on the same hospital unit and patients of the same provider. In such cases, the size $m(s)$ of a matched set s could be considered as a predictor unless it is constant.

References

Knafl, G. J., & Ding, K. (2016). *Adaptive regression for modeling nonlinear relationships*. Springer.

McCullagh, P., & Nelder, J. A. (1999). *Generalized linear models* (2nd ed.). Chapman & Hall/CRC.

Nelder, J. A., & Pregibon, D. (1987). An extended quasi-likelihood function. *Biometrika, 74*, 221–232.

Chapter 4
Fully Modified GEE Modeling of Correlated Univariate Outcomes

Abstract GEE modeling can be fully modified to account for the dependence of the likelihood on mean parameters as well as on dispersion parameters rather than using the standard GEE estimating equations for the mean parameters. General formulas are presented for gradient vectors and Hessian matrices as well as detailed formulas under alternate regression types and link functions, covering commonly used distributions including the normal, Poisson, Bernoulli, exponential, and inverse Gaussian distributions. Adjustments to the estimation process are provided to account for maximizing the likelihood rather than minimizing the absolute value of the gradient. The special case of singleton univariate outcomes, that is, independent measurements, is addressed. It can be used to generate initial estimates for parameter estimation. Standard generalized linear modeling can be used to generate initial estimates of mean parameters for standard GEE modeling. Handling of initial estimates of both mean and dispersion parameters as needed for partially modified and fully modified GEE can be addressed using extended quasi-likelihood methods. Alternately, standard linear modeling of singleton continuous univariate outcomes can be extended to address singleton categorical univariate outcomes.

Keywords Correlated outcomes · Extended quasi-likelihoods · Extended linear modeling · Generalized estimating equations · Newton's method · Non-constant dispersions

Introduction GEE modeling can be fully modified to account for the dependence of the likelihood on both mean and dispersion parameters rather than using the standard GEE estimating equations for the mean parameters combined with maximum likelihood for dispersion parameters. General formulas are presented in Sect. 4.1, while Sect. 4.2 provides detailed formulas under alternate regression types and link functions, covering commonly used distributions including the normal, Poisson, Bernoulli, exponential, and inverse Gaussian distributions. Section 4.3 addresses

---

Supplementary Information The online version contains supplementary material available at https://doi.org/10.1007/978-3-031-41988-1_4.

G. J. Knafl, *Modeling Correlated Outcomes Using Extensions of Generalized Estimating Equations and Linear Mixed Modeling*,
https://doi.org/10.1007/978-3-031-41988-1_4

adjustments to the estimation process of Sect. 3.7. Section 4.4 covers the singleton univariate outcome case used to generate initial estimates for parameter estimation.

4.1 Estimating Equations for Means and Dispersions Based on the Likelihood

Using the notation of Sect. 2.1, as in Sect. 3.2, let

$$\boldsymbol{\theta} = \begin{pmatrix} \boldsymbol{\beta} \\ \boldsymbol{\gamma} \end{pmatrix}$$

be the $(r + q) \times 1$ vector composed of the mean and dispersion parameter vectors $\boldsymbol{\beta}$ and $\boldsymbol{\gamma}$ with r and q entries (as defined in Sects. 2.2 and 3.1), respectively. As before, the correlation parameter vector $\boldsymbol{\rho}$ (as defined in Sect. 2.3) has not been included in $\boldsymbol{\theta}$ because it is a function of $\boldsymbol{\beta}$ and $\boldsymbol{\gamma}$ (see Sect. 3.3). As in Sect. 2.5, define the likelihood function $L(SC;\boldsymbol{\theta})$ as the product of the terms $L(O_s;\boldsymbol{\theta})$ satisfying

$$\ell(O_s;\boldsymbol{\theta}) = \log L(O_s;\boldsymbol{\theta}) = -\boldsymbol{e}_s^{\mathrm{T}} \cdot \boldsymbol{\Sigma}_s^{-1} \cdot \boldsymbol{e}_s/2 - (\log|\boldsymbol{\Sigma}_s|)/2 - (m(s) \cdot \log(2 \cdot \pi))/2$$

for $s \in S$, where $\boldsymbol{e}_s$ is the residual vector (as defined in Sect. 2.2), O_s denotes an observation (as defined in Sect. 3.2), $\boldsymbol{\Sigma}_s$ is the $m(s) \times m(s)$ covariance matrix satisfying

$$\boldsymbol{\Sigma}_s = \boldsymbol{DIAG}(\boldsymbol{\sigma}_s) \cdot \boldsymbol{R}_s(\boldsymbol{\rho}) \cdot \boldsymbol{DIAG}(\boldsymbol{\sigma}_s),$$

$|\boldsymbol{\Sigma}_s|$ is the determinant of $\boldsymbol{\Sigma}_s$, and π is the usual constant. The same approach as for partially modified GEE modeling given in Sect. 3.3 is used to estimate the correlation parameter vector $\boldsymbol{\rho}$ allowing for non-constant dispersions. However, now the likelihood $L(SC;\boldsymbol{\theta})$ is maximized in the coefficient parameter vector $\boldsymbol{\theta}$ holding the correlation vector $\boldsymbol{\rho}$ constant in $\boldsymbol{\theta}$. Specifically, use Newton's method as adjusted in Sect. 4.3 to solve the estimating equations

$$\boldsymbol{E}(\boldsymbol{\theta}) = \sum_{s \in S} \boldsymbol{E}_s(\boldsymbol{\theta}) = \sum_{s \in S} \frac{\partial_0 \ell(O_s;\boldsymbol{\theta})}{\partial_0 \boldsymbol{\theta}} = \frac{\partial_0 \ell(SC;\boldsymbol{\theta})}{\partial_0 \boldsymbol{\theta}} = \boldsymbol{0}$$

where as in Sect. 3.2 the operator notation $\frac{\partial_0}{\partial_0 \boldsymbol{\theta}}$ is used to indicate that this is not a full partial derivative in $\boldsymbol{\theta}$ due to not considering the effect of $\boldsymbol{\theta}$ on $\boldsymbol{\rho}$. The associated Hessian matrix is

$$\boldsymbol{E}'(\boldsymbol{\theta}) = \frac{\partial_0 \boldsymbol{E}(\boldsymbol{\theta})}{\partial_0 \boldsymbol{\theta}}.$$

Note that

$$\log|\boldsymbol{\Sigma}_s| = \log|\boldsymbol{R}_s(\boldsymbol{\rho})| + \sum_{c \in C(s)} \boldsymbol{v}_{sc}^{\mathrm{T}} \cdot \boldsymbol{\gamma} + \sum_{c \in C(s)} \log V(\mu_{sc}),$$

$$\varphi_{sc} = \exp\left(\boldsymbol{v}_{sc}^{\mathrm{T}} \cdot \boldsymbol{\gamma}\right), \text{and}$$

$$\boldsymbol{e}_s^{\mathrm{T}} \cdot \boldsymbol{\Sigma}_s^{-1} \cdot \boldsymbol{e}_s = \boldsymbol{stde}_s^{\mathrm{T}} \cdot \boldsymbol{R}_s^{-1}(\boldsymbol{\rho}) \cdot \boldsymbol{stde}_s$$

where $\boldsymbol{stde}_s$ is defined in Sect. 3.1 and examples of the variance function $V(\mu_{sc})$ depending on the means μ_{sc} are provided in Sects. 4.2.1–4.2.5. Consequently,

$$\boldsymbol{E}(\boldsymbol{\theta}) = \begin{pmatrix} \boldsymbol{E}(\boldsymbol{\beta}) \\ \boldsymbol{E}(\boldsymbol{\gamma}) \end{pmatrix}$$

where

$$\boldsymbol{E}(\boldsymbol{\beta}) = \frac{\partial_0 \ell(SC; \boldsymbol{\theta})}{\partial_0 \boldsymbol{\beta}}$$

is a $r \times 1$ vector and

$$\boldsymbol{E}(\boldsymbol{\gamma}) = \frac{\partial_0 \ell(SC; \boldsymbol{\theta})}{\partial_0 \boldsymbol{\gamma}}$$

is a $q \times 1$ vector. $\boldsymbol{E}(\boldsymbol{\beta})$ is the sum over $s \in S$ of $\boldsymbol{E}_s(\boldsymbol{\beta})$ with entries

$$E_{s,j}(\boldsymbol{\beta}) = \boldsymbol{xstde}_{s,j}^{\mathrm{T}} \cdot \boldsymbol{R}_s^{-1}(\boldsymbol{\rho}) \cdot \boldsymbol{stde}_s - \sum_{c \in C(s)} W_j(\mu_{sc})/2$$

where

$$W_j(\mu_{sc}) = \frac{\frac{\partial V(\mu_{sc})}{\partial \beta_j}}{V(\mu_{sc})}$$

and $\boldsymbol{xstde}_{s,j}$ is the $m(s) \times 1$ vector with entries $xstde_{sc,j}$ for $sc \in SC$ and $1 \leq j \leq r$ changing with the outcome distribution and link function (see Sect. 4.2 for examples). $\boldsymbol{E}(\boldsymbol{\gamma})$ is the sum over $s \in S$ of $\boldsymbol{E}_s(\boldsymbol{\gamma})$ with entries

$$E_{s,j}(\gamma) = \boldsymbol{vstde}_{s,j}^{\mathrm{T}} \cdot \boldsymbol{R}_s^{-1}(\rho) \cdot \boldsymbol{stde}_s - \sum_{c \in C(s)} v_{sc,j}/2$$

where $\boldsymbol{vstde}_{s,j}$ is the $m(s) \times 1$ vector with entries

$$vstde_{sc,j} = v_{sc,j} \cdot stde_{sc}/2$$

for $sc \in SC$ and $1 \leq j \leq q$ as also in Sect. 3.2. The predictor values $v_{sc,j}$ for the dispersions are defined in Sect. 3.1. The standardized residuals $stde_{sc}$ are defined in Sect. 3.1 with detailed formulations of $\boldsymbol{xstde}_{s,j}$ for alternate regression type provided in Sects. 4.2.1–4.2.5.

$\boldsymbol{E}'(\boldsymbol{\theta})$ has four component matrices: the $r \times r$ matrix

$$\boldsymbol{E}'(\boldsymbol{\beta}) = \frac{\partial_0 \boldsymbol{E}(\boldsymbol{\beta})}{\partial_0 \boldsymbol{\beta}}$$

for the mean parameters, the $q \times q$ matrix

$$\boldsymbol{E}'(\boldsymbol{\gamma}) = \frac{\partial_0 \boldsymbol{E}(\boldsymbol{\gamma})}{\partial_0 \boldsymbol{\gamma}}$$

for the dispersion parameters, the $r \times q$ matrix

$$\boldsymbol{E}'(\boldsymbol{\beta}, \boldsymbol{\gamma}) = \frac{\partial_0 \boldsymbol{E}(\boldsymbol{\beta})}{\partial_0 \boldsymbol{\gamma}},$$

and its transpose $\boldsymbol{E}'(\boldsymbol{\gamma}, \boldsymbol{\beta}) = \boldsymbol{E}'^{\mathrm{T}}(\boldsymbol{\beta}, \boldsymbol{\gamma})$. $\boldsymbol{E}'(\boldsymbol{\beta})$ is the sum over $s \in S$ of $\boldsymbol{E}'_s(\boldsymbol{\beta})$ with entries

$$E'_{s,j,j'}(\boldsymbol{\beta}) = -\boldsymbol{xxstde}_{s,j,j'}^{\mathrm{T}} \cdot \boldsymbol{R}_s^{-1}(\rho) \cdot \boldsymbol{stde}_s - \boldsymbol{xstde}_{s,j}^{\mathrm{T}} \cdot \boldsymbol{R}_s^{-1}(\rho) \cdot \boldsymbol{xstde}_{s,j'} - \sum_{c \in C(s)} W_{j,j'}(\mu_{sc})/2$$

where

$$W_{j,j'}(\mu_{sc}) = \frac{\partial W_j(\mu_{sc})}{\partial \beta_{j'}}$$

and $\boldsymbol{xxstde}_{s,j,j'}$ is the $m(s) \times 1$ vector with entries $xxstde_{sc,j,j'}$ for $sc \in SC$ and $1 \leq j, j' \leq r$ changing with the outcome distribution and link function (see Sect. 4.2 for examples). $\boldsymbol{E}'(\boldsymbol{\gamma})$ is the sum over $s \in S$ of $\boldsymbol{E}'_s(\boldsymbol{\gamma})$ with entries

$$E'_{s,j,j'}(\boldsymbol{\gamma}) = -\boldsymbol{vvstde}^{\mathrm{T}}_{s,j,j'} \cdot \boldsymbol{R}_s^{-1}(\rho) \cdot \boldsymbol{stde}_s - \boldsymbol{vstde}^{\mathrm{T}}_{s,j} \cdot \boldsymbol{R}_s^{-1}(\rho) \cdot \boldsymbol{vstde}_{s,j'}$$

where $\boldsymbol{vvstde}_{s,j,j'}$ is the $m(s) \times 1$ vector with entries

$$vvstde_{sc,j,j'} = v_{sc,j} \cdot v_{sc,j'} \cdot stde_{sc}/4$$

for $sc \in SC$ and $1 \le j, j' \le q$ as also in Sect. 3.2. $\boldsymbol{E}'(\boldsymbol{\beta},\boldsymbol{\gamma})$ is the sum over $s \in S$ of $\boldsymbol{E}'_s(\boldsymbol{\beta},\boldsymbol{\gamma})$ with entries

$$E'_{s,j,j'}(\boldsymbol{\beta},\boldsymbol{\gamma}) = -\boldsymbol{vxstde}^{\mathrm{T}}_{s,j,j'} \cdot \boldsymbol{R}_s^{-1}(\rho) \cdot \boldsymbol{stde}_s - \boldsymbol{xstde}^{\mathrm{T}}_{s,j} \cdot \boldsymbol{R}_s^{-1}(\rho) \cdot \boldsymbol{vstde}_{s,j'}$$

where $\boldsymbol{vxstde}_{s,j,j'}$ is the $m(s) \times 1$ vector with entries

$$vxstde_{sc,j,j'} = xstde_{sc,j} \cdot v_{sc,j'}/2$$

for $sc \in SC$, $1 \le j \le r$, and $1 \le j' \le q$.

Let

$$\boldsymbol{\theta}(SC) = \begin{pmatrix} \boldsymbol{\beta}(SC) \\ \boldsymbol{\gamma}(SC) \end{pmatrix}$$

denote the estimate of the coefficient vector $\boldsymbol{\theta}$ obtained by solving the fully modified GEE equations $\boldsymbol{E}(\boldsymbol{\theta}) = \boldsymbol{0}$ using the observations with indexes in SC. As in Sect. 2.4.2 for standard GEE and Sect. 3.4 for partially modified GEE, two estimates of the covariance matrix for the estimated parameter vector $\boldsymbol{\theta}(SC)$ can be computed: the model-based and robust empirical estimates. The model-based estimate is

$$\Sigma_{\mathrm{MB}}(\boldsymbol{\theta}(SC)) = -\boldsymbol{E}'^{-1}(\boldsymbol{\theta}(SC)).$$

The robust empirical estimate is

$$\Sigma_{\mathrm{RE}}(\boldsymbol{\theta}(SC)) = \boldsymbol{E}'^{-1}(\boldsymbol{\theta}(SC)) \cdot \boldsymbol{G}(\boldsymbol{\theta}(SC)) \cdot \boldsymbol{G}^{\mathrm{T}}(\boldsymbol{\theta}(SC)) \cdot \boldsymbol{E}'^{-1}(\boldsymbol{\theta}(SC))$$

where $\boldsymbol{G}(\boldsymbol{\theta}(SC))$ is the $(r+q) \times m(SC)$ matrix with $(r+q) \times m(s)$ component matrices $\boldsymbol{G}_s(\boldsymbol{\theta}(SC))$ for $s \in S$ satisfying

$$\boldsymbol{G}_s(\boldsymbol{\theta}(SC)) = \begin{pmatrix} \boldsymbol{G}_s(\boldsymbol{\beta}(SC)) \\ \boldsymbol{G}_s(\boldsymbol{\gamma}(SC)) \end{pmatrix}.$$

$\boldsymbol{G}_s(\boldsymbol{\beta}(SC))$ is the $r \times m(s)$ matrix with rows $\boldsymbol{G}_{s,j}(\boldsymbol{\beta}(SC))$ for $1 \le j \le r$ satisfying

$$G_{s,j}(\beta(SC)) = \left(\mathbf{xstde}_{s,j}^{\mathrm{T}} \cdot \mathbf{R}_s^{-1}(\rho)\right) \circ \mathbf{stde}_s^{\mathrm{T}} - \mathbf{W}_{s,j}^{\mathrm{T}}/2$$

where $\circ$ denotes elementwise multiplication and $\mathbf{W}_{s,j}$ is the $m(s) \times 1$ vector with entries $W_j(\mu_{sc})$ for $c \in C(s)$. $\mathbf{G}_s(\gamma(SC))$ is the $q \times m(s)$ matrix with rows $\mathbf{G}_{s,j}(\gamma(SC))$ for $1 \leq j \leq q$ satisfying

$$G_{s,j}(\gamma(SC)) = \left(\mathbf{vstde}_{s,j}^{\mathrm{T}} \cdot \mathbf{R}_s^{-1}(\rho)\right) \circ \mathbf{stde}_s^{\mathrm{T}} - \mathbf{v}_{s,j}^{\mathrm{T}}/2$$

where $\mathbf{v}_{s,j}$ is the $m(s) \times 1$ vector with entries $v_{sc,j}$ for $c \in C(s)$. Note that $\mathbf{E}(\boldsymbol{\theta}(\mathrm{SC}))$ equals the $(r + q) \times 1$ vector generated by summing the rows of $\mathbf{G}(\boldsymbol{\theta}(SC))$. The diagonal entries of $\boldsymbol{\Sigma}_{\mathrm{MB}}(\boldsymbol{\theta}(SC))$ and $\boldsymbol{\Sigma}_{\mathrm{RE}}(\boldsymbol{\theta}(SC))$ are estimates of variances for the parameter estimates given by the entries of $\boldsymbol{\theta}(SC)$. These can be used to generate z tests of zero coefficient parameter values. Results of such tests are not reported in example adaptive analyses because adaptively determined models have parameters that are usually significant as a consequence of the adaptive modeling process.

The formulation for LCV scores of Sect. 2.6, LCV ratio tests of Sect. 2.6.2, the adaptive regression modeling process of Sect. 2.7, estimation of the correlation structure in Sect. 3.3, and handling degeneracy in Sect. 3.6 generalize to the fully modified GEE case in the same ways as for the partially modified case. The estimation process is a modification of the partially modified approach of Sect. 3.7 as described later in Sect. 4.3. Examples of alternate regression types including those of Sects. 2.2.1–2.2.4 are provided next in Sect. 4.2.

4.2 Alternate Regression Types

This section provides formulas for the quantities needed to compute the gradient vector $\mathbf{E}(\boldsymbol{\beta})$ and the Hessian matrix $\mathbf{E}'(\boldsymbol{\beta})$ for fully modified GEE modeling under alternative distributions and link functions. Details on the computation of these formulas are not provided for brevity. The commonly considered cases for generalized linear modeling (see Table 2.1 in McCullagh & Nelder, 1999) are addressed including the four cases of Sects. 2.2.1–2.2.4 (with the gamma case of McCullagh & Nelder (1999) replaced by the equivalent exponential case) together with the inverse Gaussian case.

4.2.1 Linear Regression with Identity Link Function

As in Sect. 2.2.1, outcomes y_{sc} are continuous real-valued and are treated as normally distributed. The link function is the identity function $g(\mu) = \mu$ for $-\infty < \mu < \infty$ with derivative

$$\frac{dg(\mu)}{d\mu} = 1.$$

This is the canonical choice for the link function for the normal distribution. The variance function is $V(\mu) = 1$ with derivative

$$\frac{dV(\mu)}{d\mu} = 0.$$

The extended variances are

$$\sigma_{sc}^2 = \varphi_{sc} \cdot V(\mu_{sc}) = \varphi_{sc}$$

(the same as the variances), the extended standard deviations are $\sigma_{sc} = \varphi_{sc}^{1/2}$, and the standardized residuals are

$$stde_{sc} = \frac{y_{sc} - \mu_{sc}}{\varphi_{sc}^{1/2}}.$$

The means satisfy $\mu_{sc} = \boldsymbol{x}_{sc}^{\mathrm{T}} \cdot \boldsymbol{\beta}$ with partial derivatives

$$\frac{\partial \mu_{sc}}{\partial \beta_j} = \frac{x_{sc,j}}{\frac{dg(\mu_{sc})}{d\mu}} = x_{sc,j}$$

for $sc \in SC$ and $1 \leq j \leq r$. Notation for predictor values $x_{sc,j}$ for the means is defined in Sect. 2.2.

Using notation defined in Sect. 4.1, formulas for computing the gradient vector and Hessian matrix for fully modified GEE modeling satisfy for $sc \in SC$, $1 \leq j, j' \leq r$, and $1 \leq j'', j''' \leq q$

$$W_j(\mu_{sc}) = \frac{\partial V(\mu_{sc})}{\partial \beta_j} / V(\mu_{sc}) = 0,$$

$$W_{j,j'}(\mu_{sc}) = \frac{\partial W_j(\mu_{sc})}{\partial \beta_{j'}} = 0,$$

$$xstde_{sc,j} = x_{sc,j} / \varphi_{sc}^{1/2},$$

$$vstde_{sc,j''} = v_{sc,j''} \cdot stde_{sc}/2,$$

$$xxstde_{sc,j,j'} = 0,$$

$$vvstde_{sc,j'',j'''} = v_{sc,j''} \cdot v_{sc,j'''} \cdot stde_{sc}/4,$$

$$vxstde_{sc,j,j''} = xstde_{sc,j} \cdot v_{sc,j''}/2.$$

For $1 \leq j \leq r$,

$$E_{s,j}(\boldsymbol{\beta}) = \boldsymbol{xstde}_{s,j}^{\mathrm{T}} \cdot \boldsymbol{R}_s^{-1}(\rho) \cdot \boldsymbol{stde}_s$$

so that under the above settings

$$E_{s,j}(\boldsymbol{\beta}) = \boldsymbol{X}_s^{\mathrm{T}} \cdot \boldsymbol{\Sigma}_s^{-1} \cdot \boldsymbol{e}_s = \boldsymbol{D}_s^{\mathrm{T}} \cdot \boldsymbol{\Sigma}_s^{-1} \cdot \boldsymbol{e}_s$$

where

$$\boldsymbol{D}_s = \frac{\partial \boldsymbol{\mu}_s}{\partial \boldsymbol{\beta}}$$

as in Sect. 2.4. Consequently, the estimating equations for the means are the same as for standard and partially modified GEE. Moreover,

$$E'_{s,j,j'}(\boldsymbol{\beta}) = -\boldsymbol{xstde}_{s,j}^{\mathrm{T}} \cdot \boldsymbol{R}_s^{-1}(\rho) \cdot \boldsymbol{xstde}_{s,j'}$$

for $1 \leq j, j' \leq r$ so that

$$\boldsymbol{E}'_s(\boldsymbol{\beta}) = -\boldsymbol{D}_s^{\mathrm{T}} \cdot \boldsymbol{\Sigma}_s^{-1} \cdot \boldsymbol{D}_s,$$

and so solutions to the partially modified GEE and fully modified GEE estimating equations are the same in the linear regression case. Example analyses for this case are provided in Chap. 6.

4.2.2 *Poisson Regression with Natural Log Link Function*

As in Sect. 2.2.2, outcomes y_{sc} are count-valued, that is, nonnegative integer-valued, and are treated as Poisson distributed. The link function is the natural log function $g(\mu) = \log \mu$ for $0 < \mu < \infty$ with derivative

$$\frac{dg(\mu)}{d\mu} = \frac{1}{\mu}.$$

This is the canonical choice for the link function for the Poisson distribution. The variance function is $V(\mu) = \mu$ with derivative

$$\frac{dV(\mu)}{d\mu} = 1.$$

The means satisfy $\mu_{sc} = \exp\left(\boldsymbol{x}_{sc}^{\mathrm{T}} \cdot \boldsymbol{\beta}\right)$ with partial derivatives

$$\frac{\partial \mu_{sc}}{\partial \beta_j} = \frac{x_{sc,j}}{\frac{dg(\mu_{sc})}{d\mu}} = x_{sc,j} \cdot \mu_{sc}$$

for $sc \in SC$ and $1 \leq j \leq r$. The extended variances are

$$\sigma_{sc}^2 = \varphi_{sc} \cdot V(\mu_{sc}) = \varphi_{sc} \cdot \mu_{sc},$$

the extended standard deviations are

$$\sigma_{sc} = (\varphi_{sc} \cdot \mu_{sc})^{1/2},$$

and the standardized residuals are

$$stde_{sc} = \frac{y_{sc} - \mu_{sc}}{\sigma_{sc}}$$

for $sc \in SC$. An offset variable o_{sc} can be added to the model for the means as in Sect. 2.2.2 and to the model for the dispersions as in Sect. 3.1 to convert these models into models for associated rates.

Using notation defined in Sect. 4.1, formulas for computing the gradient vector and Hessian matrix for fully modified GEE modeling satisfy for $sc \in SC$, $1 \leq j, j' \leq r$, and $1 \leq j'', j''' \leq q$

$$W_j(\mu_{sc}) = \frac{\partial V(\mu_{sc})}{\partial \beta_j} / V(\mu_{sc}) = x_{sc,j},$$

$$W_{j,j'}(\mu_{sc}) = \frac{\partial W_j(\mu_{sc})}{\partial \beta_{j'}} = 0,$$

$$xstde_{sc,j} = x_{sc,j} \cdot \frac{y_{sc} + \mu_{sc}}{2 \cdot \sigma_{sc}},$$

$$vstde_{sc,j''} = v_{sc,j''} \cdot stde_{sc}/2,$$

$$xxstde_{sc,j,j'} = x_{sc,j} \cdot x_{sc,j'} \cdot stde_{sc}/4,$$

$$vvstde_{sc,j'',j'''} = v_{sc,j''} \cdot v_{sc,j'''} \cdot stde_{sc}/4,$$

$$vxstde_{sc,j,j''} = xstde_{sc,j} \cdot v_{sc,j''}/2.$$

Example analyses for this case are provided in Chap. 7.

4.2.3 Logistic Regression with Logit Link Function

As in Sect. 2.2.3, outcomes y_{sc} are dichotomous with two possible values 0 and 1 and are treated as Bernoulli distributed so that $\mu_{sc} = \mathrm{P}(y_{sc} = 1)$. The link function is the logit function

$$g(\mu) = \mathrm{logit}(\mu) = \log \frac{\mu}{1-\mu}$$

for $0 < \mu < 1$ with derivative

$$\frac{dg(\mu)}{d\mu} = \frac{1}{\mu \cdot (1-\mu)}.$$

This is the canonical choice for the link function for the Bernoulli distribution. The variance function is $V(\mu) = \mu \cdot (1 - \mu)$ with derivative

$$\frac{dV(\mu)}{d\mu} = 1 - 2 \cdot \mu.$$

The means satisfy

$$\mu_{sc} = \frac{\exp\left(\boldsymbol{x}_{sc}^{\mathrm{T}} \cdot \boldsymbol{\beta}\right)}{1 + \exp\left(\boldsymbol{x}_{sc}^{\mathrm{T}} \cdot \boldsymbol{\beta}\right)}$$

with partial derivatives

$$\frac{\partial \mu_{sc}}{\partial \beta_j} = \frac{x_{scj}}{\frac{dg(\mu_{sc})}{d\mu}} = x_{scj} \cdot \mu_{sc} \cdot (1 - \mu_{sc})$$

for $sc \in SC$ and $1 \leq j \leq r$. The extended variances are

$$\sigma_{sc}^2 = \varphi_{sc} \cdot V(\mu_{sc}) = \varphi_{sc} \cdot \mu_{sc} \cdot (1 - \mu_{sc}),$$

the extended standard deviations are

$$\sigma_{sc} = (\varphi_{sc} \cdot \mu_{sc} \cdot (1 - \mu_{sc}))^{1/2},$$

and the standardized residuals are

$$stde_{sc} = \frac{y_{sc} - \mu_{sc}}{\sigma_{sc}}$$

for $sc \in SC$.

Using notation defined in Sect. 4.1, formulas for computing the gradient vector and Hessian matrix for fully modified GEE modeling satisfy for $sc \in SC$, $1 \leq j, j^{'} \leq r$, and $1 \leq j^{''}, j^{'''} \leq q$

$$W_j(\mu_{sc}) = \frac{\partial V(\mu_{sc})}{\partial \beta_j} / V(\mu_{sc}) = x_{sc,j} \cdot (1 - 2 \cdot \mu_{sc}),$$

$$W_{j,j'}(\mu_{sc}) = \frac{\partial W_j(\mu_{sc})}{\partial \beta_{j'}} = -2 \cdot x_{sc,j} \cdot x_{sc,j'} \cdot \mu_{sc} \cdot (1 - \mu_{sc}),$$

$$xstde_{sc,j} = x_{sc,j} \cdot \frac{(1 - 2 \cdot \mu_{sc}) \cdot y_{sc} + \mu_{sc}}{2 \cdot \sigma_{sc}},$$

$$vstde_{sc,j''} = v_{sc,j''} \cdot stde_{sc}/2,$$

$$xxstde_{sc,j,j'} = x_{sc,j} \cdot x_{sc,j'} \cdot stde_{sc}/4,$$

$$vvstde_{sc,j'',j''\,'} = v_{sc,j''} \cdot v_{sc,j''\,'} \cdot stde_{sc}/4,$$

$$vxstde_{sc,j,j''} = xstde_{sc,j} \cdot v_{sc,j''}/2.$$

Example analyses for this case are provided in Chap. 8.

4.2.4 Exponential Regression with Natural Log Link Function

As in Sect. 2.2.4, outcomes y_{sc} are continuous positive-valued and are treated as exponentially distributed. The link function is the natural log function $g(\mu) = \log \mu$ for $0 < \mu < \infty$ with derivative

$$\frac{dg(\mu)}{d\mu} = \frac{1}{\mu}.$$

The variance function is $V(\mu) = \mu^2$ with derivative

$$\frac{dV(\mu)}{d\mu} = 2 \cdot \mu.$$

The means satisfy $\mu_{sc} = \exp(\boldsymbol{x}_{sc}^{\mathrm{T}} \cdot \boldsymbol{\beta})$ with partial derivatives

$$\frac{\partial \mu_{sc}}{\partial \beta_j} = \frac{x_{sc,j}}{\frac{dg(\mu_{sc})}{d\mu}} = x_{sc,j} \cdot \mu_{sc}$$

for $sc \in SC$ and $1 \leq j \leq r$. The extended variances are

$$\sigma_{sc}^2 = \varphi_{sc} \cdot V(\mu_{sc}) = \varphi_{sc} \cdot \mu_{sc}^2,$$

the extended standard deviations are $\sigma_{sc} = \varphi_{sc}^{1/2} \cdot \mu_{sc}$, and the standardized residuals are

$$stde_{sc} = \frac{y_{sc} - \mu_{sc}}{\sigma_{sc}}$$

for $sc \in SC$.

Using notation defined in Sect. 4.1, formulas for computing the gradient vector and Hessian matrix for fully modified GEE modeling satisfy for $sc \in SC$, $1 \leq j, j' \leq r$, and $1 \leq j'', j''' \leq q$

$$W_j(\mu_{sc}) = \frac{\partial V(\mu_{sc})}{\partial \beta_j} / V(\mu_{sc}) = 2 \cdot x_{sc,j},$$

$$W_{jj'}(\mu_{sc}) = \frac{\partial W_j(\mu_{sc})}{\partial \beta_{j'}} = 0,$$

$$xstde_{sc,j} = x_{sc,j} \cdot y_{sc} / \sigma_{sc},$$

$$vstde_{sc,j''} = v_{sc,j''} \cdot stde_{sc} / 2,$$

$$xxstde_{sc,j,j'} = x_{sc,j} \cdot x_{sc,j'} \cdot y_{sc} / \sigma_{sc},$$

$$vvstde_{sc,j'',j'''} = v_{sc,j''} \cdot v_{sc,j'''} \cdot stde_{sc} / 4,$$

$$vxstde_{sc,j,j''} = xstde_{sc,j} \cdot v_{sc,j''} / 2.$$

Example analyses for this case are provided in Chap. 9.

The natural log function is not the canonical choice for the link function for the exponential distribution. The canonical choice is the reciprocal function $g(\mu) = 1/\mu$ for $0 < \mu < \infty$, but that generates means $\mu_{sc} = 1/(\mathbf{x}_{sc}^{\mathrm{T}} \cdot \boldsymbol{\beta})$ so that the estimation process needs adjustment to guarantee positive values for $\mathbf{x}_{sc}^{\mathrm{T}} \cdot \boldsymbol{\beta}$ for $sc \in SC$. The natural log link function does not have this shortcoming.

4.2.5 Inverse Gaussian Regression with Natural Log Link Function

Outcomes y_{sc} are continuous positive-valued and are treated as inverse Gaussian distributed. The link function is the natural log function $g(\mu) = \log \mu$ for $0 < \mu < \infty$ with derivative

$$\frac{dg(\mu)}{d\mu} = \frac{1}{\mu}.$$

The variance function is $V(\mu) = \mu^3$ with derivative

$$\frac{dV(\mu)}{d\mu} = 3 \cdot \mu^2.$$

The means satisfy $\mu_{sc} = \exp\left(\boldsymbol{x}_{sc}^{\mathrm{T}} \cdot \boldsymbol{\beta}\right)$ with partial derivatives

$$\frac{\partial \mu_{sc}}{\partial \beta_j} = \frac{x_{sc,j}}{\frac{dg(\mu_{sc})}{d\mu}} = x_{sc,j} \cdot \mu_{sc}$$

for $sc \in SC$ and $1 \leq j \leq r$. The extended variances are

$$\sigma_{sc}^2 = \varphi_{sc} \cdot V(\mu_{sc}) = \varphi_{sc} \cdot \mu_{sc}^3,$$

the extended standard deviations are

$$\sigma_{sc} = \left(\varphi_{sc} \cdot \mu_{sc}^3\right)^{1/2},$$

and the standardized residuals are

$$stde_{sc} = \frac{y_{sc} - \mu_{sc}}{\sigma_{sc}}$$

for $sc \in SC$.

Using notation defined in Sect. 4.1, formulas for computing the gradient vector and Hessian matrix for fully modified GEE modeling satisfy for $sc \in SC$, $1 \leq j, j' \leq r$, and $1 \leq j'', j''' \leq q$

$$W_j(\mu_{sc}) = \frac{\partial V(\mu_{sc})}{\partial \beta_j} / V(\mu_{sc}) = 3 \cdot x_{sc,j},$$

$$W_{j,j'}(\mu_{sc}) = \frac{\partial W_j(\mu_{sc})}{\partial \beta_{j'}} = 0,$$

$$xstde_{sc,j} = x_{sc,j} \cdot \frac{3 \cdot y_{sc} - \mu_{sc}}{2 \cdot \sigma_{sc}},$$

$$vstde_{sc,j''} = v_{sc,j''} \cdot stde_{sc}/2,$$

$$xxstde_{sc,j,j'} = x_{sc,j} \cdot x_{sc,j'} \cdot \frac{9 \cdot y_{sc} - \mu_{sc}}{4 \cdot \sigma_{sc}},$$

$$vvstde_{sc,j'',j''\prime} = v_{sc,j''} \cdot v_{sc,j''\prime} \cdot stde_{sc}/4,$$

$$vxstde_{sc,j,j''} = xstde_{sc,j} \cdot v_{sc,j''}/2.$$

Example analyses for this case are not provided since it covers the same type of outcomes as for exponential regression covered in Sect. 4.2.4.

The natural log function is not the canonical choice for the link function for the inverse Gaussian distribution. The canonical choice is the square reciprocal function $g(\mu) = 1/\mu^2$ for $0 < \mu < \infty$, but that generates means $\mu_{sc} = 1/\left(\boldsymbol{x}_{sc}^{\mathrm{T}} \cdot \boldsymbol{\beta}\right)^{½}$ so that the estimation process needs adjustment to guarantee positive values for $\boldsymbol{x}_{sc}^{\mathrm{T}} \cdot \boldsymbol{\beta}$ for $sc \in SC$. The natural log link function does not have this shortcoming.

4.3 The Parameter Estimation Process

The estimation process presented in detail in Sect. 3.7 with its steps 0–2 is still used in the fully modified GEE case. However, now there is a log-likelihood function $\ell(SC;\boldsymbol{\theta})$ to control that process in place of $\max(|\boldsymbol{E}(\boldsymbol{\theta})|)$. Consequently, inequalities used in that process are reversed because the goal is to maximize the real-valued function $\ell(SC;\boldsymbol{\theta})$ rather than to minimize the real-valued function $\max(|\boldsymbol{E}(\boldsymbol{\theta})|)$ of a gradient vector. Also, the fact that $\ell(SC;\boldsymbol{\theta})$ need not be always positive as is the case for $\max(|\boldsymbol{E}(\boldsymbol{\theta})|)$ has to be taken into account. For example, using notation defined in Sect. 3.7, the step 2 adjustment is skipped if

$$\ell(SC;\boldsymbol{\theta}_{i+1,1}(d')) < \ell(SC;\boldsymbol{\theta}_i) + \tau_2 \cdot \mathrm{abs}(\ell(SC;\boldsymbol{\theta}_i))$$

or $\max(|\boldsymbol{E}(\boldsymbol{\theta}_{i+1,0})|) < \tau_3$ for tolerances τ_2 and τ_3. This is one exception where the maximum absolute value of the gradient entries is still used. Note that the step 1 adjustment has no need to compute the gradient $\boldsymbol{E}(\boldsymbol{\theta}_{i+1,1}(d'))$, but a gradient is needed to compute $\boldsymbol{\theta}_{i+1,0}$, and so $\max(|\boldsymbol{E}(\boldsymbol{\theta}_{i+1,0})|)$ is compared to τ_3 in place of $\max(|\boldsymbol{E}(\boldsymbol{\theta}_{i+1,1}(d'))|)$. Another exception where the maximum absolute value of the gradient entries is used is in deciding whether to stop the estimation process that is still based on $\max(|\boldsymbol{E}(\boldsymbol{\theta}_i)|) < \tau_6$. Complete details for this adjusted estimation process are not presented for brevity.

4.3.1 Revised Stopping Criteria

Stopping the estimation process is now based on proportional increases in $\ell(SC;\boldsymbol{\theta})$ rather than on proportional decreases in $\max(|\boldsymbol{E}(\boldsymbol{\theta})|)$. However, convergence is typically faster so that the stopping criteria are simpler. Still set a maximum number i^* of iterations, but use an alternative stop count equal to the number times the proportional increase has been small. For $i > 1$, the current proportional increase in $\ell(SC;\boldsymbol{\theta})$ is

$$PI_i = \frac{\ell(SC;\boldsymbol{\theta}_i) - \ell(SC;\boldsymbol{\theta}_{i-1})}{\mathrm{abs}(\ell(SC;\boldsymbol{\theta}_{i-1}))}.$$

Set a tolerance τ_7 for a small proportional increase and a maximum number *maxPI* (with recommended value 2) for small increases. Let

$$stopcnt(i) = \sum_{i'=2}^{i} I(PI_{i'} \le \tau_7)$$

and stop the search when $stopcnt(i) \ge maxPI$. Also, stop the search if $\max(|\boldsymbol{E}(\boldsymbol{\theta}_i)|) < \tau_6$ (as in Sect. 3.7.3). Altogether, the search stops when a small proportional increase in the log-likelihood occurs a sufficient number of times, the maximum gradient entry is small, or the number of iterations gets too large. The same recommended maximum numbers of iterations and tolerances are used except that τ_2 and τ_7 are both changed to 0.00001.

4.3.2 Initial Estimates

Initial estimates for starting the computation of parameter estimates for correlated outcomes can be generated by treating outcomes as independent as in Sect. 3.7.4 for partially modified GEE. The estimation process adjusted to use the log-likelihood can be applied to the computation of these initial estimates. The associated likelihood functions are those used in the generalized linear modeling context (see Knafl & Ding, 2016) and so are not based on the multivariate normal distribution (but see Sect. 4.4). These initial estimate searches start at zero parameter vectors.

4.4 Singleton Univariate Outcomes

Singleton univariate outcomes correspond to the special case with each measurement in its own separate matched set, that is, with $m = 1$ and all condition sets consisting of the single index $c = 1$. In this case, the notation can be simplified by removing the index c. The observed outcome values are y_s with expected values or means $\mathrm{E}y_s = \mu_s$, residuals $e_s = y_s - \mu_s$, non-constant dispersions φ_s, extended variances satisfying $\sigma_s^2 = \varphi_s \cdot V(\mu_s)$, standardized residuals $stde_s = e_s/\sigma_s$, and Pearson residuals

$$Pres_s = \frac{e_s}{V^{1/2}(\mu_s)}$$

for $s \in S$. Predictors for the means and dispersion are combined respectively into the vectors $\boldsymbol{x}_s$ and $\boldsymbol{v}_s$, while the observations are $O_s = \{y_s, \boldsymbol{x}_s, \boldsymbol{v}_s\}$ (also include $\boldsymbol{o}_s$ if offsets are used in the Poisson regression case) and the likelihood is the product of terms $L(O_s; \boldsymbol{\theta})$ satisfying

$$L(S;\boldsymbol{\theta}) = \exp(\ell(S;\boldsymbol{\theta}))$$

$$\begin{aligned}\ell(O_s;\boldsymbol{\theta}) = \log L(O_s;\boldsymbol{\theta}) &= -stde_s^2/2 - (\log \sigma_s^2)/2 - (\log 2\cdot\pi)/2 \\ &= -stde_s^2/2 - (\log \varphi_s)/2 - (\log V(\mu_s))/2 - (\log(2\cdot\pi))/2\end{aligned}$$

for $s \in S$. This likelihood can be maximized in $\boldsymbol{\theta}$ to generate parameter estimates $\boldsymbol{\theta}(S)$. This is reasonably called extended linear modeling.

However, extended linear modeling is different from the usual approach of generalized linear modeling of a singleton univariate outcome. Under generalized linear modeling, mean parameters are estimated using maximum likelihood estimation for an exact likelihood. For example, under the Poisson distribution, the contribution to the log-likelihood for $s \in S$ is

$$y_s \cdot \log \mu_s - \mu_s + \log y_s!$$

where $y_s!$ is the usual factorial notation, while it is

$$y_s \cdot \log \mu_s + (1 - y_s) \cdot \log(1 - \mu_s)$$

under the Bernoulli distribution. The dispersion is treated as a constant, set to either the fixed value of 1 or to a bias-adjusted or bias-unadjusted estimate. Generalized linear modeling can be extended to handle estimation of dispersion parameters as well as mean parameters by maximizing the extended quasi-likelihood function $Q^{+}(S;\boldsymbol{\theta})$ equaling the sum of terms $Q^{+}(O_s;\boldsymbol{\theta})$ satisfying

$$-2\cdot Q^{+}(O_s;\boldsymbol{\theta}) = -\frac{d(y_s,\mu_s)}{2\cdot\varphi_s} - \frac{\log\varphi_s}{2} - \frac{\log V(y_s)}{2} - \frac{\log 2\cdot\pi}{2}$$

where $d(y_s, \mu_s)$ is the deviance function satisfying

$$d(y_s, \mu_s) = 2 \cdot \int_{\mu_s}^{y_s} \frac{y_s - t}{V(t)} dt$$

(Eq. 10.3, McCullagh & Nelder, 1999). When $V(\mu) = 1$, the deviance is

$$d(y_s, \mu_s) = \frac{e_s^2}{V(\mu_s)} = e_s^2,$$

$\sigma_s^2 = \varphi_s$, $\log V(y_s) = 0$, and the extended quasi-likelihood is the same as $\ell(O_s; \boldsymbol{\theta})$. This does not hold in general. In the case of the gamma distribution covered in McCullagh and Nelder (1999), the deviance function is the same as for the exponential distribution because they have the same variance function.

The terms $-\log V(y_s)/2$ in the extended quasi-likelihood are problematic in cases where $V(y_s) = 0$. Nelder and Pregibon (1987) redefine $V(y_s)$ in certain cases of this kind to avoid this problem (see their Table 1). However, for the five cases of Sect. 4.2, $V(y_s)$ does not depend on any unknown parameters and so can be dropped without affecting parameter estimation, thereby avoiding problems with $V(y_s) = 0$. The terms $-(\log(2 \cdot \pi))/2$ can also be dropped. This is the approach used in Knafl and Ding (2016).

In the five cases of Sect. 4.2, extended quasi-likelihood modeling involves solving the estimating equations for the mean parameter vector $\boldsymbol{\beta}$ given by $\boldsymbol{E}(\boldsymbol{\beta}) = \boldsymbol{0}$ where $\boldsymbol{E}(\boldsymbol{\beta})$ is the sum over $s \in S$ of $\boldsymbol{E}_s(\boldsymbol{\beta})$ with entries

$$E_{s,j}(\boldsymbol{\beta}) = \frac{\partial \mu_s}{\partial \beta_j} \cdot stde_s$$

for $1 \leq j \leq r$ (Eq. 10.4 in McCullagh & Nelder, 1999) and the estimating equations for the dispersion parameter vector $\boldsymbol{\gamma}$ given by $\boldsymbol{E}(\boldsymbol{\gamma}) = \boldsymbol{0}$ where $\boldsymbol{E}(\boldsymbol{\gamma})$ is the sum $s \in S$ of $\boldsymbol{E}_s(\boldsymbol{\gamma})$ with entries

$$E_{s,j}(\boldsymbol{\gamma}) = \frac{\partial \varphi_s}{\partial \gamma_j} \cdot \left(\frac{d(y_s, \mu_s)}{\varphi_s^2} - \frac{1}{\varphi_s} \right)$$

for $1 \leq j \leq q$ (Eq. 10.5 in McCullagh & Nelder, 1999). As in the standard GEE context, differentiating the terms e_s of the above univariate log-likelihood $\ell(S; \boldsymbol{\theta})$ holding the terms $V(\mu_s)$ fixed generates the same estimating equations $\boldsymbol{E}(\boldsymbol{\beta}) = \boldsymbol{0}$ for the mean parameters as for extended quasi-likelihood modeling. Extended linear modeling, on the other hand, generates estimating equations for mean parameters that account for the dependence of $L(S; \boldsymbol{\theta})$ on the variances $V(\mu_s)$ as well as on the residuals e_s, as is also the case for fully modified GEE modeling. The terms $-(\log V(\mu_s))/2$ in the log-likelihood $\ell(S; \boldsymbol{\theta})$ are similar to the terms $-(\log V(y_s))/2$ of the extended quasi-likelihood $Q^+(S; \boldsymbol{\theta})$ but are well-defined since $V(\mu_s) > 0$. However, extended linear modeling generates different estimating equations $\boldsymbol{E}(\boldsymbol{\gamma}) = \boldsymbol{0}$ for the dispersion parameters than extended quasi-likelihood modeling with $\boldsymbol{E}(\gamma)$ equaling the sum over $s \in S$ of $\boldsymbol{E}_s(\gamma)$ with entries

$$E_{s,j}(\gamma) = \frac{\partial \varphi_s}{\partial \gamma_j} \cdot \left(\frac{Pres_s}{\varphi_s^2} - \frac{1}{\varphi_s} \right),$$

and so with the Pearson residuals replacing the deviances.

References

Knafl, G. J., & Ding, K. (2016). *Adaptive regression for modeling nonlinear relationships*. Springer.

McCullagh, P., & Nelder, J. A. (1999). *Generalized linear models* (2nd ed.). Chapman & Hall/CRC.

Nelder, J. A., & Pregibon, D. (1987). An extended quasi-likelihood function. *Biometrika, 74*, 221–232.

Chapter 5
Extended Linear Mixed Modeling of Correlated Univariate Outcomes

Abstract Extended linear mixed modeling (ELMM) is based on full maximum likelihood estimation, maximizing the likelihood in the correlation parameters as well as in the mean and dispersion parameters. Revised formulations are provided for estimating equations, gradient vectors, and Hessian matrices. Adjustments to the estimation process are provided. Formulations are also provided for estimating exchangeable (EC), spatial autoregressive order 1 (AR1), and unstructured (UN) correlation parameters. The formulations for the EC and spatial AR1 cases provide for efficient correlation parameter estimation without storing associated correlation matrices. How to verify gradient and Hessian formulations and their software implementations is addressed. Direct variance modeling is defined, using only general dispersions to model variances rather than using extended variance modeling also considering distribution-specific variances based on the means.

Keywords Correlated outcomes · Direct variance modeling · Extended linear mixed modeling · Newton's method · Non-constant dispersions

Introduction Full maximum likelihood estimation is possible, maximizing the likelihood in the correlation parameters as well as in the mean and dispersion parameters. In this chapter, revised estimating equations are formulated in Sect. 5.1 and adjustments to the estimation process are addressed in Sect. 5.2. Formulations are also provided for estimating EC, spatial AR1, and UN correlation parameters in Sects. 5.3–5.5, respectively. Section 5.6 addresses how to verify gradient and Hessian formulations and their software implementations. Section 5.7 addresses direct variance modeling using only general dispersions to model variances rather than using extended variance modeling also considering distribution-specific variances based on the variance function $V(\mu)$.

Supplementary Information The online version contains supplementary material available at https://doi.org/10.1007/978-3-031-41988-1_5.

G. J. Knafl, *Modeling Correlated Outcomes Using Extensions of Generalized Estimating Equations and Linear Mixed Modeling*,
https://doi.org/10.1007/978-3-031-41988-1_5

5.1 Estimating Equations for Means, Dispersions, and Correlations Based on the Likelihood

Using the notation of Sect. 2.1, as in Sect. 4.1, define the likelihood function $L(SC;\boldsymbol{\theta})$ as the product over $s \in S$ of the terms $L(O_s;\boldsymbol{\theta})$ satisfying

$$\ell(O_s;\boldsymbol{\theta}) = \log L(O_s;\boldsymbol{\theta}) = -\boldsymbol{e}_s^{\mathrm{T}} \cdot \boldsymbol{\Sigma}_s^{-1} \cdot \boldsymbol{e}_s/2 - (\log|\boldsymbol{\Sigma}_s|)/2 - (m(s) \cdot \log(2 \cdot \pi))/2$$

for $s \in S$, where $\boldsymbol{e}_s$ is the residual vector (as defined in Sect. 2.2), O_s denotes an observation (as defined in Sect. 3.2), $\boldsymbol{\Sigma}_s$ is the $m(s) \times m(s)$ covariance matrix satisfying

$$\boldsymbol{\Sigma}_s = \boldsymbol{DIAG}(\boldsymbol{\sigma}_s) \cdot \boldsymbol{R}_s(\boldsymbol{\rho}) \cdot \boldsymbol{DIAG}(\boldsymbol{\sigma}_s),$$

$|\boldsymbol{\Sigma}_s|$ is the determinant of $\boldsymbol{\Sigma}_s$, and π is the usual constant. However, the parameter vector is now

$$\boldsymbol{\theta} = \begin{pmatrix} \boldsymbol{\beta} \\ \boldsymbol{\gamma} \\ \boldsymbol{\rho} \end{pmatrix},$$

the $(r + q + p) \times 1$ vector composed of the mean, dispersion, and correlation parameter vectors $\boldsymbol{\beta}$, $\boldsymbol{\gamma}$, and $\boldsymbol{\rho}$ with r, q, and p entries as defined in Sects. 2.2, 3.1, and 2.3, respectively. The likelihood $L(SC;\boldsymbol{\theta})$ is maximized in the coefficient parameter vector $\boldsymbol{\theta}$. This is extended linear mixed modeling. In the linear regression case, the correlated outcomes are exactly multivariate normally distributed and then this is linear mixed modeling. Specifically, use Newton's method adjusted in Sects. 4.3 and 5.2 to solve the estimating equations

$$\boldsymbol{E}(\boldsymbol{\theta}) = \sum_{s \in S} \boldsymbol{E}_s(\boldsymbol{\theta}) = \sum_{s \in S} \frac{\partial \ell(O_s;\boldsymbol{\theta})}{\partial \boldsymbol{\theta}} = \frac{\partial \ell(SC;\boldsymbol{\theta})}{\partial \boldsymbol{\theta}} = \boldsymbol{0}$$

where the operator notation $\frac{\partial}{\partial \boldsymbol{\theta}}$ is used to indicate that this is the full partial derivative in $\boldsymbol{\theta}$. The associated Hessian matrix is

$$\boldsymbol{E}'(\boldsymbol{\theta}) = \frac{\partial \boldsymbol{E}(\boldsymbol{\theta})}{\partial \boldsymbol{\theta}}.$$

In this case, $\boldsymbol{E}(\boldsymbol{\theta})$ is a true gradient vector and $\boldsymbol{E}'(\boldsymbol{\theta})$ a true Hessian matrix.

Note that

$$\log|\boldsymbol{\Sigma}_s| = \log|\boldsymbol{R}_s(\boldsymbol{\rho})| + \sum_{c\in C(s)} \boldsymbol{v}_{sc}^{\mathrm{T}} \cdot \boldsymbol{\gamma} + \sum_{c\in C(s)} \log V(\mu_{sc}),$$

$$\rho_{\mathrm{sc}} = \exp\left(\boldsymbol{v}_{sc}^{\mathrm{T}} \cdot \boldsymbol{\gamma}\right), \text{ and}$$

$$\boldsymbol{e}_s^{\mathrm{T}} \cdot \boldsymbol{\Sigma}_s^{-1} \cdot \boldsymbol{e}_s = \boldsymbol{stde}_s^{\mathrm{T}} \cdot \boldsymbol{R}_s^{-1}(\boldsymbol{\rho}) \cdot \boldsymbol{stde}_s$$

where $\boldsymbol{stde}_s$ is defined in Sect. 3.1 and examples of the variance function $V(\mu_{sc})$ are provided in Sects. 4.2.1–4.2.5. Consequently,

$$\boldsymbol{E}(\boldsymbol{\theta}) = \begin{pmatrix} \boldsymbol{E}(\boldsymbol{\beta}) \\ \boldsymbol{E}(\boldsymbol{\gamma}) \\ \boldsymbol{E}(\boldsymbol{\rho}) \end{pmatrix}$$

where

$$\boldsymbol{E}(\boldsymbol{\beta}) = \frac{\partial \ell(SC;\boldsymbol{\theta})}{\partial \boldsymbol{\beta}}$$

is a $r \times 1$ vector,

$$\boldsymbol{E}(\boldsymbol{\gamma}) = \frac{\partial \ell(SC;\boldsymbol{\theta})}{\partial \boldsymbol{\gamma}}$$

is a $q \times 1$ vector, and

$$\boldsymbol{E}(\boldsymbol{\rho}) = \frac{\partial \ell(SC;\boldsymbol{\theta})}{\partial \boldsymbol{\rho}}$$

is a $p \times 1$ vector.

$\boldsymbol{E}(\boldsymbol{\beta})$ is the sum over $s \in S$ of $\boldsymbol{E}_s(\boldsymbol{\beta})$ with entries

$$E_{s,j}(\boldsymbol{\beta}) = \boldsymbol{xstde}_{s,j}^{\mathrm{T}} \cdot \boldsymbol{R}_s^{-1}(\boldsymbol{\rho}) \cdot \boldsymbol{stde}_s - \sum_{c\in C(s)} W_j(\mu_{sc})/2$$

where

$$W_j(\mu_{sc}) = \frac{\frac{\partial V(\mu_{sc})}{\partial \beta_j}}{V(\mu_{sc})}$$

and $\boldsymbol{xstde}_{s,j}$ is the $m(s) \times 1$ vector with entries $xstde_{sc,j}$ for $sc \in SC$ and $1 \le j \le r$ changing with the outcome distribution and link function (see Sect. 4.2 for examples). $\boldsymbol{E}(\boldsymbol{\gamma})$ is the sum over $s \in S$ of $\boldsymbol{E}_s(\boldsymbol{\gamma})$ with entries

$$E_{s,j}(\gamma) = \boldsymbol{vstde}_{s,j}^{\mathrm{T}} \cdot \boldsymbol{R}_s^{-1}(\boldsymbol{\rho}) \cdot \boldsymbol{stde}_s - \sum_{c \in C(s)} v_{sc,j}/2$$

where $\boldsymbol{vstde}_{s,j}$ is the $m(s) \times 1$ vector with entries

$$vstde_{sc,j} = v_{sc,j} \cdot stde_{sc}/2$$

for $sc \in SC$ and $1 \leq j \leq q$ as also in Sects. 3.2 and 4.1. The predictor values $v_{sc,j}$ for the non-constant dispersions are defined in Sect. 3.1. The standardized residual $stde_{sc}$ is defined in Sect. 3.1 with detailed formulations for alternate regression types provided in Sects. 4.2.1–4.2.5. With the entries of $\boldsymbol{\rho}$ denoted by ρ_j for $1 \leq j \leq p$, $\boldsymbol{E}(\boldsymbol{\rho})$ has entries

$$\boldsymbol{E}_j(\boldsymbol{\rho}) = \frac{\partial \ell(SC;\boldsymbol{\theta})}{\partial \rho_j}$$

equal to the sum over $s \in S$ of

$$E_{s,j}(\boldsymbol{\rho}) = -\boldsymbol{stde}_s^{\mathrm{T}} \cdot \frac{\partial \boldsymbol{R}_s^{-1}(\boldsymbol{\rho})}{\partial \rho_j} \cdot \boldsymbol{stde}_s/2 - \frac{\partial \log|\boldsymbol{R}_s(\boldsymbol{\rho})|}{\partial \rho_j}/2$$

where $\boldsymbol{R}_s(\boldsymbol{\rho})$ changes with the correlation structure but does not depend on the mean and dispersion parameters.

$\boldsymbol{E}'(\boldsymbol{\theta})$ has nine component matrices: the $r \times r$ matrix

$$\boldsymbol{E}'(\boldsymbol{\beta}) = \frac{\partial \boldsymbol{E}(\boldsymbol{\beta})}{\partial \boldsymbol{\beta}}$$

for r the mean coefficients, the $q \times q$ matrix

$$\boldsymbol{E}'(\boldsymbol{\gamma}) = \frac{\partial \boldsymbol{E}(\boldsymbol{\gamma})}{\partial \boldsymbol{\gamma}}$$

for the q dispersion coefficients, the $p \times p$ matrix

$$\boldsymbol{E}'(\boldsymbol{\rho}) = \frac{\partial \boldsymbol{E}(\boldsymbol{\rho})}{\partial \boldsymbol{\rho}}$$

for the p correlation coefficients, the $r \times q$ matrix

$$\boldsymbol{E}'(\boldsymbol{\beta},\boldsymbol{\gamma}) = \frac{\partial \boldsymbol{E}(\boldsymbol{\beta})}{\partial \boldsymbol{\gamma}}$$

and its transpose $\boldsymbol{E}'(\boldsymbol{\gamma},\boldsymbol{\beta}) = \boldsymbol{E}'^{\mathrm{T}}(\boldsymbol{\beta},\boldsymbol{\gamma})$, the $r \times p$ matrix

$$\boldsymbol{E}'(\boldsymbol{\beta},\boldsymbol{\rho}) = \frac{\partial \boldsymbol{E}(\boldsymbol{\beta})}{\partial \boldsymbol{\rho}}$$

and its transpose $\boldsymbol{E}'(\boldsymbol{\rho},\boldsymbol{\beta}) = \boldsymbol{E}'^{\mathrm{T}}(\boldsymbol{\gamma},\boldsymbol{\rho})$, the $q \times p$ matrix

$$\boldsymbol{E}'(\boldsymbol{\gamma},\boldsymbol{\rho}) = \frac{\partial \boldsymbol{E}(\boldsymbol{\gamma})}{\partial \boldsymbol{\rho}}$$

and its transpose $\boldsymbol{E}'(\boldsymbol{\rho},\boldsymbol{\gamma}) = \boldsymbol{E}'^{\mathrm{T}}(\boldsymbol{\gamma},\boldsymbol{\rho})$. $\boldsymbol{E}'(\boldsymbol{\beta})$ is the sum over $s \in S$ of $\boldsymbol{E}'_s(\boldsymbol{\beta})$ with entries

$$E'_{s,j,j'}(\boldsymbol{\beta}) = -\boldsymbol{xxstde}^{\mathrm{T}}_{s,j,j'} \cdot \boldsymbol{R}_s^{-1}(\boldsymbol{\rho}) \cdot \boldsymbol{stde}_s - \boldsymbol{xstde}^{\mathrm{T}}_{s,j} \cdot \boldsymbol{R}_s^{-1}(\boldsymbol{\rho}) \cdot \boldsymbol{xstde}_{s,j'} - \sum_{c \in C(s)} W_{j,j'}(\mu_{sc})/2$$

where

$$W_{j,j'}(\mu_{sc}) = \frac{\partial W_j(\mu_{sc})}{\partial \beta_{j'}}$$

and $\boldsymbol{xxstde}_{s,j,j'}$ is the $m(s) \times 1$ vector with entries $xxstde_{sc,j,j'}$ for $sc \in SC$ and $1 \leq j, j' \leq r$ changing with the outcome distribution and link function as also in Sect. 4.1 (see Sect. 4.2 for examples). $\boldsymbol{E}'(\boldsymbol{\gamma})$ is the sum over $s \in S$ of $\boldsymbol{E}'_s(\boldsymbol{\gamma})$ with entries

$$E'_{s,j,j'}(\boldsymbol{\gamma}) = -\boldsymbol{vvstde}^{\mathrm{T}}_{s,j,j'} \cdot \boldsymbol{R}_s^{-1}(\boldsymbol{\rho}) \cdot \boldsymbol{stde}_s - \boldsymbol{vstde}^{\mathrm{T}}_{s,j} \cdot \boldsymbol{R}_s^{-1}(\boldsymbol{\rho}) \cdot \boldsymbol{vstde}_{s,j'}$$

where $\boldsymbol{vvstde}_{s,j,j'}$ is the $m(s) \times 1$ vector with entries

$$vvstde_{sc,j,j'} = v_{sc,j} \cdot v_{sc,j'} \cdot stde_{sc}/4$$

for $sc \in SC$ and $1 \leq j, j' \leq q$ as also in Sects. 3.2 and 4.1. $\boldsymbol{E}'(\boldsymbol{\beta},\boldsymbol{\gamma})$ is the sum over $s \in S$ of $\boldsymbol{E}'_s(\boldsymbol{\beta},\boldsymbol{\gamma})$ with entries

$$E'_{s,j,j'}(\boldsymbol{\beta},\boldsymbol{\gamma}) = -\boldsymbol{vxstde}^{\mathrm{T}}_{s,j,j'} \cdot \boldsymbol{R}_s^{-1}(\boldsymbol{\rho}) \cdot \boldsymbol{stde}_s - \boldsymbol{xstde}^{\mathrm{T}}_{s,j} \cdot \boldsymbol{R}_s^{-1}(\boldsymbol{\rho}) \cdot \boldsymbol{vstde}_{s,j'}$$

where $\boldsymbol{vxstde}_{s,j,j'}$ is the $m(s) \times 1$ vector with entries

$$vxstde_{sc,j,j'} = xstde_{sc,j} \cdot v_{sc,j'}/2$$

for $sc \in SC$, $1 \leq j \leq r$, and $1 \leq j' \leq q$ as also in Sect. 4.1. $\boldsymbol{E}'(\boldsymbol{\rho})$ is the sum over $s \in S$ of $\boldsymbol{E}'_s(\boldsymbol{\rho})$ with entries

$$E'_{s,j,j'}(\boldsymbol{\rho}) = -\boldsymbol{stde}_s^{\mathrm{T}} \cdot \frac{\partial^2 \boldsymbol{R}_s^{-1}(\boldsymbol{\rho})}{\partial \rho_{j'} \partial \rho_j} \cdot \boldsymbol{stde}_s/2 - \frac{\partial^2 \log|\boldsymbol{R}_s(\boldsymbol{\rho})|}{\partial \rho_{j'} \partial \rho_j}/2$$

for $1 \leq j, j' \leq p$. $\boldsymbol{E}'(\boldsymbol{\beta},\boldsymbol{\rho})$ is the sum over $s \in S$ of $\boldsymbol{E}'_s(\boldsymbol{\beta},\boldsymbol{\rho})$ with entries

$$E'_{s,j,j'}(\boldsymbol{\beta},\boldsymbol{\rho}) = \boldsymbol{xstde}_{s,j}^{\mathrm{T}} \cdot \frac{\partial \boldsymbol{R}_s^{-1}(\boldsymbol{\rho})}{\partial \rho_{j'}} \cdot \boldsymbol{stde}_s$$

for $sc \in SC$, $1 \leq j \leq r$, and $1 \leq j' \leq p$. $\boldsymbol{E}'(\boldsymbol{\gamma},\boldsymbol{\rho})$ is the sum over $s \in S$ of $\boldsymbol{E}'_s(\boldsymbol{\gamma},\boldsymbol{\rho})$ with entries

$$E'_{s,j,j'}(\boldsymbol{\gamma},\boldsymbol{\rho}) = \boldsymbol{vstde}_{s,j}^{\mathrm{T}} \cdot \frac{\partial \boldsymbol{R}_s^{-1}(\boldsymbol{\rho})}{\partial \rho_{j'}} \cdot \boldsymbol{stde}_s$$

for $sc \in SC$, $1 \leq j \leq q$, and $1 \leq j' \leq p$. Formulations for first and second partial derivatives of $\boldsymbol{R}_s^{-1}(\boldsymbol{\rho})$ and $\log|\boldsymbol{R}_s(\boldsymbol{\rho})|$ with respect to $\boldsymbol{\rho}$ needed to compute $\boldsymbol{E}(\boldsymbol{\rho})$, $\boldsymbol{E}'(\boldsymbol{\rho})$, $\boldsymbol{E}'(\boldsymbol{\beta},\boldsymbol{\rho})$, and $\boldsymbol{E}'(\gamma,\boldsymbol{\rho})$ are provided in Sects. 5.3–5.5 for the EC, spatial AR1, and UN structures, respectively. These partial derivatives are dropped for the IND correlation structure.

Let

$$\boldsymbol{\theta}(SC) = \begin{pmatrix} \beta(SC) \\ \gamma(SC) \\ \rho(SC) \end{pmatrix}$$

denote the estimate of the coefficient vector $\boldsymbol{\theta}$ obtained by solving the ELMM estimating equations $\boldsymbol{E}(\boldsymbol{\theta}) = \boldsymbol{0}$ using the measurements with indexes in SC. As in Sect. 2.4.2 for standard GEE, Sect. 3.4 for partially modified GEE, and Sect. 4.1 for fully modified GEE, two estimates of the covariance matrix for the estimated parameter vector $\boldsymbol{\theta}(SC)$ can be computed: the model-based and robust empirical estimates. The model-based estimate is

$$\Sigma_{\mathrm{MB}}(\boldsymbol{\theta}(SC)) = -\boldsymbol{E}'^{-1}(\boldsymbol{\theta}(SC)).$$

The robust empirical estimate is

$$\Sigma_{\mathrm{RE}}(\boldsymbol{\theta}(SC)) = \boldsymbol{E}'^{-1}(\boldsymbol{\theta}(SC)) \cdot \boldsymbol{G}(\boldsymbol{\theta}(SC)) \cdot \boldsymbol{G}^{\mathrm{T}}(\boldsymbol{\theta}(SC)) \cdot \boldsymbol{E}'^{-1}(\boldsymbol{\theta}(SC))$$

where $\boldsymbol{G}(\boldsymbol{\theta}(SC))$ is the $(r + q + p) \times m(SC)$ matrix with $(r + q + p) \times m(s)$ component matrices $\boldsymbol{G}_s(\boldsymbol{\theta}(SC))$ for $s \in S$ satisfying

$$\boldsymbol{G}_s(\boldsymbol{\theta}(SC)) = \begin{pmatrix} \boldsymbol{G}_s(\boldsymbol{\beta}(SC)) \\ \boldsymbol{G}_s(\boldsymbol{\gamma}(SC)) \\ \boldsymbol{G}_s(\boldsymbol{\rho}(SC)) \end{pmatrix}.$$

$\boldsymbol{G}_s(\boldsymbol{\beta}(SC))$ is the $r \times m(s)$ matrix with rows $\boldsymbol{G}_{s,j}(\boldsymbol{\beta}(SC))$ for $1 \leq j \leq r$ satisfying

$$\boldsymbol{G}_{s,j}(\boldsymbol{\beta}(SC)) = \left(\boldsymbol{xstde}_{s,j}^{\mathrm{T}} \cdot \boldsymbol{R}_s^{-1}(\boldsymbol{\rho})\right) \circ \boldsymbol{stde}_s^{\mathrm{T}} - \boldsymbol{W}_{s,j}^{\mathrm{T}}/2$$

where $\circ$ denotes elementwise multiplication and $\boldsymbol{W}_{s,j}$ is the $m(s) \times 1$ vector with entries $W_j(\mu_{sc})$ for $c \in C(s)$. $\boldsymbol{G}_s(\boldsymbol{\gamma}(SC))$ is the $q \times m(s)$ matrix with rows $\boldsymbol{G}_{s,j}(\boldsymbol{\gamma}(SC))$ for $1 \leq j \leq q$ satisfying

$$\boldsymbol{G}_{s,j}(\boldsymbol{\gamma}(SC)) = \left(\boldsymbol{vstde}_{s,j}^{\mathrm{T}} \cdot \boldsymbol{R}_s^{-1}(\boldsymbol{\rho})\right) \circ \boldsymbol{stde}_s^{\mathrm{T}} - \boldsymbol{v}_{s,j}^{\mathrm{T}}/2$$

where $\boldsymbol{v}_{s,j}$ is the $m(s) \times 1$ vector with entries $v_{sc,j}$ for $c \in C(s)$. $\boldsymbol{G}_s(\boldsymbol{\rho}(SC))$ is the $p \times m(s)$ matrix with rows $\boldsymbol{G}_{s,j}(\boldsymbol{\rho}(SC))$ for $1 \leq j \leq p$ satisfying

$$\boldsymbol{G}_{s,j}(\boldsymbol{\rho}(SC)) = -\left(\boldsymbol{stde}_{s,j}^{\mathrm{T}} \cdot \frac{\partial \boldsymbol{R}_s^{-1}(\boldsymbol{\rho})}{\partial \rho_j}\right) \circ \boldsymbol{stde}_s^{\mathrm{T}}/2 - \boldsymbol{W}'^{\mathrm{T}}_{s,j}/2$$

where $\boldsymbol{W}'_{s,j}$ is the $m(s) \times 1$ vector with entries equal to the diagonal entries of

$$\boldsymbol{R}_s^{-1}(\boldsymbol{\rho}) \cdot \frac{\partial \boldsymbol{R}_s^{-1}(\boldsymbol{\rho})}{\partial \rho_j}$$

for $c \in C(s)$ because

$$\frac{\partial \log|\boldsymbol{R}_s(\boldsymbol{\rho})|}{\partial \rho_j} = \mathrm{tr}\left(\boldsymbol{R}_s^{-1}(\boldsymbol{\rho}) \cdot \frac{\partial \boldsymbol{R}_s^{-1}(\boldsymbol{\rho})}{\partial \rho_j}\right)$$

(Sect. 9.4 in Schott, 2005; Wolfinger et al., 1994), where tr denotes the trace of a matrix, that is, the sum of its diagonal elements. Note that $\boldsymbol{E}(\boldsymbol{\theta}(\mathrm{SC}))$ equals the $(r + q + p) \times 1$ vector generated by summing the rows of $\boldsymbol{G}(\boldsymbol{\theta}(SC))$. The diagonal entries of $\boldsymbol{\Sigma}_{\mathrm{MB}}(\boldsymbol{\theta}(SC))$ and $\boldsymbol{\Sigma}_{\mathrm{RE}}(\boldsymbol{\theta}(SC))$ are estimates of variances for the parameter estimates given by the entries of $\boldsymbol{\theta}(SC)$. These can be used to generate z tests of zero coefficient parameter values. Results of such tests are not reported in example adaptive analyses because adaptively determined models have parameters that are usually significant as a consequence of the adaptive modeling process.

The formulations for LCV scores of Sect. 2.6, LCV ratio tests of Sect. 2.6.2, and the adaptive regression modeling process of Sect. 2.7 generalize to ELMM in the same ways as for the partially and fully modified GEE cases. The four correlation structures of Sect. 2.3 can still be considered. In all cases, there is just one alternative estimate of the correlation vector and not bias-adjusted and bias-unadjusted alternatives. The parameter estimation process of Sect. 3.7 as adjusted in Sect. 4.3 for fully modified GEE extends to the ELMM case (Sect. 5.2). The EC and spatial AR1 cases can be handled without storing associated correlation matrices (Sects. 5.3 and 5.4), providing efficient computation of associated estimates for data with relatively large numbers m of conditions.

5.2 Adjustments to the Estimation Process

The estimation process of Sect. 3.7 as adjusted in Sect. 4.3 and based on the log-likelihood is used in ELMM. However, it needs to be adjusted further to handle the estimation of correlation parameters along with mean and dispersion parameters. Handling of the IND correlation structure is trivial. The EC and spatial AR1 cases require adjusting estimates of the scalar correlation parameter ρ to fall within appropriate bounds $[\rho_{\mathrm{Lo}}, \rho_{\mathrm{Hi}}]$ as defined in Sect. 3.6. Assume the current value ρ_{i} falls within those bounds. When the next value $\rho_{\mathrm{i}\,+\,1}$ for that parameter is too small, that is, when $\rho_{\mathrm{i+1}} < \rho_{\mathrm{Lo}}$, change $\rho_{\mathrm{i+1}}$ to $(\rho_{\mathrm{Lo}} + \rho_{\mathrm{i}})/2$. When the next value $\rho_{\mathrm{i+1}}$ for that parameter determined by the estimation process is too large, that is, when $\rho_{\mathrm{i+1}} > \rho_{\mathrm{Hi}}$, change $\rho_{\mathrm{i+1}}$ to $(\rho_{\mathrm{Hi}} + \rho_{\mathrm{i}})/2$. Otherwise, use $\rho_{\mathrm{i+1}}$ unchanged. This approach generates correlation estimates that are less extreme than using the closer of the two endpoints of $[\rho_{\mathrm{Lo}}, \rho_{\mathrm{Hi}}]$. For the UN correlation structure, set $\rho_{\mathrm{Lo}} = -1 + \delta_1$ and $\rho_{\mathrm{Hi}} = 1 - \delta_1$ with δ_1 some small positive number like 0.0001 as in Sect. 3.6. Then adjust each of the UN correlation parameters proportionally as in Sect. 3.6 to lie within $[\rho_{\mathrm{Lo}}, \rho_{\mathrm{Hi}}]$. This guarantees appropriate values for these parameters but not necessarily that they generate a positive definite correlation matrix. However, the correlation matrix possibly adjusted to have values within bounds can be further adjusted, if necessary, to be positive definite with smallest eigenvalue at least a small positive value as in Sect. 3.6.

Initial estimates of the mean and dispersion parameters can be generated in the same way as for fully modified GEE of Sect. 4.2.3. These can be used to generate initial estimates of the correlation parameters using the approach of Sect. 3.3 as used with fully modified GEE or any similar approach. To be consistent with ELMM maximization, only bias-unadjusted initial estimates are used. Initial estimates in the EC and AR1 cases can be readily computed without storing associated correlation matrices (as addressed in Sects. 5.3 and 5.4). These correlation estimates might need adjustments to avoid degenerate estimates as described in Sect. 3.6.

5.3 Exchangeable Correlation Structure Computations

This section describes how EC correlation structure computations can be conducted without storing the full correlation matrix and its inverse. Results are presented for the $m \times m$ working correlation matrix $\boldsymbol{R}(\rho)$ but apply as well to the $m(s) \times m(s)$ submatrices $\boldsymbol{R}_s(\rho)$ for $s \in S$.

5.3.1 A General Class of Symmetric Matrices

Let $\boldsymbol{A}$ be an $m \times m$ matrix with constant diagonal entries $a_{c,c} = a_1$ and constant off-diagonal entries $a_{c,c'} = a_2$ for $1 \leq c \neq c' \leq m$. Let $\boldsymbol{u}$ and $\boldsymbol{u}'$ denote arbitrary $m \times 1$ vectors. Then

$$\boldsymbol{A} \cdot \boldsymbol{u} = (a_1 - a_2) \cdot \boldsymbol{u} + a_2 \cdot \boldsymbol{u}[+] \cdot \mathbf{1}_{1:m}$$

where $\boldsymbol{u}[+]$ denotes the sum of the entries of $\boldsymbol{u}$ and $\mathbf{1}_{1\,:\,m}$ is the $m \times 1$ vector with all entries equal to 1. Also,

$$\boldsymbol{u}'^{\mathrm{T}} \cdot \boldsymbol{A} \cdot \boldsymbol{u} = (a_1 - a_2) \cdot \boldsymbol{u}'^{\mathrm{T}} \cdot \boldsymbol{u} + a_2 \cdot \boldsymbol{u}'[+] \cdot \boldsymbol{u}[+].$$

Consequently, $\boldsymbol{A} \cdot \boldsymbol{u}$ and $\boldsymbol{u}'^{\mathrm{T}} \cdot \boldsymbol{A} \cdot \boldsymbol{u}$ can be computed without storing the full matrix $\boldsymbol{A}$, which can substantially reduce the amount of memory used for large values of m.

Let $\boldsymbol{B}$ be the $m \times m$ matrix with constant diagonal values $b_{c,c} = b_1$ and constant off-diagonal values $b_{c,c'} = b_2$ for $1 \leq c \neq c' \leq m$ where

$$b_2 = -\frac{a_2}{d},$$

$$d = a_1^2 + a_1 \cdot a_2 \cdot (m-2) - a_2^2 \cdot (m-1) = (a_1 - a_2) \cdot (a_1 + a_2 \cdot (m-1)),$$

$$b_1 = \frac{1 + a_2^2 \cdot (m-1)/d}{a_1} = \frac{a_1^2 + a_1 \cdot a_2 \cdot (m-2)}{a_1 \cdot d} = \frac{a_1 + a_2 \cdot (m-2)}{d}.$$

assuming $a_1 \neq 0$ and $d \neq 0$. The values for b_1 and b_2 have been chosen so that $\boldsymbol{B} \cdot \boldsymbol{A} = \boldsymbol{I}$ where $\boldsymbol{I}$ is the $m \times m$ identity matrix and so $\boldsymbol{B} = \boldsymbol{A}^{-1}$. Consequently, when $\boldsymbol{A}$ has constant diagonal entries and constant off-diagonal entries, so does its inverse.

5.3.2 Eigenvalues of the EC Correlation Matrix

Under the $m \times m$ EC correlation structure with constant correlation ρ, the working correlation matrix $\boldsymbol{R}(\rho)$ has entries $r_{c,c'}(\rho) = \rho$ for $1 \le c \neq c' \le m$. The matrices $\boldsymbol{A} = \boldsymbol{R}(\rho) - \lambda \cdot \boldsymbol{I}$ for real λ are special cases of the class defined in Sect. 5.3.1 with $a_1 = 1 - \lambda$ and $a_2 = \rho$. The inverse matrices $\boldsymbol{A} = (\boldsymbol{R}(\rho) - \lambda \cdot \boldsymbol{I})^{-1}$ also have this form with

$$b_2 = -\frac{\rho}{d},$$

$$d = (1-\lambda-\rho)\cdot(1-\lambda+\rho\cdot(m-1)),$$

$$b_1 = \frac{1-\lambda+\rho\cdot(m-2)}{d}$$

assuming $\lambda \neq 1$ and $d \neq 0$.

The derivative

$$\frac{\partial(\boldsymbol{R}(\rho)-\lambda\cdot\boldsymbol{I})}{\partial\rho} = \boldsymbol{J}$$

where $\boldsymbol{J}$ is matrix with diagonal entries 0 and off-diagonal entries 1. The log-determinant function.

$h(\rho,\lambda) = \log|\boldsymbol{R}(\rho) - \lambda \cdot \boldsymbol{I}|$ has derivative (Corollary 9.1 in Schott, 2005)

$$\frac{\partial h(\rho,\lambda)}{\partial\rho} = \mathrm{tr}\left((\boldsymbol{R}(\rho)-\lambda\cdot\boldsymbol{I})^{-1}\cdot\boldsymbol{J}\right)$$

where tr denotes the trace function so that

$$\frac{\partial h(\rho,\lambda)}{\partial\rho} = 2\cdot\sum_{c=1}^{m-1}\sum_{c'=c+1}^{m} b_2 = -\frac{m\cdot(m-1)\cdot\rho}{(1-\lambda-\rho)\cdot(1-\lambda+\rho\cdot(m-1))}.$$

Let

$$g(\rho,\lambda) = (1-\lambda-\rho)^{m-1}\cdot(1-\lambda+\rho\cdot(m-1))\cdot G$$

where G is constant in ρ, then

$$\frac{\partial \log g(\rho,\lambda)}{\partial\rho} = (m-1)\cdot\frac{-1}{1-\lambda-\rho} + \frac{m-1}{1-\lambda+\rho\cdot(m-1)}$$

$$= (m-1) \cdot \frac{-(1-\lambda+\rho\cdot(m-1))+1-\lambda-\rho}{(1-\lambda-\rho)\cdot(1-\lambda+\rho\cdot(m-1))}$$

$$= (m-1) \cdot \frac{-\rho\cdot m}{(1-\lambda-\rho)\cdot(1-\lambda+\rho\cdot(m-1))}$$

$$= \frac{\partial h(\rho,\lambda)}{\partial\rho}$$

so that $|\boldsymbol{R}(\boldsymbol{\rho}) - \lambda \cdot \boldsymbol{I}| = g(\rho,\lambda)$ for some constant G. When $\rho = 0$, $|\boldsymbol{R}(\boldsymbol{\rho}) - \lambda \cdot \boldsymbol{I}| = (1 - \lambda)^m$ and $g(\rho,\lambda) = (1-\lambda)^m \cdot G$ so that $G = 1$ and

$$|\boldsymbol{R}(\boldsymbol{\rho}) - \lambda\cdot\boldsymbol{I}| = (1-\lambda-\rho)^{m-1}\cdot(1-\lambda+\rho\cdot(m-1)).$$

Consequently, the eigenvalues of $\boldsymbol{R}(\boldsymbol{\rho})$ are $\lambda = 1 - \rho$ (repeated $m - 1$ times) and $\lambda = 1 - \rho \cdot (m - 1)$ so that $\boldsymbol{R}(\boldsymbol{\rho})$ with $\lambda = 0$ is positive definite when its lowest eigenvalue

$$\lambda = 1-\rho\cdot(m-1) > 0$$

or when

$$\rho > -\frac{1}{(m-1)}.$$

Moreover, its determinant satisfies

$$|\boldsymbol{R}(\boldsymbol{\rho})| = (1-\rho)^{m-1}\cdot(1+\rho\cdot(m-1)).$$

5.3.3 *Inverse of the EC Correlation Matrix*

Using the results of Sect. 5.3.1 applied to the special case with $\lambda = 0$, the working correlation matrix $\boldsymbol{A} = \boldsymbol{R}(\boldsymbol{\rho})$ has inverse $\boldsymbol{B} = \boldsymbol{A}^{-1}$ where

$$b_2 = -\frac{\rho}{d},$$

$$d = (1-\rho)\cdot(1+\rho\cdot(m-1)),$$

$$b_1 = \frac{1+\rho\cdot(m-2)}{d}$$

when $d \neq 0$ or, equivalently, when $\rho \neq 1$ and $\rho \neq -1/(m-1)$. So, while $\boldsymbol{R}(\rho)$ is not positive definite for $1 \leq \rho \leq -1/(m-1)$, it is nonsingular when $1 \leq \rho < -1/(m-1)$.

5.3.4 Square Root of the EC Correlation Matrix

Let $\boldsymbol{U}$ be the $m \times m$ upper triangular matrix with entries $u_{c,c'}$ and columns $\boldsymbol{u}_c$ defined as follows. Let $g_1 = 0$ and, for $1 < c \leq m$,

$$g_c = g_{c-1} + \frac{(\rho - g_{c-1})^2}{1 - g_{c-1}} = \sum_{c'=1}^{c-1} \frac{(\rho - g_{c'-1})^2}{1 - g_{c'-1}}$$

assuming $1 - g_c > 0$. Let $u_{c,c} = (1 - g_c)^{½}$ and

$$u_{c,c'} = \frac{\rho - g_c}{(1 - g_c)^{½}}$$

for $c' > \mathrm{c}$. Note that $u_{c,c'}$ is constant for $c' > \mathrm{c}$. Then

$$\boldsymbol{u}_{c'}^{\mathrm{T}} \cdot \boldsymbol{u}_c = \boldsymbol{u}_{c'}^{\mathrm{T}} \cdot \boldsymbol{u}_{c'} = \rho - g_{c'} + \sum_{c''=1}^{c'-1} \frac{(\rho - g_{c''-1})^2}{1 - g_{c''-1}} = \rho$$

for $c' < \mathrm{c}$ and

$$\boldsymbol{u}_c^{\mathrm{T}} \cdot \boldsymbol{u}_c = 1 - g_c + \sum_{c'=1}^{c-1} \frac{(\rho - g_{c'-1})^2}{1 - g_{c'-1}} = 1$$

so that $\boldsymbol{R}(\rho) = \boldsymbol{U}^{\mathrm{T}} \cdot \boldsymbol{U}$. Also,

$$\log|\boldsymbol{R}(\rho)| = \sum_{c=2}^{m(s)} \log(1 - g_c)$$

provides an alternate way to compute the log-determinant.

5.3.5 Inverse of the Square Root of the EC Correlation Matrix

Let $\boldsymbol{W}$ be the $m \times m$ upper triangular matrix with entries

$$w_{c,c'} = 0, c' < \mathrm{c},$$

$$w_{c,c} = \frac{1}{u_{c,c}}, c' = \mathrm{c},$$

$$w_{c,c+1} = -\frac{u_{c,c+1}}{u_{cc} \cdot u_{c+1,c+1}}, c' = \mathrm{c} + 1,$$

$$w_{c,c'} = w_{c,c'-1} \cdot \frac{u_{c'-1,c'-1} - u_{c'-1,c'}}{u_{c',c'}}, c' > \mathrm{c} + 1,$$

for $1 \le c \le m$. Let $\boldsymbol{w}_c$ denote the rows of $\boldsymbol{W}$. Note that $w_{c,c''} \cdot u_{c'',c'} = 0$ for $c'' < \mathrm{c}$ because then $w_{c,c''} = 0$ and $w_{c,c''} \cdot u_{c'',c'} = 0$ and for $c'' > \mathrm{c}$ because then $u_{c'',\mathrm{c}} = 0$. The matrix $\boldsymbol{W} \cdot \boldsymbol{U}$ has entries

$$\boldsymbol{w}_c \cdot \boldsymbol{u}_{c'} = \sum_{c''=1}^{m} w_{c,c''} \cdot u_{c'',c'}$$

for $1 \le c$, $c' \le m$ satisfying

$$\boldsymbol{w}_c \cdot \boldsymbol{u}_{c'} = 0, c' < \mathrm{c},$$

$$\boldsymbol{w}_c \cdot \boldsymbol{u}_c = w_{c,c} \cdot u_{c,c} = 1, c' = \mathrm{c},$$

$$\boldsymbol{w}_c \cdot \boldsymbol{u}_{c+1} = w_{c,c} \cdot u_{c,c+1} + w_{c,c+1} \cdot u_{c+1,c+1}$$

$$= \frac{u_{c,c+1}}{u_{c,c}} - \frac{u_{c,c+1} \cdot u_{c+1,c+1}}{u_{c,c} \cdot u_{c+1,c+1}} = 0, c' = \mathrm{c} + 1.$$

Assume that $\boldsymbol{w}_c \cdot \boldsymbol{u}_{c'+1} = 0$ for $c' > \mathrm{c} + 1$, then

$$\boldsymbol{w}_c \cdot \boldsymbol{u}_{c'} = \sum_{c''=\mathrm{c}}^{\mathrm{c}'} w_{c,c''} \cdot u_{c'',c'}$$

$$= \sum_{c''=\mathrm{c}}^{\mathrm{c}'-2} \left(w_{c,c''} \cdot u_{c'',c'}\right) + w_{c,c'-1} \cdot u_{c'-1,c} + w_{c,c'} \cdot u_{c',c'}$$

$$= \sum_{c''=\mathrm{c}}^{\mathrm{c}'-2} \left(w_{c,c''} \cdot u_{c'',c'-1}\right) + w_{c,c'-1} \cdot u_{c'-1,c} + w_{c,c'} \cdot u_{c',c'}$$

because $u_{c'',c'}$ is constant for $c' > c''$. Since $\boldsymbol{w}_c \cdot \boldsymbol{u}_{c'+1} = 0$,

$$\boldsymbol{w}_c \cdot \boldsymbol{u}_{c'} = -w_{c,c'-1} \cdot u_{c'-1,c'-1} + w_{c,c'-1} \cdot u_{c'-1,c} + w_{c,c'} \cdot u_{c',c'}$$

$$= w_{c,c'-1} \cdot (-u_{c'-1,c'-1} + u_{c'-1,c}) + w_{c,c'-1} \cdot \frac{u_{c'-1,c'-1} - u_{c'-1,c}}{u_{c',c'}} \cdot u_{c',c'}$$

$$= 0.$$

Consequently, $\boldsymbol{W} = \boldsymbol{U}^{-1}$ and so $\boldsymbol{R}(\boldsymbol{\rho}) = \boldsymbol{U}^{\mathrm{T}} \cdot \boldsymbol{U}$ has inverse $\boldsymbol{R}^{-1}(\rho) = \boldsymbol{W} \cdot \boldsymbol{W}^{\mathrm{T}}$.

5.3.6 Derivatives with Respect to the Constant EC Correlation

Using results of Sect. 5.3.3, $\boldsymbol{A} = \boldsymbol{R}(\boldsymbol{\rho})$ has inverse $\boldsymbol{B} = \boldsymbol{R}^{-1}(\boldsymbol{\rho})$ satisfying

$$b_2 = -\frac{\rho}{d},$$

$$d = (1-\rho) \cdot (1 + \rho \cdot (m-1)) = 1 + \rho \cdot (m-2) - \rho^2 \cdot (m-1),$$

$$b_1 = \frac{1 + \rho \cdot (m-2)}{d} = 1 + \rho^2 \cdot \frac{m-1}{d}$$

assuming $d \neq 0$ or, equivalently, when $\rho \neq 1$ and $\rho \neq -1/(m-1)$. Differentiating with respect to ρ gives

$$\frac{\partial b_1}{\partial \rho} = \frac{2 \cdot \rho \cdot (m-1)}{d} - \rho^2 \cdot (m-1) \cdot \frac{m-2-2 \cdot \rho \cdot (m-1)}{d^2}$$

$$= \rho \cdot (m-1) \cdot \frac{2 \cdot (1 + \rho \cdot (m-2) - \rho^2 \cdot (m-1)) - \rho \cdot (m-2-2 \cdot \rho \cdot (m-1))}{d^2}$$

$$= \rho \cdot (m-1) \cdot \frac{2 + \rho \cdot (m-2)}{d^2}$$

and

$$\frac{\partial b_2}{\partial \rho} = -\frac{1}{d} - (-\rho) \cdot \frac{m-2-2 \cdot \rho \cdot (m-1)}{d^2}$$

$$= \frac{-(1 + \rho \cdot (m-2) - \rho^2 \cdot (m-1)) + \rho \cdot (m-2-2 \cdot \rho \cdot (m-1))}{d^2}$$

$$= -\frac{1 + \rho^2 \cdot (m-1)}{d^2}.$$

The second derivatives with respect to ρ are

$$\frac{\partial^2 b_1}{\partial \rho^2} = \frac{(m-1)\cdot(2+\rho\cdot(m-2))}{d^2} + \frac{\rho\cdot(m-1)\cdot(m-2)}{d^2}$$
$$+\frac{\rho\cdot(m-1)\cdot(2+\rho\cdot(m-2))\cdot(-2)\cdot(m-2-2\cdot\rho\cdot(m-1))}{d^3}$$
$$=\frac{(m-1)\cdot(2+\rho\cdot(m-2)+\rho\cdot(m-2))}{d^2}$$
$$-\frac{2\cdot\rho\cdot(m-1)\cdot(2+\rho\cdot(m-2))\cdot(m-2-2\cdot\rho\cdot(m-1))}{d^3}$$
$$=\frac{2\cdot(m-1)\cdot(1+\rho\cdot(m-2))}{d^2}$$
$$-\frac{2\cdot\rho\cdot(m-1)\cdot(2+\rho\cdot(m-2))\cdot(m-2-2\cdot\rho\cdot(m-1))}{d^3}$$
$$=2\cdot(m-1)\cdot\left(\frac{1+\rho\cdot(m-2)}{d^2}-\frac{\rho\cdot(2+\rho\cdot(m-2))\cdot(m-2-2\cdot\rho\cdot(m-1))}{d^3}\right)$$

and

$$\frac{\partial^2 b_2}{\partial \rho^2} = -\frac{2\cdot\rho\cdot(m-1)}{d^2} - \frac{(1+\rho^2\cdot(m-1))\cdot(-2)\cdot(m-2-2\cdot\rho\cdot(m-1))}{d^3}$$
$$=-2\cdot\left(\frac{\rho\cdot(m-1)}{d^2}-\frac{(1+\rho^2\cdot(m-1))\cdot(m-2-2\cdot\rho\cdot(m-1))}{d^3}\right).$$

These formulas can be used to compute first and second derivatives of $\boldsymbol{R}^{-1}(\rho)$. Note that

$$\frac{\partial \boldsymbol{R}(\rho)}{\partial \rho} = \boldsymbol{J}$$

where $\boldsymbol{J}$ is matrix with all diagonal entries 0 and all off-diagonal entries 1. Consequently,

$$\boldsymbol{R}^{-1}(\rho)\cdot\frac{\partial \boldsymbol{R}(\rho)}{\partial \rho} = \boldsymbol{R}^{-1}(\rho)\cdot\boldsymbol{J}$$

is the $m \times m$ matrix with all diagonal entries equal to $(m-1)\cdot b_2$ so that

$$\frac{\partial \log|\boldsymbol{R}(\rho)|}{\partial \rho} = \mathrm{tr}\left(\boldsymbol{R}^{-1}(\rho)\cdot\frac{\partial \boldsymbol{R}(\rho)}{\partial \rho}\right) = m\cdot(m-1)\cdot b_2.$$

(Sect. 9.4 in Schott, 2005; Wolfinger et al., 1994) and

$$\frac{\partial^2 \log|\boldsymbol{R}(\rho)|}{\partial \rho^2} = m \cdot (m-1) \cdot \frac{\partial b_2}{\partial \rho}.$$

Using the above formulas, entries of the gradient vector $\boldsymbol{E}(\boldsymbol{\theta})$ and the Hessian matrix $\boldsymbol{E}'(\boldsymbol{\theta})$ for the EC correlation structure corresponding to first and second partial derivatives with respect to the constant correlation parameter ρ can be computed without storing the correlation matrix.

5.4 Spatial Autoregressive Order 1 Correlation Structure Computations

This section describes how spatial AR1 correlation structure computations can be conducted without storing the full correlation matrix and its inverse.

5.4.1 *Square Root and Determinant of the Spatial AR1 Correlation Matrix*

Let $t(i)$ for $1 \leq i \leq m(s)$ denote the ordered values of $t(c)$ over $c \in C(s)$. Let the entries of $\boldsymbol{R}_s(\rho)$ be denoted as $r_{i,i'}(\rho) = \rho^{|t(i') - t(i)|}$. Let $\boldsymbol{U}_s$ be the $m(s) \times m(s)$ upper triangular matrix with entries $u_{i,i'}$ and columns $\boldsymbol{u}_i$ defined as follows. Let $g_1 = 1$ and

$$g_{\mathrm{i}} = \left(1 - \rho^{2 \cdot (t(i) - t(i-1))}\right)^{½}$$

for $1 < i \leq m(s)$ so that

$$g_i^2 + \rho^{2 \cdot (t(i) - t(i-1))} = 1$$

and $g_{\mathrm{i}} > 0$ for $0 \leq \rho < 1$ (as assumed in Sect. 2.3.3). Define

$$u_{i,i'} = g_{\mathrm{i}} \cdot \rho^{t(i') - t(i)}$$

for $1 \leq i \leq i' \leq m(s)$. For $i' \geq 1$,

$$\boldsymbol{u}_1^{\mathrm{T}} \cdot \boldsymbol{u}_{i'} = g_1^2 \cdot \rho^{t(i') - t(1)} = \rho^{t(i') - t(1)} = r_{1,i'}(\rho).$$

For $i' \geq 2$,

$$\begin{aligned}\boldsymbol{u}_2^{\mathrm{T}} \cdot \boldsymbol{u}_{i'} &= g_1^2 \cdot \rho^{t(2)-t(1)} \cdot \rho^{t(i')-t(1)} + g_2^2 \cdot \rho^{t(i')-t(2)} \\ &= \rho^{t(i')-t(2)} \cdot \left(\rho^{2\cdot(t(2)-t(1))} + g_2^2\right) = r_{2,i'}(\rho)\end{aligned}$$

by definition of g_2. For $i > 2$, assume that

$$\begin{aligned}\boldsymbol{u}_{i-1}^{\mathrm{T}} \cdot \boldsymbol{u}_{i'} &= \sum_{i''=1}^{i-1} (u_{i'',i-1} \cdot u_{i'',i'}) = \sum_{i''=1}^{i-1} \left(g_{i''}^2 \cdot \rho^{t(i-1)-t(i'')} \cdot \rho^{t(i')-t(i'')}\right) \\ &= \rho^{t(i')-t(i-1)} \cdot \sum_{i''=1}^{i-1} \left(g_{i''}^2 \cdot \rho^{2\cdot(t(i-1)-t(i''))}\right) = r_{i-1,i'}(\rho)\end{aligned}$$

holds for $i' \geq \mathrm{i} - 1$ because

$$\sum_{i''=1}^{i-1} \left(g_{i''}^2 \cdot \rho^{2\cdot(t(i-1)-t(i''))}\right) = 1.$$

Then for $i' \geq \mathrm{i}$

$$\begin{aligned}\boldsymbol{u}_i^{\mathrm{T}} \cdot \boldsymbol{u}_{i'} &= \sum_{i''=1}^{i} u_{i'',i} \cdot u_{i'',i'} = \sum_{i''=1}^{i} \left(g_{i''}^2 \cdot \rho^{t(i)-t(i'')} \cdot \rho^{t(i')-t(i'')}\right) \\ &= \rho^{t(i')-t(i)} \cdot \sum_{i''=1}^{i} \left(g_{i''}^2 \cdot \rho^{2\cdot(t(i)-t(i''))}\right) = r_{i,i'}(\rho)\end{aligned}$$

because

$$\begin{aligned}\sum_{i''=1}^{i} \left(g_{i''}^2 \cdot \rho^{2\cdot(t(i)-t(i''))}\right) &= \rho^{2\cdot(t(i)-t(i-1))} \cdot \sum_{i''=1}^{i-1} \left(g_{i''}^2 \cdot \rho^{2\cdot(t(i-1)-t(i''))}\right) + g_i^2 \\ &= \rho^{2\cdot(t(i)-t(i-1))} + g_i^2 = 1.\end{aligned}$$

Consequently,

$$\log|\boldsymbol{R}(\rho)| = \sum_{i=2}^{m(s)} \log g_i^2$$

and $\boldsymbol{R}_s(\rho) = \boldsymbol{U}_s^{\mathrm{T}} \cdot \boldsymbol{U}_s$ so that it is positive definite when $0 \leq \rho < 1$.

5.4.2 Inverse of the Square Root of the Spatial AR1 Correlation Matrix

Let $\boldsymbol{W}_s$ be the $m(s) \times m(s)$ matrix with entries $w_{i,i'}$ that are all zero except for the following:

$$w_{i,i} = \frac{1}{g_{\mathrm{i}}}$$

for $1 \leq i \leq m(s)$ and

$$w_{i-1,i} = -\frac{\rho^{t(i)-t(i-1)}}{g_{\mathrm{i}}}$$

for $1 < i \leq m(s)$ and let $\boldsymbol{w}_i$ denote the rows of $\boldsymbol{W}_s$. The matrix $\boldsymbol{W}_s \cdot \boldsymbol{U}_s$ has entries

$$\boldsymbol{w}_i \cdot \boldsymbol{u}_i = w_{i,i} \cdot u_{i,i} = \frac{1}{g_{\mathrm{i}}} \cdot g_{\mathrm{i}} = 1$$

for $1 \leq i \leq m(s)$ and

$$\boldsymbol{w}_i \cdot \boldsymbol{u}_{i'} = w_{i,i} \cdot u_{i,i'} + w_{i,i+1} \cdot u_{i+1,i'} = \frac{1}{g_{\mathrm{i}}} \cdot g_{\mathrm{i}} \cdot \rho^{t(i')-t(i)}$$
$$+ \left(\frac{-\rho^{t(i+1)-t(i)}}{g_{\mathrm{i+1}}} \right) \cdot g_{\mathrm{i+1}} \cdot \rho^{t(i')-t(i+1)} = 0$$

for $1 \leq i < m(s)$ and $i < i' \leq m(s)$. Consequently, $\boldsymbol{W}_s = \boldsymbol{U}_s^{-1}$ and $\boldsymbol{R}(\rho) = \boldsymbol{U}^{\mathrm{T}} \cdot \boldsymbol{U}$ has inverse $\boldsymbol{R}^{-1}(\rho) = \boldsymbol{W} \cdot \boldsymbol{W}^{\mathrm{T}}$.

5.4.3 Derivatives with Respect to the Spatial Autocorrelation

As demonstrated in Sect. 5.4.1,

$$\log|\boldsymbol{R}(\rho)| = \sum_{i=2}^{m(s)} \log h_i$$

where $h_i = g_i^2 = 1 - \rho^{2 \cdot \Delta(i)}$ and $\Delta(i) = t(i) - t(i-1)$ so that

$$\frac{\partial \log|\boldsymbol{R}(\rho)|}{\partial \rho} = -2 \cdot \sum_{i=2}^{m(s)} \frac{\Delta(i) \cdot \rho^{2 \cdot \Delta(i) - 1}}{h_i}$$

and

$$\frac{\partial^2 \log|\boldsymbol{R}(\rho)|}{\partial \rho^2} = -2 \cdot \sum_{i=2}^{m(s)} \frac{\Delta(i) \cdot (2 \cdot \Delta(i) - 1) \cdot \rho^{2 \cdot \Delta(i) - 2}}{h_i} - 2 \cdot \sum_{i=2}^{m(s)} \frac{2 \cdot \Delta^2(i) \cdot \rho^{4 \cdot \Delta(i) - 2}}{h_i^2}$$

$$= -2 \cdot \sum_{i=2}^{m(s)} \frac{\Delta(i) \cdot \left((2 \cdot \Delta(i) - 1) \cdot h_i + 2 \cdot \Delta(i) \cdot \rho^{2 \cdot \Delta(i)}\right) \cdot \rho^{2 \cdot \Delta(i) - 2}}{h_i^2}$$

$$= -2 \cdot \sum_{i=2}^{m(s)} \frac{\Delta(i) \cdot \left(2 \cdot \Delta(i) - 1 + \rho^{2 \cdot \Delta(i)}\right) \cdot \rho^{2 \cdot \Delta(i) - 2}}{h_i^2}.$$

As demonstrated in Sect. 5.4.2,

$$\boldsymbol{a}'^{\mathrm{T}} \cdot \boldsymbol{R}^{-1}(\rho) \cdot \boldsymbol{a} = \boldsymbol{a}'^{\mathrm{T}} \cdot \boldsymbol{W} \cdot \boldsymbol{W}^{\mathrm{T}} \cdot \boldsymbol{a} = \boldsymbol{b}'^{\mathrm{T}} \cdot \boldsymbol{b}$$

where $\boldsymbol{b} = \boldsymbol{W}^{\mathrm{T}} \cdot \boldsymbol{a}$, $\boldsymbol{b}' = \boldsymbol{W}^{\mathrm{T}} \cdot \boldsymbol{a}'$, and $\boldsymbol{a}$ and $\boldsymbol{a}'$ are arbitrary $m(s) \times 1$ vectors with entries a_i and a'_i, respectively, for $1 \leq i \leq m(s)$. The entries of $\boldsymbol{b}$ are

$$b_1 = w_{1,1} \cdot a_1 = a_1.$$

and

$$b_i = w_{i-1,i} \cdot a_{i-1} + w_{i,i} \cdot a_i$$

for $1 < i \leq m(s)$ so that

$$\frac{\partial b_1}{\partial \rho} = \frac{\partial w_{1,1}}{\partial \rho} \cdot a_1 = 0$$

and

$$\frac{\partial b_i}{\partial \rho} = \frac{\partial w_{i-1,i}}{\partial \rho} \cdot a_{i-1} + \frac{\partial w_{i,i}}{\partial \rho} \cdot a_i$$

for $1 < i \leq m(s)$ with

$$\frac{\partial w_{i,i}}{\partial \rho} = -\frac{-2 \cdot \Delta(i) \cdot \rho^{2 \cdot \Delta(i) - 1}}{2 \cdot h_i^{3/2}} = \frac{\Delta(i) \cdot \rho^{2 \cdot \Delta(i) - 1}}{h_i^{3/2}}.$$

By definition,

$$w_{i-1,i} = -\rho^{t(i) - t(i-1)} / g_i = -\rho^{\Delta(i)} \cdot w_{i,i}$$

so that

$$\frac{\partial w_{i-1,i}}{\partial \rho} = -\rho^{\Delta(i)} \cdot \frac{\partial w_{i,i}}{\partial \rho} - \Delta(i) \cdot \rho^{\Delta(i) - 1} \cdot w_{i,i}$$

for $1 < i \leq m(s)$. First partial derivatives $\frac{\partial b'_i}{\partial \rho}$ are computed similarly. These can be used to compute the second partial derivatives with respect to ρ and with respect to a mean or dispersion parameter of terms involving $\boldsymbol{a}' \neq \boldsymbol{a}$. Otherwise, $\boldsymbol{a} = \boldsymbol{a}' = \boldsymbol{stde}_s$ and then

$$\boldsymbol{b}'^{\mathrm{T}} \cdot \boldsymbol{b} = \boldsymbol{b}^{\mathrm{T}} \cdot \boldsymbol{b} = \sum_{i=1}^{m(s)} b_i^2$$

where

$$b_i^2 = \frac{c_i^2}{h_i}$$

with $c_1 = a_1$, $h_1 = 1$, and

$$c_i = -\rho^{\Delta(i)} \cdot a_{i-1} + a_i$$

for $1 < i \leq m(s)$. Hence,

$$\frac{\partial b_1^2}{\partial \rho} = 0,$$

$$\frac{\partial b_i^2}{\partial \rho} = d_1 + d_2,$$

$$d_1 = -2 \cdot \Delta(i) \cdot \rho^{\Delta(i) - 1} \cdot a_{i-1} \cdot \frac{c_i}{h_i},$$

$$d_2 = 2 \cdot \Delta(i) \cdot \rho^{2 \cdot \Delta(i) - 1} \cdot \frac{c_i^2}{h_i^2}$$

for $1 < i \le m(s)$. This can be used to compute the first partial derivative of $\boldsymbol{stde}_s^{\mathrm{T}} \cdot \boldsymbol{R}_s^{-1}(\boldsymbol{\rho}) \cdot \boldsymbol{stde}_s$ with respect to ρ. Its second partial with respect to ρ can be computed using

$$\frac{\partial^2 b_1^2}{\partial \rho^2} = 0,$$

$$\frac{\partial^2 b_i^2}{\partial \rho^2} = \frac{\partial d_1}{\partial \rho} + \frac{\partial d_2}{\partial \rho},$$

$$\frac{\partial d_1}{\partial \rho} = -2 \cdot \Delta(i) \cdot (\Delta(i) - 1) \cdot \rho^{\Delta(i)-2} \cdot a_{i-1} \cdot \frac{c_i}{h_i} + 2 \cdot \Delta^2(i) \cdot \rho^{2 \cdot \Delta(i) - 2} \cdot \frac{a_{i-1}^2}{h_i} - 4 \cdot \Delta^2(i) \cdot \rho^{3 \cdot \Delta(i) - 2} \cdot a_{i-1} \cdot \frac{c_i}{h_i^2},$$

$$\frac{\partial d_2}{\partial \rho} = 2 \cdot \Delta(i) \cdot (2 \cdot \Delta(i) - 1) \cdot \rho^{2 \cdot \Delta(i) - 2} \cdot \frac{c_i^2}{h_i^2} - 4 \cdot \Delta^2(i) \cdot \rho^{3 \cdot \Delta(i) - 2} \cdot a_{i-1} \cdot \frac{c_i}{h_i^2} + 8 \cdot \Delta^2(i) \cdot \rho^{4 \cdot \Delta(i) - 2} \cdot \frac{c_i^2}{h_i^3}$$

for $1 < i \le m(s)$. Using the above formulas, entries of the gradient vector $\boldsymbol{E}(\boldsymbol{\theta})$ and the Hessian matrix $\boldsymbol{E}'(\boldsymbol{\theta})$ for the spatial AR1 correlation structure corresponding to first and second partial derivatives with respect to the constant correlation parameter ρ can be computed without storing the correlation matrix.

5.5 Unstructured Correlation Structure Computations

In general, computation of the determinants $|\boldsymbol{R}_s(\boldsymbol{\rho})|$ and the inverses $\boldsymbol{R}_s^{-1}(\boldsymbol{\rho})$ for the correlation matrices $\boldsymbol{R}_s(\boldsymbol{\rho})$ requires specialized software; for example, PROC IML of SAS provides matrix functions for generating these quantities. Derivatives of these quantities are based on established formulas (Sect. 9.4 in Schott, 2005; Wolfinger et al., 1994). In the casse of UN correlations, for $c < c'$ with $c, c' \in C(s)$, the first partial derivative of $\boldsymbol{R}_s(\boldsymbol{\rho})$ with respect to $\rho_{c,\ c'}$ satisfies

$$\frac{\partial \boldsymbol{R}_s(\boldsymbol{\rho})}{\partial \rho_{c,c'}} = \boldsymbol{J}_{s,c,c'}$$

where $\boldsymbol{J}_{s,c,c'}$ is the $m(s) \times m(s)$ matrix with entries equal to 1 for the entry at row c and column c′, 1 for the entry at row c′ and column c, and equal to 0 for the other entries. The first partial derivative of $\log|\boldsymbol{R}_s(\boldsymbol{\rho})|$ with respect to $\rho_{c,c'}$ satisfies

$$\frac{\partial \log|\boldsymbol{R}_s(\boldsymbol{\rho})|}{\partial \rho_{c,c'}} = \mathrm{tr}\left(\boldsymbol{R}_s^{-1}(\boldsymbol{\rho}) \cdot \frac{\partial \boldsymbol{R}_s(\boldsymbol{\rho})}{\partial \rho_{c,c'}}\right) = \mathrm{tr}\left(\boldsymbol{R}_s^{-1}(\boldsymbol{\rho}) \cdot \boldsymbol{J}_{s,c,c'}\right).$$

The derivative of $\boldsymbol{R}_s^{-1}(\boldsymbol{\rho})$ with respect to $\rho_{c,c'}$ satisfies

$$\frac{\partial \boldsymbol{R}_s^{-1}(\boldsymbol{\rho})}{\partial \rho_{c,c'}} = -\boldsymbol{R}_s^{-1}(\boldsymbol{\rho}) \cdot \frac{\partial \boldsymbol{R}_s(\boldsymbol{\rho})}{\partial \rho_{c,c'}} \cdot \boldsymbol{R}_s^{-1}(\boldsymbol{\rho}) = -\boldsymbol{R}_s^{-1}(\boldsymbol{\rho}) \cdot \boldsymbol{J}_{s,c,c'} \cdot \boldsymbol{R}_s^{-1}(\boldsymbol{\rho}).$$

For $c < c'$ and $d < d'$ with $c, c', d, d' \in C(s)$, the second partial derivatives of $\boldsymbol{R}_s(\boldsymbol{\rho})$, $\boldsymbol{R}_s^{-1}(\boldsymbol{\rho})$, and $\log|\boldsymbol{R}_s(\boldsymbol{\rho})|$ with respect to $\rho_{c,c'}$ and $\rho_{d,d'}$ satisfy

$$\frac{\partial^2 \boldsymbol{R}_s(\boldsymbol{\rho})}{\partial \rho_{d,d'}\,\partial \rho_{c,c'}} = 0,$$

$$\begin{aligned}\frac{\partial^2 \boldsymbol{R}_s^{-1}(\boldsymbol{\rho})}{\partial \rho_{d,d'}\,\partial \rho_{c,c'}} &= 2 \cdot \boldsymbol{R}_s^{-1}(\boldsymbol{\rho}) \cdot \frac{\partial \boldsymbol{R}_s(\boldsymbol{\rho})}{\partial \rho_{d,d'}} \cdot \boldsymbol{R}_s^{-1}(\boldsymbol{\rho}) \cdot \frac{\partial \boldsymbol{R}_s(\boldsymbol{\rho})}{\partial \rho_{c,c'}} \cdot \boldsymbol{R}_s^{-1}(\boldsymbol{\rho}) \\ &\quad - \boldsymbol{R}_s^{-1}(\boldsymbol{\rho}) \cdot \frac{\partial^2 \boldsymbol{R}_s(\boldsymbol{\rho})}{\partial \rho_{d,d'}\,\partial \rho_{c,c'}} \cdot \boldsymbol{R}_s^{-1}(\boldsymbol{\rho}) \\ &= 2 \cdot \boldsymbol{R}_s^{-1}(\boldsymbol{\rho}) \cdot \boldsymbol{J}_{s,d,d'} \cdot \boldsymbol{R}_s^{-1}(\boldsymbol{\rho}) \cdot \boldsymbol{J}_{s,c,c'} \cdot \boldsymbol{R}_s^{-1}(\boldsymbol{\rho}),\end{aligned}$$

and

$$\begin{aligned}\frac{\partial^2 \log|\boldsymbol{R}_s(\boldsymbol{\rho})|}{\partial \rho_{d,d'}\,\partial \rho_{c,c'}} &= -\,\mathrm{tr}\left(\boldsymbol{R}_s^{-1}(\boldsymbol{\rho}) \cdot \frac{\partial \boldsymbol{R}_s(\boldsymbol{\rho})}{\partial \rho_{d,d'}} \cdot \boldsymbol{R}_s^{-1}(\boldsymbol{\rho}) \cdot \frac{\partial \boldsymbol{R}_s(\boldsymbol{\rho})}{\partial \rho_{c,c'}}\right) \\ &\quad + \mathrm{tr}\left(\boldsymbol{R}_s^{-1}(\boldsymbol{\rho}) \cdot \frac{\partial^2 \boldsymbol{R}_s(\boldsymbol{\rho})}{\partial \rho_{d,d'}\,\partial \rho_{c,c'}}\right) \\ &= -\,\mathrm{tr}\left(\boldsymbol{R}_s^{-1}(\boldsymbol{\rho}) \cdot \boldsymbol{J}_{s,d,d'} \cdot \boldsymbol{R}_s^{-1}(\boldsymbol{\rho}) \cdot \boldsymbol{J}_{s,c,c'}\right)\end{aligned}$$

Entries of the gradient vector $\boldsymbol{E}(\boldsymbol{\theta})$ and the Hessian matrix $\boldsymbol{E}'(\boldsymbol{\theta})$ for the UN correlation structure corresponding to partial derivatives with respect to the correlation parameters $\rho_{c,c'}$ can be computed using the above formulas. Similar formulations can be used to compute these partial derivatives for general correlation structures.

5.6 Verifying Gradient and Hessian Computations

Formulations for the gradient vector $\boldsymbol{E}(\boldsymbol{\theta})$ and the Hessian matrix $\boldsymbol{E}'(\boldsymbol{\theta})$ are complex. The effectiveness of the parameter estimation process of Sect. 3.7 and its adjustments of Sects. 4.3 and 5.2 require that these formulations and their software implementations be correct. They can be verified by comparing results generated by software implementations to results generated by finite difference approximations. Specifically, in the ELMM case, for $1 \leq j \leq r + p + q$ let $\mathbf{1}_j$ denote the $(r + q + p) \times 1$ vector with j^{th} entry equal to 1 and all other entries equal to 0 and let ε be a small non-zero value such as 10^{-5}. For $1 \leq j \leq r + p + q$, estimate the jth entry $E_j(\boldsymbol{\theta})$ of $\boldsymbol{E}(\boldsymbol{\theta})$ using the central difference approximation

$$d\ell_j = \frac{\ell(SC; \boldsymbol{\theta} + \varepsilon \cdot \mathbf{1}_j) - \ell(SC; \boldsymbol{\theta} - \varepsilon \cdot \mathbf{1}_j)}{2 \cdot \varepsilon}$$

and then compare these approximations to values of $E_j(\boldsymbol{\theta})$ generated by software implementations of the associated formulation for $\boldsymbol{E}(\boldsymbol{\theta})$. When the software implementations are correct, the parameter estimation process is likely to generate values for $E_j(\boldsymbol{\theta})$ smaller than can be verified through approximations. This can be circumvented by setting the maximum number i^* of iterations for the estimation process to a very small number such as 3. Once implementations of $\boldsymbol{E}(\boldsymbol{\theta})$ are verified, the columns $\boldsymbol{E}'_j(\boldsymbol{\theta})$ of the Hessian matrix $\boldsymbol{E}'(\boldsymbol{\theta})$ can be similarly verified using the central difference approximations

$$d\boldsymbol{E}'_j = \frac{\boldsymbol{E}(\boldsymbol{\theta} + \varepsilon \cdot \mathbf{1}_j) - \boldsymbol{E}(\boldsymbol{\theta} - \varepsilon \cdot \mathbf{1}_j)}{2 \cdot \varepsilon}.$$

The fully modified GEE case can be handled similarly, but then $\boldsymbol{\theta}$ has $r + p$ entries and the approximations need to be based on values of $\ell(SC; \boldsymbol{\theta} \pm \varepsilon \cdot \mathbf{1}_j)$ and $\boldsymbol{E}(\boldsymbol{\theta} \pm \varepsilon \cdot \mathbf{1}_j)$ computed using the fixed value $\boldsymbol{\rho}(\boldsymbol{\theta})$ for the correlation parameter vector. In the partially modified GEE case, computations for first and second partial derivatives based solely on the dispersion parameters can be verified similarly. Formulations of the second partial derivative matrix $\boldsymbol{E}'(\boldsymbol{\beta}, \boldsymbol{\gamma})$ based on both the mean and dispersion parameters of Sect. 3.2 mainly use formulations also used in computing other partial derivatives and so should be implemented by reusing verified formulations used to compute the other partial derivatives so that they are likely to also be correct. Computations for first and second partial derivatives based solely on the mean parameters can be verified by comparing them to results generated by existing software for standard GEE (e.g., PROC GENMOD of SAS), but this only applies to cases implemented by that existing software. However, these computations only require correct implementations of the first partial derivative matrices

$$\boldsymbol{D}_s = \frac{\partial \boldsymbol{\mu}_s}{\partial \boldsymbol{\beta}}$$

that are also computed as part of the fully modified and ELMM computations, and so results can be compared across alternate modeling procedures.

5.7 Direct Variance Modeling

Partially modified GEE, fully modified GEE, and ELMM use extended variances based on both dispersions and the variance function $V(\mu)$. In the GEE context, this serves to extend standard GEE to provide for non-constant variances based on the assumed distribution. The dispersions cannot do this in the standard GEE case because they are assumed to be constant. However, for partially modified GEE, fully modified GEE, and ELMM, dispersions can be non-constant and so might be sufficient for modeling non-constant variances without including $V(\mu)$. This is equivalent to changing the variance function to the unit function $V(\mu) = 1$ as for the linear regression case of Sect. 4.2.1. Formally, model the extended variances as $\sigma_{sc}^2 = \varphi_{sc}$ where $\log \varphi_{sc} = \boldsymbol{v}_{sc}^{\mathrm{T}} \cdot \boldsymbol{\gamma}$. This is direct variance modeling. It is trivial in the linear regression case since that is already based on the unit variance function.

Direct variance modeling might provide competitive models for regression types other than linear regression or even distinctly better models when the usual assumed variance function is not a good fit for a given data set. On the other hand, the assumed variance function may be so appropriate that direct variance modeling might not even generate a competitive model. While direct variance modeling applies to partially and fully modified GEE modeling, example analyses provided later only consider direct variance modeling in the most general case of ELMM, and so the following formulation addresses only the ELMM case. Only formulations involving the vector $\boldsymbol{\beta}$ of mean parameters are provided here. Formulations involving only $\boldsymbol{\gamma}$ and $\boldsymbol{\rho}$ are the same as before. Formulations involving $\boldsymbol{\beta}$ combined with either $\boldsymbol{\gamma}$ or $\boldsymbol{\rho}$ are the same as before but use the revised formulations for $\boldsymbol{\beta}$ as provided next.

Direct variance modeling has the advantage of having a simpler gradient sub-vector

$$\boldsymbol{E}(\boldsymbol{\beta}) = \frac{\partial \ell(SC;\boldsymbol{\theta})}{\partial \boldsymbol{\beta}}$$

and Hessian submatrix

$$\boldsymbol{E}'(\boldsymbol{\beta}) = \frac{\partial \boldsymbol{E}(\boldsymbol{\theta})}{\partial \boldsymbol{\beta}}.$$

Determinants of covariance matrices now satisfy

$$\log|\boldsymbol{\Sigma}_s| = \log|\boldsymbol{R}_s(\boldsymbol{\rho})| + \sum_{c \in C(s)} \boldsymbol{v}_{sc}^{\mathrm{T}} \cdot \boldsymbol{\gamma}$$

so that, using the notation used in Sects. 3.2, 4.1, and 5.1,

$$W_j(\mu_{sc}) = 0,$$
$$W_{j,j'}(\mu_{sc}) = 0$$

for $1 \leq j, j' \leq r$. It always is the case that

$$vstde_{sc,j''} = v_{sc,j''} \cdot stde_{sc}/2,$$
$$vvstde_{sc,j'',j'''} = v_{sc,j''} \cdot v_{sc,j'''} \cdot stde_{sc}/4,$$
$$vxstde_{sc,j,j''} = xstde_{sc,j} \cdot v_{sc,j''}/2,$$

for $1 \leq j'', j''' \leq q$ and $1 \leq j \leq r$. Consequently, only $xstde_{sc,j}$ determining $\boldsymbol{E}(\boldsymbol{\beta})$ and $xxstde_{sc,j,j'}$ determining $\boldsymbol{E}'(\boldsymbol{\beta})$ can change for $1 \leq j, j' \leq r$. Since the standardized residuals $stde_{sc}$ no longer depend on the non-unit variance function $V(\mu_{sc})$,

$$\boldsymbol{E}(\boldsymbol{\beta}) = \sum_{s \in S} \boldsymbol{E}_s(\boldsymbol{\beta}) = \sum_{s \in S} \boldsymbol{D}_s^{\mathrm{T}} \cdot \boldsymbol{\Sigma}_s^{-1} \cdot \boldsymbol{e}_s,$$

where

$$\boldsymbol{D}_s = \frac{\partial \boldsymbol{\mu}_s}{\partial \boldsymbol{\beta}}$$

is a $m(s) \times r$ matrix for $s \in S$. In other words, using a unit variance function generates analogous estimating equations for the means as for standard GEE modeling, but the matrices $\boldsymbol{\Sigma}_s$ are now computed with $V(\mu_{sc}) = 1$. Consequently, the estimating equations for the means under direct variance estimation in conventional cases have the same formulation as for standard GEE modeling but use simplified covariance matrices $\boldsymbol{\Sigma}_s$. Moreover,

$$\boldsymbol{E}'(\boldsymbol{\beta}) = -\sum_{s \in S} \boldsymbol{D}_s^{\mathrm{T}} \cdot \boldsymbol{\Sigma}_s^{-1} \cdot \boldsymbol{D}_s.$$

is also analogous with the same formulation as for standard GEE modeling but also using simplified covariance matrices. This formulation addresses direct variance modeling in the correlated univariate outcome context, but it holds as well for extended linear modeling in the singleton univariate outcome context of Sect. 4.4.

In the case of Poisson regression with log link function of Sect. 4.2.2,

$$xstde_{sc,j} = x_{sc,j'} \cdot \mu_{sc} / \varphi_{sc}^{1/2},$$

$$xxstde_{sc,j,j'} = -x_{sc,j} \cdot x_{sc,j'} \cdot \mu_{sc} / \varphi_{sc}^{1/2},$$

for $sc \in SC$ and $1 \leq j, j' \leq r$. In the case of logistic regression with logit link function of Sect. 4.2.3,

$$xstde_{sc,j} = x_{sc,j'} \cdot \mu_{sc} \cdot (1 - \mu_{sc}) / \varphi_{sc}^{1/2},$$

$$xxstde_{sc,j,j'} = -x_{sc,j} \cdot x_{sc,j'} \cdot \mu_{sc} \cdot (1 - \mu_{sc}) \cdot (1 - 2 \cdot \mu_{sc}) / \varphi_{sc}^{1/2},$$

for $sc \in SC$ and $1 \leq j, j' \leq r$. In the case of exponential regression with log link function of Sect. 4.2.4,

$$xstde_{sc,j} = x_{sc,j'} \cdot \mu_{sc} / \varphi_{sc}^{1/2},$$

$$xxstde_{sc,j,j'} = -x_{sc,j} \cdot x_{sc,j'} \cdot \mu_{sc} / \varphi_{sc}^{1/2},$$

for $sc \in SC$ and $1 \leq j, j' \leq r$. In the case of inverse Gaussian regression with log link function of Sect. 4.2.5,

$$xstde_{sc,j} = x_{sc,j'} \cdot \mu_{sc} / \varphi_{sc}^{1/2},$$

$$xxstde_{sc,j,j'} = -x_{sc,j} \cdot x_{sc,j'} \cdot \mu_{sc} / \varphi_{sc}^{1/2},$$

for $sc \in SC$ and $1 \leq j, j' \leq r$.

In the case of Poisson regression with log link function of Sect. 4.2.2 when an offset variable $o_{sc} = \log T_{sc}$ is included, the mean rates still satisfy

$$\mu'_{sc} = Ey'_{sc} = \frac{\mu_{sc}}{T_{sc}} = \exp\left(\mathbf{x}_{sc}^{\mathrm{T}} \cdot \boldsymbol{\beta}\right)$$

as in Sect. 2.2.2. On the other hand, using the same offset variable for the dispersions means that the variances for the counts/rates change from those given in Sect. 3.1. The variances for the counts become

$$\sigma_{sc}^2 = \varphi_{sc} = \exp\left(\mathbf{v}_{sc}^{\mathrm{T}} \cdot \boldsymbol{\gamma}\right) \cdot \exp(o_{sc}) = \exp\left(\mathbf{v}_{sc}^{\mathrm{T}} \cdot \boldsymbol{\gamma}\right) \cdot T_{sc}$$

so that the variances for the rates are

$$\sigma'^2_{sc} = \frac{\sigma^2_{sc}}{T^2_{sc}} = \frac{\varphi'_{sc}}{T_{sc}}$$

where $\varphi'_{sc} = \exp\left(\boldsymbol{v}_{sc}^{\mathrm{T}} \cdot \boldsymbol{\beta}\right)$ is defined in Sect. 3.1. Models for rates based on this kind of direct variances are not comparable to models for rates based on extended variances. This problem is rectified by changing the offsets $o_{sc} = \log T_{sc}$ for the dispersions to $o'_{sc} = \log T^2_{sc}$ so that

$$\sigma^2_{sc} = \varphi_{sc} = \exp\left(\boldsymbol{v}_{sc}^{\mathrm{T}} \cdot \gamma\right) \cdot \exp(o'_{sc}) = \exp\left(\boldsymbol{v}_{sc}^{\mathrm{T}} \cdot \gamma\right) \cdot T^2_{sc}$$

and then

$$\sigma'^2_{sc} = \frac{\sigma^2_{sc}}{T^2_{sc}} = \varphi'_{sc}.$$

References

Schott, J. R. (2005). *Matrix analysis for statistics* (2nd ed.). Wiley.

Wolfinger, R., Tobias, R., & Sall, J. (1994). Computing gaussian likelihoods and their derivatives for general linear mixed models. *SIAM Journal on Scientific Computing, 6*, 1294–1310.

Chapter 6
Example Analyses of the Dental Measurement Data

Abstract Adaptive analyses are presented of dental measurements for children at 8, 10, 12, and 14 years old using linear regression with the identity link function. The choice of the number k of folds for computing likelihood cross-validation (LCV) scores is addressed as well as the choice of the correlation structure. Results are compared for partially modified generalized estimating equations (GEE), fully modified GEE, and linear mixed modeling (LMM). Linearity of means in child age with constant variances is addressed as well as a comparison to standard GEE modeling and the dependence of means and variances on child age. Adaptive additive and adaptive moderation models are generated for child age and child gender. A comparison to the standard linear moderation model is provided. A summary of the analysis results is provided as well. SAS code is described for generating these analyses along with output generated by that code.

Keywords Generalized estimating equations · Likelihood cross-validation · Linear mixed modeling · Linear regression · Moderation · Non-constant variances

Introduction Adaptive analyses are presented in this chapter of the dental measurement data of Sect. 2.8.1 (Potthoff & Roy, 1964). All LCV scores are computed using matched-set-wise deletion since there are no missing measurements. The cutoff using DF = 1 for a distinct percent decrease in LCV scores for these data is 1.76%. Section 6.1 addresses choosing the number k of folds as described in Sect. 2.6.1 and choosing the correlation structure from among those described in Sect. 2.3. Results are compared for partially modified GEE, fully modified GEE, and LMM. Section 6.2 addresses linearity of means in child age with constant variances, while Sect. 6.3 provides a comparison to standard GEE modeling and Sect. 6.4 addresses the dependence of means and variances on child age. Adaptive additive and adaptive moderation models are generated for child age and child gender in Sects. 6.5 and 6.6, respectively. A comparison to the standard linear moderation model is provided in

Supplementary Information The online version contains supplementary material available at https://doi.org/10.1007/978-3-031-41988-1_6.

G. J. Knafl, *Modeling Correlated Outcomes Using Extensions of Generalized Estimating Equations and Linear Mixed Modeling*,
https://doi.org/10.1007/978-3-031-41988-1_6

Sect. 6.7. Section 6.8 provides a summary of the analysis results described in prior sections, while Sect. 6.9 provides example SAS code for generating such analyses and descriptions of output generated by that code.

The primary purpose of Chap. 6 is to compare adaptive modeling results for partially modified GEE, fully modified GEE, and LMM applied to continuous real-valued correlated outcomes using linear regression models. Partially modified GEE (see Chap. 3 for details) extends standard GEE (see Chap. 2 for details) by adding extra estimating equations for variance parameters to the standard GEE estimating equations for mean parameters. Fully modified GEE (see Chap. 4 for details) extends standard GEE further by providing alternative estimating equations for mean parameters while utilizing the same estimating equations for the variances used by partially modified GEE. These new estimating equations are based on minimizing a likelihood function. Both partially modified and fully modified GEE use the standard GEE method of estimating correlation parameters using residuals. LMM (see Chap. 5 for more details) is based on estimating equations for mean, variance, and correlation parameters determined by maximizing the likelihood. The estimating equations for the means and variances are the same as for fully modified GEE.

6.1 Choosing the Number of Folds and the Correlation Structure

Linear regression analyses reported in this section assume constant variances. The effects of the number k of folds and of the correlation structure on estimation by partially modified GEE, fully modified GEE, and LMM are assessed.

Table 6.1 contains results for adaptive models for mean dental measurements with constant variances generated for 36 cases corresponding to each of the 3 modeling approaches partially modified GEE, fully modified GEE, and LMM; each of the 4 correlation structures IND, spatial AR1, EC, and UN; and each of the 3 numbers k of folds 5, 10, and 15. Note that equivalent results would be generated for non-spatial AR1 correlations as for spatial AR1 correlations since outcome measurements are equally spaced at 2-year intervals. The best LCV score of 0.12014 for the 12 partially modified GEE models is achieved at $k = 10$ under EC correlations. The best LCV score of 0.11880 for the 12 fully modified GEE models is achieved at $k = 5$ under EC correlations. The best LCV score of 0.11880 for the 12 LMM models is achieved at $k = 5$ under EC correlations. Consequently, all three modeling approaches select EC as the most appropriate of the four correlation structures for the dental measurement data.

The best score of Table 6.1 for partially modified GEE is achieved using $k = 10$ folds. The other two modeling approaches generate the same model for the means as each other but using $k = 5$ folds. A 5-fold LCV score should not be compared using a LCV ratio test to a 10-fold LCV score. However, partially modified GEE generates the same model using $k = 5$, as it does using $k = 10$ folds. The 5-fold LCV score for

Table 6.1 Adaptive models of mean dental measurements in child age for alternate modeling approaches, correlation structures, and numbers of folds assuming constant variances

		5 folds			10 folds			15 folds		
Modeling approach	Correlation	Powers of age[a]	LCV score	Clock time (min)	Powers of age[a]	LCV score	Clock time (min)	Powers of age[a]	LCV score	Clock time (min)
Partially modified GEE	IND	0.29	0.09010	0.1	0.3	0.09172	0.2	0.3	0.08921	0.3
	AR1	0, 2	0.11545	1.5	0.3	0.11778	2.9	0.3	0.11636	4.0
	EC	0.31	0.11952	0.8	0.31	0.12014	1.2	0.31	0.11864	1.5
	UN	0.6.1	0.10592	2.3	0, 5	0.10582	3.4	0, 5	0.10509	4.4
Fully modified GEE	IND	0.29	0.09010	0.1	0.3	0.09172	0.2	0.3	0.08921	0.3
	AR1	0.29	0.10311	0.8	0.29	0.10414	1.1	0.28	0.10289	2.1
	EC	0.2	0.11880	0.3	0.2	0.11875	0.6	0.31	0.11864	0.5
	UN	0.32	0.10649	1.4	0.33	0.11041	2.6	0.33	0.10872	3.6
LMM	IND	0.29	0.09010	0.02	0.3	0.09172	0.03	0.3	0.08921	0.03
	AR1	0.3	0.10552	0.1	0.2	0.10487	0.6	0.2	0.10395	0.7
	EC	0, 2	0.11880	0.1	0, 2	0.11875	0.2	0.31	0.11864	0.2
	UN	0.39	0.07800	0.7	0.399	0.08829	1.1	0.4	0.08807	1.4

AR1 spatial autoregressive order 1, *EC* exchangeable correlations, *GEE* generalized estimating equations, *IND* independent, *LCV* likelihood cross-validation, *LMM* linear mixed modeling, *UN* unstructured

[a]A power of 0 corresponds to an intercept parameter; otherwise, the model has a zero intercept

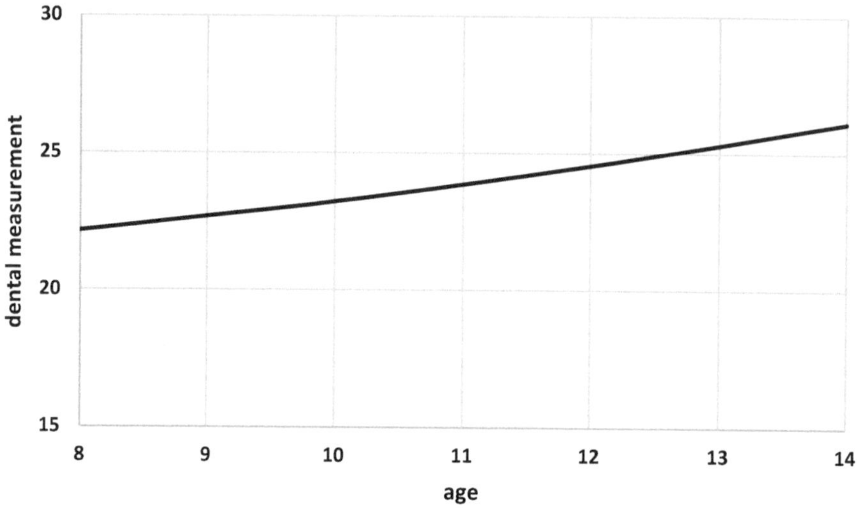

Fig. 6.1 Estimated means for dental measurements for children as they age from 8 to 14 years old assuming constant variances

the partially modified GEE model computed using ELMM is 0.11952. The model generated by fully modified GEE and ELMM has 5-fold LCV score 0.11880 with non-distinct percent decrease (PD) of 0.60% (i.e., less than or equal to the cutoff 1.76% for a distinct PD in the LCV score). Consequently, all three modeling approaches generate competitive models.

Table 6.1 also contains clock times for generated models. Clock times for partially modified GEE range from 0.1 to 4.4 min with a total over all 12 cases of about 0.4 h, for fully modified GEE from 0.3 to 3.6 min for a total of about 0.2 h, and for LMM from 0.02 to 1.4 min for a total of about 0.1 h (totals not reported in Table 6.1). Note that clock times are rounded to 1 decimal digit, but sums are based on unrounded values and so may not be the same as the sum of the rounded values. Consequently, LMM requires less time, with partially modified GEE requiring about 4.0 times as much and fully modified GEE requiring about 2.0 times as much.

Subsequent models use $k = 5$ folds and EC correlations since those choices generate the best LCV score for LMM in Table 6.1 and LMM generates the same model as fully modified GEE and a competitive model to the one generated by partially modified GEE. LMM also requires less time. The adaptive model generated by LMM has means based on age^2 with an intercept, estimated constant standard deviation 2.5 mm, and estimated exchangeable correlation 0.68. Estimated mean dental measurements are plotted in Fig. 6.1 and increase from 22.1 mm at age 8 to 26.1 mm at age 14.

6.2 Assessing Linearity of Means in Child Age

Using LMM with constant variances, $k = 5$ folds, and EC correlations identified as an appropriate choice in Sect. 6.1, the linear polynomial model in child age has LCV = 0.11840 with non-distinct PD of 0.34% compared to the adaptive model in child age with LCV score 0.11880. Consequently, mean dental measurements are reasonably treated as linear in child age when the variances are treated as constant.

6.3 Comparison to Standard GEE Modeling

When dispersions are treated as constant, the only difference between partially modified GEE and standard GEE is how the constant dispersion parameter is estimated. Partially modified GEE uses a bias-unadjusted estimate (Sect. 3.5), while standard GEE uses a bias-adjusted estimate (Sect. 2.4). Standard GEE is thus a possible alternative to partially modified GEE for modeling means with constant dispersions. For the dental measurement data, the adaptively generated standard GEE model for the means assuming unit dispersions (to reduce the computations; see Sect. 3.5) is based on $\text{age}^{0.31}$ without an intercept and with LCV score 0.11974. In contrast, the associated partially modified GEE model has the same model for the means and LCV score 0.11952 with non-distinct PD 0.18%, indicating that in this case standard GEE modeling and partially modified GEE generate competitive models. However, standard GEE requires 1.2 min of clock time, compared to 0.8 min for the partially modified GEE model, or about 1.5 times as much. On the other hand, the model for the means generated by standard GEE modeling run using LMM and constant dispersions has LCV score 0.11952 and the associated LMM model has LCV score of 0.11880 (Table 7.1) with non-distinct PD 0.60%, and so these are competitive models. However, the standard GEE model requires about 12.0 times more clock time than the 0.1 min for LMM.

6.4 Modeling Means and Variances in Child Age

Adaptive analyses of dental measurements are presented in this section using $k = 5$ folds and the EC correlation structure as determined in Sect. 6.1. Adaptive models for means and non-constant variances in child age are generated to assess the usual assumption of constant variances. Table 6.2 provides results for adaptive models for means and variances in child age compared to adaptive models for means with constant variances (from Table 6.1). The three modeling approaches partially modified GEE, fully modified GEE, and LMM are considered.

For each of the three modeling approaches, models for the means are the same or very close with constant and with non-constant variances. Also, models generated

Table 6.2 Adaptive models of dental measurements for means and variances in child age compared to adaptive models for means in child age with constant variances[a]

Modeling approach	Modeling means and variances: Transforms for means[b]	Transforms for variances[b]	LCV score	Clock time (min)	Modeling means with constant variances: Transforms for means[b]	LCV score	Clock time (min)
Partially modified GEE	$age^{0.32}$	1	0.11951	6.6	$age^{0.31}$	0.11952	0.8
Fully modified GEE	$1, age_2^b$	1	0.11880	2.8	$1, age_2^b$	0.11880	0.3
LMM	$1, age_2^b$	$age^{0.1}$	0.11881	0.4	$1, age_2^b$	0.11880	0.1

GEE generalized estimating equations, *LCV* likelihood cross-validation, *LMM* linear mixed modeling

[a]Computed with exchangeable correlations and 5 folds

[b]A value of 1 corresponds to an intercept parameter; otherwise, the model has a zero intercept

assuming constant variances have only slightly different LCV scores than models allowing for non-constant variances, differing in the fifth decimal digit. Consequently, the common assumption of constant variances is reasonable for modeling the dependence of dental measurements on child age.

The model generated by partially modified GEE has LCV score 0.11937 when computed using LMM so that the model generated by LMM generates a non-distinct PD 0.47% (not reported in Table 6.2). The model generated by fully modified GEE has LCV score 0.11880 when computed using LMM and a non-distinct PD 0.01% compared to the model generated by LMM. Consequently, using LMM, the models generated by the three modeling approaches are competitive alternatives.

Table 6.2 also contains clock times for generated models for means and variances in child age. Partially and fully modified GEE require longer clock times of 6.6 and 2.8 min, respectively, compared to 0.4 min, so about 13.2 and 7.0 times longer. As would be expected, computation times are shorter when variances are treated as constant.

6.5 Adaptive Additive Models in Child Age and Child Gender

Table 6.3 contains results for adaptive additive models for mean dental measurements in terms of child age and the indicator for the child being male with constant variances based on partially modified GEE, fully modified GEE, and LMM. The indicator for being male is included in all three of these models for the means. PDs for LCV score of associated models in child age from Table 6.2 using EC

Table 6.3 Adaptive additive models of mean dental measurements in child age and child gender[a]

	Modeling means and variances				Modeling means with constant variances		
Modeling approach	Transforms for means[b]	Transforms for variances[b]	LCV score	Clock time (min)	Transforms for means[b]	LCV score	Clock time (min)
Partially modified GEE	$\text{age}^{0.334}$, male	1	0.12257	12.9	$\text{age}^{0.33}$, male	0.12257	1.2
Fully modified GEE	1, $\text{age}^{1.3}$	male, $\text{age}^{0.6}$	0.12775	7.7	1, age_2^{b}, male	0.12216	0.5
LMM	$\text{age}^{0.27}$	1, male	0.12577	0.7	1, age_2^{b}, male	0.12216	0.1

GEE generalized estimating equations, *LCV* likelihood cross-validation, *LMM* linear mixed modeling
[a]Computed with exchangeable correlations and 5 folds
[b]A value of 1 corresponds to an intercept parameter; otherwise, the model has a zero intercept. The variable male is the indicator for being a male child

correlations and $k = 5$ folds and assuming constant variances are, respectively, 2.49%, 2.75%, and 2.75% (not reported in Table 6.3). All three of these PDs are distinct, indicating that mean dental measurements are reasonably considered to change additively with child gender when variances are treated as constant.

The model generated by partially modified GEE has LCV score 0.12257 computed using LMM so that the common model generated by fully modified GEE and LMM has a competitive LCV score 0.12216 with non-distinct PD 0.33% (not reported in Table 6.3). Consequently, using LMM, the models generated by the three modeling procedures are competitive alternatives.

Table 6.3 also contains clock times for generated models for the means assuming constant variances. LMM requires the shortest clock time of 0.1 min for generating the adaptive additive model. On the other hand, partially modified GEE requires 1.2 min or about 12.0 times more than LMM, while fully modified GEE requires 0.5 min or about 5.0 times more than for LMM.

Table 6.3 also contains results for adaptive additive models for both dental measurement means and variances in terms of child age and the indicator for the child being male based on partially modified GEE, fully modified GEE, and LMM. Partially modified GEE generates almost the same model as for constant variances and with the same LCV score. On the other hand, the indicator for the child being male is included in the model for the variances for models generated by fully modified GEE and LMM rather than in the model for the means. The adaptive model for the means and variances in child age and the indicator male generated by fully modified GEE has LCV score 0.12775, while the associated constant variances model has LCV score 0.12216 with distinct PD 4.38%. The adaptive model for the means and variances in child age and the indicator male generated by LMM has LCV score 0.12577, while the associated constant variances model has LCV score 0.12216 with distinct PD 2.87%. Consequently, fully modified GEE and LMM both indicate that child gender has a distinct additive effect on the variances. Moreover, the usual assumption of constant variances leads to the misleading conclusion that child gender has a distinct additive effect on the means when it actually has a distinct additive effect on the variances and not on the means.

The model generated by fully modified GEE has LCV score 0.12729 computed using LMM so that the model generated by LMM has competitive LCV score 0.12577 with non-distinct PD 1.19% (not reported in Table 6.2). The model generated by partially modified GEE has LCV score 0.12257 computed using LMM and distinct PD 2.54%. Consequently, using LMM, models generated by fully modified GEE and LMM are competitive alternatives, while the model generated by partially modified GEE is distinctly inferior.

Table 6.3 also contains clock times for generated models for the means and variances. LMM requires the shortest clock time of 0.7 min for generating the adaptive additive model. On the other hand, partially modified GEE requires 12.9 min or about 18.4 times more than LMM, while fully modified GEE requires 7.7 min or about 11.0 times more than for LMM.

6.6 Adaptive Moderation of the Effect of Child Age by Child Gender

Table 6.4 contains results for an assessment of adaptive moderation of the effect of child age by child gender on means of dental measurements assuming constant variances based on the three modeling approaches partially modified GEE, fully modified GEE, and LMM. Geometric combinations based on child age and the indicator male are generated by each of these three modeling approaches. However, this is not enough to establish moderation. For moderation to hold, these models need to outperform associated adaptive additive models with constant variances of Table 6.3. PDs for these additive models (not reported in Table 6.4) compared to the

Table 6.4 Adaptive moderation models for means of dental measurements in child age, child gender, and geometric combinations with constant variances[a]

Modeling approach	Mean transforms[b]	LCV score	Clock time (min)
Partially modified GEE	$\mathrm{age}^{0.21}$, $\mathrm{age}_2^{b}\cdot\mathrm{male}$	0.12985	31.3
Fully modified GEE	$\mathrm{age}^{0.21}$, $(\mathrm{age}_2^{b}\cdot\mathrm{male})^{0.903}$	0.12975	5.3
LMM	1, age^2, $\mathrm{age}^2\cdot\mathrm{male}$	0.12863	0.7

GEE generalized linear modeling, *LCV* likelihood cross-validation, *LMM* linear mixed modeling
[a]Computed with exchangeable correlations and 5 folds
[b]A value of 1 corresponds to an intercept; otherwise, the model has a zero intercept. The variable male is the indicator for being a male child

Table 6.5 Adaptive moderation models for means and variances of dental measurements in child age, child gender, and geometric combinations[a]

Modeling approach	Mean transforms[b]	Variance transforms[b]	LCV score	Clock time (min)
Partially modified GEE	$age^{0.21}$, $(age^2 \cdot male)^{1.003}$	1	0.12981	109.5
Fully modified GEE	$age^{0.23}$, $(age^2 \cdot male)^{1.003}$	1, male	0.13576	44.1
LMM	$age^{0.23}$, $age^2 \cdot male$	1, male	0.13570	4.7

GEE generalized linear modeling, *LCV* likelihood cross-validation, *LMM* linear mixed modeling
[a]Computed with exchangeable correlations and 5 folds
[b]A value of 1 corresponds to an intercept; otherwise, the model has a zero intercept. The variable male is the indicator for being a male child

moderation models of Table 6.4 are distinct at 5.61%, 5.85%, and 5.03% for partially modified GEE, fully modified GEE, and LMM, respectively. Consequently, moderation is established using all three modeling approaches assuming constant variances.

The partially modified GEE model computed with LMM has LCV score of 0.12971. The model generated using LMM has LCV score of 0.12863 with non-distinct PD of 0.83%. The fully modified GEE model computed with LMM has LCV score of 0.12975, while the model generated using LMM has LCV score of 0.12863 with non-distinct PD of 0.86%. Consequently, all three modeling approaches generate competitive moderation models assuming constant variances.

Table 6.4 also contains clock times for generated models. LMM requires 0.7 min compared to 31.3 min or about 44.7 times more for partially modified GEE and 5.3 min or about 7.6 times more for fully modified GEE.

Table 6.5 contains results for an assessment of adaptive moderation of the effect of child age by child gender on means and variances of dental measurements based on three modeling approaches partially modified GEE, fully modified GEE, and LMM. Geometric combinations based on child age and the indicator male are generated for the means by each of these three modeling approaches but not for the variances. However, this is not enough to establish moderation. For moderation to hold, these models need to outperform associated adaptive additive models for means and variances of Table 6.3. PDs for these additive models compared to the moderation models of Table 6.4 are distinct at 5.58%, 5.90%, and 7.32% for partially modified GEE, fully modified GEE, and LMM, respectively (not reported in Table 6.5). Consequently, moderation is established for all three modeling approaches allowing for non-constant variances.

Partially modified GEE generates a constant variances model, while fully modified GEE and LMM generate almost the same model for the means and the same non-constant model for the variances. The partially modified GEE model computed with LMM has LCV score of 0.12971 with distinct PD of 4.41% compared to the LMM model. The fully modified GEE model computed with LMM has LCV score of 0.13570, which is the same as the LCV score for the LMM model. Moreover, the

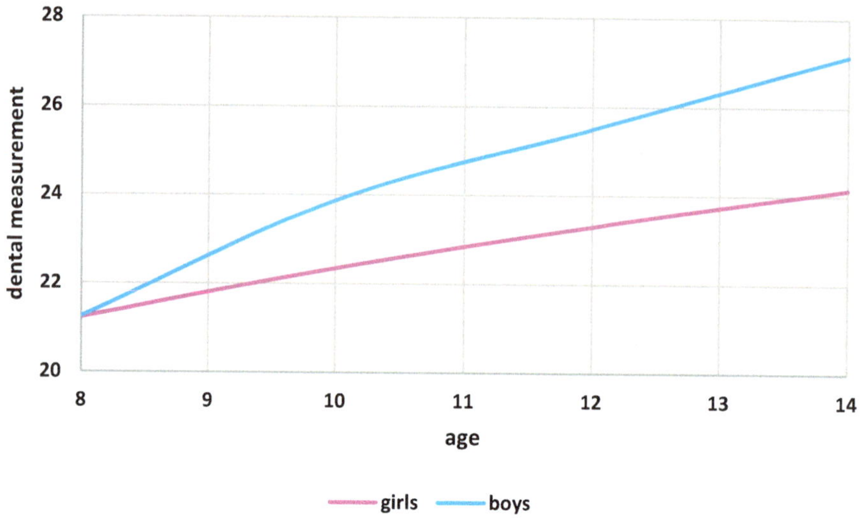

Fig. 6.2 Estimated means for dental measurements for girls and for boys as they age from 8 to 14 years old

non-constant variances moderation models for fully modified GEE and for LMM outperform associated constant variances moderation models of Table 6.4 with distinct PDs of 4.43% and 5.21%, respectively (not reported in Table 6.5). Consequently, partially modified GEE generates a distinctly inferior model suggesting variances are constant when allowing for moderation models for the means and variances in the child age and child gender, while fully modified GEE and LMM generate competitive models to each other that outperform the partially modified GEE model and indicate that not only does child gender moderate the impact of child age on mean dental measurements but it also has an additive effect on the variances.

Table 6.5 also contains clock times for generated models. LMM requires 4.7 min compared to 109.5 min or about 23.3 times more for partially modified GEE and 44.1 min or about 9.4 times more for fully modified GEE.

The LMM model of Table 6.5 is a competitive alternative to the fully modified GEE model of Table 6.5 and requires less time, and so is a reasonable choice to use to describe the dental measurement data. The estimated standard deviation for girls is 1.7 mm and increases to 2.9 mm for boys. Figure 6.2 displays mean dental measurements over child age and child gender. Mean dental measurements increase as children age from a common value of 22.2 mm at age 8 for boys and girls but to a higher level by age 14 for boys of 27.1 mm than the level for girls at age 14 of 24.2 mm. Figure 6.3 displays standardized residuals for dental measurements by child age and child gender. There are two outlying measurements. A mild outlier with standardized residual −2.78 is generated for a girl (subject ID 10) with dental measurement 16.5 mm at age 8. This is the smallest dental measurement for girls at age 8; the other girls have dental measurements at age 8 ranging from 20.0 to

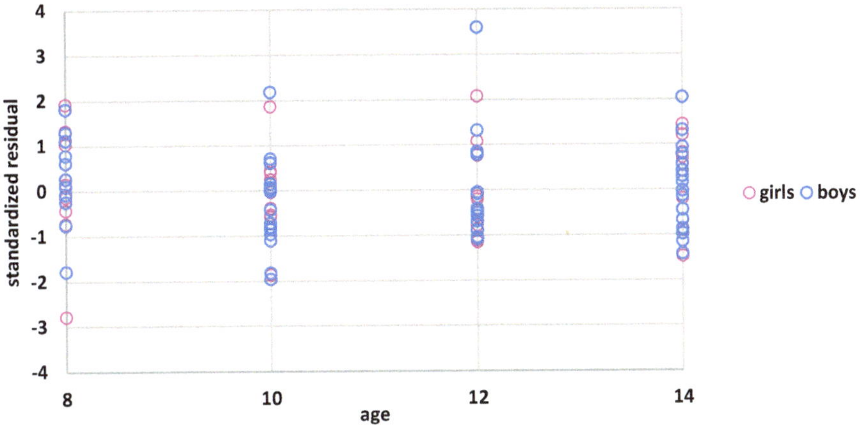

Fig. 6.3 Standardized residuals for dental measurements for girls and for boys as they age from 8 to 14 years old

24.5 mm. The second outlier with standardized residual 3.60 is generated for a boy (subject ID 20) with dental measurement 31.0 mm at age 12. This is the largest dental measurement for boys at age 12; the other boys have dental measurements at age 12 ranging from 22.5 to 29.0 mm. Also, this boy's dental measurements vary from 23.0 mm at age 8 to 20.5 mm at age 10, 31.0 mm at age 12, and 26.0 mm at age 14, and so these dental measurements are highly variable as the boy aged.

6.7 Comparison to Standard Linear Moderation

The standard linear moderation model has means based on an intercept, main effects to untransformed child age and child gender, and the interaction between untransformed child age and child gender along with constant variances. This model computed using LMM has LCV score 0.12539 with distinct PD 2.52% compared to the adaptive moderation model assuming constant variances of Table 6.4, indicating that in this case moderation is distinctly nonlinear.

The assumption of constant variances for linear moderation can be assessed using LMM by starting with the linear moderation model for the means with constant variances, expanding the model for the variances allowing for main effects to child age and child gender as well as geometric combinations in child age and child gender, and then contracting the model for the variances while holding the model for the means unchanged. The resulting model has variances based on an intercept and a main effect to child gender with LCV score 0.13071. The linear moderation model with constant variances generates a distinct PD of 4.07%, indicating that the assumption of constant variances is not appropriate in this case for a standard moderation assessment for the mean dental measurements. On the other hand, the linear moderation model with non-constant variances generates a distinct PD of 3.68% compared to the adaptive LMM moderation model of Table 6.5, indicating that moderation of the mean dental measurements is distinctly nonlinear even after allowing for non-constant variances.

6.8 Analysis Summary

A summary of the results of analyses of the dental measurement data is provided broken down into six categories of results.

1. Models for Means in Child Age Assuming Constant Variances

The preferable model for the dental measurement data has EC correlations with LCV score based on $k = 5$ folds. Models selected by partially modified GEE, fully modified GEE, and LMM are all competitive alternatives. Estimated mean dental measurements are plotted in Fig. 6.1 and are reasonably treated as linear in child age assuming constant variances. The model generated by standard GEE is a competitive alternative to the model generated by partially modified GEE. LMM requires less time with partially modified GEE requiring about 4.0 times as much and fully modified GEE requiring about 2.0 times as much.

2. Models for Means and Variances in Child Age

Models selected by partially modified GEE, fully modified GEE, and LMM are all competitive alternatives. Variances are reasonably treated as constant in child age. LMM requires less time with partially modified GEE requiring about 13.2 times as much and fully modified GEE requiring about 7.0 times as much.

3. Additive Models in Child Age and Child Gender

Models selected by partially modified GEE, fully modified GEE, and LMM assuming constant variances are all competitive alternatives. Mean dental measurements are reasonably considered to change additively with child gender when variances are treated as constant. LMM requires less time with partially modified GEE requiring about 12.0 times as much and fully modified GEE requiring about 5.0 times as much.

Models selected by fully modified GEE and LMM allowing for non-constant variances are competitive alternatives, while the model generated by partially modified GEE is distinctly inferior. Variances for dental measurements are reasonably considered to change additively with child gender, while means are reasonably considered to change only with child age. The usual assumption of constant variances leads to the misleading conclusion that child gender has a distinct additive effect on the means when it actually has a distinct additive effect on the variances and not the means. LMM requires less time with partially modified GEE requiring about 18.4 times as much and fully modified GEE requiring about 11.0 times as much.

4. Moderation Models in Child Age and Child Gender

Models selected by partially modified GEE, fully modified GEE, and LMM assuming constant variances are all competitive alternatives. The effect of child age on mean dental measurements is reasonably considered to be moderated by child gender when variances are treated as constant. This moderation effect is distinctly nonlinear in child age. LMM requires less time with partially modified GEE requiring about 44.7 times as much and fully modified GEE requiring about 7.6 times as much.

Models selected by fully modified GEE and LMM allowing for non-constant variances are competitive alternatives, while the model generated by partially modified GEE is distinctly inferior. The effect of child age on mean dental measurements is reasonably considered to be moderated by child gender, while variances are reasonably treated as depending on child gender but not child age. This moderation effect is distinctly nonlinear in child age. LMM requires less time with partially modified GEE requiring about 23.3 times as much and fully modified GEE requiring about 9.4 times as much.

5. All Models for Dental Measurements in Child Age and Child Gender

In all cases, fully modified GEE and LMM generate competitive models, while partially modified GEE generates competitive models in all but two cases for which its model is distinctly inferior. Over all clock times reported in Tables 6.1, 6.2, 6.3, 6.4 and 6.5, LMM requires about 0.2 h compared to about 3.1 h or about 15.5 times as much for partially modified GEE and about 1.2 h or about 6.0 times as much for fully modified GEE.

6. Selected Model for Dental Measurements in Child Age and Child Gender

Under the most appropriate model for dental measurements, estimated means are plotted in Fig. 6.2. Estimated mean dental measurements are the same for girls and boys at 8 years old and increase with child age at higher levels for boys than for girls over ages 10–14 years with higher constant levels of variability for boys than for girls. The moderation effect on the means is distinctly nonlinear and the estimated variances are distinctly non-constant. Standardized residuals for this model are plotted in Fig. 6.3 with one mild outlier for a measurement for a girl and one distinct outlier for a measurement for a boy.

6.9 Example SAS Code for Analyzing the Dental Measurement Data

Example SAS code is presented in this section for conducting analyses of dental measurements as a function of child age and child gender. The code assumes that a data set called dentdata has been created in the SAS default library containing the dental measurement data (Sect. 2.8.1) in long format, that is, with one measurement (or row) for each dental measurement at each age for each child. This data set contains variables (or columns) called subject loaded with unique identifiers for different children; dentmeas loaded with dental measurements in mm; age loaded with child ages of 8, 10, 12, and 14 years; and the indicator male set to 1 for male children and to 0 for female children. Altogether, there are 4 dental measurements at different ages for each of 27 different children, 16 boys and 11 girls, for a total of 108 measurements.

The code also assumes that a %include statement has been executed to load in the current version of the genreg macro for use in conducting adaptive analyses. The genreg macro supports a wide variety of macro parameters, some of which are described here. The interface for this macro contains the complete list of macro parameters along with their default settings. Default settings are used by the macro if a value for the macro parameter has not been specified in the code invoking the macro. Macro parameter settings are case insensitive. The cutoff for a distinct percent decrease in LCV scores (Sect. 2.6.2) using DF $=$ 1 for these data with 108 measurements is 1.76%.

6.9.1 *Modeling Means in Child Age Assuming Constant Variances*

The following code uses the genreg macro to generate the adaptive constant variances model for dental measurement means as a possibly nonlinear function of child age using $k = 5$ folds, exchangeable correlations (EC), and linear mixed modeling (LMM) as selected in Sect. 6.1 assuming constant variances.

```
%genreg(modtype=norml,datain=dentdata,yvar=dentmeas,
matchvar=subject,withinvr=age,foldcnt=5,corrtype=EC,GEE=n,
srchtype=logL,expand=y,expxvars=age,contract=y);
```

The modtype macro parameter specifies the model type; in this case "modtype=norml" means treat the outcome variable as normally distributed with identity link function, that is, use linear regression (Sect. 2.2.1). The datain macro parameter indicates that the data to be analyzed are contained in the dentmeas data set loaded in the SAS default library. The yvar macro parameter specifies the name of the outcome variable, in this case the variable dentmeas. The matchvar and withinvr macro parameters specify, respectively, the variable containing unique identifiers for different matched sets, in this case the variable subject identifying different children, and the variable containing within matched set values, in this case the variable age. The corrtype macro parameter specifies the correlation structure, in this case the EC structure. The other possible corrtype settings are "corrtype=IND", "corrtype=AR1", and "corrtype=UN" for independent, spatial autoregressive order 1, and unstructured correlations, respectively. To request that the clock time for an invocation of the macro be printed in the output, add the setting "rprttime=y" where the value "y" is short for "yes", while the default setting is "rprttime=n" with "n" short for "no".

The modeling approach used by genreg is determined by the combination of the GEE and srchtype macro parameters. In this case, "GEE=n" means use LMM, while "srchtype=logL" means base estimation on maximizing the log-likelihood (as described in Sects. 4.3 and 5.2). These are the default settings for these two macro parameters. Setting "GEE=y" requests GEE modeling. Combining "GEE=y" with "srchtype=GEE" requests partially modified GEE with estimation based on the minimizing the maximum absolute value of the gradient (as described in Sect. 3.7). Combining "GEE=y" with "srchtype=logL" requests fully modified GEE. By default, partially modified and fully modified GEE use bias-unadjusted dispersion estimates. Bias-adjusted dispersion estimates, as used in standard GEE modeling (Sect. 2.4), are requested by adding the setting "biasadj=y".

Adaptive modeling is requested using "expand=y" together with "contract=y" meaning first expand the base model and then contract the expanded model. In this case, the base model has constant means and constant variances based on only intercept parameters (but this can be changed). The expxvars macro parameter specifies the primary predictor variables for the means to consider in the expansion. In this case, the expansion grows the model for the means by systematically adding in power transforms of the single variable age while holding the variances constant. The maximum number of transforms added by the expansion to the model for the means is controlled by the expxmax parameter with default value "expxmax=5" meaning at most five transforms can be added to the means. Changing to the empty setting "expxmax=" removes the restriction on the number of such transforms.

The contraction systematically removes transforms from the expanded model for the means, possibly the constant transform corresponding to the intercept, and adjusts the powers of the remaining transforms to increase the LCV score, which in this case is computed with 5 folds as specified by the setting of the foldcnt macro parameter. It is also computed using matched-set-wise deletion corresponding to the default setting "measdlte=n". Measurement-wise deletion is requested using "measdlte=y". The contraction can optionally be restricted not to remove the intercept for the means in order to generate a non-zero intercept model. An LCV ratio test is used to decide when to stop the contraction. The contraction also stops when there is only one transform remaining in the model for the means. When the contraction leaves the expanded model unchanged, that expanded model has its powers adjusted to increase the LCV score.

The following code directly generates the above adaptive model selected with $k = 5$ folds, EC correlations, and LMM, including parameter estimates and LCV score.

```
%genreg(modtype=norml,datain=dentdata,yvar=dentmeas,
matchvar=subject,withinvr=age,foldcnt=5,corrtype=EC,GEE=n,
srchtype=logL,xintrcpt=y,xvars=age,xpowers=2);
```

The xintrcpt macro parameter specifies whether or not the base model for the means includes an intercept, the xvars macro parameter provides the list of primary predictors for the base model for the means, and the xpowers macro parameter provides the powers for transforming those primary predictors. In this case, the model for the means includes an intercept along with the transform age^2. The default values for these macro parameters are “xintrcpt=y”, “xvars=”, and “xpowers=” requesting constant means. An empty setting for the xvars macro parameter means include no transforms for the means, and an empty setting for the xpowers macro parameter means power transform xvars variables if any with the power 1 (and so include them untransformed). The model for the variances is based on macro parameters vintrcpt, vvars, and vpowers with analogous meanings and with the same default settings requesting constant variances. The xvalid macro parameter is not set in the above code and so has its default setting “xvalid=y” meaning to compute the LCV score for the requested model. In this case, the model has LCV score 0.11880. Adding the setting “xvalid=n” means compute only parameter estimates for the requested model and not the LCV score.

The above code can be changed to generate the standard linear polynomial model for the means based on untransformed age in two ways. Either change the setting for the xpowers macro parameter to “xpowers=1” or remove the setting for the xpowers macro parameter so that it has its default empty value, which means to use the power 1 to transform all variables listed in the setting of the xvars macro parameter. To request the standard quadratic polynomial model for the means, change the xvars setting to “xvars=age age” and the xpowers setting to “xpowers=1 2”.

6.9.2 Modeling Means and Variances in Child Age

The following code uses the genreg macro to generate the adaptive non-constant variances model for dental measurement means and variances as possibly nonlinear functions of child age using $k = 5$ folds, EC correlations, and LMM.

```
%genreg(modtype=norml,datain=dentdata,yvar=dentmeas,
matchvar=subject,withinvr=age,foldcnt=5,corrtype=EC,GEE=n,
srchtype=logL,expand=y,expxvars=age,expvvars=age,contract=y);
```

As before, adaptive modeling is requested using “expand=y” together with “contract=y”, meaning first expand the base model with constant means and constant variances and then contract the expanded model. The expxvars and expvvars macro parameters specify the primary predictor variables to consider in the expansion for the means and variances, respectively. In this case, the same set of primary predictors is used for the means and for the variances, but different sets of primary predictors can be specified. The expansion grows the model for the means and the variances in combination by systematically adding in power transforms of the single variable age one-at-a-time to either the means or to the variances, whichever generates the better LCV score. Similar to the expxmax parameter, the expvmax parameter specifies the maximum number of transforms added by the expansion to the model for the variances with default value “expvmax=5” meaning at most five transforms can be added to the variances. Changing to the empty setting “expvmax=” removes the restriction on the number of such transforms.

The contraction systematically removes transforms from the expanded model for the means and variances in combination, possibly the constant transforms corresponding to intercepts, and adjusts the powers of the remaining transforms to increase the LCV score. Transforms are removed one-at-a-time from either the means or from the variances, whichever generates the better LCV score after adjusting all the powers of the remaining transforms for both the means and the dispersions. An LCV ratio test is used to decide when to stop the contraction. The contraction stops removing transforms from the means when there is only one transform remaining in the model for the means. Also, by default, the contraction stops removing transforms from the variances when there is only one transform remaining in the model for the variances. Unit variances models can be considered in the contraction by changing the setting of the cnvzero parameter from its default setting of "cnvzero=n" to "cnvzero=y". When the contraction leaves the expanded model unchanged, that expanded model has its powers adjusted to increase the LCV score.

The following code directly generates the above adaptive model selected with $k = 5$ folds, EC correlations, and LMM, including parameter estimates and LCV score.

```
%genreg(modtype=norml,datain=dentdata,yvar=dentmeas,
matchvar=subject,withinvr=age,foldcnt=5,corrtype=EC,GEE=n,
srchtype=logL,xintrcpt=y,xvars=age,xpowers=2,vintrcpt=n,
vvars=age,vpowers=0:1);
```

In this case, the model for the means is the same as generated assuming constant variances, while the model for the variances is based on a zero intercept and the single transform $\text{age}^{0.1}$. The LCV score is 0.11881, while the associated model assuming constant variances has LCV score 0.11880 with non-distinct percent decrease (PD) 0.01%. Consequently, the variances are reasonably treated as constant when the means are modeled in terms of only child age.

6.9.3 Additive Models in Child Age and Child Gender

The following code uses the genreg macro to generate the adaptive additive model for dental measurement means and variances as possibly nonlinear functions of child age and child gender using $k = 5$ folds, EC correlations, and LMM.

```
%genreg(modtype=norml,datain=dentdata,yvar=dentmeas,
matchvar=subject,withinvr=age,foldcnt=5,corrtype=EC,GEE=n,
srchtype=logL,expand=y,expxvars=age male,
expvvars=age male,contract=y);
```

In this case, the expxvars and expvvars macro parameters specify the variables age and male to be the primary predictor variables to consider in the expansion for the means and variances, respectively. The expansion grows the model for the means and the variances in combination by systematically adding in power transforms of age or the indicator variable male one-at-a-time to either the means or to the variances, whichever generates the better LCV score. Note that indicator variables like male are not transformed and are included at most once in the model for the means and at most once in the model for the variances. The contraction then systematically removes transforms from the expanded model for the means and variances in combination, possibly the constant transforms corresponding to intercepts, and adjusts the powers of the remaining transforms to increase the LCV score. The model is additive because by default geometric combinations are not considered in the expansion. An adaptive additive model for the means in age and male assuming constant variances can be generated by changing the expvvars macro parameter to have an empty setting, that is, "expvvars=", or by removing its setting from the above code, because the empty setting is its default setting.

The following code directly generates the adaptive additive model assuming constant variances.

```
%genreg(modtype=norml,datain=dentdata,yvar=dentmeas,
matchvar=subject,withinvr=age,foldcnt=5,corrtype=EC,GEE=n,
srchtype=logL,xintrcpt=y,xvars=age male,xpowers=2 1,vintrcpt=y);
```

In this case, the model for the means is based on an intercept, age^2, and the indicator male. The LCV score is 0.12216, while the associated constant variances model based on only age has LCV score 0.11880 with distinct PD 2.75%. Consequently, child age and child gender are reasonably considered to have additive effects on the means assuming constant variances.

The following code directly generates the adaptive additive model for means and variances.

```
%genreg(modtype=norml,datain=dentdata,yvar=dentmeas,
matchvar=subject,withinvr=age,foldcnt=5,corrtype=EC,GEE=n,
srchtype=logL,xintrcpt=y,xvars=age,xpowers=2,vintrcpt=y,
vvars=male);
```

In this case, the means are based on an intercept and age^2 and the variances are based on an intercept and the indicator male. The LCV score is 0.12577, while the associated constant variances model has LCV score 0.12216 with distinct PD 2.87%. Consequently, the means are reasonably considered to depend only on child age, while the variances are reasonably considered to depend only on child gender when child age and child gender are considered to have additive effects.

6.9.4 Moderation Models in Child Age and Child Gender

The following code uses the genreg macro to generate the adaptive moderation model for dental measurement means and variances as possibly nonlinear functions of child age, child gender, and geometric combinations in child age and child gender using $k = 5$ folds, EC correlations, and LMM.

```
%genreg(modtype=norml,datain=dentdata,yvar=dentmeas,
matchvar=subject,withinvr=age,foldcnt=5,corrtype=EC,GEE=n,
srchtype=logL,expand=y,expxvars=age male,expvvars=age male,
geomcmbn=y,contract=y);
```

In this case, the expxvars and expvvars macro parameters specify the variables age and male to be the primary predictor variables to consider in the expansion for the means and variances, respectively. The expansion grows the model for the means and the variances in combination by systematically adding in power transforms of age, the indicator variable male, or geometric combinations in age and male one-at-a-time to either the means or to the variances, whichever generates the better LCV score. Geometric combinations are considered due to adding the setting "geomcmbn=y" to the code for generating the associated additive model in age and male. The default setting for the geomcmbn macro parameter is "geomcmbn=n" meaning to restrict the expansion to an additive model in the variables specified in the expxvars and expvvars settings. The contraction systematically removes transforms from the expanded model for the means and variances in combination, possibly the constant transforms corresponding to intercepts, and adjusts the powers of the remaining transforms to increase the LCV score. Note that when a geometric combination of the form $(\text{age}^p \cdot \text{male})^q$ or $(\text{male} \cdot \text{age}^p)^q$ is generated by the expansion, the contraction only adjusts the power q and leaves the power p unchanged. When there are more than two primary predictors for the means and/or variances, geometric combinations can be generated based on any number of two or more of those primary predictors. An adaptive moderation model for the means in age, male, and geometric combinations in age and male assuming constant variances can be generated by changing the expvvars macro parameter to have an empty setting, that is, "expvvars=", or by removing its setting from the above code, because the empty setting is its default setting.

The following code directly generates the adaptive moderation model assuming constant variances.

```
%genreg(modtype=norml,datain=dentdata,yvar=dentmeas,
matchvar=subject,withinvr=age,foldcnt=5,corrtype=EC,GEE=n,
srchtype=logL,xintrcpt=y,xvars=age,xpowers=2,xgcs=age 2 male 1,
xgcpowrs=1,vintrcpt=y);
```

In this case, the model for the means is based on an intercept, age^2, and the geometric combination

$$\left(\text{age}^2 \cdot \text{male}\right)^1 = \text{age}^2 \cdot \text{male}.$$

The LCV score is 0.12863, while the associated additive model assuming constant variances has LCV score 0.12216 with distinct PD 5.03%. Consequently, child gender is reasonably considered to moderate the effect of child age on the means assuming constant variances.

The macro parameters xgcs and xgcpowrs are used to specify geometric combinations for the means. The setting "xgcs=age 2 male 1" specifies the untransformed geometric combination age^2. male, while the setting "xgcpowrs=1" means to transform age^2. male to the power 1. The xgcpowrs setting is not needed in this case because its default empty setting "xgcpowrs=" means to leave all the geometric combinations specified by the xgcs macro parameter untransformed. Multiple geometric combinations are specified by separating them by colons (:). For example, use the following code to generate the model with means based on an intercept and the two geometric combinations $(age^2 \cdot male)^{0.1}$ and $(age^{0.5} \cdot male)^{0.5}$ along with constant variances.

```
%genreg(modtype=norml,datain=dentdata,yvar=dentmeas,
matchvar=subject,withinvr=age,foldcnt=5,corrtype=EC,GEE=n,
srchtype=logL,xintrcpt=y,xgcs=age 2 male 1 : age 0.5 male 1,
xgcpowrs=0.1 0.5,vintrcpt=y);
```

The macro parameters vgcs and vgcpowrs are used in the same way to specify geometric combinations for the variances.

The following code directly generates the adaptive moderation model for means and variances.

```
%genreg(modtype=norml,datain=dentdata,yvar=dentmeas,
matchvar=subject,withinvr=age,foldcnt=5,corrtype=EC,GEE=n,
srchtype=logL,xintrcpt=n,xvars=age,xpowers=0.23,
xgcs=age 2 male 1,vintrcpt=y,vvars=male);
```

In this case, the model for the means is based on a zero intercept, $age^{0.23}$, and the geometric combination $age^2 \cdot male$, while the variances are based on an intercept and the indicator male. The LCV score is 0.13570, while the associated moderation model for only the means has LCV score 0.12863 with distinct PD 5.21%. Consequently, child gender is reasonably considered to moderate the effect of child age on the means, while the variances are reasonably considered to change with child gender but not with child age.

The standard linear moderation model has means based on an intercept, age, male, and the interaction age. male with constant variances. This can be generated using LMM with the following code.

```
%genreg(modtype=norml,datain=dentdata,yvar=dentmeas,
matchvar=subject,withinvr=age,foldcnt=5,corrtype=EC,GEE=n,
srchtype=logL,xintrcpt=y,xvars=age male,xgcs=age 1 male 1,
vintrcpt=y);
```

The LCV score is 0.12539 with distinct PD 2.52% compared to the adaptive moderation model assuming constant variances with LCV score 0.12863, indicating that moderation is distinctly nonlinear assuming constant variances.

However, linear moderation of the means may be reasonable allowing for nonconstant variances. This can be assessed using the following code.

```
%genreg(modtype=norml,datain=dentdata,yvar=dentmeas,
matchvar=subject,withinvr=age,foldcnt=5,corrtype=EC,GEE=n,
srchtype=logL,xintrcpt=y,xvars=age male,xgcs=age 1 male 1,
vintrcpt=y,expand=y,expvvars=age male,geomcmbn=y,
contract=y,nocnxbas=y,notrxbas=y);
```

The base model for the means is the standard linear moderation model based on an intercept, age, and the interaction age · male with constant variances. The expansion has no effect on the means because the expxvars macro parameter has its default empty setting "expxvars=". The expansion systematically adds transforms of age, the indicator male, or geometric combinations in age and male, but only to the model for the variances. The contraction removes transforms from the model for the variances but not from the model for the means because of the setting "nocnxbas=y", meaning do not contract the base model for the means. However, the base model for the means might have its powers adjusted. This is avoided by adding in the setting "notrxbas=y", meaning do not transform the base model for the means. Under the default settings "nocnxbas=n" and "notrxbas=n", the contraction would consider removal of terms from the model for the means and possibly nonlinearly transforming the other terms in the model for the means.

The following code directly generates the linear moderation model for means with non-constant variances.

```
%genreg(modtype=norml,datain=dentdata,yvar=dentmeas,
matchvar=subject,withinvr=age,foldcnt=5,corrtype=EC,GEE=n,
srchtype=logL,xintrcpt=y,xvars=age male,xgcs=age 1 male 1,
xgcpowrs=1,vintrcpt=y,vvars=male);
```

The variances are based on an intercept and the indicator male and has LCV score 0.13071. The linear moderation model with constant variances has LCV score 0.12539 with distinct PD 4.07%, indicating that the usual assumption of constant variances for linear moderation is inappropriate for the dental measurements. Furthermore, the nonlinear moderation model for means and variances has LCV score 0.13570 so that the linear moderation model for the means with non-constant variances generates a distinct PD 3.68%, indicating that not only is moderation of the means nonlinear but the variances are also non-constant.

6.9.5 Example Output

As also considered in Sect. 6.9.4, the following code uses the genreg macro to generate the adaptive moderation model for dental measurement means and variances as possibly nonlinear functions of child age, child gender, and geometric combinations in child age and child gender.

Table 6.6 Part of the SAS listing output describing the base model for generation of the adaptive moderation model

```
                    base expectation component

                 predictor      power     estimate

                 XINTRCPT           1    24.023148

                   base log variance component

                 predictor      power     estimate

                 VINTRCPT           1    2.1397307

estimated correlation:                                      0.4198308
mth root of the likelihood using deleted predictions:       0.0869076
```

Table 6.7 Part of the SAS listing output describing the expanded model for the generation of the adaptive moderation model

```
          geometric combination expectation variables:
                    XGC_1     age**(2)*male
                    XGC_2     age**(2)*male
                    XGC_3     male*age**(10)
                    XGC_4     male*age**(9)

         geometric combination log variance variables:
                    VGC_1     age**(10)*male

                   expanded expectation component

        predictor      power     estimate        score    order

        XINTRCPT           1    19.926086    0.0869076        0
        age                2    0.0218181     0.118796        1
        XGC_1              1    10.645037    0.1286256        2
        XGC_2          1.003    -10.49183    0.1345347        6
        XGC_3              1    -1.72E-10    0.1339358        7
        XGC_4              1    2.6947E-9    0.1316497        8

                  expanded log variance component

        predictor      power     estimate        score    order

        VINTRCPT           1    0.9567318    0.0869076        0
        male               1    1.2536665    0.1339893        3
        VGC_1              1    -2.09E-12    0.1342822        4
        age               10    1.023E-12    0.1344942        5

estimated correlation:                                      0.7274581
mth root of the likelihood using deleted predictions:       0.1316497
```

```
%genreg(modtype=norml,datain=dentdata,yvar=dentmeas,
matchvar=subject,withinvr=age,foldcnt=5,corrtype=EC,GEE=n,
srchtype=logL,expand=y,expxvars=age male,expvvars=age male,
geomcmbn=y,contract=y);
```

The output generated by this code starts with descriptions of settings controlling what kind of model has been generated including the cutoff for a distinct percent decrease in LCV scores followed by a description of the base model. Table 6.6 contains SAS listing output describing the base model. The means (i.e., the expectation component) are based only on an intercept parameter XINTRCPT with estimated value 24.02, while the variances (i.e., the log variance component) are also based only on an intercept parameter VINTRCPT with estimated value 2.14. The estimated correlation is 0.42 and the LCV score rounds to 0.08691 (called the "mth root of the likelihood using deleted predictions" in the output).

The output then describes the parameters controlling the expansion followed by the expanded model as described in Table 6.7. The output uses the SAS double asterisk power operator (**). The base model (order 0) has LCV score 0.08691. First, the transform age^2 (order 1) is added to the means generating LCV score 0.11880, then the geometric combination

$$\text{XGC\_1}^1 = \text{age}^2 \cdot \text{male (order 2)}$$

is added to the means generating LCV score 0.12863. Next, three terms are added to the variances: male (order 3),

$$\text{VGC\_1}^1 = \text{age}^{10} \cdot \text{male (order 4)},$$

and age^{10} (order 5) with LCV scores 0.13399, 0.13428, and 0.13449. Finally, three geometric combinations are added to the means:

$$\text{XGC\_2}^{1.003} = \left(\text{age}^2 \cdot \text{male}\right)^{1.003} = \text{age}^{2.006} \cdot \text{male (order 6)}$$

$$\text{XGC\_3}^1 = \text{male} \cdot \text{age}^{2.006} \text{ (order 7)}$$

and

$$\text{XGC\_4}^1 = \text{male} \cdot \text{age}^9 \text{ (order 8)}$$

with LCV scores 0.13453, 0.13394, and 0.13165, which is the LCV score for the expanded model. Each transform is added to the model without adjusting the powers for previously added transforms. The LCV score is allowed to decrease, and so expanded models usually require contraction. However, in cases where the contraction leaves the expanded model unchanged, a conditional transformation step is executed to adjust the powers of the expanded model to improve its LCV score. The estimated correlation is 0.73.

The output then describes the parameters controlling the contraction followed by the contracted model as described in Table 6.8. The expanded model (order 0) has LCV score 0.13165. First, the geometric combination XGC_4^1 (order 1) is removed from the means generating the LCV score 0.13416, followed by removal from the means of XGC_3^1 (order 2) with LCV score 0.13476 and of the intercept XINTRCPT (order 3) with LCV score 0.13682. Next, age^{10} (order 4) is removed from the variances generating LCV score 0.13660 followed by VGC_1^1 (order 5) with LCV score 0.13648. Finally, $\text{XGC\_2}^{1.003}$ (order 6) is removed from the means

Table 6.8 Part of the SAS listing output describing the contracted model for the generation of the adaptive moderation model

```
                contracted expectation component

            predictor old power new power     estimate

            age                 2      0.23   13.158476
            XGC_1               1         1   0.0152611

            discarded    old power          score order

                                .  0.1316497      0
            XGC_4               1  0.1341643      1
            XGC_3               1  0.1347578      2
            XINTRCPT            1  0.1368165      3
            XGC_2           1.003  0.1357043      6

              contracted log variance component

            predictor old power new power     estimate

            VINTRCPT           1          1   1.0605443
            male               1          1   1.0854864

            discarded    old power          score order

                                .  0.1316497      0
            age                10  0.1365954      4
            VGC_1               1  0.1364847      5

estimated correlation:                                      0.7240222
mth root of the likelihood using deleted predictions:       0.1357043
```

generating the LCV score 0.13570, which is the LCV score for the contracted model. With the removal of each transform from the model, the powers for the other transforms are adjusted to improve the LCV score. Only changes in powers from the expanded model to the contracted model are presented in the contraction output. In this case, the power for age in the means changes from 2 to 0.23, while the other powers are unchanged. Details on how the powers change at each step of the contraction are not provided in the contraction output, but are available in the SAS log output if that is of interest. Note that the LCV score increases with the removal of the first three transforms and then decreases with the removal of the next three transforms. In this way, a parsimonious model is generated by the contraction. The contraction stopped because the removal of the next transform would have generated a model with a distinct PD in the LCV score using an LCV ratio test. The estimated correlation is 0.72.

Reference

Potthoff, R. F., & Roy, S. N. (1964). A generalized multivariate analysis of variance model useful especially for growth curve problems. *Biometrika, 51*, 313–326.

Chapter 7
Example Analyses of the Epilepsy Seizure Rate Data

Abstract Adaptive analyses are presented in this chapter of epilepsy seizure rates per week over a baseline and four subsequent clinic visits using Poisson regression with the natural log link function. The choice of the number of folds is addressed as well as the choice of the correlation structure. Results are compared for partially modified generalized estimating equations (GEE), fully modified GEE, and extended linear mixed modeling (ELMM). Linearity of the log of the means in visit with constant dispersions, a comparison to standard GEE modeling, and the dependence of means and dispersions on visit are addressed. Adaptive additive and adaptive moderation models are generated for visit and the indicator for being in the intervention group. An assessment of linear additive and moderation effects for the means with constant dispersions is provided as well as of direct variance modeling of seizure rates. A summary of the analysis results is also provided. SAS code for generating these analyses is described along with output generated by that code.

Keywords Direct variance modeling · Extended linear mixed modeling · Generalized estimating equations · Poisson regression · Moderation · Non-constant dispersions

Introduction Adaptive analyses are presented in this chapter of the epilepsy seizure rate data of Sect. 2.8.2 (Thall & Vail, 1990). All likelihood cross-validation (LCV) scores are computed using matched-set-wise deletion since there are no missing measurements. The cutoff using DF $= 1$ for a distinct percent decrease in LCV scores for these data is 0.65%. Section 7.1 addresses choosing the number k of folds as described in Sect. 2.6.1 and choosing the correlation structure from among those described in Sect. 2.3. Results are compared for partially modified GEE, fully modified GEE, and ELMM. Section 7.2 addresses linearity of the log of the means in visit with constant dispersions, Sect. 7.3 provides a comparison to standard GEE modeling, while Sect. 7.4 addresses the dependence of means and dispersions on

---

Supplementary Information The online version contains supplementary material available at https://doi.org/10.1007/978-3-031-41988-1_7.

G. J. Knafl, *Modeling Correlated Outcomes Using Extensions of Generalized Estimating Equations and Linear Mixed Modeling*,
https://doi.org/10.1007/978-3-031-41988-1_7

visit. Adaptive additive and adaptive moderation models are generated for visit and the indicator for being in the intervention group in Sects. 7.5 and 7.6, respectively. Section 7.7 provides an assessment of linear additive and moderation effects for the means with constant dispersions, while Sect. 7.8 addresses direct variance modeling of seizure rates. Section 7.9 provides a summary of the analysis results described in prior sections, while Sect. 7.10 provides example SAS code for generating such analyses and descriptions of output generated by that code.

The primary purpose of Chap. 7 is to compare adaptive modeling results for partially modified GEE, fully modified GEE, and ELMM applied to count/rate correlated outcomes using Poisson regression models. Partially modified GEE (see Chap. 3 for details) extends standard GEE (see Chap. 2 for details) by adding extra estimating equations for dispersion parameters to the standard GEE estimating equations for mean parameters. Fully modified GEE (see Chap. 4 for details) extends standard GEE further by providing alternative estimating equations for mean parameters while utilizing the same estimating equations for the dispersions used by partially modified GEE. These new estimating equations are based on minimizing an extended likelihood function, treated as a likelihood function for brevity in what follows. Both partially modified and fully modified GEE use the standard GEE method of estimating correlation parameters using residuals. ELMM (see Chap. 5 for more details) is based on estimating equations for mean, dispersion, and correlation parameters determined by maximizing the likelihood. The estimating equations for the means and dispersions are the same as for fully modified GEE.

7.1 Choosing the Number of Folds and the Correlation Structure

Poisson regression analyses reported in this section assume constant dispersions. The effects of the number k of folds and of the correlation structure on estimation by partially modified GEE, fully modified GEE, and ELMM are assessed.

Table 7.1 contains results for adaptive models for mean seizure rates with constant dispersions generated for 36 cases corresponding to each of the 3 modeling approaches partially modified GEE, fully modified GEE, and ELMM; each of the 4 correlation structures IND, spatial AR1, EC, and UN; and each of the 3 numbers k of folds 5, 10, and 15. Note that equivalent results would be generated for non-spatial AR1 correlations as for spatial AR1 correlations since outcome measurements are equally spaced over visits. The best LCV score of 0.022845 for the 12 partially modified GEE models is achieved at $k = 15$ under EC correlations. The best LCV score of 0.023187 for the 12 fully modified GEE models is achieved at $k = 5$ under EC correlations. The best LCV score of 0.023204 for the 12 ELMM models is achieved at $k = 5$ under EC correlations. Consequently, all three modeling approaches select EC as the most appropriate of the four correlation structures for the dental measurement data.

Table 7.1 Adaptive models of mean seizure rates in visit with constant dispersions for alternate modeling approaches, correlation structures, and numbers of folds assuming constant dispersions

		5 folds			10 folds			15 folds		
Modeling approach	Correlation	Powers of visit[a]	LCV score	Clock time (min)	Powers of visit[a]	LCV score	Clock time (min)	Powers of visit[a]	LCV score	Clock time (min)
Partially modified GEE	IND	−0.41	0.013574	1.3	−0.39	0.013641	2.6	−0.4	0.013172	3.4
	AR1	−1.3	0.019790	8.5	8, 0.079	0.022748	25.7	0.003	0.021712	41.9
	EC	−0.596	0.021711	11.0	−1.274, 18	0.022599	15.6	−1.285, 18	0.022845	25.7
	UN	−0.2798	0.018859	6.0	−0.992	0.019306	13.4	−0.233	0.018919	16.6
Fully modified GEE	IND	−0.4	0.013579	1.7	−0.4	0.013496	3.2	−0.4	0.013055	5.1
	AR1	0.08, 4.9	0.020655	9.7	4.96, 0.19	0.020189	21.4	0.12, 6.01	0.019948	30.5
	EC	−0.02, 12.3	0.023187	4.4	0.03, 14.1	0.022543	10.1	0.01, 14	0.022332	15.8
	UN	0, 8.9, −0.1101	0.022514	80.3	7, −0.07	0.022004	134.5	7, −0.088	0.021920	231.3
ELMM	IND	−0.4	0.013579	0.1	−0.4	0.013496	0.2	−0.4	0.013055	0.3
	AR1	0.06, 7	0.020638	0.9	0.13, 6	0.020210	1.6	0.1, 8	0.019944	2.6
	EC	−0.04, 19	0.023204	0.6	0.02, 17	0.022556	1.2	0.02, 19	0.022346	1.8
	UN	18, −0.169	0.018710	5.5	−0.09, 20	0.020388	9.4	−0.11, 20	0.019964	13.3

AR1 spatial autoregressive order 1, *EC* exchangeable correlations, *ELMM* extended linear mixed modeling, *GEE* generalized estimating equations, *IND* independent, *LCV* likelihood cross-validation, *UN* unstructured

[a]A power of 0 corresponds to an intercept parameter; otherwise, the model has a zero intercept

The best overall score for ELMM of Table 7.1 of 0.023204 is achieved using $k = 5$ folds. The best LCV score for fully modified GEE is also achieved using $k = 5$ folds. The 5-fold LCV score for this fully modified GEE model using ELMM is 0.023189 with non-distinct percent decrease (PD) of 0.06% (i.e., less than or equal to the cutoff 0.65% for a distinct PD in the LCV score) compared to the ELMM model, indicating that these are competitive models. The best LCV score for partially modified GEE is achieved using $k = 15$ folds. The 5-fold LCV score for this partially modified GEE model using ELMM is 0.020540 with distinct PD of 11.48% compared to the ELMM model, indicating that this partially modified GEE model is distinctly inferior.

Table 7.1 also contains clock times for generated models. Clock times for partially modified GEE range from 1.3 to 41.9 min with a total over all 12 cases of about 2.9 h, for fully modified GEE from 1.7 to 231.3 min for a total of about 9.1 h, and for ELMM from 0.1 to 13.3 min for a total of about 0.6 h (totals not reported in Table 7.1). Note that clock times are rounded to one decimal digit, but sums are based on unrounded values and so may not be the same as the sum of the rounded values. Consequently, ELMM requires less computation time, with partially modified GEE taking about 4.8 times as much and fully modified GEE about 15.7 times as much.

Subsequent models use $k = 5$ folds and EC correlations since those choices generate the best LCV score for ELMM in Table 7.1 and ELMM generates a competitive model in less time. The associated adaptive model has means based on $\text{visit}^{-0.04}$ and visit^{19} without an intercept, estimated constant dispersions 23.4, and estimated exchangeable correlation 0.81.

Figure 7.1 provides the plot of estimated mean seizure counts over visits 0–4, which decrease from visit 0 to visit 1, stay relatively constant from visit 1 to visit

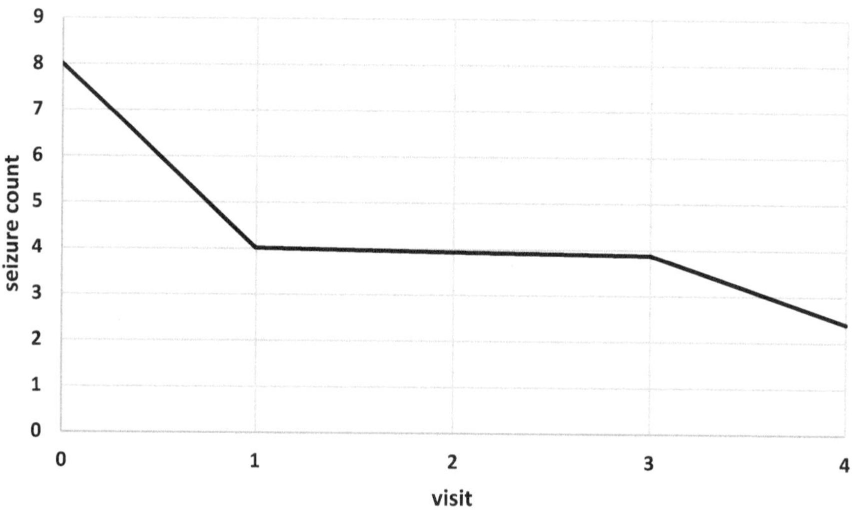

Fig. 7.1 Mean seizure counts over visits 0–4 under the ELMM model in visit with constant dispersions

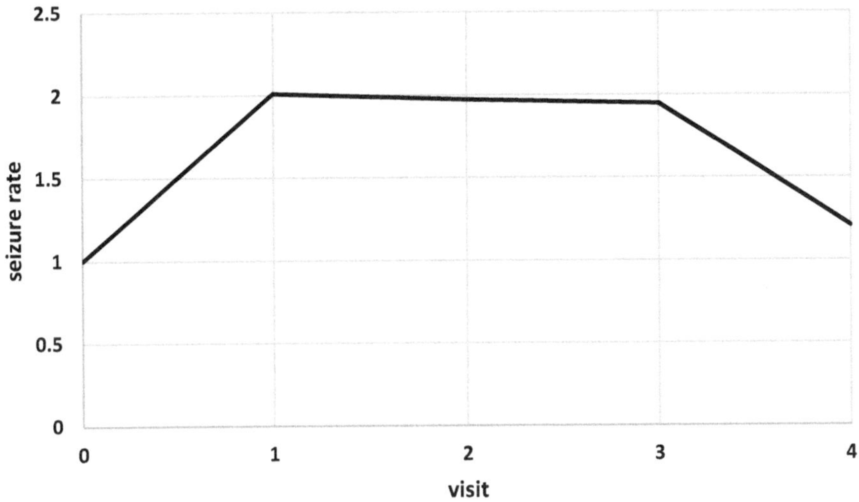

Fig. 7.2 Mean seizure rates per week over visits 0–4 under the ELMM model in visit with constant dispersions

3, and then decrease more to visit 4. Figure 7.2 provides the plot of estimated mean seizure rates per week over visits 0–4, which increase from visit 0 to visit 1, stay relatively constant over visits 2 and 3, and then decrease at visit 4.

7.2 Assessing Linearity of the Log of the Means in Visit

Using ELMM with constant dispersions, $k = 5$ folds, and EC correlations identified as an appropriate choice in Sect. 7.1, the linear polynomial model in visit has LCV = 0.020532 with distinct PD of 11.52% compared to the adaptive model in visit with LCV score 0.023204. Consequently, the log of the mean seizure rates is distinctly nonlinear in visit when the dispersions are treated as constant.

7.3 Comparison to Standard GEE Modeling

When dispersions are treated as constant, the only difference between partially modified GEE and standard GEE is how the constant dispersion parameter is estimated. Partially modified GEE uses a bias-unadjusted estimate (Sect. 3.5), while standard GEE uses a bias-adjusted estimate (Sect. 2.4). Standard GEE is thus a possible alternative to partially modified GEE for modeling means with constant dispersions. For the epilepsy seizure rate data, the adaptively generated standard GEE model for the means assuming unit dispersions (to reduce the computations; see Sect. 3.5) is based on $\text{visit}^{-0.2}$ and visit^{18} without an intercept and LCV score 0.022858. In contrast, the associated partially modified GEE model has LCV score 0.021711 with distinct PD 5.02%, indicating that in this case standard GEE modeling outperforms partially modified GEE. Moreover, it requires 2.8 min of clock time compared to 11.0 or about 3.9 times as much minutes for the partially modified GEE model. On the other hand, the model for the means generated by standard GEE modeling run using ELMM and constant dispersions has LCV score 0.023084 with non-distinct PD 0.52% compared to the LCV score of 0.023204 for the associated ELMM model (Table 7.1), and so these are competitive models. However, the standard GEE model requires about 3.1 times more than the 0.9 min required by ELMM.

It is important to note that what is called standard GEE modeling above is based on offset variables for both the means and the dispersions. As usually implemented, standard GEE modeling supports the use of an offset variable for only the means and not for the dispersions. Consequently, the above results are technically not for standard GEE modeling, but are more appropriate to compare to results for partially modified GEE, which are based on offset variables for both the means and the dispersions.

7.4 Modeling Means and Dispersions in Visit

Adaptive analyses of seizure rates are presented in this section using $k = 5$ folds and the EC correlation structure as determined in Sect. 7.1. Adaptive models for means and non-constant dispersions in visit are generated to assess the common assumption of constant dispersions. Table 7.2 provides results for adaptive models for means and dispersions in visit compared to adaptive models for means with constant dispersions. The three modeling approaches partially modified GEE, fully modified GEE, and ELMM are considered.

Table 7.2 contains a comparison of models generated by the three modeling approaches allowing for non-constant dispersions. The LCV score for the model generated by ELMM of the means and dispersions is 0.024437. The model generated by fully modified GEE computed using ELMM has LCV score 0.024413 with non-distinct PD of 0.10% (not reported in Table 7.2). The model generated by partially modified GEE computed using ELMM has LCV score 0.024400 with non-distinct PD of 0.15%. Consequently, all three modeling approaches generate competitive models.

Table 7.2 contains a comparison of models allowing for non-constant dispersions and models assuming constant dispersions (from Table 7.1). For partially modified GEE, fully modified GEE, and ELMM, models generated assuming constant dispersions have LCV scores with distinct PDs of 9.80%, 5.00%, and 5.05%, respectively (not reported in Table 7.2), compared to LCV scores for associated models allowing for non-constant dispersions. Consequently, the common assumption of

Table 7.2 Adaptive models of seizure rates for means and dispersions in visit compared to adaptive models for means in visit with constant dispersions[a]

	Modeling means and dispersions				Modeling means with constant dispersions		
Modeling approach	Transforms of visit for means[b]	Transforms of visit for dispersions[b]	LCV score	Clock time (min)	Transforms of visit for means[b]	LCV score	Clock time (min)
Partially modified GEE	1, $visit^{19.1}$	1, $visit^{-0.07}$	0.024071	25.1	$visit^{-0.596}$	0.021711	11.0
Fully modified GEE	1	1, $visit^{0.07}$ $visit^{7}$	0.024408	23.8	$visit^{-0.02}$, $visit^{12.3}$	0.023187	4.4
ELMM	1, $visit^{19}$	1, $visit^{-0.01}$	0.024437	4.0	$visit^{-0.04}$, $visit^{19}$	0.023204	0.9

ELMM extended linear mixed modeling, *GEE* generalized linear modeling, *LCV* likelihood cross-validation
[a]Computed with exchangeable correlations and 5 folds
[b]A value of 1 corresponds to an intercept parameter; otherwise, the model has a zero intercept

constant dispersions is inappropriate for modeling the dependence of seizure rates on visit.

Table 7.2 also contains clock times for generated models allowing for non-constant dispersions. ELMM requires 4.0 min. Partially and fully modified GEE require longer clock times than ELMM of 25.1 and 23.8 min, so about 6.3 and 6.0 times longer, respectively. Not surprisingly, clock times for constant dispersions models are shorter.

7.5 Additive Models in Visit and Being in the Intervention Group

Table 7.3 contains results for adaptive additive models for mean seizure rates in terms of visit and the indicator int for being in the intervention group with constant dispersions based on partially modified GEE, fully modified GEE, and ELMM. The indicator for being in the intervention group is included in none of these three models for the means. All three of these models are the same as the associated models of Table 7.2 for the means in only visit assuming constant dispersions. These results indicate that mean seizure rates are reasonably considered not to depend additively on being in the intervention group when dispersions are treated as constant. The three constant dispersions models of Table 7.3 are demonstrated to be competitive alternatives to each other in Sect. 7.4.

Table 7.3 also contains results for adaptive additive models for both seizure rate means and dispersions in terms of visit and the indicator int for being in the intervention group based on partially modified GEE, fully modified GEE, and ELMM. The indicator for being in the intervention group is included in none of these three models for the means and dispersions. All three of these models are the same as the associated models of Table 7.2 for the means and dispersions in only visit. These results indicate that seizure rate means and dispersions are reasonably considered not to depend additively on being in the intervention group. The three non-constant dispersions models of Table 7.3 are demonstrated in Sect. 7.4 to be competitive alternatives to each other and to distinctly outperform the constant dispersions models of Table 7.3.

Table 7.3 also contains clock times for generated models. For constant dispersions models, ELMM generates the shortest clock time of 0.7 min, while partially modified GEE requires 11.2 min or about 16.0 times longer and fully modified GEE requires 4.7 min or about 6.7 times longer. For non-constant dispersions models, ELMM generates the shortest clock time of 3.6 min, while partially modified GEE requires 26.3 min or about 7.3 times longer and fully modified GEE requires 23.8 min or about 6.6 times longer.

Table 7.3 Adaptive additive models of seizure rates in visit and the indicator for being in the intervention group[a]

	Modeling means and dispersions				Modeling means with constant dispersions		
Modeling approach	Transforms for means[b]	Transforms for dispersions[b]	LCV score	Clock time (min)	Transforms for means[b]	LCV score	Clock time (min)
Partially modified GEE	1, $visit^{19.1}$	1, $visit^{-0.07}$	0.024071	26.3	$visit^{-0.596}$	0.021711	11.2
Fully modified GEE	1	1, $visit^{0.07}$, $visit^{7}$	0.024408	23.8	$visit^{-0.02}$, $visit^{12.3}$	0.023187	4.7
ELMM	1, $visit^{19}$	1, $visit^{-0.01}$	0.024437	3.6	$visit^{-0.04}$, $visit^{19}$	0.023204	0.7

ELMM extended linear mixed modeling, *GEE* generalized estimating equations, *LCV* likelihood cross-validation

[a]Computed with exchangeable correlations and 5 folds

[b]A value of 1 corresponds to an intercept parameter; otherwise, the model has a zero intercept

7.6 Adaptive Moderation of the Effect of Visit by Being in the Intervention Group

Table 7.4 contains results for an assessment of adaptive moderation of the effect of visit on seizure rate means assuming constant dispersions based on the three modeling approaches partially modified GEE, fully modified GEE, and ELMM. Neither main effects to the indicator int nor geometric combinations based on visit and the indicator int are generated for the means by each of the three modeling approaches, indicating that being in the intervention group is reasonably considered not to affect mean seizure rates assuming constant dispersions.

Table 7.4 also contains clock times for generated models with constant dispersions. ELMM generated the shortest clock time of 1.5 min, while partially modified GEE requires 20.8 min or about 13.9 times longer and fully modified GEE requires 6.2 min or about 10.8 times longer.

Table 7.5 contains results for an assessment of adaptive moderation of the effect of visit on seizure rate means and dispersions by being in the intervention group based on the three modeling approaches partially modified GEE, fully modified GEE, and ELMM. The non-constant dispersions models of Table 7.5 outperform

Table 7.4 Adaptive moderation models for means of seizure rates in visit, being in the intervention group, and geometric combinations with constant dispersions[a]

Modeling approach	Mean transforms[b]	LCV Score	Clock time (min)
Partially modified GEE	1, $\mathrm{visit}^{-0.2}$, visit^{18}	0.021900	20.8
Fully modified GEE	$\mathrm{visit}^{-0.02}$, $\mathrm{visit}^{12.3}$	0.023187	6.2
ELMM	$\mathrm{visit}^{-0.02}$, visit^{19}	0.023203	1.5

ELMM extended linear mixed modeling, *GEE* generalized linear modeling, *LCV* likelihood cross-validation

[a]Computed with exchangeable correlations and 5 folds

[b]A value of 1 corresponds to an intercept; otherwise, the model has a zero intercept. Int is the indicator for being in the intervention group

Table 7.5 Adaptive moderation models for means and dispersions of seizure rates in visit, being in the intervention group, and geometric combinations[a]

Modeling approach	Mean transforms[b]	Dispersion transforms[b]	LCV Score	Clock time (min)
Partially modified GEE	$(\mathrm{int}\cdot\mathrm{visit}^{2.8})^{0.611}$, $(\mathrm{int}\cdot\mathrm{visit}^{14})_2^{b}$	1, $\mathrm{visit}^{-0.0987}$	0.025086	123.5
Fully modified GEE	1	1, $\mathrm{visit}^{0.07}$, visit^{7}	0.024408	28.2
ELMM	1, visit^{19}	1, $\mathrm{visit}^{-0.01}$	0.024437	4.7

ELMM extended linear mixed modeling, *GEE* generalized linear modeling, *LCV* likelihood cross-validation

[a]Computed with exchangeable correlations and 5 folds

[b]A value of 1 corresponds to an intercept; otherwise, the model has a zero intercept. The variable int is the indicator for being in the intervention group

associated constant dispersions models of Table 7.4 with distinct PDs of 12.70%, 5.00%, and 5.05% (not reported in Table 7.5) for partially modified GEE, fully modified GEE, and ELMM, respectively. These results indicate that, as before, dispersions for seizure rates are non-constant.

Geometric combinations based on visit and the indicator int are generated by the partially modified GEE model of Table 7.5. However, this is not enough to establish moderation, which requires that this model outperforms the associated adaptive additive model with constant dispersions of Table 7.3. The LCV score of 0.024071 for this additive model given in Table 7.3 has distinct PD of 4.05% compared to the partially modified GEE moderation model of Table 7.5 (not reported in Table 7.5). Consequently, moderation is established for partially modified GEE. On the other hand, the adaptive moderation models of Table 7.5 for fully modified GEE and for ELMM are the same as the associated additive models of Table 7.3 and do not depend on the indicator int, supporting the opposite conclusion that moderation of the means does not hold.

The fully modified GEE model computed using ELMM has LCV score 0.024427 with non-distinct PD 0.04% compared to the ELMM model. On the other hand, the partially modified GEE model computed using ELMM has LCV score 0.022647 with distinct PD 7.32% compared to the ELMM model. Consequently, the fully modified GEE and ELMM models are competitive alternatives, while the partially modified GEE model is distinctly inferior. Hence, means and dispersions for seizure rates are reasonably considered not to depend on main effects to the indicator for being in the intervention group or on geometric combinations in visit and that indicator.

Table 7.5 also contains clock times for generated models with non-constant dispersions. ELMM generated the shortest clock time of 4.7 min, while partially modified GEE requires 123.5 min or about 2.1 h and 26.3 times longer and fully modified GEE requires 28.2 min or about 0.5 h and about 6.0 times longer.

The ELMM model of Table 7.5 for the means and dispersions of seizure rates is the same as associated models in Tables 7.3 and 7.4 and has means based on an intercept and visit^{19}, dispersions based on an intercept and $\text{visit}^{-0.01}$, and estimated exchangeable correlation 0.79. Estimated means for this model are plotted in Fig. 7.3 and are relatively constant over visits 0–3 and then decrease to visit 4. Note that these estimated means allowing for non-constant dispersions are larger than those for the model of Fig. 7.2 assuming constant dispersions. Estimated extended standard deviations for this model are plotted in Fig. 7.4 and increase from visit 0 to visit 1, are relatively constant over visits 1–3, and then decrease to visit 4. Note that these estimated standard deviations allowing for non-constant dispersions have a similar pattern to those for the model for the means of Fig. 7.2 assuming constant dispersions.

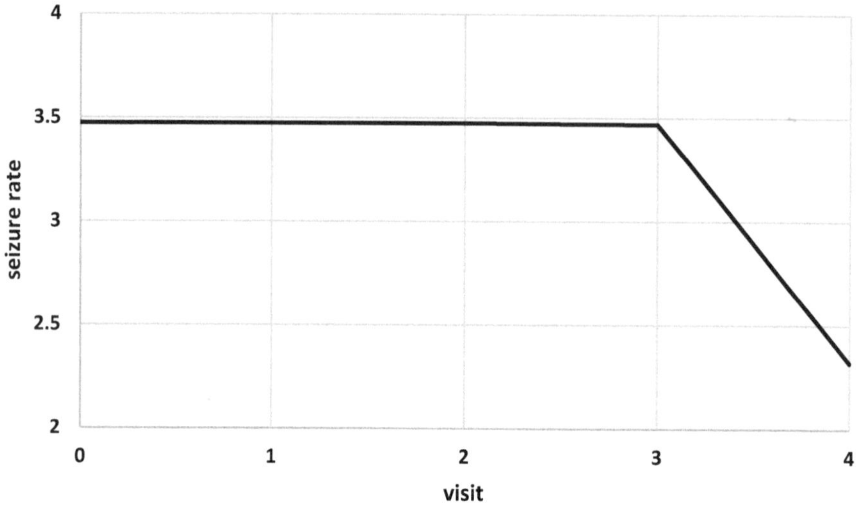

Fig. 7.3 Estimated means for seizure rates per week over visits

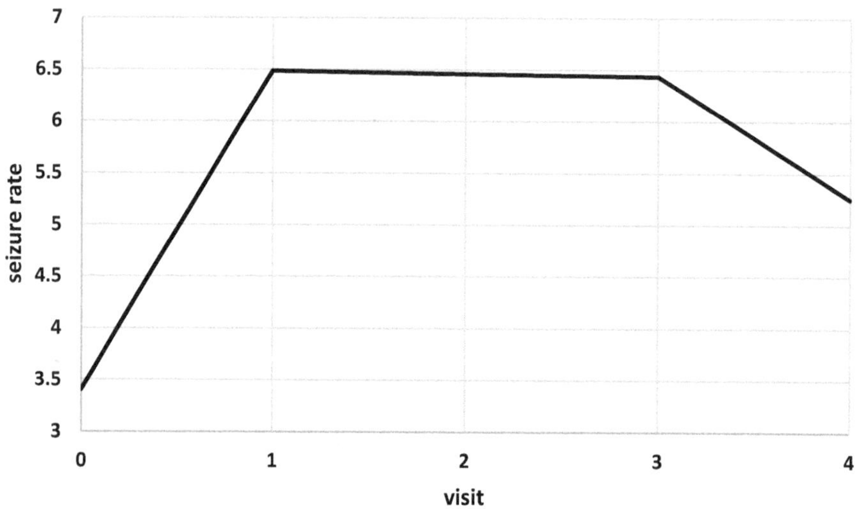

Fig. 7.4 Estimated extended standard deviations for seizure rates per week over visits

7.7 Comparison of Linear Additive and Moderation Models with Constant Dispersions

The standard linear moderation model has the log of the means based on an intercept, main effects to untransformed visit and int, and the interaction between untransformed visit and int along with constant dispersions. This model computed using ELMM has LCV score 0.021575. The associated additive model in untransformed visit and int has larger LCV score 0.021771, indicating that linear moderation does not hold. The associated model linear in only untransformed visit has LCV score 0.020532 (as reported in Sect. 7.2) and distinct PD 5.69%, indicating that there is a distinct additive effect to being in the intervention group assuming linearity in the log of the means and constant dispersions. However, the linear additive model generates a distinct PD 6.18% compared to the LCV score 0.023204 for the adaptive additive model in untransformed visit and int with constant dispersions (reported in Sect. 7.5). Consequently, the log of the means is distinctly nonlinear in visit. Moreover, this adaptive model does not include an additive effect to being in the intervention group.

7.8 Direct Variance Modeling of Epilepsy Seizure Rates

Direct variance modeling treats the variance function as $V(\mu) = 1$ so that the extended variances are the same as the dispersions. Using ELMM, the adaptive model for the means and dispersions of seizure rates in visit using direct variance modeling has constant means based on only an intercept along with dispersions, and so also variances, based on an intercept, $\text{visit}^{0.06}$, and visit^{9}. The direct variance adaptive additive model in visit and the indicator int is this same model as is also the direct variance adaptive moderation model allowing for both main effects and geometric combinations in visit and int. This direct variance model has LCV score 0.024414 with non-distinct PD 0.09% compared to the associated extended variance model of Table 7.5 with LCV score, indicating that these are competitive models. The direct variance model is based on four parameters, one for the means and three for the dispersions, the same number as for the extended variance model with two for the means and two for the dispersions. However, the direct variance model indicates that mean seizure rates are constant over visits 0–5 rather than decreasing from visit 3 to visit 4 as in Fig. 7.3.

Under direct variance modeling, clock times are 2.3 min to generate the adaptive model for the means and dispersions of seizure rates in visit, 2.5 min to generate the associated adaptive additive model in visit and the indicator int, and 5.5 min to generate the associated adaptive moderation model allowing for both main effects and geometric combinations in visit and int for a total of 10.3 min. Associated models based on extended variances depending on means are 4.0 min to generate the adaptive model for the means and dispersions of seizure rates in visit of Table 7.2, 3.6 min to generate the associated adaptive additive model in visit and the indicator int of Table 7.3, and 4.7 min to generate the associated adaptive model allowing for both main effects and geometric combinations in visit and int of Table 7.5 for a total of 12.3 min or about 1.2 times more than using direct variance modeling. The first two models are generated in less time using direct variance modeling, the last in more time, and all three models together in less time. These results indicate that direct variance modeling in this case sometimes requires less time, sometimes more

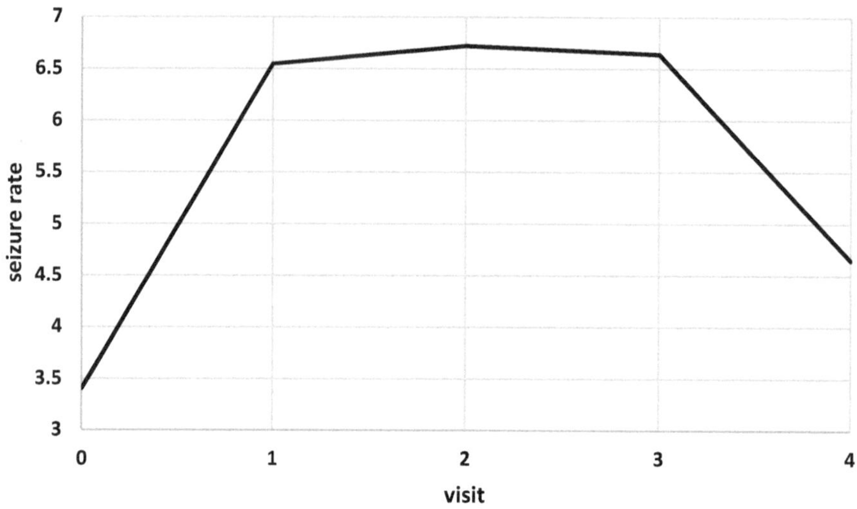

Fig. 7.5 Estimated standard deviations for seizure rates per week over visits based only on dispersions

time, but it requires less time overall, and so time to compute models is not a limitation.

Since the direct variance model has constant means, the associated extended variance model with the same dispersion transforms and constant means is equivalent because it adjusts the variances by a constant value (i.e., the estimated mean). Under these equivalent constant means models, the mean seizure rates per week have the constant value 3.6 at all visits or about the same value as for the means of Fig. 7.3 at visits 0–3. The estimated exchangeable correlation is 0.80, about the same as for the model generating Fig. 7.3. Figure 7.5 provides the plot for estimated standard deviations for seizure rates. The plot is similar to the one of Fig. 7.4. Estimated standard deviations start at about the same point at visit 0 as for Fig. 7.4, increase to a higher level at visit 1, increase a little from visit 1 to visit 3 to a little more than the value as in Fig. 7.4, and then decrease to a lower level than in Fig. 7.4 by visit 4.

Figure 7.6 displays the plot of standardized residuals by visit for the direct variance model. The standardized residuals are highly skewed in the positive direction for each visit. There are seven measurements with standardized residuals larger than 3.00. The patient with ID 18 has standardized residual 3.06 at visit 0 corresponding to an observed seizure rate 13.875, the second largest observed seizure rate at visit 0. The patient with ID 25 has standardized residual 5.24 at visit 3 corresponding to an observed seizure rate 38.0, the largest observed seizure rate at visit 3. The patient with ID 49 has standardized residuals 4.55, 7.07, 4.31, 4.93, and 6.00 at visits 0–4 corresponding to observed seizure rates 18.875, 51, 32.5, 36, and 31.5, the largest observed seizure rates at visits 0–2 and 4 and the second largest observed seizure rate at visit 3.

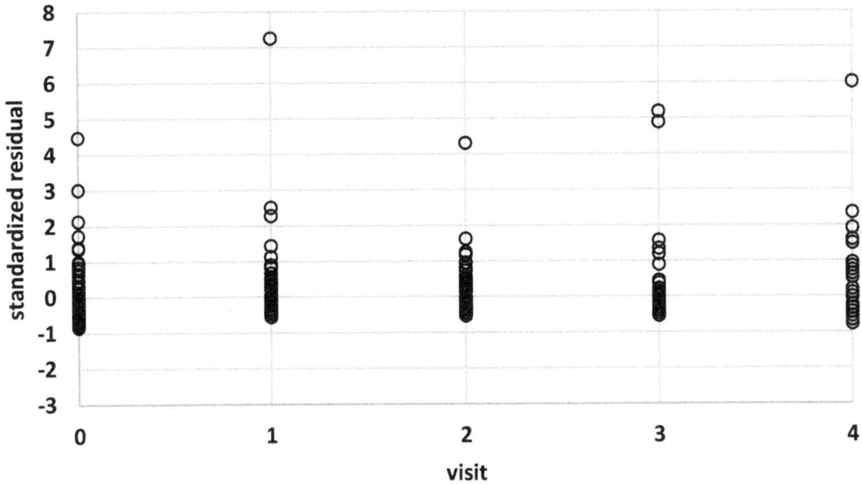

Fig. 7.6 Standardized residuals for seizure rates over visits based only on dispersions

7.9 Analysis Summary

A summary of the results of analyses of the epilepsy seizure rate data is provided broken down into seven categories of results.

1. Models for Means in Visit Assuming Constant Dispersions

The preferable model for the epilepsy seizure rate data has EC correlations with LCV score based on $k = 5$ folds. Models selected by fully modified GEE and ELMM are competitive alternatives, but distinctly outperform the model selected by partially modified GEE. Estimated mean seizure counts are plotted in Fig. 7.1 and estimated mean seizure rates in Fig. 7.2. The log of the mean seizure rates is distinctly nonlinear in visit assuming constant dispersions. The model generated by standard GEE distinctly outperforms the model generated by partially modified GEE, but is competitive with the ELMM model. ELMM requires less time with partially modified GEE requiring about 4.8 times as much and fully modified GEE requiring about 15.7 times as much.

2. Models for Means and Dispersions in Visit

Models selected by partially modified GEE, fully modified GEE, and ELMM are all competitive alternatives. Dispersions are distinctly non-constant in visit. ELMM requires less time with partially modified GEE requiring about 6.3 times as much and fully modified GEE requiring about 6.0 times as much.

3. Additive Models in Visit and Being in the Intervention Group

Models selected by partially modified GEE, fully modified GEE, and ELMM assuming constant dispersions are all the same as non-additive models for the means in visit assuming constant dispersions. Mean seizure rates are reasonably considered not to change additively with being in the intervention group when dispersions are treated as constant. ELMM requires less time with partially modified GEE requiring about 16.0 times as much and fully modified GEE requiring about 6.7 times as much.

Models selected by partially modified GEE, fully modified GEE, and ELMM allowing for non-constant dispersions are both the same as non-additive models for the means in visit allowing for non-constant dispersions. Dispersions for seizure rates are reasonably considered not to change additively with being in the intervention group and means are also reasonably considered not to change additively with being in the intervention group. ELMM requires less time with partially modified GEE requiring about 7.3 times as much and fully modified GEE requiring about 6.6 times as much.

4. Moderation Models in Visit and Being in the Intervention Group

Models selected by partially modified GEE, fully modified GEE, and ELMM assuming constant dispersions are all competitive alternatives. The effect of visit on mean seizure rates is reasonably considered not to be moderated by being in the intervention group when dispersions are treated as constant. ELMM requires less time with partially modified GEE requiring about 13.9 times as much and fully modified GEE requiring about 10.8 times as much.

Models selected by fully modified GEE and ELMM allowing for non-constant dispersions are the same and outperform the model generated by partially modified GEE. The effect of visit on mean seizure rates is reasonably considered not to be moderated by being in the intervention group, while dispersions are reasonably treated as depending on only visit. Estimated means for this model are plotted in Fig. 7.3 and estimated extended standard deviations in Fig. 7.4. A standard linear moderation effect is also not supported. ELMM requires less time with partially modified GEE requiring about 26.3 times as much and fully modified GEE requiring about 6.0 times as much.

5. Direct Variance Models for Seizure Rates

The same direct variance model is generated accounting only for the effect to visit, allowing also for an additive effect to being in the intervention group, and allowing for moderation of the effect of visit by being in the intervention group. Altogether, these models require less time to compute than extended variance models treating variances as a function of the means and dispersions, which require 1.2 times more. This model is a competitive alternative to the extended variance model treating dispersions as a function of the means and dispersions. It has the same number of parameters, but it has constant means, and so is equivalent to the associated extended variance model assuming constant means, and so seems the more appropriate model for the epilepsy seizure rate data.

6. All Models for Seizure Rates in Visit and Being in the Intervention Group

In all cases, fully modified GEE and ELMM generate competitive models, while partially modified GEE generates competitive models in all but two cases for which its model is distinctly inferior. Over all clock times reported in Tables 7.1, 7.2, 7.3, 7.4 and 7.5, ELMM requires about 0.9 h compared to about 6.3 h or about 7.0 times as much for partially modified GEE and about 10.6 h or about 11.8 times as much for fully modified GEE.

7. Selected Model for Seizure Rates in Visit and Being in the Intervention Group

Under the appropriate model for the seizure rates, estimated means are constant and estimated standard deviations are plotted in Fig. 7.5. Standardized residuals for this model are plotted in Fig. 7.6 and are highly skewed in the positive direction with seven outlying measurements.

7.10 Example SAS Code for Analyzing the Epilepsy Seizure Rate Data

Example SAS code is presented in this section for conducting analyses of epilepsy seizure counts/rates as a function of clinic visit and treatment group, that is, either the intervention group taking the antiepileptic drug progabide or the control group taking a placebo. The code assumes that a data set called longseiz has been created in the SAS default library containing the epilepsy seizure rate data (Sect. 2.8.2) in long format, that is, with one measurement (or row) for each seizure count at each clinic visit for each patient. This data set contains variables (or columns) called id loaded with unique identifiers for patients, count loaded with seizure counts, visit loaded with visit indexes of 0–4, the indicator int set to 1 for patients in the intervention group and to 0 for patients in the control group, dltatime loaded with the number of weeks over which counts were collected for each visit (8 weeks prior to clinic visit 0 and 2 weeks between subsequent clinic visits), xoffset loaded with the natural log of dltatime for converting means of counts to means of rates (Sect. 2.2.2), voffset also loaded with the natural log of dltatime for converting dispersions of counts to dispersions of rates for extended variance models (Sect. 3.1), and voffset2 loaded with two times the natural log of dltatime for converting dispersions of counts to dispersions of rates for direct variance models (Sect. 5.7). Altogether, there are 5 seizure counts at different clinic visits for each of 59 patients, 31 in the intervention group and 28 in the control group, for a total of 295 measurements.

The code also assumes that a %include statement has been executed to load in the current version of the genreg macro for use in conducting adaptive analyses. The genreg macro supports a wide variety of macro parameters, some of which are described here. The interface for this macro contains the complete list of macro parameters along with their default settings. Default settings are used by the macro if a value for the macro parameter has not been specified in the code invoking the macro. Macro parameter settings are case insensitive. The cutoff for a distinct percent decrease in LCV scores (Sect. 2.6.2) using DF $= 1$ for these data with 295 measurements is 0.65%.

7.10.1 Modeling Means in Visit Assuming Constant Dispersions

The following code uses the genreg macro to generate the adaptive model for epilepsy seizure rate means as a possibly nonlinear function of visit using $k = 5$ folds, exchangeable correlations (EC), and extended linear mixed modeling (ELMM) as selected in Sect. 7.1 assuming constant dispersions.

```
%genreg(modtype=poiss,datain=longseiz,yvar=count,matchvar=id,
withinvr=visit,foldcnt=5,corrtype=EC,GEE=y,srchtype=logL,
xoffstvr=xoffset,voffstvr=voffset,expand=y,expxvars=visit,
contract=y;
```

The modtype macro parameter specifies the model type; in this case "modtype=poiss" means treat the outcome variable as Poisson distributed with natural log link function, that is, use Poisson regression (Sect. 2.2.2). The datain macro parameter indicates that the data to be analyzed is contained in the longseiz data set loaded in the SAS default library. The yvar macro parameter specifies the name of the outcome variable, in this case the variable count. The matchvar and withinvr macro parameters specify, respectively, the variable containing unique identifiers for different matched sets, in this case the variable id identifying different patients, and the variable containing within matched set values, in this case the variable visit. The corrtype macro parameter specifies the correlation structure, in this case the EC structure. The other possible corrtype settings are "corrtype=IND", "corrtype=AR1", and "corrtype=UN" for independent, spatial autoregressive order 1, and unstructured correlations, respectively. To request that the clock time for an invocation of the macro be printed in the output, add the setting "rprttime=y" where the value "y" is short for "yes", while the default setting is "rprttime=n" with "n" short for "no".

The xoffstvr and voffstvr macro parameters specify the offset variables for adjusting means and dispersions, respectively, for counts to those for rates. Separate macro parameters are provided to allow for different offset variables for the means and the dispersions. The offset variables would usually be the same as in this case. One common example with different offset variables is the case with an offset variable for the means but no offset variable for the dispersions (using the default empty setting "voffstvr=") as used in standard implementations of GEE modeling (e.g., SAS PROC GENMOD).

The modeling approach used by genreg is determined by the combination of the GEE and srchtype macro parameters. In this case, "GEE=n" means use ELMM, while "srchtype=logL" means base estimation on maximizing the log-likelihood (as described in Sects. 4.3 and 5.2). These are the default settings for these two macro parameters. Setting "GEE=y" requests GEE modeling. Combining "GEE=y" with "srchtype=GEE" requests partially modified GEE with estimation based on the minimizing the maximum absolute value of the gradient (as described in Sect. 3.7). Combining "GEE=y" with "srchtype=logL" requests fully modified GEE.

By default, partially modified and fully modified GEE use bias-unadjusted dispersion estimates. Bias-adjusted dispersion estimates, as used in standard GEE modeling (Sect. 2.4), are requested by adding the setting "biasadj=y".

Adaptive modeling is requested using "expand=y" together with "contract=y" meaning first expand the base model and then contract the expanded model. In this case, the base model has constant means and constant dispersions based on only intercept parameters (but this can be changed). The expxvars macro parameter specifies the primary predictor variables for modeling the means to consider in the expansion. In this case, the expansion grows the model for the means by systematically adding in power transforms of the single variable visit while holding the dispersions constant. The maximum number of transforms added by the expansion to the model for the means is controlled by the expxmax parameter with default value "expxmax=5" meaning at most five transforms can be added to the means. Changing to the empty setting "expxmax=" removes the restriction on the number of such transforms.

The contraction systematically removes transforms from the expanded model for the means, possibly the constant transform corresponding to the intercept, and adjusts the powers of the remaining transforms to increase the LCV score, which in this case is computed with 5 folds as specified by the setting of the foldcnt macro parameter. It is also computed using matched-set-wise deletion corresponding to the default setting "measdlte=n". Measurement-wise deletion is requested using "measdlte=y". The contraction can optionally be restricted not to remove the intercept for the means in order to generate a non-zero intercept model. An LCV ratio test is used to decide when to stop the contraction. The contraction also stops when there is only one transform remaining in the model for the means. When the contraction leaves the expanded model unchanged, that expanded model has its powers adjusted to increase the LCV score.

The following code directly generates the above adaptive model selected with $k = 5$ folds, EC correlations, and ELMM, including parameter estimates and LCV score.

```
%genreg(modtype=poiss,datain=longseiz,yvar=count,matchvar=id,
withinvr=visit,foldcnt=5,corrtype=EC,GEE=y,srchtype=logL,
xoffstvr=xoffset,voffstvr=voffset,xintrcpt=n,xvars=visit visit,
xpowers=−0.04 19);
```

The xintrcpt macro parameter specifies whether or not the base model for the means includes an intercept, the xvars macro parameter provides the list of primary predictors for the base model for the means, and the xpowers macro parameter provides the powers for transforming those primary predictors. In this case, the model for the means has a zero intercept along with the two transforms $\text{visit}^{-0.04}$ and visit^{19}. The default values for these macro parameters are "xintrcpt=y", "xvars=", and "xpowers=" requesting constant means. An empty setting for the xvars macro parameter means include no transforms for the means, and an empty setting for the xpowers macro parameter means power transform xvars variables if any with the power 1 (and so include them untransformed). The model for the dispersions is based on macro parameters vintrcpt, vvars, and vpowers with analogous meanings and with the same default settings requesting constant dispersions. The xvalid macro parameter is not set in the above code and so has its default setting "xvalid=y" meaning to compute the LCV score for the requested model. In this case, the model has LCV score 0.023204. Adding the setting "xvalid=n" means compute only parameter estimates for the requested model and not the LCV score.

The above code can be changed to generate the standard linear polynomial model for the means based on untransformed visit as follows. First change the settings for the xintrcpt and xvars macro parameters to "xintrcpt=y" and "xvars=visit". Then change the setting for the xpowers macro parameter to "xpowers=1" or remove the setting for the xpowers macro parameter so that it has its default empty value, which means to use the power 1 to transform all variables listed in the setting of the xvars macro parameter. Note that the log of the means is linear in visit, but the means are nonlinear due to using the natural log link function. To request the standard quadratic polynomial model for the means, use the settings "xintrcpt=y", "xvars=visit visit", and "xpowers=1 2".

7.10.2 Modeling Means and Dispersions in Visit

The following code uses the genreg macro to generate the adaptive non-constant dispersions model for epilepsy seizure rate means and dispersions as possibly nonlinear functions of visit using $k = 5$ folds, EC correlations, and ELMM.

```
%genreg(modtype=poiss,datain=longseiz,yvar=count,matchvar=id,
withinvr=visit,foldcnt=5,corrtype=EC,GEE=n,srchtype=logL,
xoffstvr=xoffset,voffstvr=voffset,expand=y,expxvars=visit,
expvvars=visit,contract=y);
```

As before, adaptive modeling is requested using "expand=y" together with "contract=y" meaning first expand the base model with constant means and constant dispersions and then contract the expanded model. The expxvars and expvvars macro parameters specify the primary predictor variables to consider in the expansion for the means and dispersions, respectively. In this case, the same set of primary predictors is used for the means and for the dispersions, but different sets of primary predictors can be specified. The expansion grows the model for the means and the dispersions in combination by systematically adding in power transforms of the single variable visit one-at-a-time to either the means or to the dispersions, whichever generates the better LCV score. Similar to the expxmax parameter, the expvmax parameter specifies the maximum number of transforms added by the expansion to the model for the dispersions with default value "expvmax=5" meaning at most five transforms can be added to the dispersions. Changing to the empty setting "expvmax=" removes the restriction on the number of such transforms.

The contraction systematically removes transforms from the expanded model for the means and dispersions in combination, possibly the constant transforms corresponding to intercepts, and adjusts the powers of the remaining transforms to increase the LCV score. Transforms are removed one-at-a-time from either the means or from the dispersions, whichever generates the better LCV score after adjusting all the powers of the remaining transforms for both the means and the dispersions. An LCV ratio test is used to decide when to stop the contraction. The contraction stops removing transforms from the means when there is only one transform remaining in the model for the means. Also, by default, the contraction stops removing transforms from the dispersions when there is only one transform remaining in the model for the dispersions. Unit dispersions models can be considered in the contraction by changing the setting of the cnvzero parameter from its default setting of "cnvzero=n" to "cnvzero=y". When the contraction leaves the expanded model unchanged, that expanded model has its powers adjusted to increase the LCV score.

The following code directly generates the above adaptive model selected with $k = 5$ folds, EC correlations, and ELMM, including parameter estimates and LCV score.

```
%genreg(modtype=poiss,datain=longseiz,yvar=count,matchvar=id,
withinvr=visit,foldcnt=5,corrtype=EC,GEE=n,srchtype=logL,
xoffstvr=xoffset,voffstvr=voffset,xintrcpt=y,xvars=visit,xpowers=19,
vintrcpt=y,vvars=visit,vpowers=−0.01);
```

In this case, the model for the means is based on an intercept and the single transform visit^{19}, while the model for the dispersions is based on an intercept and the single transform $\text{visit}^{-0.1}$. The LCV score is 0.024437, while the associated model assuming constant dispersions has LCV score 0.023204 with distinct percent decrease (PD) 5.05%. Consequently, the dispersions are reasonably treated as non-constant in visit when the means are modeled in terms of only visit.

7.10.3 Additive Models in Visit and Being in the Intervention Group

The following code uses the genreg macro to generate the adaptive additive model for epilepsy seizure rate means and dispersions as possibly nonlinear functions of visit and being in the intervention group using $k = 5$ folds, EC correlations, and ELMM.

```
%genreg(modtype=poiss,datain=longseiz,yvar=count,matchvar=id,
withinvr=visit,foldcnt=5,corrtype=EC,GEE=n,srchtype=logL,xoffstvr=xoffset,
voffstvr=voffset,expand=y,expxvars=visit int,expvvars=visit int,
contract=y);
```

In this case, the expxvars and expvvars macro parameters specify the variables visit and int to be the primary predictor variables to consider in the expansion for the means and dispersions, respectively. The expansion grows the model for the means and the dispersions in combination by systematically adding in power transforms of visit or the indicator variable int one-at-a-time to either the means or to the dispersions, whichever generates the better LCV score. Note that indicator variables like int are not transformed and are included at most once in the model for the means and at most once in the model for the dispersions. The contraction then systematically removes transforms from the expanded model for the means and dispersions in combination, possibly the constant transforms corresponding to intercepts, and adjusts the powers of the remaining transforms to increase the LCV score. The model is additive because by default geometric combinations are not considered in the expansion. An adaptive additive model for the means in visit and int assuming constant dispersions can be generated by changing the expvvars macro parameter to have an empty setting, that is, "expvvars=", or by removing its setting from the above code, because the empty setting is its default setting.

The adaptively generated additive model for means assuming constant dispersions is the same as the adaptively generated model in only visit with constant dispersions. The adaptively generated additive model for means and dispersions is the same as the adaptively generated model for means and dispersions in only visit. Consequently, being in the intervention group is reasonably considered not to have an additive effect on the means or on the dispersions.

7.10.4 Moderation Models in Visit and Being in the Intervention Group

The following code uses the genreg macro to generate the adaptive moderation model for epilepsy seizure rate means and dispersions as possibly nonlinear functions of visit, being in the intervention group, and geometric combinations in visit and being in the intervention group using $k = 5$ folds, EC correlations, and ELMM.

```
%genreg(modtype=poiss,datain=longseiz,yvar=count,matchvar=id,
withinvr=visit,foldcnt=5,corrtype=EC,GEE=n,srchtype=logL,
xoffstvr=xoffset,voffstvr=voffset,expand=y,expxvars=visit int,
expvvars=visit int,geomcmbn=y,contract=y);
```

In this case, the expxvars and expvvars macro parameters specify the variables visit and int to be the primary predictor variables to consider in the expansion for the means and dispersions, respectively. The expansion grows the model for the means and the dispersions in combination by systematically adding in power transforms of visit, the indicator variable int, or geometric combinations in visit and int one-at-a-time to either the means or to the dispersions, whichever generates the better LCV score. Geometric combinations are considered due to adding the setting "geomcmbn=y" to the code for generating the associated additive model in visit and int. The default setting for the geomcmbn macro parameter is "geomcmbn=n" meaning to restrict the expansion to an additive model in the variables specified in the expxvars and expvvars settings. The contraction systematically removes transforms from the expanded model for the means and dispersions in combination, possibly the constant transforms corresponding to intercepts, and adjusts the powers of the remaining transforms to increase the LCV score. Note that when a geometric combination of the form $(\text{visit}^p \cdot \text{int})^q$ or $(\text{int} \cdot \text{visit}^p)^q$ is generated by the expansion, the contraction only adjusts the power q and leaves the power p unchanged. When there are more than two primary predictors for the means and/or dispersions, geometric combinations can be generated based on any number of two or more of those primary predictors. An adaptive moderation model for the means in visit, int, and geometric combinations in visit and int assuming constant dispersions can be generated by changing the expvvars macro parameter to have an empty setting, that is, "expvvars=", or by removing its setting from the above code, because the empty setting is its default setting.

The following code directly generates the adaptive moderation model assuming constant dispersions.

```
%genreg(modtype=poiss,datain=longseiz,yvar=count,matchvar=id,
withinvr=visit,foldcnt=5,corrtype=EC,GEE=n,srchtype=logL,
xoffstvr=xoffset,voffstvr=voffset,xintrcpt=n,xvars=visit visit,
xpowers=−0.02 19,vintrcpt=y);
```

In this case, the model for the means is based on a zero intercept and the two transforms $\text{visit}^{-0.02}$ and visit^{19}, but with no geometric combinations. The LCV score is 0.023203, while the associated additive model assuming constant dispersions has almost the same LCV score 0.023204. Consequently, being in the intervention group is reasonably considered not to moderate the effect of visit on the means and not to have an additive effect on the means assuming constant dispersions.

The macro parameters xgcs and xgcpowrs are used to specify geometric combinations for the means although they are not needed here. The setting "xgcs=visit 2 int 1" specifies the untransformed geometric combination $\text{visit}^2 \cdot \text{int}$, while the setting "xgcpowrs=0.5" means to transform $\text{visit}^2 \cdot \text{int}$ to the power 0.5. The xgcpowrs setting is needed in this case because its default empty setting "xgcpowrs=" means to leave all the geometric combinations specified by the xgcs macro parameter untransformed. Multiple geometric combinations are specified by separating them by colons (:). For example, use the following code to generate the model with means based on an intercept and the two geometric combinations $(\text{visit}^2 \cdot \text{int})^{0.1}$ and $(\text{visit}^{0.5} \cdot \text{int})^{0.5}$ along with constant dispersions.

```
%genreg(modtype=poiss,datain=longseiz,yvar=count,matchvar=id,
withinvr=visit,foldcnt=5,corrtype=EC,GEE=n,srchtype=logL,
xoffstvr=xoffset,voffstvr=voffset,xintrcpt=y,
xgcs=visit 2 int 1 :visit 0.5int 1,xgcpowrs=0.1 0.5,vintrcpt=y);
```

The macro parameters vgcs and vgcpowrs are used in the same way to specify geometric combinations for the dispersions.

The adaptive moderation model for means and dispersions is the same as the model for means and dispersions in visit by itself. Consequently, being in the intervention group is reasonably considered not to moderate the effect of visit on the means and on the dispersions as well as not to have an additive effect on the means and dispersions (Sect. 7.10.3).

The standard linear moderation model has means based on an intercept, visit, int, and the interaction visit · int with constant dispersions. This can be generated using ELMM with the following code.

```
%genreg(modtype=poiss,datain=longseiz,yvar=count,matchvar=id,
withinvr=visit,foldcnt=5,corrtype=EC,GEE=n,srchtype=logL,
xoffstvr=xoffset,voffstvr=voffset,xintrcpt=y,xvars=visit int,
xgcs=visit 1 int 1,vintrcpt=y);
```

The LCV score is 0.021575, which is smaller than the LCV score 0.021771 for the standard additive model, indicating that linear moderation is not supported assuming constant dispersions.

7.10.5 Direct Variance Modeling

The dirctvar macro parameter controls whether or not variances are directly modeled. The default setting "dirctvar=n" means use extended variances based on both the dispersions and the variance function, which in this case is $V(\mu) = \mu$. Adding the setting "dirctvar=y" treats the variance function as $V(\mu) = 1$ so that the extended variances are the same as the dispersions. The following code uses the genreg macro to generate the adaptive direct variance ELMM model for epilepsy seizure rate means and dispersions as possibly nonlinear functions of visit.

```
%genreg(modtype=poiss,datain=longseiz,yvar=count,matchvar=id,
withinvr=visit,foldcnt=5,corrtype=EC,GEE=n,srchtype=logL,
xoffstvr=xoffset,voffstvr=voffset2,expand=y,expxvars=visit,
expvvars=visit,contract=y,dirctvar=y);
```

The voffstvr setting is changed to "voffsetvr=voffset2" so that the adjustment of variances for counts to variance for rates using direct variance modeling is equivalent to the associated adjustment using extended variance modeling (see Sect. 5.7).

The following code directly generates the above direct variance model.

```
%genreg(modtype=poiss,datain=longseiz,yvar=count,matchvar=id,
withinvr=visit,foldcnt=5,corrtype=EC,GEE=n,srchtype=logL,
xoffstvr=xoffset,voffstvr=voffset2,xintrcpt=y,vintrcpt=y,
vvars=visit visit,vpowers=0.06 9,dirctvar=y);
```

This model has constant means based on only an intercept along with dispersions, and so also variances, based on an intercept, $\text{visit}^{0.06}$, and visit^{9}. It has LCV score 0.024414 with non-distinct PD compared to the associated extended variance model with LCV score 0.024437. Both models have the same number of parameters, but the direct variance model has constant means. The associated adaptive extended variance model with constant means can be generated using the following code.

```
%genreg(modtype=poiss,datain=longseiz,yvar=count,matchvar=id,
withinvr=visit,foldcnt=5,corrtype=EC,GEE=n,srchtype=logL,
xoffstvr=xoffset,voffstvr=voffset,expand=y,expvvars=visit,
contract=y);
```

The default model for the means is based on an intercept and no transforms and so are constant in visit. The setting "expvvars=visit" means that the model for the dispersions is expanded in transforms of visit but not the model for the means because expxvars has its default empty setting. This model is equivalent to the associated direct variance model assuming constant means.

7.10.6 Example Output

The following code uses the genreg macro to generate the adaptive moderation model for epilepsy seizure rate means and variances as possibly nonlinear functions of visit, being in the intervention group, and geometric combinations in visit and being in the intervention group using direct variance modeling.

```
%genreg(modtype=poiss,datain=longseiz,yvar=count,matchvar=id,
withinvr=visit,foldcnt=5,corrtype=EC,GEE=n,srchtype=logL,
xoffstvr=xoffset,voffstvr=voffset2,expand=y,expxvars=visit int,
expvvars=visit int,geomcmbn=y,contract=y,dirctvar=y);
```

The output generated by this code starts with descriptions of settings controlling what kind of model is generated including the cutoff for a distinct percent decrease in LCV scores followed by a description of the base model. Table 7.6 contains SAS listing output describing the base model. The means (i.e., the log expectation component) are based only on an intercept parameter XINTRCPT with estimated value 1.41, while the dispersions (i.e., the log dispersion component) are also based

Table 7.6 Part of the SAS listing output describing the base model for the generation of the adaptive moderation model using direct variance modeling

```
               base log expectation component

              predictor     power    estimate

              XINTRCPT          1   1.4083999

               base log dispersion component

              predictor     power    estimate

              VINTRCPT          1   3.4849524

estimated correlation:                                   0.7411696
mth root of extended likelihood using deleted predictions:   0.0212652
```

Table 7.7 Part of the SAS listing output describing the expanded model for the generation of the adaptive moderation model using direct variance modeling

```
geometric combination log expectation variables:
              XGC_1     int*visit**(6)

          expanded log expectation component

predictor      power     estimate         score    order

XINTRCPT           1    1.3526202    0.0212652        0
visit           -0.5    0.1180817    0.0241909        3
XGC_1              2    -1.193E-8    0.0240573        4

          expanded log dispersion component

predictor      power     estimate         score    order

VINTRCPT           1    2.4415388    0.0212652        0
visit           -0.1    1.4207977    0.0237761        1
visit              9    -2.307E-6    0.0241997        2

estimated correlation:                                 0.7965699
mth root of extended likelihood using deleted predictions: 0.0240573
```

only on an intercept parameter VINTRCPT with estimated value 3.48. The estimated correlation is 0.74 and the LCV score rounds to 0.021265 (called the "mth root of the extended likelihood using deleted predictions" in the output).

The output then describes the parameters controlling the expansion followed by the expanded model as described in Table 7.7. The output uses the SAS double asterisk power operator (**). The base model (order 0) has LCV score 0.021265. First, the transform $\text{visit}^{-0.1}$ (order 1) is added to the dispersions generating the LCV score 0.023776, and then the transform visit^9 (order 2) is added to the dispersions generating the LCV score 0.024200. Next, the transform $\text{visit}^{-0.5}$ (order 3) is added to the dispersions generating the LCV score 0.024191. Finally, the geometric combination

$$\text{XGC\_1}^2 = \left(\text{int} \cdot \text{visit}^6\right)^2 = \text{int} \cdot \text{visit}^{12} \text{ (order 4)}$$

is added to the means with LCV score 0.024057, which is the LCV score for the expanded model. Each transform is added to the model without adjusting the powers for previously added transforms. The LCV score is allowed to decrease, and so expanded models usually require contraction. However, in cases where the contraction leaves the expanded model unchanged, a conditional transformation step is executed to adjust the powers of the expanded model to improve its LCV score. The estimated correlation is 0.80.

The output then describes the parameters controlling the contraction followed by the contracted model as described in Table 7.8. The expanded model (order 0) has LCV score 0.024057. First, the geometric combination XGC_1^2 (order 1) is removed from the means generating the LCV score 0.024403, followed by removal from the means of the transform $\text{visit}^{-0.5}$ (order 2) with LCV score 0.024414, which is the LCV score for the contracted model. With the removal of each transform from

Table 7.8 Part of the SAS listing output describing the contracted model for the generation of the adaptive moderation model using direct variance modeling

```
    contracted log expectation component

  predictor old power new power    estimate

  XINTRCPT          1         1  1.2859604

 discarded   old power       score   order

                    .   0.0240573       0
 XGC_1              2   0.0244029       1
 visit           -0.5   0.0244139       2

    contracted log dispersion component

  predictor old power new power    estimate

  VINTRCPT          1         1  2.4502106
  visit          -0.1      0.06  1.3063222
  visit             9         9  -3.044E-6

  discarded   old power       score order

                     .   0.0240573     0

estimated correlation:                             0.7956065
mth root of extended likelihood using deleted predictions: 0.0244139
```

the model, the powers for the other transforms are adjusted to improve the LCV score. In this case, only the transform visit$^{-0.1}$ for the dispersions is changed to visit$^{0.06}$. Details on how the powers change at each step of the contraction are not provided in the contraction output, but are available in the SAS log output if that is of interest. In this case, the LCV score increased with the removal of each of the two transforms and never decreased. Decreases are possible in general so that a parsimonious model is generated by the contraction. The contraction stopped because the removal of the next transform would have generated a model with a distinct PD in the LCV score using an LCV ratio test. The estimated correlation is 0.80.

Reference

Thall, P. F., & Vail, S. C. (1990). Some covariance models for longitudinal count data with overdispersion. *Biometrics, 46*, 657–671.

Chapter 8
Example Analyses of the Dichotomous Respiratory Status Data

Abstract Adaptive analyses are presented of dichotomous respiratory status levels over a baseline and four subsequent clinic visits using logistic regression with the logit link function. The choice of the number of folds is addressed as well as the choice of the correlation structure. Results are compared for partially modified generalized estimating equations (GEE), fully modified GEE, and extended linear mixed modeling (ELMM). Linearity of the logits of the means in visit with constant dispersions is addressed as well as whether unit dispersions are appropriate for these data, a comparison to standard GEE, and the dependence of means and dispersions on visit. Adaptive additive and adaptive moderation models are generated for visit and being on active treatment. A comparison to the standard linear moderation model is provided as well as direct variance modeling of dichotomous respiratory status levels. A summary of the analysis results is also provided. SAS code for generating these analyses is described along with output generated by that code.

Keywords Direct variance modeling · Extended linear mixed modeling · Generalized estimating equations · Logistic regression · Moderation · Non-constant dispersions

Introduction Adaptive analyses are presented in this chapter of the dichotomous respiratory status data of Sect. 2.8.3 (Stokes et al., 2012). All likelihood cross-validation (LCV) scores are computed using matched-set-wise deletion since there are no missing measurements. The cutoff using DF = 1 for a distinct percent decrease in LCV scores for these data is 0.35%. Section 8.1 addresses choosing the number k of folds as described in Sect. 2.6.1 and choosing the correlation structure from among those described in Sect. 2.3. Results are compared for partially modified GEE, fully modified GEE, and ELMM. Section 8.2 addresses linearity of the logits of the means in visit with constant dispersions, while Sect. 8.3 addresses whether unit dispersions are appropriate for these data, Sect. 8.4 a comparison to

Supplementary Information The online version contains supplementary material available at https://doi.org/10.1007/978-3-031-41988-1_8.

G. J. Knafl, *Modeling Correlated Outcomes Using Extensions of Generalized Estimating Equations and Linear Mixed Modeling*,
https://doi.org/10.1007/978-3-031-41988-1_8

standard GEE, and Sect. 8.5 the dependence of means and dispersions on visit. Adaptive additive and adaptive moderation models are generated for visit and being on active treatment in Sects. 8.6 and 8.7, respectively. A comparison to the standard linear moderation model is provided in Sect. 8.8. Section 8.9 addresses direct variance modeling of the dichotomous respiratory status data. Section 8.10 provides a summary of the analysis results described in prior sections, while Sect. 8.11 provides example SAS code for generating such analyses and descriptions of output generated by that code.

The primary purpose of Chap. 8 is to compare adaptive modeling results for partially modified GEE, fully modified GEE, and ELMM applied to dichotomous correlated outcomes using logistic regression models. Partially modified GEE (see Chap. 3 for details) extends standard GEE (see Chap. 2 for details) by adding extra estimating equations for dispersion parameters to the standard GEE estimating equations for mean parameters. Fully modified GEE (see Chap. 4 for details) extends standard GEE further by providing alternative estimating equations for mean parameters while utilizing the same estimating equations for the dispersions used by partially modified GEE. These new estimating equations are based on minimizing an extended likelihood function, treated as a likelihood function for brevity in what follows. Both partially modified and fully modified GEE use the standard GEE method of estimating correlation parameters using residuals. ELMM (see Chap. 5 for more details) is based on estimating equations for mean, dispersion, and correlation parameters determined by maximizing the likelihood. The estimating equations for the means and dispersions are the same as for fully modified GEE.

8.1 Choosing the Number of Folds and the Correlation Structure

Logistic regression analyses reported in this section assume constant dispersions. The effects of the number k of folds and of the correlation structure on estimation by partially modified GEE, fully modified GEE, and ELMM are assessed.

Table 8.1 contains results for adaptive models for mean dichotomous respiratory with constant dispersions generated for 36 cases corresponding to each of the 3 modeling approaches partially modified GEE, fully modified GEE, and ELMM; each of the 4 correlation structures IND, spatial AR1, EC, and UN; and each of the 3 numbers k of folds 5, 10, and 15. Note that equivalent results would be generated for non-spatial AR1 correlations as for spatial AR1 correlations since outcome measurements are equally spaced in visit. The best LCV score of 0.56527 for the 12 partially modified GEE models is achieved at $k = 10$ under EC correlations. The best LCV score of 0.56524 for the 12 fully modified GEE models is achieved at $k = 10$ under EC correlations. The best LCV score of 0.56511 for the 12 ELMM models is achieved at $k = 10$ under EC correlations. Consequently, all three modeling approaches select EC as the most appropriate of the four correlation

Table 8.1 Adaptive models of mean dichotomous respiratory status in power transforms of visit assuming constant dispersions for alternate modeling approaches, correlation structures, and numbers of folds

		5 folds			10 folds			15 folds		
Modeling approach	Correlation	Powers of visit[a]	LCV score	Clock time (min)	Powers of visit[a]	LCV score	Clock time (min)	Powers of visit[a]	LCV score	Clock time (min)
Partially modified GEE	IND	−1.2	0.48540	2.4	−1.2	0.48522	4.2	−1.3	0.48486	5.7
	AR1	−0.7	0.55676	30.6	−0.6	0.55568	16.0	−1.3	0.55481	21.0
	EC	−0.1	0.56389	8.6	−0.2	0.56527	12.9	−0.3	0.56473	17.8
	UN	−0.3	0.55772	46.2	−0.3	0.55759	18.3	−0.6	0.55803	26.8
Fully modified GEE	IND	−1.2	0.48543	1.3	−1.2	0.48527	2.3	−1.3	0.48491	3.5
	AR1	−0.8	0.55674	12.6	−0.3	0.55542	4.4	−0.4	0.55481	6.6
	EC	−0.1	0.56384	2.6	−0.2	0.56524	4.4	−0.3	0.56472	6.5
	UN	−0.3	0.55780	12.0	−0.2	0.55755	5.8	−0.5	0.55816	8.5
ELMM	IND	−1.2	0.48543	0.1	−1.2	0.48527	0.2	−1.3	0.48491	0.3
	AR1	−0.8	0.55670	2.3	−1.3	0.55554	1.0	−1.4	0.55491	1.4
	EC	−0.1	0.56366	0.5	−0.2	0.56511	0.8	−0.3	0.56459	1.1
	UN	−0.3	0.55698	5.0	−0.5	0.55688	4.6	−0.6	0.55763	6.3

AR1 spatial autoregressive order 1, *EC* exchangeable correlations, *ELMM* extended linear mixed modeling, *GEE* generalized estimating equations, *IND* independent, *LCV* likelihood cross-validation, *UN* unstructured

[a]A power of 0 corresponds to an intercept parameter; otherwise, the model has a zero intercept

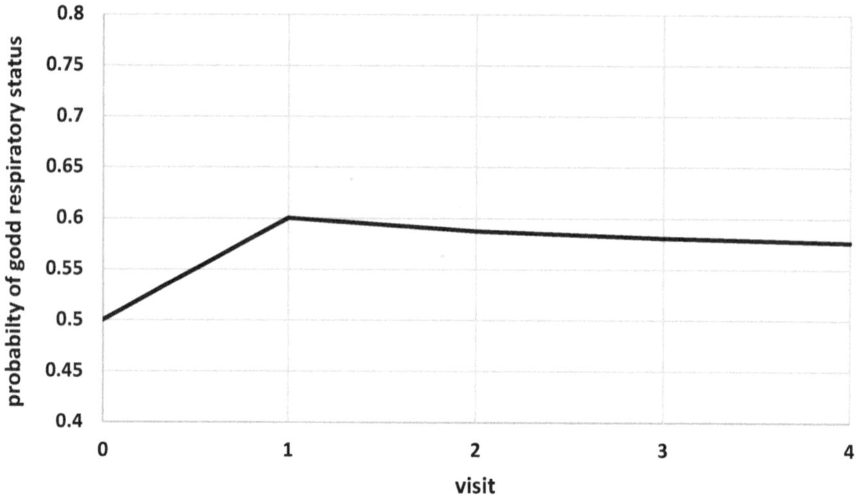

Fig. 8.1 Estimated probability of good respiratory status over visits 0–4 under the ELMM model in visit with constant dispersions

structures for the respiratory status data. They also select $k = 10$ as the most appropriate of the three numbers of folds.

The same model for the means based on visit$^{-0.2}$ without an intercept is selected by all three modeling approaches. Hence, the models generated by partially and fully modified GEE computed using ELMM generate the same LCV score as the model generated by ELMM, indicating that the choice of the model for the means assuming constant dispersions is reasonably robust to the choice of modeling approach.

Table 8.1 also contains clock times for generated models. Clock times for partially modified GEE range from 2.4 to 46.2 min with a total over all 12 cases of about 3.5 h, for fully modified GEE from 1.3 to 12.6 min for a total of about 1.2 h, and for ELMM from 0.1 to 6.3 min for a total of about 0.4 h (totals not reported in Table 8.1). Note that clock times are rounded to one decimal digit, but sums are based on unrounded values and so may not be the same as the sum of the rounded values. Consequently, ELMM requires less computation time, with partially modified GEE taking about 8.8 times as much and fully modified GEE about 3.0 times as much.

Subsequent models use $k = 10$ folds and EC correlations since those choices generate the best LCV score for ELMM in Table 8.1 and ELMM generates a competitive model in less time. The associated adaptive model has means based on visit$^{-0.2}$ without an intercept, estimated constant dispersion 1.02, and estimated exchangeable correlation 0.48. Figure 8.1 provides the plot of estimated mean dichotomous respiratory status, that is, the estimated probability of good respiratory status, over visits 0–4. The probability of good respiratory status increases from 0.5 at visit 0 to 0.60 at visit 1 and then remains relatively constant after that decreasing a little to 0.58 by visit 4.

8.2 Assessing Linearity of the Logits of the Means in Visit

Using ELMM with constant dispersions, $k = 10$ folds, and EC correlations as identified as an appropriate alternative in Sect. 8.1, the linear polynomial model in visit has LCV $= 0.56133$ with distinct percent decrease (PD) of 0.67% (i.e., greater than the cutoff 0.35% for a distinct PD in the LCV score) compared to the adaptive model in visit with LCV score 0.56511. Consequently, the logits of mean dichotomous respiratory status are distinctly nonlinear in visit when the dispersions are treated as constant.

8.3 Assessing Unit Versus Constant Dispersions

The adaptive model using ELMM has estimated constant dispersions of 1.02, very close to having unit dispersions. The adaptive model using ELMM for the means in visit with unit dispersions can be used to assess the appropriateness of unit dispersions. The generated unit dispersions model has means depending on visit$^{-0.2}$ without an intercept, estimated exchangeable correlation 0.48, and LCV score 0.56523. This is the same model for the means as for the associated constant dispersions model with the same estimated correlation and little larger LCV score. These results indicate that unit dispersion models are appropriate alternatives to constant dispersion models for these data, but more complex dispersion models may be appropriate as well. Consequently, unless otherwise indicated, subsequent adaptive analyses start with constant dispersions, allow for more complex dispersions, but also allow for contraction to unit dispersion models (as opposed to the default contraction that stops removing dispersion transforms when there is one such transform remaining in the model).

8.4 Comparison to Standard GEE Modeling

When dispersions are treated as constant, the only difference between partially modified GEE and standard GEE is how the constant dispersion parameter is estimated. Partially modified GEE uses a bias-unadjusted estimate (Sect. 3.5), while standard GEE uses a bias-adjusted estimate (Sect. 2.4). Standard GEE is thus a possible alternative to partially modified GEE for modeling means with constant dispersions. For the dichotomous respiratory status data, the adaptively generated standard GEE model assuming unit dispersions (to reduce the computations; see Sect. 3.5) has means based on visit$^{-0.2}$ without an intercept, LCV score 0.56494, and non-distinct PD 0.06% compared to the associated partially modified GEE model of Table 8.1. This is the same model for the means as generated by partially modified GEE, fully modified GEE, and ELMM assuming constant dispersions ($k = 10$ cases of Table 8.1). Standard GEE modeling requires 2.2 min to generate this model compared to 12.9 min for partially modified GEE and 0.8 min for ELMM (Table 8.1). Consequently, standard GEE modeling requires less time or about 0.2 shorter than partially modified GEE, but more time or about 2.8 times longer than ELMM. It also requires about 4.4 times more than the 0.5 min required for the unit dispersion ELMM model of Sect. 8.3 (not reported in Sect. 8.3).

8.5 Modeling Means and Dispersions in Visit

Adaptive analyses of dichotomous respiratory status are presented in this section using $k = 10$ folds and the EC correlation structure as determined in Sect. 8.1. Adaptive models for means and non-constant dispersions in visit are generated to assess the usual assumption of constant dispersions. Analyses start with constant dispersions but allow for contraction to unit dispersions when warranted. Table 8.2 provides results for adaptive models for means and dispersions in visit. The three modeling approaches partially modified GEE, fully modified GEE, and ELMM are considered. The same model for the means with unit dispersions is generated in all three cases, indicating that an assumption of unit dispersions is reasonable for these data. Since the same models are generated in all three cases, the choice of the model for the means starting with constant dispersions and allowing for unit dispersion is reasonably robust to the modeling approach used to generate it. Moreover, this is the same model selected in Sect. 8.3 assuming unit dispersions.

Table 8.2 also contains clock times for generated models. The clock time is 41.5 min for partially modified GEE, 13.1 min for fully modified GEE, and 3.1 min for ELMM. Consequently, ELMM requires less computation time, with partially modified GEE taking about 13.4 times as much and fully modified GEE about 4.2 times as much.

Table 8.2 Adaptive models of dichotomous respiratory status for means and dispersions in visit[a]

Modeling approach	Transforms of visit for means[b]	Transforms of visit for dispersions[c]	LCV score	Clock time (min)
Partially modified GEE	$\text{visit}^{-0.2}$	–	0.56494	41.5
Fully modified GEE	$\text{visit}^{-0.2}$	–	0.56506	13.1
ELMM	$\text{visit}^{-0.2}$	–	0.56523	3.1

ELMM extended linear mixed modeling, *GEE* generalized estimating equations, *LCV* likelihood cross-validation

[a]Computed with exchangeable correlations and 10 folds

[b]A power of 0 corresponds to an intercept parameter; otherwise, the model has a zero intercept

[c]All models have unit dispersions

8.6 Additive Models in Visit and Being on Active Treatment

Table 8.3 contains results for adaptive additive models for mean dichotomous respiratory status in terms of visit and the indicator active for being on active treatment starting with constant dispersions and allowing for unit dispersions based on partially modified GEE, fully modified GEE, and ELMM. The partially modified GEE model computed using ELMM has LCV score 0.56750, and so the associated ELMM model with LCV score 0.56523 generates a PD of 0.40%. While this is greater than the cutoff of 0.35% for a distinct PD, that cutoff is based on DF = 1 and the partially modified GEE model has two more parameters than the ELMM model. The partially modified GEE model for the means along with unit dispersions is generated as part of the contraction step using ELMM modeling with LCV score 0.56750. The contraction removes next the intercept from the dispersions with decreased LCV score of 0.56569 and non-distinct PD 0.32% compared to the prior contracted model and then removes the intercept for the means with LCV score 0.56523 and non-distinct PD of 0.08%. Consequently, the model generated by ELMM is a competitive alternative to the model generated by partially modified GEE and is simpler. The fully modified GEE model is the same as the partially modified GEE model and so is also a competitive alternative to the ELMM model.

Table 8.3 also contains clock times for adaptive additive models for the means generated starting with constant dispersions and allowing for unit dispersions. The clock times are 18.6 min for partially modified GEE, 7.6 min for fully modified GEE, and 1.3 min for ELMM. Consequently, ELMM requires less computation time, with

Table 8.3 Adaptive additive models of dichotomous respiratory status in visit and the indicator for being on active treatment[a]

	Modeling means and dispersions				Modeling means with unit dispersions[b]		
Modeling approach	Transforms for means[c]	Transforms for dispersions[d]	LCV score	Clock time (min)	Transforms for means[c]	LCV score	Clock time (min)
Partially modified GEE	1, $\text{visit}^{-0.2}$, active	–	0.56730	95.8	1, $\text{visit}^{-0.2}$, active	0.56730	18.6
Fully modified GEE	1, $\text{visit}^{-0.2}$, active	–	0.56745	29.8	1, $\text{visit}^{-0.2}$, active	0.56745	7.6
ELMM	$\text{visit}^{-0.2}$	–	0.56523	4.1	$\text{visit}^{-0.2}$	0.56523	1.3

ELMM extended linear mixed modeling, *GEE* generalized estimating equations, *LCV* likelihood cross-validation

[a]Computed with exchangeable correlations and 10 folds

[b]Computed starting with constant dispersions and allowing contraction to unit dispersions. Unit dispersions selected in all cases

[c]A value of 1 corresponds to an intercept parameter; otherwise, the model has a zero intercept. The variable active is the indicator for being on active treatment

[d]All models based on unit dispersions

partially modified GEE taking about 14.3 times as much and fully modified GEE about 5.8 times as much.

Table 8.3 also contains results for adaptive additive models for dichotomous respiratory status means and dispersions in terms of visit and the indicator for being on active treatment based on partially modified GEE, fully modified GEE, and ELMM. All three generated models have unit dispersions and are the same as associated models starting with constant dispersions and allowing for unit dispersions also reported in Table 8.3. Consequently, as for models generated starting with constant dispersions and allowing for unit dispersions, the ELMM model is a competitive alternative to the other two models. These results indicate that means and dispersions for dichotomous respiratory status are reasonably considered not to differ by type of treatment when considering only additive effects to being on active treatment.

Table 8.3 also contains clock times for adaptive additive models for means and dispersions. The clock times are 95.8 min for partially modified GEE, 29.8 min for fully modified GEE, and 4.1 min for ELMM. Consequently, ELMM requires less computation time, with partially modified GEE taking about 23.4 times as much and fully modified GEE about 7.3 times as much.

8.7 Adaptive Moderation of the Effect of Visit by Being on Active Treatment

Table 8.4 contains results for an assessment of adaptive moderation of the effect of visit on mean dichotomous respiratory status starting with constant dispersions and allowing for unit dispersions based on the three modeling approaches: partially modified GEE, fully modified GEE, and ELMM. Unit dispersions are generated by all three approaches. Also, geometric combinations based on visit and the indicator active are generated by all three modeling approaches. However, this is not enough to establish moderation, which requires that these models outperform the associated adaptive additive models with unit dispersions of Table 8.3. PDs for these

Table 8.4 Adaptive moderation models for means of dichotomous respiratory status in visit, being on active treatment, and geometric combinations with unit dispersions[a]

Modeling approach	Mean transforms[b]	LCV score	Clock time (min)
Partially modified GEE	$(\text{active}\cdot\text{visit}^{-2})^{0.08}$	0.57305	130.8
Fully modified GEE	$(\text{active}\cdot\text{visit}^{-3})^{0.05}$	0.57341	64.2
ELMM	$(\text{visit}^{3}\cdot\text{active})^{-0.05}$	0.57350	8.6

ELMM extended linear mixed modeling, *GEE* generalized linear modeling, *LCV* likelihood cross-validation

[a]Computed with exchangeable correlations and 10 folds, starting with constant dispersions and allowing for unit dispersions; all models have unit dispersions

[b]A value of 1 corresponds to an intercept parameter; otherwise, the model has a zero intercept. The variable active is the indicator for being on active treatment

Table 8.5 Adaptive moderation models for means and dispersions of dichotomous respiratory status in visit, being on active treatment, and geometric combinations[a]

Modeling approach	Mean transforms[b]	Dispersion transforms[c]	LCV score	Clock time (min)
Partially modified GEE	$(\text{active}\cdot\text{visit}^{-2})^{0.08}$	–	0.57305	653.6
Fully modified GEE	$(\text{visit}^{4}\cdot\text{active})^{-0.03}$	–	0.57341	277.0
ELMM	$(\text{visit}^{10}\cdot\text{active})^{-0.011}$	–	0.57348	65.1

ELMM extended linear mixed modeling, *GEE* generalized linear modeling, *LCV* likelihood cross-validation

[a]Computed with exchangeable correlations and 10 folds

[b]A value of 1 corresponds to an intercept parameter; otherwise, the model has a zero intercept. The variable active is the indicator for being on active treatment

[c]All models based on unit dispersions

additive models compared to associated adaptive moderation models of Table 8.4 are distinct at 1.00%, 1.04%, and 1.44% for partially modified GEE, fully modified GEE, and ELMM, respectively (not reported in Table 8.4). Consequently, moderation is established using each of the three modeling approaches.

The partially modified GEE model computed using ELMM has LCV score 0.57341 with non-distinct PD less the 0.01% compared to the associated ELMM. The fully modified GEE model is the same model as for ELMM, only the powers for visit and for the geometric combination are reversed, and so has the same LCV score 0.57350 computed using ELMM. Consequently, all three of these models are competitive alternatives.

Table 8.4 also contains clock times for adaptive moderation models generated starting with constant dispersions and allowing for unit dispersions. The clock times are 130.8 min for partially modified GEE, 64.2 min for fully modified GEE, and 8.6 min for ELMM. Consequently, ELMM requires less computation time, with partially modified GEE taking about 15.2 times as much and fully modified GEE about 7.5 times as much.

Table 8.5 contains results for an assessment of adaptive moderation of the effect of visit on dichotomous respiratory status means and dispersions based on three modeling approaches: partially modified GEE, fully modified GEE, and ELMM. Geometric combinations based on visit and the indicator active are generated for the means by each of the three modeling approaches. However, this is not enough to establish moderation, which requires that these models outperform the associated adaptive additive models of Table 8.3. PDs for these additive models compared to the adaptive moderation models of Table 8.5 are distinct at 1.00%, 1.45%, and 1.44% for partially modified GEE, fully modified GEE, and ELMM, respectively (not reported in Table 8.5). Consequently, moderation of the means is established using each of the three modeling approaches. On the other hand, all three models of Table 8.5 are based on unit dispersion and, while not all the same as associated models of Table 8.4, their LCV scores are either the same or close. These results

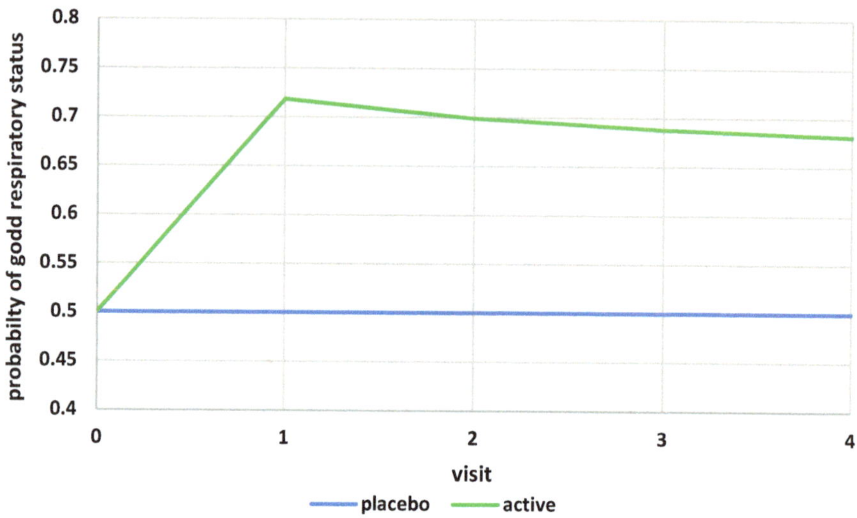

Fig. 8.2 Estimated probability of good respiratory status over visits for patients on active versus placebo treatment

indicate that dispersions are reasonably considered to be unit dispersions for dichotomous respiratory status and not depend on main effects or geometric combinations based on visit and the indicator active.

The partially modified GEE model computed using ELMM has LCV score 0.57349 and the fully modified GEE model computed using ELMM has the same LCV score 0.57349. The ELMM model has smaller LCV score 0.57348 with non-distinct PD less than 0.01%. Consequently, all three of these models are competitive alternatives.

Table 8.5 also contains clock times for adaptive moderation models for means and dispersions generated starting with constant dispersions and allowing for unit dispersions. The clock times are 653.6 min or about 10.9 h for partially modified GEE, 277.0 min or about 4.6 h for fully modified GEE, and 65.1 min or about 1.1 h for ELMM. Consequently, ELMM requires less computation time, with partially modified GEE taking about 10.0 times as much and fully modified GEE about 4.3 times as much. Clock times are relatively long because the expansion step adds in multiple transforms to the dispersions and then the contraction step removes all those transforms as well as the intercept and also some transforms for the means.

The ELMM model of Table 8.4 has the better LCV score than the ELMM moderation model of Table 8.5. This model has means based on

$$\left(\text{visit}^3 \cdot \text{active}\right)^{-0.05} = \text{visit}^{-0.15} \cdot \text{active}$$

without an intercept, unit dispersions, and estimated exchangeable correlation 0.47. Figure 8.2 displays estimated probabilities for good respiratory status over visits for

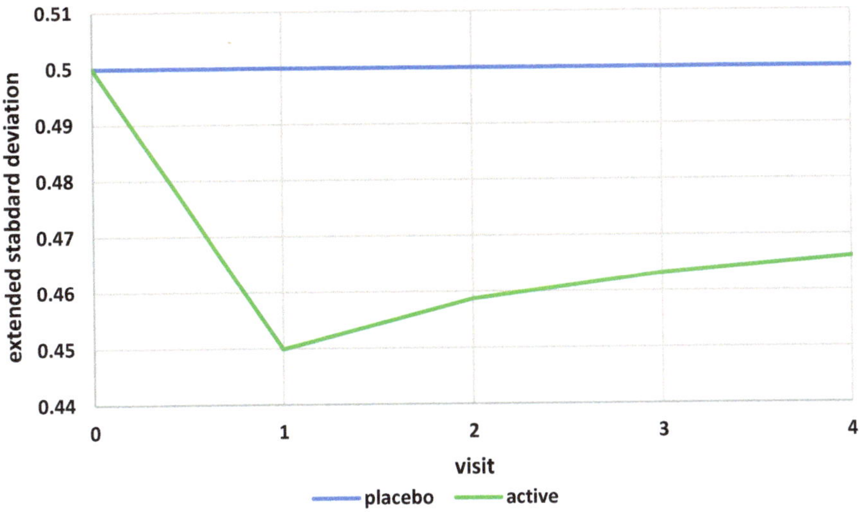

Fig. 8.3 Estimated extended standard deviations for good respiratory status over visits for patients on active versus placebo treatment

patients on active and placebo treatment. There is no effect to visit for patients on placebo treatment with estimated probabilities of good respiratory status constant at 0.5 over all visits. On the other hand, the estimated probabilities of good respiratory status increase from 0.50 at baseline to about 0.72 at visit 1 and then decrease slowly over time to 0.68 at visit 4. Figure 8.3 displays estimated extended standard deviations for good respiratory status over visits for patients on active and placebo treatment. There is no effect to visit for patients on placebo treatment with estimated extended standard deviations of good respiratory status constant at 0.5 over all visits. On the other hand, the estimated extended standard deviations of good respiratory status decrease from 0.50 at baseline to about 0.45 at visit 1 and then increase slowly over time to about 0.47 at visit 4. Figure 8.4 displays the standardized residuals for this model, which range from −2.56 to 2.23, and so there are no distinctly outlying measurements.

8.8 Comparison to Standard Linear Moderation

The standard linear moderation model has means based on an intercept, main effects to untransformed visit and the indicator active, and the interaction between visit and active. Assuming unit dispersions as justified above, the standard linear moderation model computed using ELMM has LCV score 0.56339 with distinct PD 1.76% compared to the adaptive moderation model with unit dispersions of Table 8.4, indicating that in this case moderation is distinctly nonlinear.

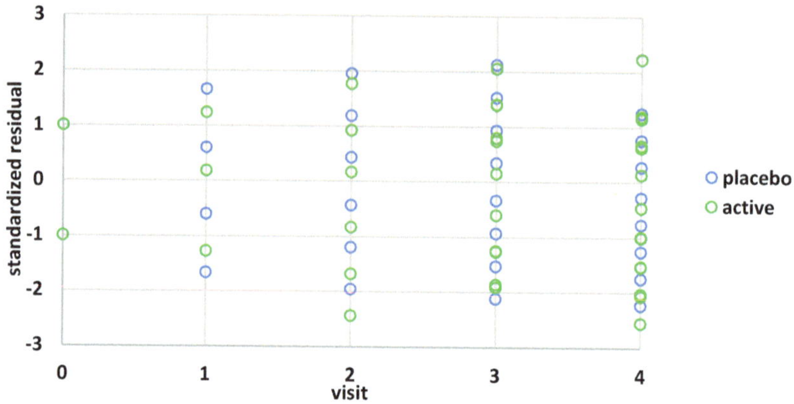

Fig. 8.4 Standardized residuals for dichotomous respiratory status levels by being on active treatment versus on a placebo and based on unit dispersions

8.9 Direct Variance Modeling of Dichotomous Respiratory Status

Direct variance modeling treats the variance function as $V(\mu) = 1$ so that the variances are the same as the dispersions. Table 8.6 provides an assessment of direct variance modeling using ELMM applied to dichotomous respiratory status in terms of only visit, additive in visit and the indicator active, and moderation in visit, active, and geometric combinations based on visit and active.

The adaptive model for the means and dispersions of dichotomous respiratory status in visit using direct variance modeling has means based on $\text{visit}^{-0.3}$ without an intercept along with dispersions, and so also variances, based on $\text{visit}^{10.2}$ without an intercept and LCV score 0.51245. The associated extended variance model of Table 8.2 has LCV score 0.56523, and so the direct variance model generates a

Table 8.6 Adaptive models of dichotomous respiratory status for means and dispersions using direct variance modeling[a]

Predictors[b]	Transforms of visit for means[b]	Transforms of visit for dispersions	LCV score	Clock time (min)
visit	$\text{visit}^{-0.3}$	$\text{visit}^{10.2}$	0.51245	32.3
visit, active	$\text{visit}^{-0.11}$	$\text{visit}^{19.6}$	0.51243	39.6
visit, active, GCs	$(\text{active}\cdot\text{visit})^{-0.1}$	$(\text{active}\cdot\text{visit}^5)^{-1}$	0.51741	79.1

ELMM linear mixed modeling, *GCs* geometric combinations, *GEE* generalized estimating equations, *LCV* likelihood cross-validation

[a]Computed with extended linear mixed modeling, exchangeable correlations, and 10 folds

[b]A value of 1 corresponds to an intercept parameter; otherwise, the model has a zero intercept. The variable active is the indicator for being on active treatment

distinct PD 9.34% (not reported in Table 8.6), indicating that direct variance modeling in visit generates a distinctly inferior model.

The adaptive additive model in visit and the indicator active has means based on $\text{visit}^{-0.11}$ without an intercept along with dispersions, and so also variances, based on $\text{visit}^{19.6}$ without an intercept and LCV score 0.51243. The associated model of Table 8.3 has LCV score 0.56523, and so the direct variance model generates a distinct PD 9.34% (not reported in Table 8.6), indicating that direct variance additive modeling in visit and active generates a distinctly inferior model.

The adaptive moderation model in visit, the indicator active, and geometric combinations in visit and active has means based on

$$(\text{active} \cdot \text{visit})^{-0.1} = \text{active} \cdot \text{visit}^{-0.1}$$

without an intercept along with dispersions, and so also variances, based on

$$\left(\text{active} \cdot \text{visit}^5\right)^{-1} = \text{active} \cdot \text{visit}^{-5}$$

without an intercept and LCV score 0.51741. The associated direct variance additive model has LCV score 0.51243 and distinct PD 0.96%, supporting moderation of the effect of visit on means and dispersions by active. However, the associated model of Table 8.5 has LCV score 0.57348, and so the direct variance model generates a distinct PD 9.78% (not reported in Table 8.6), indicating that direct variance moderation modeling in visit and active generates a distinctly inferior model.

Under direct variance modeling, clock times as reported in Table 8.6 are 32.3 min to generate the adaptive model for the means and dispersions of dichotomous respiratory status levels in visit, 39.6 min to generate the associated adaptive additive model in visit and the indicator active, and 79.1 min to generate the associated adaptive model allowing for both main effects and geometric combinations in visit and active for a total of 151.0 min or about 2.5 h. Associated models with extended variances depending on means are 3.1 min to generate the adaptive model for the means and dispersions of dichotomous respiratory status levels in visit of Table 8.2, 4.1 min to generate the associated adaptive additive model in visit and the indicator active of Table 8.3, and 65.1 min to generate the associated adaptive model allowing for both main effects and geometric combinations in visit and active of Table 8.5 for a total of 72.3 min or about 1.2 h. All three models are generated in more time using direct variance modeling while requiring a total time of about 2.1 times more. These results and the earlier results indicate that direct variance modeling in this case generates distinctly inferior models while also requiring more time overall.

8.10 Analysis Summary

A summary of the results of analyses of the dichotomous respiratory status data is provided broken down into seven categories of results.

1. Models for Means in Visit Assuming Constant Dispersions

The preferable model for the dichotomous respiratory status data has EC correlations with LCV score based on $k = 10$ folds. Models selected by partially modified GEE, fully modified GEE, and ELMM are not only competitive alternatives but are exactly the same model. Estimated mean dichotomous respiratory status levels, that is, estimated probabilities of good respiratory status, are plotted in Fig. 8.1. The logits of the mean dichotomous respiratory status levels are distinctly nonlinear in visit assuming constant dispersions. The unit dispersions model is a competitive, simpler model. The model for the means generated by standard GEE assuming unit dispersions is the same as the model for the means generated by partially modified GEE assuming constant dispersions. ELMM requires less time with partially modified GEE requiring about 8.8 times as much and fully modified GEE requiring about 3.0 times as much.

2. Models for Means and Dispersions in Visit

Models selected by partially modified GEE, fully modified GEE, and ELMM are not only all competitive alternatives but are also the same model. This model has unit dispersions and is the same as the model generated assuming unit dispersions. ELMM requires less time with partially modified GEE requiring about 13.4 times as much and fully modified GEE requiring about 4.2 times as much.

3. Additive Models in Visit and Being on Active Treatment

Models selected by partially modified GEE, fully modified GEE, and ELMM starting with constant dispersions and allowing for unit dispersions are all competitive alternatives and have unit dispersions. Mean dichotomous respiratory status levels are reasonably considered not to change additively with being on active treatment when dispersions are treated as constant. Although partially modified GEE does generate a model with an additive effect to being on active treatment, this model computed using ELMM is a competitive alternative to the associated ELMM model after accounting for the partially modified GEE model having two more parameters. ELMM requires less time with partially modified GEE requiring about 14.3 times as much and fully modified GEE requiring about 5.8 times as much.

Models selected by fully modified GEE and ELMM allowing for non-constant dispersions have unit dispersions, are all the same as associated additive models starting with constant dispersions and allowing for unit dispersions, and so are all competitive alternatives. ELMM requires less time with partially modified GEE requiring about 23.4 times as much and fully modified GEE requiring about 7.3 times as much.

4. Moderation Models in Visit and Being on Active Treatment

Models selected by partially modified GEE, fully modified GEE, and ELMM starting with constant dispersions and allowing for unit dispersions are all competitive alternatives and have unit dispersions. The effect of visit on mean dichotomous respiratory status is reasonably considered to be moderated by being on active treatment and is distinctly nonlinear in visit. ELMM requires less time with partially modified GEE requiring about 15.2 times as much and fully modified GEE requiring about 7.5 times as much.

Models selected by partially modified GEE, fully modified GEE, and ELMM allowing for non-constant dispersions are all competitive alternatives, have unit dispersions, and are competitive alternatives to associated models starting with constant dispersions and allowing for unit dispersions. The effect of visit on mean dichotomous respiratory status levels is reasonably considered to be moderated by being on active treatment allowing for non-constant dispersions. ELMM requires less time with partially modified GEE requiring about 10.0 times as much and fully modified GEE requiring about 4.3 times as much.

5. Direct Variance Models for Dichotomous Respiratory Status Levels

The direct variance model generated accounting for the effect to visit on means and dispersions is distinctly inferior to the associated model treating variances as a function of the means and dispersions. This is also the case for both additive and moderation models in visit and being on active treatment. These direct variance models require more overall time than the associated three extended variance models. Extended variance models are preferable to models based on direct variance modeling.

6. All Models for Dichotomous Respiratory Status Levels in Visit and Being on Active Treatment

In all cases, partially modified GEE, fully modified GEE, and ELMM generate competitive models. In all cases, unit dispersions are the appropriate choice. Over all clock times reported in Tables 8.1, 8.2, 8.3, 8.4 and 8.5, ELMM requires about 1.8 h compared to about 19.2 h or about 10.7 times as much for partially modified GEE and about 7.7 h or about 4.2 times as for fully modified GEE.

7. Selected Model for Dichotomous Respiratory Status in Visit and Being on Active Treatment

Under the most appropriate model for dichotomous respiratory status, estimated means are plotted in Fig. 8.2 and change differently over visits for patients on a placebo and patients on active treatment. Estimated extended standard deviations are plotted in Fig. 8.3 and also change differently over visits for patients on a placebo and patients on active treatment. Standardized residuals for this model are plotted in Fig. 8.4, and there are no outlying measurements.

8.11 Example SAS Code for Analyzing the Dichotomous Respiratory Status Data

Example SAS code is presented in this section for conducting analyses of dichotomous respiratory status levels as a function of clinic visit and treatment group (either on active treatment or taking a placebo). The code assumes that a data set called longresp has been created in the SAS default library containing the dichotomous respiratory status data (Sect. 2.8.3) in long format, that is, with one measurement (or row) for each dichotomous respiratory status level at each clinic visit for each patient. This data set contains variables (or columns) called id loaded with unique identifiers for patients, status0_1 loaded with dichotomous respiratory status levels coded as 0:poor or 1:good, visit loaded with visit indexes of 0–4, and the indicator active set to 1 for patients on active treatment and to 0 for patients in the control group. Altogether, there are 5 dichotomous respiratory status levels at different clinic visits for each of 111 different patients, 54 on active treatment and 57 on a placebo, for a total of 555 measurements.

The code also assumes that a %include statement has been executed to load in the current version of the genreg macro for use in conducting adaptive analyses. The genreg macro supports a wide variety of macro parameters, some of which are described here. The interface for this macro contains the complete list of macro parameters along with their default settings. Default settings are used by the macro if a value for the macro parameter has not been specified in the code invoking the macro. Macro parameter settings are case insensitive. The cutoff for a distinct percent decrease in LCV scores (Sect. 2.6.2) using DF = 1 for these data with 555 measurements is 0.35%.

8.11.1 *Modeling Means in Visit Assuming Constant Dispersions*

The following code uses the genreg macro to generate the adaptive model for dichotomous respiratory status means as a possibly nonlinear function of visit using $k = 10$ folds, exchangeable correlations (EC), and extended linear mixed modeling (ELMM) as selected in Sect. 8.1 assuming constant dispersions.

```
%genreg(modtype=logis,datain=longresp,yvar=status0_1,
matchvar=id,withinvr=visit,foldcnt=10,corrtype=EC,GEE=n,
srchtype=logL,expand=y,expxvars=visit,contract=y);
```

The modeling approach used by genreg is determined by the combination of the GEE and srchtype macro parameters. In this case, “GEE=n” means use ELMM, while “srchtype=logL” means base estimation on maximizing the log-likelihood (as described in Sects. 4.3 and 5.2). These are the default settings for these two macro parameters. Setting "GEE=y" requests GEE modeling. Combining "GEE=y" with "srchtype=GEE" requests partially modified GEE with estimation based on minimizing the maximum absolute value of the gradient (as described in Sect. 3.7). Combining "GEE=y" with "srchtype=logL" requests fully modified GEE. By default, partially modified and fully modified GEE use bias-unadjusted dispersion estimates. Bias-adjusted dispersion estimates, as used in standard GEE modeling (Sect. 2.4), are requested by adding the setting "biasadj=y".

Adaptive modeling is requested using "expand=y" together with "contract=y", meaning first expand the base model and then contract the expanded model. In this case, the base model has constant means and constant dispersions based on only intercept parameters (but this can be changed). The expxvars macro parameter specifies the primary predictor variables for modeling the means to consider in the expansion. In this case, the expansion grows the model for the means by systematically adding in power transforms of the single variable visit while holding the dispersions constant. The maximum number of transforms added by the expansion to the model for the means is controlled by the expxmax parameter with default value "expxmax=5" meaning at most five transforms can be added to the means. Changing to the empty setting "expxmax=" removes the restriction on the number of such transforms.

The contraction systematically removes transforms from the expanded model for the means, possibly the constant transform corresponding to the intercept, and adjusts the powers of the remaining transforms to increase the LCV score, which in this case is computed with 10 folds as specified by the setting of the foldcnt macro parameter. It is also computed using matched-set-wise deletion corresponding to the default setting "measdlte=n". Measurement-wise deletion is requested using "measdlte=y". The contraction can optionally be restricted not to remove the intercept for the means in order to generate a non-zero intercept model. An LCV ratio test is used to decide when to stop the contraction. The contraction also stops when there is only one transform remaining in the model for the means. When the contraction leaves the expanded model unchanged, that expanded model has its powers adjusted to increase the LCV score.

The following code directly generates the above adaptive model selected with $k = 10$ folds, EC correlations, and ELMM, including parameter estimates and LCV score.

```
%genreg(modtype=logis,datain=longresp,yvar=status0_1,
matchvar=id,withinvr=visit,foldcnt=10,corrtype=EC,GEE=n,
srchtype=logL,xintrcpt=n,xvars=visit,xpowers=−0.2);
```

The xintrcpt macro parameter specifies whether or not the base model for the means includes an intercept, the xvars macro parameter provides the list of primary predictors for the base model for the means, and the xpowers macro parameter provides the powers for transforming those primary predictors. In this case, the model for the means has a zero intercept along with the single transform $\text{visit}^{-0.2}$. The default values for these macro parameters are "xintrcpt=y", "xvars=", and "xpowers=" requesting constant means. An empty setting for the xvars macro parameter means include no transforms for the means, and an empty setting for the xpowers macro parameter means power transform xvars variables if any with the power 1 (and so include them untransformed). The model for the dispersions is based on macro parameters vintrcpt, vvars, and vpowers with analogous meanings and with the same default settings requesting constant dispersions. The xvalid macro parameter is not set in the above code and so has its default setting "xvalid=y" meaning to compute the LCV score for the requested model. In this case, the model has LCV score 0.56511. Adding the setting "xvalid=n" means compute only parameter estimates for the requested model and not the LCV score.

The above code can be changed to generate the standard linear polynomial model for the means based on untransformed visit as follows. First change the settings for the xintrcpt and xvars macro parameters to "xintrcpt=y" and "xvars=visit". Then change the setting for the xpowers macro parameter to "xpowers=1" or remove the setting for the xpowers macro parameter so that it has its default empty value, which means to use the power 1 to transform all variables listed in the setting of the xvars macro parameter. Note that the logits of the means are linear in visit, but the means are nonlinear due to using the logit link function. To request the standard quadratic polynomial model for the means, use the settings "xintrcpt=y", "xvars=visit visit", and "xpowers=1 2".

As reported in Sect. 8.3, the above model has estimated constant dispersions equal to 1.02, suggesting that unit dispersions might be appropriate for the dichotomous respiratory status levels. The following code uses the genreg macro to generate the adaptive model for dichotomous respiratory status means as a possibly nonlinear function of visit using $k = 10$ folds, EC correlations, and ELMM as selected in Sect. 8.1 assuming unit dispersions.

```
%genreg(modtype=logis,datain=longresp,yvar=status0_1,
matchvar=id,withinvr=visit,foldcnt=10,corrtype=EC,GEE=n,
srchtype=logL,vintrcpt=n,expand=y,expxvars=visit,contract=y);
```

The base model for the dispersions has a zero intercept, due to the setting "vintrcpt=n" along with default empty settings for the vvars and vpowers macro parameters, and it remains that way because the model for the dispersions does not change. Since the dispersions are modeled using the natural log link function, all models generated as part of the adaptive process have unit dispersions. The generated unit dispersions model has the same model for the means as generated assuming constant dispersions with a better LCV score, indicating that dispersions are reasonably treated as having value 1 when means are modeled in terms of only visit. The following code directly generates the adaptive unit dispersions model.

```
%genreg(modtype=logis,datain=longresp,yvar=status0_1,
matchvar=id,withinvr=visit,foldcnt=10,corrtype=EC,GEE=n,
srchtype=logL,xintrcpt=n,xvars=visit,xpowers=-0.2,vintrcpt=n);
```

8.11.2 Modeling Means and Dispersions in Visit

The following code uses the genreg macro to generate the adaptive non-constant dispersions model for dichotomous respiratory level means and dispersions as possibly nonlinear functions of visit using $k = 10$ folds, EC correlations, and ELMM, starting from constant dispersions and allowing for unit dispersions.

```
%genreg(modtype=logis,datain=longresp,yvar=status0_1,
matchvar=id,withinvr=visit,foldcnt=10,corrtype=EC,GEE=n,
srchtype=logL,expand=y,expxvars=visit,expvvars=visit,
contract=y,cnvzero=y);
```

Adaptive modeling is requested using "expand=y" together with "contract=y" meaning first expand the base model with constant means and constant dispersions and then contract the expanded model. The expxvars and expvvars macro parameters specify the primary predictor variables to consider in the expansion for the means and dispersions, respectively. In this case, the same set of primary predictors is used for the means and for the dispersions, but different sets of primary predictors can be specified. The expansion grows the model for the means and the dispersions in combination by systematically adding in power transforms of the single variable visit one-at-a-time to either the means or to the dispersions, whichever generates the better LCV score. Similar to the expxmax parameter, the expvmax parameter specifies the maximum number of transforms added by the expansion to the model for the dispersions with default value "expvmax=5" meaning at most five transforms can be added to the dispersions. Changing to the empty setting "expvmax=" removes the restriction on the number of such transforms.

The contraction systematically removes transforms from the expanded model for the means and dispersions in combination, possibly the constant transforms corresponding to intercepts, and adjusts the powers of the remaining transforms to increase the LCV score. Transforms are removed one-at-a-time from either the means or from the dispersions, whichever generates the better LCV score after adjusting all the powers of the remaining transforms for both the means and the dispersions. An LCV ratio test is used to decide when to stop the contraction. By default, the contraction stops removing transforms from the means when there is only one transform remaining in the model for the means. However, in this case the contraction is allowed to remove all the transforms from the dispersions due to the setting "cnvzero=y". This does not happen otherwise because the default setting is "cnvzero=n". When the contraction leaves the expanded model unchanged, that expanded model has its powers adjusted to increase the LCV score.

As reported in Sect. 8.5, not only does the generated model have unit dispersions, but it has the same model for the means as generated assuming unit dispersions. Consequently, the dispersions are reasonably treated as having value 1 when both the means and dispersions are modeled in terms of only visit.

8.11.3 Additive Models in Visit and Being on Active Treatment

The following code uses the genreg macro to generate the adaptive additive model for dichotomous respiratory status means and dispersions as possibly nonlinear functions of visit and being on active treatment using $k = 10$ folds, EC correlations, and ELMM allowing for unit dispersions.

```
%genreg(modtype=logis,datain=longresp,yvar=status0_1,
matchvar=id,withinvr=visit,foldcnt=10,corrtype=EC,GEE=n,
srchtype=logL,expand=y,expxvars=visit active,contract=y,cnvzero=y);
```

In this case, the expxvars and expvvars macro parameters specify the variables visit and active to be the primary predictor variables to consider in the expansion for the means and dispersions, respectively. The expansion grows the model for the means and the dispersions in combination by systematically adding in power transforms of visit or the indicator variable active one-at-a-time to either the means or to the dispersions, whichever generates the better LCV score. Note that indicator variables like active are not transformed and are included at most once in the model for the means and at most once in the model for the dispersions.

The contraction then systematically removes transforms from the expanded model for the means and dispersions in combination, possibly the constant transforms corresponding to intercepts, and adjusts the powers of the remaining transforms to increase the LCV score. The model is additive because by default geometric combinations are not considered in the expansion. An adaptive additive model for the means in visit and active assuming constant dispersions can be generated by changing the expvvars macro parameter to have an empty setting, that is, "expvvars=", or by removing its setting from the above code, because the empty setting is its default setting.

The base model has constant dispersions because that is the default base dispersions model (corresponding to "vintrcpt=y", "vvars=", and "vpowers="). The expansion considers adding transforms based on visit and the indicator active to the dispersions model, and then the contraction considers removing those transforms if any and the intercept from the dispersions model. By default, the contraction of the dispersions model stops if that model is based on a single transform. The setting "cnvzero=y" overrides that default (corresponding to "cnvzero=n") so that the contraction considers removal of a single remaining dispersion transform should the contraction generate such a dispersions model. When the last dispersion transform is removed, the dispersions are based on a zero intercept with no transforms, which corresponds to unit dispersions since these are based on the log link function.

The adaptively generated additive model for means assuming constant dispersions and allowing for unit dispersions is the same as the adaptively generated model in only visit assuming constant dispersions and allowing for unit dispersions. The adaptively generated additive model for means and dispersions allowing for unit dispersion is also this same model. Consequently, being on active treatment is reasonably considered not to have an additive effect on the means or on the dispersions.

8.11.4 Moderation Models in Visit and Being on Active Treatment

The following code uses the genreg macro to generate the adaptive moderation model for dichotomous respiratory status means and dispersions as possibly nonlinear functions of visit, being on active treatment, and geometric combinations in visit and being on active treatment using $k = 10$ folds, EC correlations, and ELMM allowing for unit dispersions.

```
%genreg(modtype=logis,datain=longresp,yvar=status0_1,
matchvar=id,withinvr=visit,foldcnt=10,corrtype=EC,GEE=n,
srchtype=logL,expand=y,expxvars=visit active,
expvvars=visit active,geomcmbn=y,contract=y,cnvzero=y);
```

In this case, the expxvars and expvvars macro parameters specify the variables visit and active to be the primary predictor variables to consider in the expansion for the means and dispersions, respectively. The expansion grows the model for the means and the dispersions in combination by systematically adding in power transforms of visit, the indicator variable active, or geometric combinations in visit and active one-at-a-time to either the means or to the dispersions, whichever generates the better LCV score. Geometric combinations are considered due to adding the setting "geomcmbn=y" to the code for generating the associated additive model in age and male. The default setting for the geomcmbn macro parameter is "geomcmbn=n" meaning to restrict the expansion to an additive model in the variables specified in the expxvars and expvvars settings. The contraction systematically removes transforms from the expanded model for the means and dispersions in combination, possibly the constant transforms corresponding to intercepts, and adjusts the powers of the remaining transforms to increase the LCV score. Note that when a geometric combination of the form $(\text{visit}^p \cdot \text{active})^q$ or $(\text{active} \cdot \text{visit}^p)^q$ is generated by the expansion, the contraction only adjusts the power q and leaves the power p unchanged. When there are more than two primary predictors for the means and/or dispersions, geometric combinations can be generated based on any number of two or more of those primary predictors. An adaptive moderation model for the means in visit, active, and geometric combinations in visit and active starting with constant dispersions and allowing for unit dispersions can be generated by changing the expvvars macro parameter to have an empty setting, that is, "expvvars=", or by removing its setting from the above code, because the empty setting is its default setting.

The following code directly generates the adaptive moderation model for the means starting with constant dispersions and allowing for unit dispersions.

```
%genreg(modtype=logis,datain=longresp,yvar=status0_1,
matchvar=id,withinvr=visit,foldcnt=10,corrtype=EC,GEE=n,
srchtype=logL,srchtype=logL,xintrcpt=n,xgcs=visit 3 active 1,xgcpowrs=-0.05,
vintrcpt=n);
```

In this case, the model for the means is based on a zero intercept and the geometric combination

$$\left(\text{visit}^3 \cdot \text{active}\right)^{-0.05} = \text{visit}^{-0.15} \cdot \text{active}.$$

The LCV score is 0.57350, while the associated additive model starting with constant dispersions and allowing for unit dispersions has LCV score 0.56523 with distinct PD 1.44%. Consequently, being on active treatment is reasonably considered to moderate the effect of visit on the means together with unit dispersions.

The macro parameters xgcs and xgcpowrs are used to specify geometric combinations for the means. The setting "xgcs=visit 3 active 1" specifies the untransformed geometric combination $\text{visit}^3 \cdot \text{active}$, while the setting "xgcpowrs=−0.05" means to transform $\text{visit}^3 \cdot \text{active}$ to the power −0.05. The xgcpowrs setting is needed in this case because its default empty setting "xgcpowrs=" means to leave all the geometric combinations specified by the xgcs macro parameter untransformed. Multiple geometric combinations are specified by separating them by colons (:). For example, use the following code to generate the model with means based on an intercept and the two geometric combinations $(\text{visit}^2 \cdot \text{active})^{0.1}$ and $(\text{visit}^{0.5} \cdot \text{active})^{0.5}$ along with unit dispersions.

```
%genreg(modtype=logis,datain=longresp,yvar=status0_1,
matchvar=id,withinvr=visit,foldcnt=10,corrtype=EC,GEE=n,
srchtype=logL,xintrcpt=n,xgcs=visit 2 active 1 : visit 0.5 active 1,
xgcpowrs=0.1 0.5,vintrcpt=n);
```

The macro parameters vgcs and vgcpowrs are used in the same way to specify geometric combinations for the dispersions.

The following code directly generates the adaptive moderation model for means and dispersions allowing for unit dispersions.

```
%genreg(modtype=logis,datain=longresp,yvar=status0_1,
matchvar=id,withinvr=visit,foldcnt=10,corrtype=EC,GEE=n,
srchtype=logL,xintrcpt=n,xgcs=visit 10 active 1,
xgcpowrs=-0.011,vintrcpt=n);
```

In this case, the model for the means is based on a zero intercept and the geometric combination

$$\left(\text{visit}^{10}\cdot\text{active}\right)^{-0.011}=\text{visit}^{-0.11}\cdot\text{active}$$

while the dispersions are based on a zero intercept. The LCV score is 0.57348, while the associated moderation model for the means has close LCV score 0.57350. Consequently, as before being on active treatment is reasonably considered to moderate the effect of visit on the means together with unit dispersions.

The standard linear moderation model has means based on an intercept, visit, active, and the interaction visit · active. While it would usually have constant dispersions, unit dispersions are more appropriate for dichotomous respiratory status. The standard linear moderation model with unit dispersions can be generated using ELMM with the following code.

```
%genreg(modtype=logis,datain=longresp,yvar=status0_1,
matchvar=id,withinvr=visit,foldcnt=10,corrtype=EC,GEE=n,
srchtype=logL,xintrcpt=y,xvars=visit active,
xgcs=visit 1 active 1,vintrcpt=n);
```

The LCV score is 0.56339 with distinct PD 1.76% compared to the adaptive moderation model with unit dispersions with LCV score 0.57350, indicating that in this case moderation is distinctly nonlinear.

8.11.5 Direct Variance Modeling

The dirctvar macro parameter controls whether or not variances are directly modeled. The default setting "dirctvar=n" means use extended variances based on both the dispersions and the variance function which in this case is $V(\mu) = \mu \cdot (1 - \mu)$. Adding the setting "dirctvar=y" treats the variance function as $V(\mu) = 1$ so that the extended variances are the same as the dispersions. The following code uses the genreg macro to generate the adaptive direct variances, ELMM model for dichotomous respiratory status means and dispersions as possibly nonlinear functions of visit.

```
%genreg(modtype=logis,datain=longresp,yvar=status0_1,
matchvar=id,withinvr=visit,foldcnt=10,corrtype=EC,GEE=n,
srchtype=logL,expand=y,expxvars=visit,expvvars=visit,
contract=y,cnvzero=y,dirctvar=y);
```

The following code directly generates the above direct variance model.

```
%genreg(modtype=logis,datain=longresp,yvar=status0_1,
matchvar=id,withinvr=visit,foldcnt=10,corrtype=EC,GEE=n,
srchtype=logL,xintrcpt=n,xvars=visit,xpowers=-0.3,
vintrcpt=n,vvars=visit,vpowers=10.2,dirctvar=y);
```

This model has means based on a zero intercept and the transform $\text{visit}^{-0.3}$ along with dispersions, and so also extended variances, based on a zero intercept and $\text{visit}^{10.2}$. It has LCV score 0.51245 with distinct PD 9.34% compared to the associated model accounting for the variance function $V(\mu) = \mu \cdot (1 - \mu)$ with LCV score 0.56523. Consequently, direct variance modeling in visit generates a distinctly inferior model. The same conclusions hold for direct variance modeling allowing for additive effects to visit and active as well as moderation effects.

8.11.6 Example Output

As also considered in Sect. 8.11.4, the following code uses the genreg macro to generate the adaptive moderation model for dichotomous respiratory status means and dispersions as possibly nonlinear functions of visit, being in the intervention group, and geometric combinations in visit and being in the intervention group.

```
%genreg(modtype=logis,datain=longresp,yvar=status0_1,
matchvar=id,withinvr=visit,foldcnt=10,corrtype=EC,GEE=n,
srchtype=logL,expand=y,expxvars=visit active,
expvvars=visit active,geomcmbn=y,contract=y,cnvzero=y);
```

The output generated by this code starts with descriptions of settings controlling what kind of model has been generated including the cutoff for a distinct percent decrease in LCV scores followed by a description of the base model. Table 8.7 contains SAS listing output describing the base model. The means or the probabilities for status0_1=1 (i.e., the logit expectation component) are based only on an intercept parameter XINTRCPT with estimated value 0.15, while the dispersions (i.e., the log dispersion component) are also based only on an intercept parameter VINTRCPT with estimated value $-2.26 \cdot 10^{-10}$. The estimated correlation is 0.47

Table 8.7 Part of the SAS listing output describing the base model for the generation of the adaptive moderation model

```
                base logit expectation component

parameter estimates for logits relative to smallest status0_1=0

              predictor     power   status0_1=1

              XINTRCPT          1     0.1480174

                base log dispersion component

                predictor     power  estimate

                VINTRCPT          1 -2.26E-10

estimated correlation:                                    0.4746102
mth root of extended likelihood using deleted predictions: 0.5612317
```

Table 8.8 Part of the SAS listing output describing the expanded model for the generation of the adaptive moderation model

```
geometric combination logit expectation variables:
          XGC_1    visit**(-0.2)*active
          XGC_2    visit**(-6)*active
          XGC_3    visit**(10)*active
          XGC_4    active*visit

 geometric combination log dispersion variables:
          VGC_1    active*visit
          VGC_2    visit**(-0.5)*active

       expanded logit expectation component

parameter estimates for logits relative to smallest status0_1=0

   predictor      power   status0_1=1        score    order

   XINTRCPT           1     -0.251142   0.5612317        0
   XGC_1            0.7     0.9142582   0.5738438        1
   XGC_2             -3      -9.4E-12   0.5733733        7
   XGC_3             -1     -0.266484   0.5729581        8
   visit             -7     0.2256186   0.5725296        9
   XGC_4              1     0.1436276   0.5715734       10

         expanded log dispersion component

    predictor      power   estimate          score    order

    VINTRCPT           1   0.0374436   0.5612317        0
    visit           -0.5   -0.043661   0.5739031        2
    visit              2   -0.003209   0.5739123        3
    VGC_1             -1   0.0933757   0.5738742        4
    VGC_2              3    -0.11426   0.5739373        5
    active             1   0.0104343   0.5738797        6

estimated correlation:                                  0.4728479
mth root of extended likelihood using deleted predictions: 0.5715734
```

and the LCV score rounds to 0.56123 (called the "mth root of the extended likelihood using deleted predictions" in the output).

The output then describes the parameters controlling the expansion followed by the expanded model as described in Table 8.8. The output uses the SAS double asterisk power operator (**). The base model (order 0) has LCV score 0.56123. First, the geometric combination

$$\mathrm{XGC\_1}^{0.7} = \left(\mathrm{visit}^{-0.2} \cdot \mathrm{active}\right)^{0.7} = \mathrm{visit}^{-0.14} \cdot \mathrm{active}\ (\mathrm{order}\ 1)$$

is added to the means generating LCV score 0.57384. Next, five terms are added to the dispersions: the two transforms $\mathrm{visit}^{-0.5}$ (order 2) and visit^{2} (order 3), the two geometric combinations

$$\mathrm{VGC\_1}^{-1} = (\mathrm{active} \cdot \mathrm{visit})^{-1} = \mathrm{active} \cdot \mathrm{visit}^{-1}\ (\mathrm{order}\ 4)$$

and

$$\text{VGC\_2}^3 = \left(\text{visit}^{-0.5} \cdot \text{active}\right)^3 = \text{visit}^{-1.5} \cdot \text{active (order 5)},$$

and the indicator active (order 6) with LCV scores 0.57390, 0.57391, 0.57387, 0.57394, and 0.57388. Finally, four more terms are added to the means: the two geometric combinations

$$\text{XGC\_2}^{-3} = \left(\text{visit}^{-6} \cdot \text{active}\right)^{-13} = \text{visit}^{18} \cdot \text{active (order 7)}$$

and

$$\text{XGC\_3}^{-1} = \left(\text{visit}^{10} \cdot \text{active}\right)^{-1} = \text{visit}^{-10} \cdot \text{active (order 8)},$$

the transform visit^{-7} (order 9), and the geometric combination

$$\text{XGC\_4}^1 = \text{active} \cdot \text{visit (order 10)}$$

with LCV scores 0.57337, 0.57296, 0.57253, and 0.57157, which is the LCV score for the expanded model. Each transform is added to the model without adjusting the powers for previously added transforms. The LCV score is allowed to decrease, and so expanded models usually require contraction. However, in cases where the contraction leaves the expanded model unchanged, a conditional transformation step is executed to adjust the powers of the expanded model to improve its LCV score. The estimated correlation is 0.47.

The output then describes the parameters controlling the contraction followed by the contracted model as described in Table 8.9. The expanded model (order 0) has LCV score 0.57157. First, two geometric combinations $\text{XGC\_1}^{0.7}$ (order 1) and XGC_2^{-3} (order 2) are removed from the means generating the LCV scores 0.57291 and 0.57401. Then four terms are removed from the dispersions: the intercept VINTRCPT (order 3), the indicator active (order 4), VGC_1^{-1} (order 5), and VGC_2^3 (order 6) with LCV scores 0.57429, 0.57452, 0.57458, and 0.57449. Next, the transform visit^{-7} (order 7) is removed from the means with LCV score 0.57439, the transform visit^2 (order 8) is removed from the dispersions with LCV score 0.57429, the geometric combination XGC_4^1 (order 9) is removed from the means with LCV score 0.57407, and the transform $\text{visit}^{-0.5}$ (order 10) is removed from the dispersions with LCV score 0.57378. Finally, the intercept XINTRCPT (order 11) is removed from the means with LCV score 0.57348, which is the LCV score for the contracted model. With the removal of each transform from the model, the powers for the other transforms are adjusted to improve the LCV score. In this case, the power for XGC_3 in the means changes from -1 to -0.011, while the other powers are unchanged. Details on how the powers change at each step of the contraction are not provided in the contraction output, but are available in the SAS log output if that is of interest. Note that the LCV score increased with the removal of the first five transforms and then decreased with

Table 8.9 Part of the SAS listing output describing the contracted model for the generation of the adaptive moderation model

```
              contracted logit expectation component

parameter estimates for logits relative to smallest status0_1=0

                 predictor old power new power

                 XGC_3              -1    -0.011

               predictor     power   status0_1=1

               XGC_3        -0.011     0.9098647

           discarded   old power        score   order

                               .   0.5715734       0
           XGC_1             0.7    0.572907       1
           XGC_2              -3    0.574011       2
           visit              -7   0.5743899       7
           XGC_4               1   0.5740662       9
           XINTRCPT            1   0.5734835      11

             contracted log dispersion component

           predictor old power new power    estimate

           VZERO             1         1           0

           discarded   old power        score   order

                               .   0.5715734       0
           VINTRCPT            1    0.574292       3
           active              1   0.5745216       4
           VGC_1              -1   0.5745845       5
           VGC_2               3   0.5744856       6
           visit               2   0.5742865       8
           visit            -0.5   0.5737789      10

estimated correlation:                                   0.4680241
mth root of extended likelihood using deleted predictions: 0.5734835
```

the removal of the next six transforms. In this way, a parsimonious model is generated by the contraction. The contraction stopped because the removal of the next transform would have generated a model with a distinct PD in the LCV score using an LCV ratio test. The estimated correlation is 0.47. Note that all six terms for the dispersion in the expanded model are removed leaving a zero dispersion intercept denoted as VZERO or, equivalently, unit dispersions.

Reference

Stokes, M. E., Davis, C. S., & Koch, G. G. (2012). *Categorical data analysis using the SAS system* (3rd ed.). SAS Institute.

Chapter 9
Example Analyses of the Blood Lead Level Data

Abstract Adaptive analyses are presented of blood lead levels for children at 0, 1, 4, and 6 weeks using exponential regression with the natural log link function. The choice of the number of folds is addressed as well as the choice of the correlation structure. Results are compared for partially modified generalized estimating equations (GEE), fully modified GEE, and extended linear mixed modeling (ELMM). Linearity of the log of the means in week with constant dispersions is addressed as well as a comparison to standard GEE modeling and the dependence of means and dispersions on week. Adaptive additive and adaptive moderation models are generated for week and the indicator for being on the chelating agent succimer. Direct variance modeling of the blood lead levels is addressed and a summary of the analysis results is provided. SAS code for generating these analyses is described along with output generated by that code.

Keywords Direct variance modeling · Extended linear mixed modeling · Generalized estimating equations · Exponential regression · Moderation · Non-constant dispersions

Introduction Adaptive analyses are presented in this chapter of the blood lead level data of Sect. 2.8.4 (Treatment of Lead-exposed Children (TLC) Trial Group, 2000). All LCV scores are computed using matched-set-wise deletion since there are no missing measurements. The cutoff using DF = 1 for a distinct percent decrease in LCV scores for these data is 0.48%. Section 9.1 addresses choosing the number k of folds as described in Sect. 2.6.1 and choosing the correlation structure from among those described in Sect. 2.3. Results are compared for partially modified GEE, fully modified GEE, and ELMM. Section 9.2 addresses linearity of the log of the means in week with constant dispersions, Sect. 9.3 provides a comparison to standard GEE modeling, and Sect. 9.4 addresses the dependence of means and dispersions on week. Adaptive additive and adaptive moderation models are generated for week

Supplementary Information The online version contains supplementary material available at https://doi.org/10.1007/978-3-031-41988-1_9.

G. J. Knafl, *Modeling Correlated Outcomes Using Extensions of Generalized Estimating Equations and Linear Mixed Modeling*,
https://doi.org/10.1007/978-3-031-41988-1_9

and the indicator succimer for being on the chelating agent succimer in Sects. 9.5–9.6, respectively. Section 9.7 addresses direct variance modeling of the blood lead level data. Section 9.8 provides a summary of the analysis results described in prior sections while Sect. 9.9 provides example SAS code for generating such analyses and descriptions of output generated by that code.

The primary purpose of Chap. 9 is to compare adaptive modeling results for partially modified GEE, fully modified GEE, and ELMM applied to continuous positive-valued correlated outcomes using exponential regression models. Partially modified GEE (see Chap. 3 for details) extends standard GEE (see Chap. 2 for details) by adding extra estimating equations for dispersion parameters to the standard GEE estimating equations for mean parameters. Fully modified GEE (see Chap. 4 for details) extends standard GEE further by providing alternative estimating equations for mean parameters while utilizing the same estimating equations for the dispersions used by partially modified GEE. These new estimating equations are based on minimizing an extended likelihood function, treated as a likelihood function for brevity in what follows. Both partially modified and fully modified GEE use the standard GEE method of estimating correlation parameters using residuals. ELMM (see Chap. 5 for more details) is based on estimating equations for mean, dispersion, and correlation parameters determined by maximizing the likelihood. The estimating equations for the means and dispersions are the same as for fully modified GEE.

9.1 Choosing the Number of Folds and the Correlation Structure

Exponential regression analyses reported in this section assume constant dispersions. The effects of the number k of folds and of the correlation structure on estimation by partially modified GEE, fully modified GEE, and ELMM are assessed.

Table 9.1 contains results for adaptive models for mean blood lead levels with constant dispersions generated for 36 cases corresponding to each of the three modeling approaches partially modified GEE, fully modified GEE, and ELMM; each of the four correlation structures IND, spatial AR1, EC, and UN; and each of the three numbers k of folds 5, 10, and 15. Note that spatial AR1 correlations are more appropriate than non-spatial AR1 correlations since outcome measurements are not equally spaced in week. The best LCV score of 0.036860 for the 12 partially modified GEE models is achieved at $k = 10$ under UN correlations. The best LCV score of 0.037437 for the 12 fully modified GEE models is achieved at $k = 10$ under UN correlations. The best LCV score of 0.037899 for the 12 ELMM models is achieved at $k = 10$ under UN correlations. Consequently, all three modeling approaches select UN as the most appropriate of the four correlation structures for the dental measurement data and also $k = 10$ folds.

Table 9.1 Adaptive models of mean blood lead levels in power transforms of week for alternate modeling approaches, correlation structures, and numbers of folds assuming constant dispersions

Modeling approach	Correlation	5 folds			10 folds			15 folds		
		Powers of week[a]	LCV score	Clock time (min)	Powers of week[a]	LCV score	Clock time (min)	Powers of week[a]	LCV score	Clock time (min)
Partially modified GEE	IND	0, −0.2	0.030104	1.9	0, −0.2	0.030373	4.1	0, −0.2	0.030353	5.8
	AR1	0, −1.32, −3	0.032950	16.3	0, −0.11	0.032996	23.0	0, −0.1	0.032949	29.9
	EC	0, −0.26	0.035447	3.8	0, −5.26, −1.7	0.036051	17.5	0, −0.26	0.035651	13.8
	UN	0, 0.5	0.036602	15.4	0, 1.52	0.036860	36.1	0, 1.41	0.036816	44.5
Fully modified GEE	IND	0, −0.3	0.030488	1.0	0, −0.3	0.030739	2.0	0, −0.2	0.030710	3.4
	AR1	0, −0.19	0.033034	4.6	0, −0.19	0.033338	8.7	0, −0.1	0.033233	13.9
	EC	0, −0.28	0.035777	3.8	0, −0.28	0.036054	11.0	0, −0.27	0.035955	78.7
	UN	0	0.036770	24.2	1, 1.99, 0.3	0.037437	37.7	0	0.036999	35.2
ELMM	IND	0, −0.3	0.030488	0.1	0, −0.3	0.030739	0.2	0, −0.2	0.030710	0.3
	AR1	0, −0.16	0.033045	0.8	0, −0.14	0.033346	4.5	0, −0.11	0.033286	2.7
	EC	0, −0.28	0.035778	0.4	0, −0.28	0.036054	0.7	0, −0.27	0.035955	1.0
	UN	0, −2.39, −7	0.037622	9.0	0, −2.65, −4.1	0.037899	12.9	0, −0.2981	0.037670	9.7

AR1 spatial autoregressive order 1, *EC* exchangeable correlations, *ELMM* extended linear mixed modeling, *GEE* generalized estimating equations, *IND* independent, *LCV* likelihood cross-validation, *UN* unstructured

[a]A power of 0 corresponds to an intercept parameter; otherwise, the model has a zero intercept

The model generated by partially modified GEE computed using ELMM has 10-fold LCV score 0.036022 with distinct percent decrease (PD) 4.95% (i.e., greater than the cutoff 0.48% for a distinct PD in the LCV score). The model generated by fully modified GEE computed using ELMM using $k = 10$ has 10-fold LCV score 0.037093 with distinct PD 2.13%. Consequently, ELMM generates a distinctly better model for the data than the two modified GEE modeling approaches.

Table 9.1 also contains clock times for generated models. Clock times for partially modified GEE range from 1.9 to 44.5 min with a total over all 12 cases of about 3.5 h, for fully modified GEE from 1.0 to 78.7 min for a total of about 3.7 h, and for ELMM from 0.1 to 12.9 min for a total of about 0.7 h (totals not reported in Table 9.1). Note that clock times are rounded to 1 decimal digit, but sums are based on unrounded values and so may not be the same as the sum of the rounded values. Consequently, ELMM requires less overall computation time, with partially modified GEE taking about 5.0 times as much and fully modified GEE about 5.3 times as much.

The use of UN correlations can increase computation times substantially. For example, the ELMM model with UN correlations based on $k = 10$ folds requires 12.9 min compared to 0.7 min or 18.4 times more than the associated model with EC correlations generating the next best 10-fold LCV score. The model with UN correlations is also more complex having 3 mean parameters, 1 dispersion parameter, and $4 \cdot (3)/2 = 6$ correlation parameters, 6 more than the associated model with EC correlations having 2 mean parameters, 1 dispersion parameter, and 1 correlation parameter. On the other hand, the model with EC correlations has LCV score 0.036054 with PD 4.87% compared to the LCV score 0.037899 for the model with UN correlations. This is a distinct PD compared to the cutoff using DF = 6 of 1.56% for the data, indicating that there is a distinct benefit in this case to the use of UN correlations.

The adaptive model using ELMM, UN correlations, and $k = 10$ folds has means based on $\text{week}^{-2.65}$ and $\text{week}^{-4.1}$ with an intercept and estimated constant dispersions 0.12. Figure 9.1 provides the plot of estimated means for blood lead levels over weeks 0–6. Mean blood lead level decreases from 24.6 μg/dL at week 0 to 10.1 μg/dL at week 2 and then increases to 22.9 μg/dL at week 6. Estimated UN correlations are provided in Table 9.2. They range from 0.26 for measurements at weeks 0 and 1 to 0.78 for measurements at weeks 1 and 4.

9.2 Assessing Linearity of the Log of the Means in Week

Using ELMM with constant dispersions, $k = 10$ folds, and UN correlations as identified as the appropriate alternative in Sect. 9.1, the linear polynomial model in week has LCV score 0.036076 with distinct PD of 4.81% compared to the adaptive model in week with LCV score 0.037899. Consequently, the log blood lead level means are distinctly nonlinear in week when the dispersions are treated as constant.

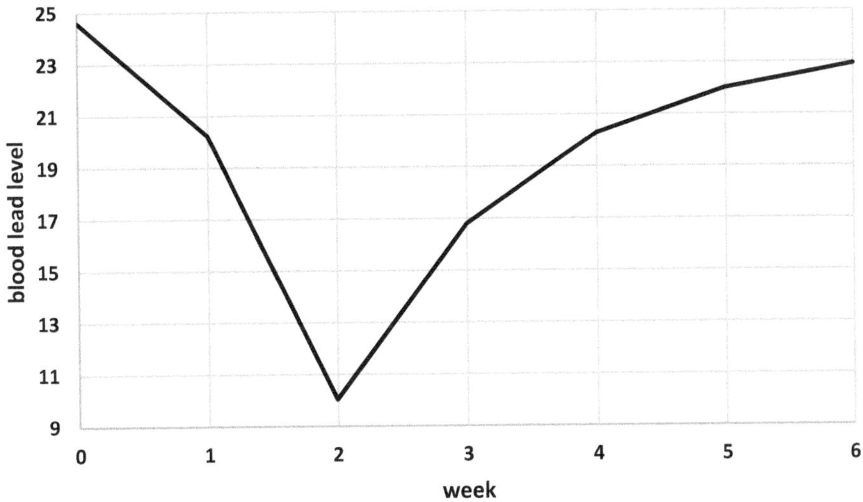

Fig. 9.1 Estimated mean blood level levels in μg/dL over 0–6 weeks under the ELMM model in week with constant dispersions

Table 9.2 Estimated unstructured correlations for blood lead levels at weeks 0, 1, 4, and 6[a]

week	1	4	6
0	0.26	0.42	0.58
1		0.78	0.47
4			0.55

[a]Using extended linear mixed modeling with 10 folds with means based on week and constant dispersions

9.3 Comparison to Standard GEE Modeling

When dispersions are treated as constant, the only difference between partially modified GEE and standard GEE is how the constant dispersion parameter is estimated. Partially modified GEE uses a bias-unadjusted estimate (Sect. 3.5) while standard GEE uses a bias-adjusted estimate (Sect. 2.4). Standard GEE is thus a possible alternative to partially modified GEE for modeling means with constant dispersions. For the blood lead level data, the adaptively generated standard GEE model for the means assuming unit dispersions (to reduce the computations; see Sect. 3.5) is based on week$^{0.05}$ without an intercept and very small LCV score 0.001878. The problem is that degenerate estimates of the UN correlation parameters can occur when combined with unit dispersions. In contrast, the adaptively generated standard GEE model for the means assuming constant dispersions is based on week^2 with an intercept and much improved LCV score 0.035595. The associated partially modified GEE model has LCV score 0.036860 so that the latter standard GEE model generates a distinct PD 3.43%, indicating that in this case partially modified GEE modeling distinctly outperforms standard GEE modeling using constant dispersions, and so this also holds using unit dispersions. On the other hand, the standard GEE model using constant dispersions requires 16.8 min of clock time compared to 32.4 min, or about 1.9 times as much, for the partially modified GEE model. However, the model for the means generated by standard GEE modeling computed using ELMM has LCV score 0.036000 with distinct PD 5.01% compared to the LCV score of 0.037899 for the associated ELMM model of Table 9.1.

9.4 Modeling Means and Dispersions in Week

Adaptive analyses of blood lead levels are presented in this section using $k = 10$ folds and the UN correlation structure as determined in Sect. 9.1. Adaptive models for means and non-constant dispersions in week are generated to assess the usual assumption of constant dispersions and are presented in Table 9.3. The three modeling approaches partially modified GEE, fully modified GEE, and ELMM are considered. All three modeling approaches generate models with dispersions based on an intercept and one transform of week. LCV scores for partially modified GEE, fully modified GEE, and ELMM are 0.042153, 0.041962, and 0.040662, respectively, while models assuming constant dispersions of Table 9.1 are 0.036860, 0.037437, and 0.037899 with distinct PDs 12.56%, 10.78%, and 6.80%, respectively. Consequently, results for all three modeling approaches indicate that dispersions are distinctly non-constant in week.

The model generated by partially modified GEE computed using ELMM has 10-fold LCV score 0.040631 with non-distinct PD 0.08%. The model generated by fully modified GEE using ELMM has 10-fold LCV score 0.040640 with non-distinct PD 0.05%. Consequently, all three modified GEE modeling approaches generate competitive models.

Table 9.3 also contains clock times for generated models. The clock time is 495.8 min or about 8.3 h for partially modified GEE, 152.2 min or about 2.5 h for fully modified GEE, and 30.7 min or about 0.5 h for ELMM. Consequently, ELMM

Table 9.3 Adaptive models of blood lead levels for means and dispersions in week[a]

Modeling approach	Transforms of week for means[b]	Transforms of week for dispersions	LCV score	Clock time (min)
Partially modified GEE	1, $\text{week}^{-0.5}$, $\text{week}^{-2.019}$	1, $\text{week}^{-0.1211}$	0.042153	495.8
Fully modified GEE	1, $\text{week}^{-0.19}$	1, $\text{week}^{-0.131}$	0.041962	152.2
ELMM	1, $\text{week}^{-0.17}$	1, $\text{week}^{-0.1}$	0.040662	30.7

ELMM extended linear mixed modeling, *GEE* generalized estimating equations, *LCV* likelihood cross-validation
[a]Computed with unstructured correlations and 10 folds
[b]A value of 1 corresponds to an intercept; otherwise, the model has a zero intercept

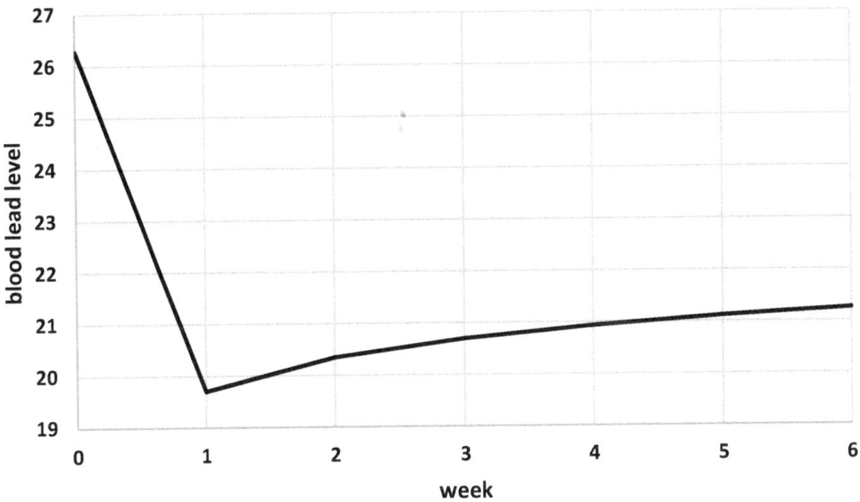

Fig. 9.2 Estimated mean blood level levels in μg/dL over 0–6 weeks under the ELMM model in week with dispersions also depending on week

requires less computation time, with partially modified GEE taking about 16.1 times as much and fully modified GEE about 5.0 times as much.

The adaptive model using ELMM and $k = 10$ folds has means based on week$^{-0.17}$ with an intercept. Figure 9.2 provides the plot of estimated means for blood lead levels over weeks 0–6. Mean blood lead levels decrease from 26.3 μg/dL at week 0 to 19.7 μg/dL at week 1 and then increase gradually to 21.2 μg/dL at week 6, and so follow a different pattern than the model for the means assuming constant dispersions of Fig. 9.1. The adaptive model using ELMM and $k = 10$ folds has dispersions based on week$^{-0.1}$ with an intercept. Figure 9.3 provides the plot of estimated standard deviations for blood lead levels over weeks 0–6. These standard deviations increase from 4.5 μg/dL at week 0 to 7.3 μg/dL at week 1 and then decreases gradually to 7.0 μg/dL at week 6. Estimated UN correlations are provided in Table 9.4. They range from 0.42 for measurements at weeks 0 and 1 to 0.84 for measurements at weeks 1 and 4, and so are stronger than those of Table 9.2.

9.5 Additive Models in Week and Being on Succimer

Table 9.5 contains results for adaptive models for mean blood lead levels in terms of week and the indicator succimer for being on the chelating agent succimer with constant dispersions based on partially modified GEE, fully modified GEE, and ELMM. None of the models contain an additive effect to the indicator succimer. They are also the same models as generated assuming constant dispersions of

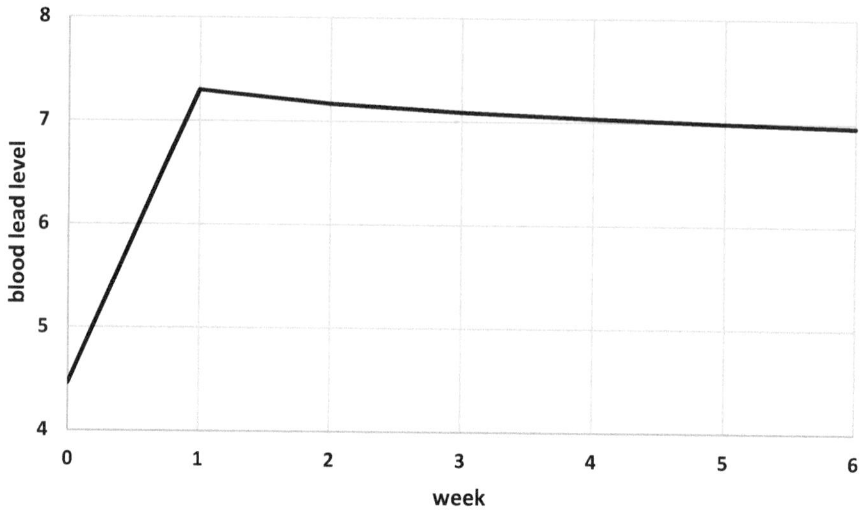

Fig. 9.3 Estimated blood lead level extended standard deviations in μg/dL over 0–6 weeks under the ELMM model in week with means and dispersions depending on week

Table 9.4 Estimated unstructured correlations for blood lead levels at weeks 0, 1, 4, and 6[a]

week	1	4	6
0	0.42	0.46	0.57
1		0.84	0.54
4			0.56

[a]Using extended linear mixed modeling with 10 folds with means and dispersions based on week

Table 9.1. Consequently, as indicated in Sect. 9.1, ELMM generates a distinctly better model for the data than the two modified GEE modeling approaches.

Table 9.5 also contains clock times for adaptive additive models generated with constant dispersions. The clock times are 33.8 min for partially modified GEE, 34.9 min for fully modified GEE, and 12.7 min for ELMM. Consequently, ELMM requires less computation time, with partially modified GEE taking about 2.7 times as much and fully modified GEE about 2.7 times as much.

Table 9.5 also contains results for adaptive additive models for blood lead level means and dispersions in terms of week and the indicator for being on succimer based on partially modified GEE, fully modified GEE, and ELMM. The generated model for partially modified GEE is not provided because of an excessively long clock time; the computation was aborted after taking over 15 h. The fully modified GEE model has LCV score 0.045121 while the ELMM model has LCV score 0.044400. In contrast, the associated constant dispersion models for fully modified GEE and ELMM of Table 9.5 have LCV scores 0.037437 and 0.037899 with distinct PDs of 17.03% and 14.64%, respectively. Consequently, additive models for dispersions in week and succimer outperform associated constant dispersion models. However, the associated models for the means do not include an additive effect to

Table 9.5 Adaptive additive models of blood lead levels in week and the indicator for being on succimer[a]

	Modeling means and dispersions				Modeling means with constant dispersions		
Modeling approach	Transforms for means[b]	Transforms for dispersions	LCV score	Clock time (min)	Transforms for means[2]	LCV score	Clock time (min)
Partially modified GEE	—[c]	—[c]	—[c]	—[c]	1, $week^{1.52}$	0.036860	33.8
Fully modified GEE	1, $week^{0.08}$	1, succimer, $week^{-0.05}$	0.045121	107.6	1, $week^{1.99}$, $week^{0.3}$	0.037437	34.9
ELMM	1, $week^{0.01}$	1, succimer, $week^{-0.03}$	0.044400	23.7	1, $week^{-2.65}$, $week^{-4.1}$	0.037899	12.7

ELMM extended linear mixed modeling, *GEE* generalized estimating equations, *LCV* likelihood cross-validation

[a]Computed with unstructured correlations and 10 folds

[b]A value of 1 corresponds to an intercept parameter; otherwise, the model has a zero intercept. The variable succimer is the indicator for being on the chelating agent succimer

[c]Adaptive generation of the model was aborted during the contraction after running over 15 h without completing

succimer, and so the distinct additive effect to being on succimer is for the dispersions. The fully modified GEE model computed using ELMM has LCV score 0.044381 with non-distinct PD 0.04%. Consequently, in this case, fully modified GEE and ELMM generate competitive models.

Table 9.5 also contains clock times for adaptive additive models for means and dispersions. The clock times are 107.6 min or about 1.8 h for fully modified GEE and 23.7 min or about 0.4 h for ELMM. Consequently, ELMM requires less computation time, with fully modified GEE about 4.5 times as much. The exact clock time for partially modified GEE is not available but it would be larger than 15 h and so more than 37 time longer than for ELMM. Also, as reported in Sect. 9.4, the partially modified GEE model of Table 9.3 required about 8.3 h or about 16.1 times longer than the associated ELMM model. These are excessively long times, and so partially modified GEE modeling is not considered in subsequent analyses.

9.6 Adaptive Moderation of the Effect of Week by Being on Succimer

Table 9.6 contains results for an assessment of adaptive moderation of the effect of week on blood lead level means assuming constant dispersions based on two modeling approaches: fully modified GEE and ELMM. Neither model contains an additive effect to the indicator succimer. The fully modified GEE model also does not contain any geometric combinations in week and succimer, but the ELMM model contains one such geometric combination. The fully modified GEE model is the same as the associated additive model. The ELMM additive model of Table 9.5 associated with the ELMM moderation model of Table 9.6 has LCV score 0.037899 with non-distinct PD 0.22%. Consequently, moderation is not supported with both fully modified GEE and ELMM assuming constant dispersions. The fully modified GEE model of Table 9.6 when run using ELMM has LCV score 0.037093 with distinct PD 2.35% compared to the Table 9.6 ELMM model, indicating that in this case ELMM distinctly outperforms fully modified GEE

Table 9.6 Adaptive moderation models for means of blood lead levels in week, being on succimer, and geometric combinations with constant dispersions[a]

Modeling approach	Mean transforms[b]	LCV score	Clock time (min)
Fully modified GEE	1, $\text{week}^{1.99}$, $\text{week}^{0.3}$	0.037437	42.9
ELMM	1, $(\text{succimer}\cdot\text{week}^{3.9})^{-2}$, $\text{week}^{0.11}$	0.037984	38.2

ELMM extended linear mixed modeling, *GEE* generalized estimating equations, *LCV* likelihood cross-validation

[a]Computed with unstructured correlations and 10 folds. Partially modified GEE not considered due to requiring excessive times in prior analyses

[b]A value of 1 corresponds to an intercept parameter; otherwise, the model has a zero intercept. The variable succimer is the indicator for being on the chelating agent succimer

Table 9.6 also contains clock times for adaptive moderation models generated assuming constant dispersions. The clock times are 42.9 min for fully modified GEE and 38.2 min for ELMM. Consequently, ELMM requires less computation time, with fully modified GEE about 1.1 times as much.

The standard linear moderation model has means based on an intercept, main effects to untransformed week and the indicator succimer, and the interaction between week and succimer along with constant dispersions. However, nonlinear moderation assuming constant dispersions is not supported, and so an assessment of whether moderation is distinctly nonlinear is not addressed.

Table 9.7 contains results for an assessment of adaptive moderation of the effect of week on blood lead level means and dispersions based on two modeling approaches: fully modified GEE and ELMM. Geometric combinations based on week and the indicator succimer are generated for the means by both of the two modeling approaches. However, this is not enough to establish moderation. That requires that these models outperform the associated adaptive additive models of Table 9.5. LCV scores for those associated additive models are 0.045185 and 0.044400 with distinct PDs 9.80% and 9.89% for fully modified GEE and ELMM, respectively. Consequently, moderation of the means is established using both of the two modeling approaches. Furthermore, associated constant moderation models of Table 9.6 have LCV scores 0.037437 and 0.037984 with distinct PDs of 25.27% and 22.91% compared to the moderation models with non-constant dispersions of Table 9.7 for fully modified GEE and ELMM, respectively. Moreover, geometric combinations based on week and the indicator succimer are also generated for the dispersions by both of the two modeling approaches indicating that the effect of succimer on the dispersions is more complex than can be modeled additively as indicated by the distinct improvement over the additive models of Table 9.5.

The fully modified GEE model computed using ELMM has LCV score 0.049597 so that the ELMM generates an LCV score with PD 0.65%. Although this PD is greater than the cutoff of 0.35% for a distinct PD, that cutoff is based on 1 degree of

Table 9.7 Adaptive moderation models for means and dispersions of blood lead levels in week, being on succimer, and geometric combinations[a]

Modeling approach	Mean transforms[b]	Dispersion transforms	LCV score	Clock time (min)
Fully modified GEE	1, $(\text{succimer}\cdot\text{week}^{-0.91})^{-2.0989}$, $\text{succimer}\cdot\text{week}^{7}$, $\text{week}^{0.21}$	1, succimer, $(\text{week}^{0.089}\cdot\text{succimer})^{-0.9}$, $\text{week}^{0.1}$	0.050096	288.3
ELMM	1, $(\text{week}^{0.06}\cdot\text{succimer})^{-3.6}$, $\text{week}^{0.22}$, $(\text{week}^{8}\cdot\text{succimer})^{2}$	1, $(\text{week}^{-0.1}\cdot\text{succimer})^{0.6}$	0.049274	82.5

ELMM extended linear mixed modeling; *GEE* generalized estimating equations; *LCV* likelihood cross-validation

[a]Computed with unstructured correlations and 10 folds. Partially modified GEE not considered due to requiring excessive times in prior analyses

[b]A value of 1 corresponds to an intercept parameter; otherwise, the model has a zero intercept. The variable succimer is the indicator for being on the chelating agent succimer

freedom while the ELMM model is based on two less transforms for the dispersions and the same number four transforms for the means as the fully modified model. The expanded model generated by ELMM has four transforms for both means and dispersions, the same as for the model selected by fully modified GEE, and LCV score 0.049450 with non-distinct PD 0.29% compared to that fully modified GEE model. The contraction step removes two dispersion transforms from the ELMM model. The PD for each contraction is less than 0.35% because otherwise the contraction would stop earlier. Consequently, fully modified GEE and ELMM generate competitive models with ELMM generating a more parsimonious model than fully modified GEE.

Table 9.7 also contains clock times for adaptive moderation models allowing for non-constant dispersions. The clock times are 288.3 min or about 4.8 h for fully modified GEE and 82.5 min or about 1.4 h for ELMM. Consequently, ELMM requires less computation time, with fully modified GEE about 3.5 times as much.

Figure 9.4 provides the plot of estimated means for blood lead levels over weeks 0–6 based on the adaptive moderation model of Table 9.7. For children on a placebo, mean blood lead levels decrease from 26.4 μg/dL at week 0 to 24.7 μg/dL at week 1 and then continue to decrease gradually to 23.9 μg/dL at week 6. For children on succimer, mean blood lead levels decrease from 26.4 μg/dL at week 0 to 13.5 μg/dL at week 1 and then increase to 31.2 μg/dL at week 6. Figure 9.5 provides the plot of estimated dispersions for blood lead levels over weeks 0–6. For children on a placebo, the estimated dispersions are constant at 0.04 μg/dL at weeks 0–6. On the other hand, for children on succimer, the estimated dispersions increase from 0.04 μg/dL at week 0 to 0.41 μg/dL at week 1 and then decrease to 0.32 μg/dL at week 6. Consequently, although post-baseline mean blood lead levels are lower over

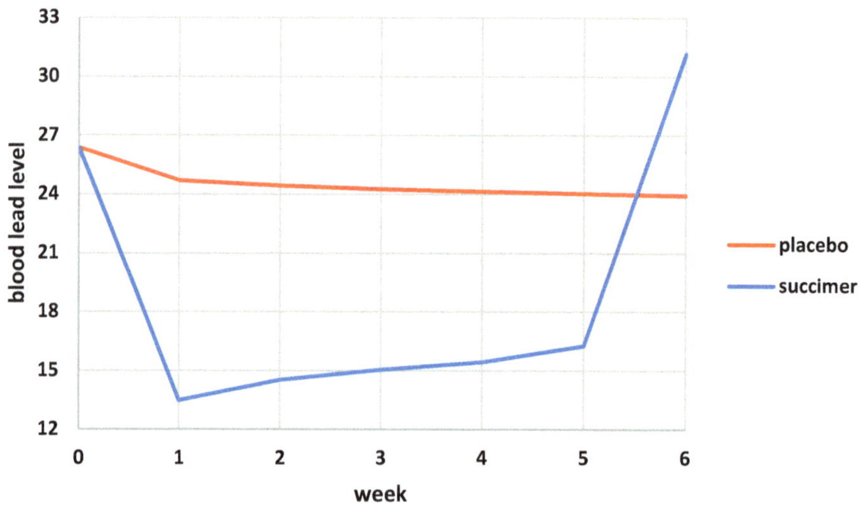

Fig. 9.4 Estimated mean blood level levels in μg/dL over 0–6 weeks under the ELMM model in week, the indicator succimer, and geometric combinations

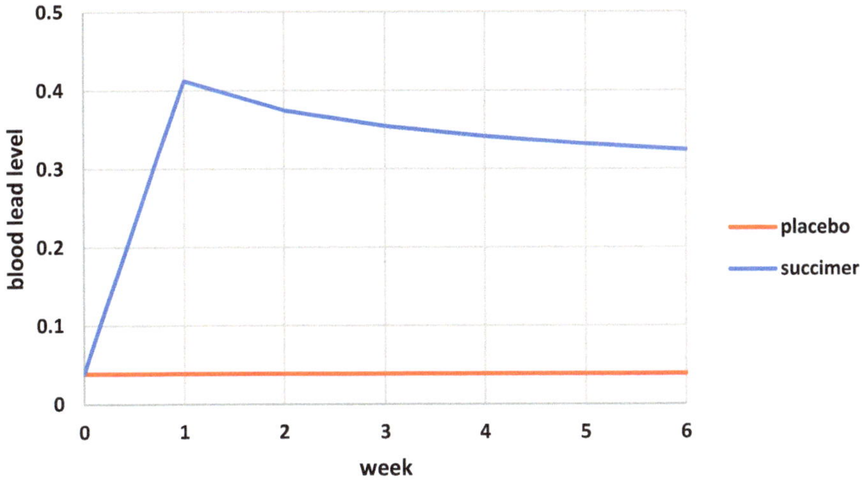

Fig. 9.5 Estimated dispersions for blood lead levels in μg/dL over 0–6 weeks under the ELMM model in week, the indicator succimer, and geometric combinations

time for children on succimer except at week 6, there is more variability in those post-baseline blood lead levels than for children on a placebo. Estimated UN correlations are provided in Table 9.8. They range from 0.64 for measurements at weeks 0 and 1, 0 and 4, and 0 and 6 to 0.81 for measurements at weeks 1 and 4.

Figure 9.6 displays the plot of standardized residuals by week and by being on succimer versus a placebo. There are three outliers with absolute value greater than 3.00. The child with ID 100 in the succimer group has blood lead levels 20.7, 8.1, 25.7, and 12.3 μg/dL at weeks 0, 1, 4, and 6 with the value at week 4 having standardized residual 3.13. The child with ID 98 in the succimer group has blood lead levels 29.4, 22.1, 25.3, and 4.1 μg/dL at weeks 0, 1, 4, and 6 with the value at week 4 having standardized residual −3.37. The child with ID 40 in the succimer group has blood lead levels 33.7, 14.9, 14.5, and 63.9 μg/dL at weeks 0, 1, 4, and 6 with the value at week 6 having the extreme standardized residual 5.34, and the value 63.9 μg/dL is the largest value at week 6 while the next largest value at week 6 is 43.3 μg/dL. This extreme value may be why there is such a large estimated mean at week 6 for the succimer, but that is not addressed further here.

Table 9.8 Estimated unstructured correlations for blood lead levels using the adaptive moderation model based on direct variance modeling at weeks 0, 1, 4, and 6[a]

week	1	4	6
0	0.64	0.64	0.64
1		0.81	0.66
4			0.72

[a]Using extended linear mixed modeling with 10 folds with means and dispersions based on week, the indicator succimer, and geometric combinations

Table 9.9 Adaptive models of blood lead levels for means and dispersions using direct variance modeling[a]

Predictors	Mean transforms[b]	Dispersion transforms[2]	LCV score	Clock time (min)
Week	1, $\text{week}^{-0.17}$	1, $\text{week}^{-0.08}$	0.040630	38.6
Week, succimer	1, $\text{week}^{0.06}$	1, succimer, $\text{week}^{-0.09}$	0.044408	32.5
Week, succimer, GCs	1, $(\text{week}^{0.08}\cdot\text{succimer})^{-2.7}$, $\text{week}^{0.3}$, $(\text{week}^{8}\cdot\text{succimer})^{2}$	1, $(\text{week}^{-0.1}\cdot\text{succimer})^{-1.4}$, succimer	0.049388	168.6

ELMM extended linear mixed modeling, *GCs* geometric combinations, *GEE* generalized estimating equations, *LCV* likelihood cross-validation

[a]Computed with extended linear mixed modeling, unstructured correlations, and 10 folds

[b]A value of 1 corresponds to an intercept parameter; otherwise, the model has a zero intercept. The variable succimer is the indicator for being on the chelating agent succimer

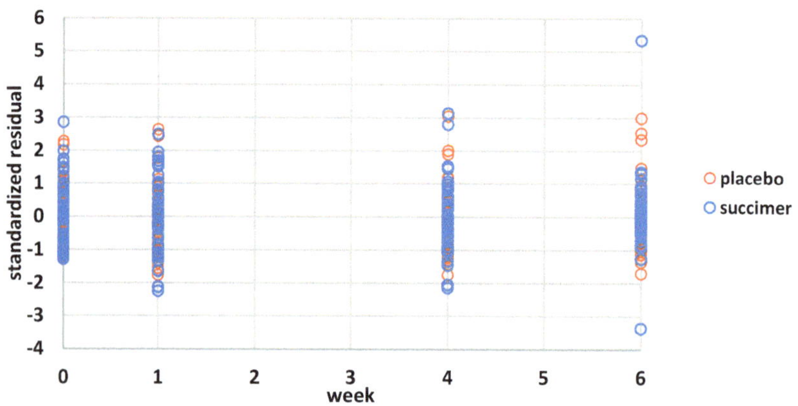

Fig. 9.6 Standardized residuals for blood lead levels by week and being on succimer versus on a placebo based on direct variance modeling

9.7 Direct Variance Modeling of Blood Lead Level Data

Direct variance modeling treats the variance function as $V(\mu) = 1$ so that the variances are the same as the dispersions. Table 9.9 contains direct variance modeling results for the blood lead level data using ELMM. The adaptive model for the means and dispersions of blood lead levels in week using direct variance modeling has LCV score 0.040630. The associated adaptive extended variance model of Table 9.3 has LCV score 0.040662, and so the direct variance model is a competitive alternative with PD 0.08%. The adaptive additive model for the means and dispersions of blood lead levels in week and succimer using direct variance modeling has LCV score 0.044408. The associated adaptive additive model of Table 9.5 has LCV score 0.044400 with non-distinct PD 0.02% and so is a competitive alternative to the direct variance model. The adaptive moderation model for the means and dispersions of blood lead levels in week, succimer, and geometric combinations using direct variance modeling has LCV score 0.049388. The adaptive additive model of Table 9.9 has distinct PD 10.08%, and so direct variance modeling supports the conclusion of a distinct moderation effect. The associated adaptive extended variance moderation model of Table 9.7 has LCV score 0.049274 with non-distinct PD 0.23% and so is a competitive alternative to the direct variance moderation model. Moreover, it is simpler with the same number of mean parameters and one less dispersion parameters. Consequently, the extended variance moderation model of Table 9.7 is the most appropriate model for the blood lead level data (Table 9.9).

Under direct variance modeling, clock times are 38.6 min to generate the adaptive model for the means and dispersions of blood lead levels in week, 32.5 min to generate the associated adaptive additive model in week and the indicator succimer, and 168.6 min to generate the associated adaptive model allowing for both main effects and geometric combinations in week and succimer for a total of 239.7 min or about 4.0 h. Associated models with extended variances depending on means are 30.7 min to generate the adaptive model for the means and dispersions of blood lead levels in week of Table 9.3, 23.7 min to generate the associated adaptive additive model in week and the indicator succimer of Table 9.5, and 82.5 min to generate the associated adaptive model allowing for both main effects and geometric combinations in week and succimer of Table 9.7 for a total of 136.9 min or about 2.3 h so that direct variance modeling requires about 1.8 times more.

9.8 Analysis Summary

A summary of the results of analyses of the blood lead level data is provided broken down into seven categories of results.

1. Models for Means in Week Assuming Constant Dispersions

The preferable model for the blood lead level data has UN correlations with LCV scores based on $k = 10$ folds. The model selected by ELMM distinctly outperforms the models selected by partially and fully modified GEE. Estimated mean blood lead levels are plotted in Fig. 9.1. The log of the mean blood lead levels is distinctly nonlinear in week assuming constant dispersions. The model generated by standard GEE using constant dispersions (because it outperforms the associated unit dispersion model) is distinctly inferior to the model generated by partially modified GEE and to the ELMM model. ELMM requires less time with partially modified GEE requiring about 5.0 times as much and fully modified GEE requiring about 5.3 times as much.

2. Models for Means and Dispersions in Week

Models selected by partially modified GEE, fully modified GEE, and ELMM are all competitive alternatives. Dispersions are distinctly non-constant in week. Estimated means for the ELMM model are plotted in Fig. 9.2 and estimated extended standard deviations in Fig. 9.3. ELMM requires less time with partially modified GEE requiring about 16.1 times as much and fully modified GEE requiring about 5.0 times as much.

3. Additive Models in Week and Being on Succimer

Models selected by partially modified GEE, fully modified GEE, and ELMM assuming constant dispersions are all the same as non-additive models for the means in week assuming constant dispersions, and so the model selected by ELMM distinctly outperforms the models selected by partially and fully modified GEE. Mean blood lead levels are reasonably considered not to change additively with being on succimer when dispersions are treated as constant. ELMM requires less time with partially modified GEE requiring about 2.7 times as much and fully modified GEE requiring about 2.7 times as much.

Models selected by fully modified GEE and ELMM allowing for non-constant dispersions are competitive alternatives. Dispersions for blood lead levels are reasonably considered to change additively with being on succimer while means are reasonably considered not to change additively with being on succimer. ELMM requires less time with fully modified GEE requiring about 4.5 times as much. The partially modified GEE model was canceled due to requiring an excessive amount of time, and so partially modified GEE is not considered further.

4. Moderation Models in Week and Being on Succimer

Assuming constant dispersions, the model selected by ELMM distinctly outperforms the model selected by fully modified GEE. The effect of week on mean blood lead levels is reasonably considered not to be moderated by being on succimer when dispersions are treated as constant. ELMM requires less time with fully modified GEE requiring about 1.1 times as much.

Models selected by fully modified GEE and ELMM allowing for non-constant dispersions are competitive alternatives, but only after accounting for the ELMM model having two less parameters. The effects of week on blood lead level means and dispersions are reasonably considered to be moderated by being on succimer. ELMM requires less time with fully modified GEE requiring about 3.5 times as much.

5. Direct Variance Models for Blood Lead Levels

The direct variance model generated accounting for the effect to visit on means and dispersions is a competitive alternative to the associated extended variance model treating variances as a function of the means and dispersions. This is also the case for additive and moderation models in visit and being on active treatment.

Altogether, these direct variance models require 2.3 times more time than associated extended variance models.

6. All Models for Blood Lead Levels in Week and Being on Succimer

In three cases, the model generated by ELMM is distinctly superior to the associated model generated by fully modified GEE. In the other cases, fully modified GEE and ELMM generate competitive models. Over all clock times reported in Tables 9.1, 9.3, and 9.5–9.7, ELMM requires about 4.7 h compared to about 16.0 h or about 3.4 times as much for fully modified GEE. Partially modified GEE can require excessive times and so is not considered in some cases. In two of the cases it is considered, it generates distinctly inferior models. The direct variance models of Table 9.8 add about 6.1 h to give a total of about 10.8 h for ELMM modeling.

7. Selected Model for Blood Lead Levels in Week and Being on Succimer

Under the most appropriate model for the blood lead levels based on extended variance modeling, estimated means are plotted in Fig. 9.4 and extended standard deviations are plotted in Fig. 9.5. Estimated correlations are provided in Table 9.8. Standardized residuals for this model are plotted in Fig. 9.6. There are three outlying measurements.

9.9 Example SAS Code for Analyzing the Blood Lead Level Data

Example SAS code is presented in this section for conducting analyses of blood lead levels as a function of week during the study and treatment group (either taking the chelating agent succimer or taking a placebo). The code assumes that a data set called longtlc has been created in the SAS default library containing the blood lead level data (Sect. 2.8.4) in long format, that is, with one measurement (or row) for each blood lead level at each week for each patient. This data set contains variables (or columns) called id loaded with unique identifiers for patients; lead loaded with blood lead levels in μg/dL; week set to weeks during the study of 0, 1, 4, 6; and the indicator succimer set to 1 for patients taking succimer and to 0 for patients taking a placebo. Altogether, there are four blood lead levels at different weeks for each of 100 different patients, 50 taking succimer and 50 taking a placebo, for a total of 400 measurements.

The code also assumes that a %include statement has been executed to load in the current version of the genreg macro for use in conducting adaptive analyses. The genreg macro supports a wide variety of macro parameters, some of which are described here. The interface for this macro contains the complete list of macro parameters along with their default settings. Default settings are used by the macro if a value for the macro parameter has not been specified in the code invoking the macro. Macro parameter settings are case insensitive. The cutoff for a distinct percent decrease in LCV scores (Sect. 2.6.2) using DF = 1 for these data with 400 measurements is 0.48%.

9.9.1 Modeling Means in Week Assuming Constant Dispersions

The following code uses the genreg macro to generate the adaptive model for blood lead level means as a possibly nonlinear function of visit using $k = 10$ folds, unstructured (UN) correlations, and extended linear mixed modeling (ELMM) as selected in Sect. 9.1 assuming constant dispersions.

```
%genreg(modtype=expon,datain=longtlc,yvar=lead,matchvar=id,
withinvr=week,foldcnt=10,corrtype=UN,GEE=n,srchtype=logL,
expand=y,expxvars=week,contract=y);
```

The modtype macro parameter specifies the model type, in this case "modtype=expon" means treat the outcome variable as exponentially distributed with natural log link function, that is, use exponential regression (Sect. 2.2.4). The datain macro parameter indicates that the data to be analyzed is contained in the longtlc data set loaded in the SAS default library. The yvar macro parameter specifies the name of the outcome variable, in this case the variable lead. The matchvar and withinvr macro parameters specify, respectively, the variable containing unique identifiers for different matched sets, in this case the variable id identifying different patients, and the variable containing within matched set values, in this case the variable week. The corrtype macro parameter specifies the correlation structure, in this case the UN structure. The other possible corrtype settings are "corrtype=IND", "corrtype=AR1", and "corrtype=EC" for independent, spatial autoregressive order 1, and exchangeable correlations, respectively. To request that the clock time for an invocation of the macro be printed in the output, add the setting "rprttime=y" where the value "y" is short for "yes" while the default setting is "rprttime=n" with "n" short for "no".

The modeling approach used by genreg is determined by the combination of the GEE and srchtype macro parameters. In this case, "GEE=n" means use ELMM while "srchtype=logL" means base estimation on maximizing the log-likelihood (as described in Sects. 4.3 and 5.2). These are the default settings for these two macro parameters. Setting "GEE=y" requests GEE modeling. Combining "GEE=y" with "srchtype=GEE" requests partially modified GEE with estimation based on the minimizing the maximum absolute value of the gradient (as described in Sect. 3.7). Combining "GEE=y" with "srchtype=logL" requests fully modified GEE. By default, partially modified and fully modified GEE use bias-unadjusted dispersion estimates. Bias-adjusted dispersion estimates, as used in standard GEE modeling (Sect. 2.4), are requested by adding the setting "biasadj=y".

Adaptive modeling is requested using "expand=y" together with "contract=y" meaning first expand the base model and then contract the expanded model. In this case, the base model has constant means and constant dispersions based on only intercept parameters (but this can be changed). The expxvars macro parameter specifies the primary predictor variables for modeling the means to consider in the expansion. In this case, the expansion grows the model for the means by systematically adding in power transforms of the single variable week while holding the dispersions constant. The maximum number of transforms added by the expansion to the model for the means is controlled by the expxmax parameter with default value "expxmax=5" meaning at most 5 transforms can be added to the means. Changing to the empty setting "expxmax=" removes the restriction on the number of such transforms.

The contraction systematically removes transforms from the expanded model for the means, possibly the constant transform corresponding to the intercept, and adjusts the powers of the remaining transforms to increase the LCV score, which in this case is computed with 10 folds as specified by the setting of the foldcnt macro parameter. It is also computed using matched-set-wise deletion corresponding to the default setting "measdlte=n". Measurement-wise deletion is requested using "measdlte=y". The contraction can optionally be restricted not to remove the intercept for the means in order to generate a non-zero intercept model. An LCV ratio test is used to decide when to stop the contraction. The contraction also stops when there is only one transform remaining in the model for the means. When the contraction leaves the expanded model unchanged, that expanded model has its powers adjusted to increase the LCV score.

The following code directly generates the above adaptive model selected with $k = 10$ folds, UN correlations, and ELMM, including parameter estimates and LCV score.

```
%genreg(modtype=expon,datain=longtlc,yvar=lead,matchvar=id,
withinvr=week,foldcnt=10,corrtype=UN,GEE=n,srchtype=logL,
xintrcpt=y,xvars=week week,xpowers=−2.65 –4.1);
```

The xintrcpt macro parameter specifies whether or not the base model for the means includes an intercept, the xvars macro parameter provides the list of primary predictors for the base model for the means, and the xpowers macro parameter the powers for transforming those primary predictors. In this case, the model for the means has an intercept along with the two transforms $\text{week}^{-2.65}$ and $\text{week}^{-4.1}$. The default values for these macro parameters are "xintrcpt=y", "xvars=", and "xpowers=" requesting constant means. An empty setting for the xvars macro parameter means includes no transforms for the means, and an empty setting for the xpowers macro parameter means power transform xvars variables if any with the power 1 (and so include them untransformed). The model for the dispersions is based on macro parameters vintrcpt, vvars, and vpowers with analogous meanings and with the same default settings requesting constant dispersions. The xvalid macro parameter is not set in the above code and so has its default setting "xvalid=y" meaning to compute the LCV score for the requested model. In this case, the model has LCV score 0.037899. Adding the setting "xvalid=n" means compute only parameter estimates for the requested model and not the LCV score.

The above code can be changed to generate the standard linear polynomial model for the means based on untransformed week as follows. First change the setting for the xvars macro parameters to "xvars=week". Then change the setting for the xpowers macro parameter to "xpowers=1" or remove the setting for the xpowers macro parameter so that it has its default empty value, which means to use the power 1 to transform all variables listed in the setting of the xvars macro parameter. Note that the log of the means is linear in week, but the means are nonlinear due to using the natural log link function. To request the standard quadratic polynomial model for the means, use the settings "xintrcpt=y", "xvars=week week", and "xpowers=1 2".

9.9.2 Modeling Means and Dispersions in Week

The following code uses the genreg macro to generate the adaptive model for blood lead level means and non-constant dispersions as possibly nonlinear functions of week using $k = 10$ folds, UN correlations, and ELMM.

```
%genreg(modtype=expon,datain=longtlc,yvar=lead,matchvar=id,
withinvr=week,foldcnt=10,corrtype=UN,GEE=n,srchtype=logL,
expand=y,expxvars=week,expvvars=week,contract=y);
```

Adaptive modeling is requested using "expand=y" together with "contract=y" meaning first expand the base model with constant means and constant dispersions and then contract the expanded model. The expxvars and expvvars macro parameters specify the primary predictor variables to consider in the expansion for the means and dispersions, respectively. In this case, the same set of primary predictors is used for the means and for the dispersions, but different sets of primary predictors can be specified. The expansion grows the model for the means and the dispersions in combination by systematically adding in power transforms of the single variable week one-at-a-time to either the means or the dispersions, whichever generates the better LCV score. Similar to the expxmax parameter, the expvmax parameter specifies the maximum number of transforms added by the expansion to the model for the dispersions with default value "expvmax=5" meaning at most 5 transforms can be added to the dispersions. Changing to the empty setting "expvmax=" removes the restriction on the number of such transforms.

The contraction systematically removes transforms from the expanded model for the means and dispersions in combination, possibly the constant transforms corresponding to intercepts, and adjusts the powers of the remaining transforms to increase the LCV score. Transforms are removed one-at-a-time from either the means or the dispersions, whichever generates the better LCV score after adjusting all the powers of the remaining transforms for both the means and the dispersions. An LCV ratio test is used to decide when to stop the contraction. The contraction stops removing transforms from the means when there is only one transform remaining in the model for the means. Also, by default, the contraction stops removing transforms from the dispersions when there is only one transform remaining in the model for the dispersions. Unit dispersion models can be considered in the contraction by changing the setting of the cnvzero parameter from its default setting of "cnvzero=n" to "cnvzero=y". When the contraction leaves the expanded model unchanged, that expanded model has its powers adjusted to increase the LCV score.

The following code directly generates the above adaptive model selected with $k = 10$ folds, UN correlations, and ELMM, including parameter estimates and the LCV score.

```
%genreg(modtype=expon,datain=longtlc,yvar=lead,matchvar=id,
withinvr=week,foldcnt=10,corrtype=UN,GEE=n,srchtype=logL,
xintrcpt=y,xvars=week,xpowers=−0.17,vintrcpt=y,vvars=week,
vpowers=−0.1);
```

In this case, the model for the means is based on an intercept and the single transform $\text{week}^{-0.17}$ while the model for the dispersions is based on an intercept and the single transform $\text{week}^{-0.1}$. The LCV score is 0.040662 while the associated model assuming constant dispersions has LCV score 0.037899 with distinct percent decrease (PD) 6.80%. Consequently, the dispersions are reasonably treated as non-constant in week when the means are modeled in terms of only week.

9.9.3 Additive Models in Week and Being on Succimer

The following code uses the genreg macro to generate the adaptive additive model for blood lead level means and dispersions as possibly nonlinear functions of week and being on succimer using $k = 10$ folds, unstructured (UN) correlations, and extended linear mixed modeling (ELMM).

```
%genreg(modtype=expon,datain=longtlc,yvar=lead,matchvar=id,
withinvr=week,foldcnt=10,corrtype=UN,GEE=n,srchtype=logL,
expand=y,expxvars=week succimer,expvvars=week succimer,
contract=y);
```

In this case, the expxvars and expvvars macro parameters specify the variables week and succimer to be the primary predictor variables to consider in the expansion for the means and dispersions, respectively. The expansion grows the model for the means and the dispersions in combination by systematically adding in power transforms of week or the indicator variable succimer one-at-a-time to either the means or the dispersions, whichever generates the better LCV score. Note that indicator variables like succimer are not transformed and are included at most once in the model for the means and at most once in the model for the dispersions. The contraction then systematically removes transforms from the expanded model for the means and dispersions in combination, possibly the constant transforms corresponding to intercepts, and adjusts the powers of the remaining transforms to increase the LCV score. The model is additive because by default geometric combinations are not considered in the expansion. An adaptive additive model for the means in week and succimer assuming constant dispersions can be generated by changing the expvvars macro parameter to have an empty setting, that is, "expvvars=", or by removing its setting from the above code, because the empty setting is its default setting.

The adaptive additive model in week and succimer assuming constant dispersions is the same as the model for the means in only week assuming constant dispersions. Consequently, being on succimer is reasonably considered not to have an additive effect on the means assuming constant dispersions.

The following code directly generates the adaptive additive model for means and dispersions.

```
%genreg(modtype=expon,datain=longtlc,yvar=lead,matchvar=id,
withinvr=week,foldcnt=10,corrtype=UN,GEE=n,srchtype=logL,
xintrcpt=y,xvars=week,xpowers=0.01,vintrcpt=y,
vvars=succimer week,vpowers=1 -0.03);
```

In this case, the model for the means is based on an intercept and week$^{0.01}$ while the dispersions are based on an intercept, the indicator succimer, and the transform week$^{-0.03}$. The LCV score is 0.044400 while the associated constant dispersion model has LCV score 0.037899 with distinct PD 14.64%. Consequently, the means are reasonably considered to depend only on week while the dispersions are reasonably considered to depend on additive effects to both week and being on succimer.

9.9.4 Moderation Models in Week and Being on Succimer

The following code uses the genreg macro to generate the adaptive moderation model for blood lead level means and dispersions as possibly nonlinear functions of week, being on succimer, and geometric combinations in week and being on succimer using $k = 10$ folds, UN correlations, and ELMM.

```
%genreg(modtype=expon,datain=longtlc,yvar=lead,matchvar=id,
withinvr=week,foldcnt=10,corrtype=UN,GEE=n,srchtype=logL,
expand=y,expxvars=week succimer,expvvars=week succimer,
geomcmbn=y,contract=y);
```

In this case, the expxvars and expvvars macro parameters specify the variables week and succimer to be the primary predictor variables to consider in the expansion for the means and dispersions, respectively. The expansion grows the model for the means and the dispersions in combination by systematically adding in power transforms of week, the indicator variable succimer, or geometric combinations in week and succimer one-at-a-time to either the means or the dispersions, whichever generates the better LCV score. Geometric combinations are considered due to adding the setting "geomcmbn=y" to the code for generating the associated additive model in week and succimer. The default setting for the geomcmbn macro parameter is "geomcmbn=n" meaning to restrict the expansion to an additive model in the variables specified in the expxvars and expvvars settings. The contraction systematically removes transforms from the expanded model for the means and dispersions in combination, possibly the constant transforms corresponding to intercepts, and adjusts the powers of the remaining transforms to increase the LCV score. Note that when a geometric combination of the form $(\text{week}^p \cdot \text{succimer})^q$ or $(\text{succimer} \cdot \text{week}^p)^q$ is generated by the expansion, the contraction only adjusts the power q and leaves the power p unchanged. When there are more than two primary predictors for the means and/or dispersions, geometric combinations can be generated based on any number of two or more of those primary predictors. An adaptive moderation model for the means in week, succimer, and geometric combinations in week and succimer assuming constant dispersions can be generated by changing the expvvars macro parameter to have an empty setting, that is, "expvvars=", or by removing its setting from the above code, because the empty setting is its default setting.

The following code directly generates the adaptive moderation model assuming constant dispersions.

```
%genreg(modtype=expon,datain= longtlc,yvar=lead,matchvar=id,
withinvr=week,foldcnt=10,corrtype=UN,GEE=n,srchtype=logL,
xintrcpt=y,xvars=week,xpowers=0.11,xgcs=succimer 1 week 3.9,
xgcpowrs=−2,vintrcpt=y);
```

In this case, the model for the means is based on an intercept, $\text{week}^{0.11}$, and the geometric combination

$$\left(\text{succimer} \cdot \text{week}^{3.9}\right)^{-2} = \text{succimer} \cdot \text{week}^{-7.8}.$$

The LCV score is 0.037984 while the associated additive model assuming constant dispersions has LCV score 0.037899 with non-distinct PD 0.22%. Consequently, being on succimer is reasonably considered not to moderate the effect of week on the means assuming constant dispersions.

The macro parameters xgcs and xgcpowrs are used to specify geometric combinations for the means. The setting "xgcs=succimer 1 week 3.9" specifies the untransformed geometric combination $\text{succimer} \cdot \text{week}^{3.9}$ while the setting "xgcpowrs=−2" means to transform $\text{succimer} \cdot \text{week}^{3.9}$ to the power -2. The xgcpowrs setting is needed in this case because its default empty setting "xgcpowrs=" means to leave all the geometric combinations specified by the xgcs macro parameter untransformed. Multiple geometric combinations are specified by separating them by colons (:). For example, use the following code to generate the model with means based on an intercept and the two geometric combinations $(\text{week}^2 \cdot \text{succimer})^{0.1}$ and $(\text{week}^{0.5} \cdot \text{succimer})^{0.5}$ along with constant dispersions.

```
%genreg(modtype=expon,datain=longtlc,yvar=lead,matchvar=id,
withinvr=week,foldcnt=10,corrtype=UN,GEE=n,srchtype=logL,
xintrcpt=y,xgcs=week 2 succimer 1: week 0.5 succimer 1,
xgcpowrs=0.1 0.5,vintrcpt=y);
```

The macro parameters vgcs and vgcpowrs are used in the same way to specify geometric combinations for the dispersions.

The following code directly generates the adaptive moderation model for means and dispersions.

```
%genreg(modtype=expon,datain=longtlc,yvar=lead,matchvar=id,
withinvr=week,foldcnt=10,corrtype=UN,GEE=n,srchtype=logL,
xintrcpt=y,xvars=week,xpowers=0.22,
xgcs=week 0.06 succimer 1: week 8 succimer 1,xgcpowrs=−3.6 2,
vintrcpt=y,vgcs=week −0.1 succimer 1,vgcpowrs=0.6);
```

In this case, the model for the means is based on an intercept, $\text{week}^{0.22}$, and the two geometric combinations

$$\left(\text{week}^{0.06}\cdot\text{succimer}\right)^{-3.6}=\text{week}^{-0.216}\cdot\text{succimer}$$

and

$$\left(\text{week}^{8}\cdot\text{succimer}\right)^{2}=\text{week}^{16}\cdot\text{succimer}$$

while the dispersions are based on an intercept and the geometric combination

$$\left(\text{week}^{-0.1}\cdot\text{succimer}\right)^{0.6}=\text{week}^{-0.06}\cdot\text{succimer}.$$

The LCV score is 0.049274 while the associated moderation model for only the means has LCV score 0.037899 with distinct PD 22.91%. Consequently, being on succimer is reasonably considered to moderate the effect of visit on both the means and the dispersions.

The standard linear moderation model has means based on an intercept, week, succimer, and the interaction week · succimer with constant dispersions. This can be generated using ELMM with the following code.

```
%genreg(modtype=expon,datain=longtlc,yvar=lead,matchvar=id,
withinvr=week,foldcnt=10,corrtype=UN,GEE=n,srchtype=logL,
xintrcpt=y,xvars=week succimer,xgcs=week 1 succimer 1,
vintrcpt=y);
```

9.9.5 *Direct Variance Modeling*

The dirctvar macro parameter controls whether or not variances are directly modeled. The default setting "dirctvar=n" means use extended variances based on both the dispersions and the variance function which in this case is $V(\mu) = \mu^2$. Adding the setting "dirctvar=y" treats the variance function as $V(\mu) = 1$ so that the extended variances are the same as the dispersions. The following code uses the genreg macro to generate the adaptive direct variance, ELMM model for blood lead level means and dispersions as possibly nonlinear functions of week.

```
%genreg(modtype=expon,datain=longtlc,yvar=lead,matchvar=id,
withinvr=week,foldcnt=10,corrtype=UN,GEE=n,srchtype=logL,
expand=y,expxvars=week,expvvars=week,contract=y,dirctvar=y);
```

The following code directly generates the above direct variance model.

```
%genreg(modtype=expon,datain=longtlc,yvar=lead,matchvar=id,
withinvr=week,foldcnt=10,corrtype=UN,GEE=n,srchtype=logL,
xintrcpt=y,xvars=week,xpowers=−0.17,vintrcpt=y,vvars=week,
vpowers=−0.08,dirctvar=y);
```

This model has means based on an intercept and the transform $\text{week}^{-0.17}$ along with dispersions, and so also extended variances, based on an intercept and $\text{week}^{-0.08}$. It has LCV score 0.040630 with non-distinct PD 0.08% compared to the associated model accounting for the variance function $V(\mu) = \mu^2$ with LCV score 0.040662. Consequently, the direct variance model is a competitive alternative. This also holds for the direct variance adaptive additive model in visit and the indicator succimer.

The following code directly generates the adaptive direct variance model allowing for effects to visit, succimer, and geometric combinations in visit and succimer.

```
%genreg(modtype=expon,datain=longtlc,yvar=lead,matchvar=id,
withinvr=week,foldcnt=10,corrtype=UN,GEE=n,srchtype=logL,
xvars=week,xpowers=0.3,xgcs=week 0.08 succimer 1 : week 8 succimer 1,
xgcpowrs=−2.7 2,vvars=succimer,vpowers=1,vgcs=week −0.1 succimer 1,
vgcpowrs=−1.4,dirctvar=y);
```

This model has means based on an intercept, the transform $\text{week}^{-0.3}$, and the two geometric combinations

$$\left(\text{week}^{0.08} \cdot \text{succimer}\right)^{-2.7} = \text{week}^{-0.216} \cdot \text{succimer}$$

and

$$\left(\text{week}^{8} \cdot \text{succimer}\right)^{2} = \text{week}^{16} \cdot \text{succimer}$$

along with dispersions, and so also extended variances, based on an intercept, succimer, and the geometric combination

$$\left(\text{week}^{-0.1} \cdot \text{succimer}\right)^{-1.4} = \text{week}^{0.14} \cdot \text{succimer}.$$

It has LCV score 0.049388. The associated adaptive moderation model accounting for the variance function $V(\mu) = \mu^2$ has LCV score 0.049274 with non-distinct PD 0.23% and so is a competitive alternative to the direct variance moderation model.

9.9.6 Example Output

As also considered in Sect. 9.9.4, the following code uses the genreg macro to generate the adaptive moderation model for blood lead level means and dispersions as possibly nonlinear functions of week, being on succimer, and geometric combinations in week and being on succimer.

```
%genreg(modtype=expon,datain=longtlc,yvar= lead,matchvar=id,
withinvr=week,foldcnt=10,corrtype=UN,GEE=n,srchtype=logL,
expand=y,expxvars=week succimer,expvvars=week succimer,
geomcmbn=y,contract=y);
```

The output generated by this code starts with descriptions of settings controlling what kind of model has been generated including the cutoff for a distinct percent decrease in LCV scores followed by a description of the base model. Table 9.10 contains SAS listing output describing the base model. The means (i.e., the log expectation component) are based only on an intercept parameter XINTRCPT with estimated value 3.12 while the dispersions (i.e., the log dispersion component) are also based only on an intercept parameter VINTRCPT with estimated value −2.12. The LCV score rounds to 0.037309 (called the "mth root of the extended likelihood using deleted predictions" in the output). The estimated correlation matrix is generated in the output but is not included in Table 9.10.

The output then describes the parameters controlling the expansion followed by the expanded model as described in Table 9.11. The output uses the SAS double asterisk power operator (**). The base model (order 0) has LCV score 0.037309. First, the geometric combination

$$\mathrm{VGC\_1}^{0.6} = \left(\mathrm{week}^{-0.1} \cdot \mathrm{succimer}\right)^{0.6} = \mathrm{week}^{-0.06} \cdot \mathrm{succimer}\ (\mathrm{order}\ 1)$$

is added to the dispersions with LCV score 0.043445. The geometric combination

Table 9.10 Part of the SAS listing output describing the base model for the generation of the adaptive moderation model

```
base log expectation component

predictor      power     estimate

XINTRCPT           1    3.1201564

base log dispersion component

predictor      power     estimate

VINTRCPT           1     -2.12151

mth root of extended likelihood using deleted predictions:   0.0373085
```

Table 9.11 Part of the SAS listing output describing the expanded model for the generation of the adaptive moderation model

```
                         expanded model

         geometric combination expectation variables:
                XGC_1    week**(0.06)*succimer
                XGC_2    week**(8)*succimer

         geometric combination log variance variables:
                VGC_1    week**(-0.1)*succimer

               expanded log expectation component

      predictor     power    estimate        score    order

      XINTRCPT          1   3.2765343    0.0373085        0
      XGC_1            -5    -0.57629    0.0474747        2
      week           0.12   -0.081377    0.0483817        3
      XGC_2             2   1.923E-13    0.0491645        4

               expanded log dispersion component

      predictor     power    estimate        score    order

      VINTRCPT          1   -3.599677    0.0373085        0
      VGC_1           0.6   1.7045119     0.043445        1
      succimer          1   0.6193394    0.0491918        5
      week            0.1   0.3275583    0.0494496        6

 mth root of extended likelihood using deleted predictions: 0.0494496
```

$$\text{XGC\_1}^{-5} = \left(\text{week}^{0.06} \cdot \text{succimer}\right)^{-5} = \text{week}^{-0.3} \cdot \text{succimer (order 2)}$$

is added next to the means with LCV score 0.047475 followed by the transform $\text{week}^{0.12}$ (order 3) and the geometric combination

$$\text{XGC\_2}^{2} = \left(\text{week}^{8} \cdot \text{succimer}\right)^{2} = \text{week}^{16} \cdot \text{succimer (order 4)}$$

also added to the means with LCV scores 0.048382 and 0.049165. Finally, the indicator succimer (order 5) and the transform $\text{week}^{0.1}$ (order 6) are added to the dispersions with LCV scores 0.049192 and 0.049450, which is the LCV score for the expanded model. Each transform is added to the model without adjusting the powers for previously added transforms. The LCV score is allowed to decrease, although that does not happen in this case, and so expanded models usually require contraction. However, in cases where the contraction leaves the expanded model unchanged, a conditional transformation step is executed to adjust the powers of the expanded model to improve its LCV score. The estimated correlation matrix is generated in the output but is not included in Table 9.11.

The output then describes the parameters controlling the contraction followed by the contracted model as described in Table 9.12. The expanded model (order 0) has LCV score 0.049450. First, the transform $\text{week}^{0.1}$ (order 1) is removed from the dispersions generating the LCV score 0.049328. Finally, the indicator succimer (order 2) is removed from the dispersions with LCV score 0.049274, which is the

Table 9.12 Part of the SAS listing output describing the contracted model for the generation of the adaptive moderation model

```
      contracted log expectation component

    predictor old power new power     estimate

    XINTRCPT          1         1    3.2718713
    XGC_1            -5      -3.6    -0.604046
    week           0.12      0.22    -0.065122
    XGC_2             2         2    2.389E-13

   discarded    old power         score    order

                        .     0.0494496        0

      contracted log dispersion component

    predictor old power new power     estimate

    VINTRCPT          1         1    -3.255561
    VGC_1           0.6       0.6       2.3701

    discarded    old power         score order

                        .     0.0494496      0
    week              0.1     0.0493284      1
    succimer            1      0.049274      2

mth root of extended likelihood using deleted predictions:  0.049274
```

Table 9.13 Part of the SAS listing output describing the estimated UN correlation matrix of the contracted model for the generation of the adaptive moderation model

```
           estimated correlation matrix:

               w1          w2          w3          w4

    w1          1  0.6385875  0.6378543  0.6404572
    w2 0.6385875           1  0.805328   0.6617385
    w3 0.6378543  0.805328            1  0.7242853
    w4 0.6404572  0.6617385  0.7242853           1

w1, w2, ... are withinvr values from smallest to largest
```

LCV score for the contracted model. With the removal of each transform from the model, the powers for the other transforms are adjusted to improve the LCV score. In this case, the powers for XGC_1 and week in the means change from -5 and 0.12 to -3.6 and 0.22, respectively, while the other powers are unchanged. Details on how the powers change at each step of the contraction are not provided in the contraction output, but are available in the SAS log output if that is of interest. Note that the LCV score decreased with the removal of the two transforms. In this way, a parsimonious model is generated by the contraction. The contraction stopped because the removal of the next transform would have generated a model with a distinct PD in the LCV score using an LCV ratio test. The estimated correlation matrix is generated but not included in Table 9.12; it is displayed in Table 9.13. Rounded values for the estimated correlations range from 0.64 to 0.81. Within values are denoted as w1, w2, w3, and w4 representing in this case week 0, 1, 4, and 6, respectively.

Reference

Treatment of Lead-exposed Children (TLC) Trial Group. (2000). Safety and efficacy of succimer in toddlers with blood lead levels of 20-44 μg/dL. *Pediatric Research, 48*, 593–599.

Part II
Polytomous Outcomes

Polytomous outcomes are commonly formulated as having a finite number of consecutive integer values 0, 1, $\cdots$, K and treated as categorically distributed. Logistic regression addresses the special case with $K = 1$ and the two outcome values 0 and 1. The outcome values represent either ordered categories as for income levels categorized into 0:under \$50,000, 1:\$50,000–\$100,000, and 2:over \$100,000 or nominal categories as for patient decision making categorized into 0:patient only, 1:provider advice only, and 2:patient–provider interaction. Three possible alternative approaches for modeling polytomous outcomes are formulated and demonstrated.

Multinomial regression (Chap. 10) applies to polytomous outcomes with either ordered or nominal outcome categories. Ordinal regression (Chap. 11) applies to polytomous outcomes with ordered categories for the two cases of individual outcomes (Sect. 11.1) and cumulative outcomes (Sect. 11.2). These three approaches replace a univariate polytomous outcome by indicators for that outcome taking on all but one of its possible values, thereby replacing each univariate polytomous outcome measurement with $K + 1$ values by K multivariate outcome measurements each with the two values 0 and 1.

Polytomous outcomes can also have an arbitrary finite number of discrete numeric values. Discrete regression (Chap. 12) treats a polytomous outcome with multiple numeric values as a single univariate outcome without considering indicators for that outcome's values. The categories are either inherently ordered, as for the income categories given above, or an order is imposed on nominal categories as for 0:don't know, 1:no, and 2:yes. The categories can also be numbers to start with, as for pain level ratings of 0–10. Patients do not always utilize all the possible pain ratings and so analyses need to allow for such an outcome utilizing arbitrary subsets of the possible rating values.

Chapters 13–14 provide example analyses of correlated polytomous outcome data using partially modified GEE, fully modified GEE, and ELMM modeling. Chapter 13 addresses such analyses in the context of multinomial and ordinal regression for polytomous outcomes under the generalized and cumulative logit link functions, respectively. Chapter 14 addresses such analyses in the context of discrete regression for discrete numeric outcomes under multinomial, ordinal, and censored Poisson probabilities.

Chapters 10–12 provide technical details for multinomial, ordinal, and discrete regression, respectively. These chapters can be skipped by readers more interested in the data analyses reported in Chaps. 13–14.

Chapter 10
Multinomial Regression

Abstract Multinomial regression modeling of correlated sets of polytomous outcomes using the generalized logit link function is addressed allowing for non-constant dispersions. Formulations are provided for standard generalized estimating equations (GEE) modeling, partially modified GEE modeling, fully modified GEE modeling, and extended linear mixed modeling (ELMM). These formulations include estimating equations, gradient vectors, and Hessian matrices. Alternate correlation structures and their estimation are also addressed.

Keywords Correlated polytomous outcomes · Extended linear mixed modeling · Generalized estimating equations · Multinomial regression · Newton's method · Non-constant dispersions

Introduction This chapter addresses multinomial regression modeling of correlated polytomous outcomes (Lipsitz et al., 1994; Miller et al., 1993). Section 10.1 provides formulations of standard GEE modeling, Sect. 10.2 partially and fully modified GEE modeling, and Sect. 10.4 ELMM. Section 10.3 addresses alternate correlation structures and their estimation. Direct variance modeling of Sect. 5.7 can be generalized to multinomial regression, but is not considered for brevity. A likelihood is defined so that the formulations for LCV scores of Sect. 2.6, LCV ratio tests of Sect. 2.6.2, and the adaptive modeling process of Sect. 2.7 generalize to the multinomial regression case. However, the removal of a predictor for the means reduces the number of parameters by K rather than by 1 (see Sect. 10.1), and so LCV ratio tests need to be revised to adjust for this difference. Furthermore, since the $m(SC)$ polytomous measurements with $K + 1$ possible values are replaced by $m(SC) \cdot K$ dichotomous measurements, LCV scores are normalized by the number $m(SC) \cdot K$ of effective measurements rather than by $m(SC)$. For brevity, some formulations are provided without details on how they were computed.

Supplementary Information The online version contains supplementary material available at https://doi.org/10.1007/978-3-031-41988-1_10.

G. J. Knafl, *Modeling Correlated Outcomes Using Extensions of Generalized Estimating Equations and Linear Mixed Modeling*,
https://doi.org/10.1007/978-3-031-41988-1_10

10.1 Standard GEE Modeling

Using the notation of Sect. 2.1, the correlated polytomous outcomes y_{sc} for $sc \in SC$ have values 0, 1, $\cdots$, K and are treated as categorically distributed for a total of $m(SC)$ polytomous measurements. For $0 \leq u \leq K$, define individual outcomes $y_{sc,u}$ to be the indicators for $y_{sc} = u$ so that

$$\mu_{sc,u} = \mathrm{E}y_{sc,u} = \mathrm{P}\left(y_{sc,u} = 1\right) = \mathrm{P}(y_{sc} = u)$$

with residuals $e_{sc,u} = y_{sc,u} - \mu_{sc,u}$. As for logistic regression, the variance function is

$$V(\mu) = \mu \cdot (1 - \mu)$$

with derivative

$$\frac{dV(\mu)}{d\mu} = 1 - 2 \cdot \mu.$$

Note that for the logistic regression case with $K = 1$ (Sect. 2.2.3), the GEE estimating equations are based only on $y_{sc} = y_{sc,1}$ and not on both $y_{sc,0}$ and $y_{sc,1}$ because $y_{sc,0} = 1 - y_{sc,1}$ is redundant. Similarly, when $K > 1$, one of the values of u is treated as the reference category and is the left out of the formulation. The value of $u = 0$ is left out in what follows. Lipsitz et al. (1994) and Miller et al. (1993) leave out the largest value K.

As in Sect. 2.2, predictor values for the means are denoted by $x_{sc,j}$ for $1 \leq j \leq r$ and $sc \in SC$. Combine these over $1 \leq j \leq r$ into $r \times 1$ vectors $\boldsymbol{x}_{sc}$, which are then combined over $c \in C(s)$ into $m(s) \times r$ predictor matrices $\boldsymbol{X}_s$ with rows $\boldsymbol{x}_{sc}^{\mathrm{T}}$.

For $sc \in SC$, combine $y_{sc,u}$, $\mu_{sc,u}$, and $e_{sc,u} = y_{sc,u} - \mu_{sc,u}$ over $1 \leq u \leq K$ into the $K \times 1$ vectors $\boldsymbol{y}_{sc}$, $\boldsymbol{\mu}_{sc}$, and $\boldsymbol{e}_{sc} = \boldsymbol{y}_{sc} - \boldsymbol{\mu}_{sc}$. Combine the vectors $\boldsymbol{y}_{sc}$, $\boldsymbol{\mu}_{sc}$, and $\boldsymbol{e}_{sc}$ over $c \in C(s)$ into the $(m(SC) \cdot K) \times 1$ vectors $\boldsymbol{y}_s$, $\boldsymbol{\mu}_s$, and $\boldsymbol{e}_s = \boldsymbol{y}_s - \boldsymbol{\mu}_s$ in the order of the values $c \in C(s)$. The link function is generalized logits. The case $u = 0$ is treated as the reference category (but any other value u could be used instead) and logits are computed for the other outcome values relative to this category. Formally, for $1 \leq u \leq K$,

$$g\left(\mu_{sc,u}\right) = \log \frac{\mu_{sc,u}}{\mu_{sc,0}} = \boldsymbol{x}_{sc}^{\mathrm{T}} \cdot \boldsymbol{\beta}_u$$

for K $r \times 1$ vectors $\boldsymbol{\beta}_u$ of coefficient parameters $\beta_{u,j}$ for $1 \leq u \leq K$ and $1 \leq j \leq r$. Altogether, there are $K \cdot r$ coefficient parameters for modeling the means, which are combined into the $(K \cdot r) \times 1$ vector $\boldsymbol{\beta}$. For $sc \in SC$, the means satisfy

$$\mu_{sc,u} = \frac{\exp\left(\boldsymbol{x}_{sc}^{\mathrm{T}} \cdot \boldsymbol{\beta}_u\right)}{1 + \sum\limits_{u'=1}^{K} \exp\left(\boldsymbol{x}_{sc}^{\mathrm{T}} \cdot \boldsymbol{\beta}_{u'}\right)}$$

for $1 \leq u \leq K$ and

$$\mu_{sc,0} = \frac{1}{1 + \sum\limits_{u'=1}^{K} \exp\left(\boldsymbol{x}_{sc}^{\mathrm{T}} \cdot \boldsymbol{\beta}_{u'}\right)}.$$

The partial derivatives $\frac{\partial \mu_{sc,u}}{\partial \beta_{w,j}}$ (computed directly) satisfy

$$\frac{\partial \mu_{sc,u}}{\partial \beta_{w,j}} = x_{sc,j} \cdot \mu_{sc,w} \cdot \left(1 - \mu_{sc,w}\right) = x_{sc,j} \cdot V\left(\mu_{sc,w}\right), w = u,$$

and

$$\frac{\partial \mu_{sc,u}}{\partial \beta_{w,j}} = -x_{sc,j} \cdot \mu_{sc,u} \cdot \mu_{sc,w}, w \neq u,$$

for $1 \leq u, w \leq K$ and $1 \leq j \leq r$.

Let φ be a constant dispersion parameter as in Sect. 2.4 so that it is constant in sc,u for $sc \in SC$ and $1 \leq u \leq K$. Define the extended variances

$$\sigma_{sc,u}^2 = \varphi \cdot V\left(\mu_{sc,u}\right),$$

the standardized residuals

$$stde_{sc,u} = e_{sc,u} / \sigma_{sc,u},$$

and the Pearson residuals

$$Pres_{sc,u} = \frac{e_{sc,u}}{V^{1/2}\left(\mu_{sc,u}\right)}$$

for $sc \in SC$ and $1 \leq u \leq K$. Combine these values over $1 \leq u \leq K$ into the $K \times 1$ vectors $\boldsymbol{\sigma}_{sc}$, $\boldsymbol{stde}_{sc}$, and $\boldsymbol{Pres}_{sc}$, and then combine these vectors into the $(m(s) \cdot K) \times 1$ vectors $\boldsymbol{\sigma}_s$, $\boldsymbol{stde}_s$, and $\boldsymbol{Pres}_s$ ordered by their values $c \in C(s)$. Model the $(m(s) \cdot K) \times (m(s) \cdot K)$ covariance matrices $\boldsymbol{\Sigma}_s$ as

$$\boldsymbol{\Sigma}_s = \boldsymbol{DIAG}(\boldsymbol{\sigma}_s) \cdot \boldsymbol{R}_s(\rho) \cdot \boldsymbol{DIAG}(\boldsymbol{\sigma}_s)$$

for appropriate choices of the $(m(s) \cdot K) \times (m(s) \cdot K)$ correlation matrices $\boldsymbol{R}_s(\boldsymbol{\rho})$ for $s \in S$.

Standard GEE modeling can be extended to the multinomial case by providing correlation structures and methods for their estimation (see Sect. 10.3). The notation of Sect. 2.4 also extends to the multinomial case. Specifically, the generalized estimating equations are given by $\boldsymbol{E}(\boldsymbol{\beta}) = \boldsymbol{0}$ where the $(K \cdot r) \times 1$ vector $\boldsymbol{E}(\boldsymbol{\beta})$ satisfies

$$\boldsymbol{E}(\boldsymbol{\beta}) = \sum_{s \in S} \boldsymbol{E}_s(\boldsymbol{\beta}) = \sum_{s \in S} \boldsymbol{D}_s^{\mathrm{T}} \cdot \boldsymbol{\Sigma}_s^{-1} \cdot \boldsymbol{e}_s,$$

and the $(m(SC) \cdot K) \times (K \cdot r)$ matrices

$$\boldsymbol{D}_s = \frac{\partial \boldsymbol{\mu}_s}{\partial \boldsymbol{\beta}}$$

for $s \in S$ have entries

$$D_{sc,u,w,j} = \frac{\partial \mu_{sc,u}}{\partial \beta_{w,j}}$$

for $sc \in SC$, $1 \le u$, $w \le K$, and $1 \le j \le r$. Let

$$\boldsymbol{E}'(\boldsymbol{\beta}) = -\sum_{s \in S} \boldsymbol{D}_s^{\mathrm{T}} \cdot \boldsymbol{\Sigma}_s^{-1} \cdot \boldsymbol{D}_s.$$

The standard GEE estimation process uses Newton's method to iteratively solve $\boldsymbol{E}(\boldsymbol{\beta}) = \boldsymbol{0}$ with $\boldsymbol{E}(\boldsymbol{\beta})$ serving in the role of the gradient vector and $\boldsymbol{E}'(\boldsymbol{\beta})$ in the role of the Hessian matrix (see Sect. 3.7 for details). The bias-adjusted estimate of the constant dispersion parameter φ for a given value of the coefficient parameter vector $\boldsymbol{\beta}$ is

$$\varphi(\boldsymbol{\beta}) = \frac{\sum_{sc \in SC} \boldsymbol{Pres}_{sc}^{\mathrm{T}}(\boldsymbol{\beta}) \cdot \boldsymbol{Pres}_{sc}(\boldsymbol{\beta})}{m(SC) \cdot K - r}$$

assuming $m(SC) \cdot K - r > 0$. Lipsitz et al. (1994) and Miller et al. (1993) assume unit dispersions and not more general constant dispersions.

The likelihood function $L(SC; \boldsymbol{\theta})$ generalizes to handle multinomial regression modeling in the standard GEE context. This is a special case of the formulation given in Sect. 10.2, and so is not provided here.

Model-based and robust empirical estimates of the covariance matrix for the standard GEE estimate $\boldsymbol{\beta}(SC)$ of the coefficient parameter vector $\boldsymbol{\beta}$ can be computed similarly to those for standard GEE modeling given in Sect. 2.4.2. These use the standard GEE versions of $\boldsymbol{E}'(\boldsymbol{\beta}(SC))$ and $\boldsymbol{G}(\boldsymbol{\beta}(SC))$ for multinomial regression.

$\boldsymbol{G}(\boldsymbol{\beta}(SC))$ is defined so that summing the entries of its rows generates $\boldsymbol{E}(\boldsymbol{\beta}(SC))$. A detailed formulation for $\boldsymbol{G}(\boldsymbol{\beta}(SC))$ is not provided for brevity.

10.2 Partially and Fully Modified GEE Modeling

As in Sect. 3.1, predictor values for non-constant dispersions are denoted by $v_{sc,j}$ for $1 \leq j \leq q$ and $sc \in SC$ and combined over $1 \leq j \leq q$ into $q \times 1$ vectors $\boldsymbol{v}_{sc}$, which are combined over $c \in C(s)$ into $m(s) \times q$ predictor matrices $\boldsymbol{V}_s$ with rows $\boldsymbol{v}_{sc}^{\mathrm{T}}$. Define $\varphi_{sc} = exp\left(\boldsymbol{v}_{sc}^{\mathrm{T}} \cdot \boldsymbol{\gamma}\right)$ as in Sect. 3.1 so that it is constant in u for $1 \leq u \leq K$. Dispersions are readily generalized to change with u, and so this is not considered for brevity. Treating dispersions as constant in u reduces the complexity of models and their computation time. Let

$$\sigma_{sc,u}^2 = \varphi_{sc} \cdot V\left(\mu_{sc,u}\right),$$

$$stde_{sc,u} = e_{sc,u} / \sigma_{sc,u},$$

and

$$Pres_{sc,u} = \frac{e_{sc,u}}{V^{1/2}\left(\mu_{sc,u}\right)},$$

for $sc \in SC$ and $1 \leq u \leq K$. Combine these over $1 \leq u \leq K$ into the $K \times 1$ vectors $\boldsymbol{\sigma}_{sc}$, $\boldsymbol{stde}_{sc}$, and $\boldsymbol{Pres}_{sc}$, and then combine these vectors, respectively, into the $(m(s) \cdot K) \times 1$ vectors $\boldsymbol{\sigma}_s$, $\boldsymbol{stde}_s$, and $\boldsymbol{Pres}_s$ in the order of the values $c \in C(s)$. Model the $(m(s) \cdot K) \times (m(s) \cdot K)$ covariance matrices $\boldsymbol{\Sigma}_s$ as

$$\boldsymbol{\Sigma}_s = \boldsymbol{DIAG}(\boldsymbol{\sigma}_s) \cdot \boldsymbol{R}_s(\boldsymbol{\rho}) \cdot \boldsymbol{DIAG}(\boldsymbol{\sigma}_s)$$

for appropriate choices of the $(m(s) \cdot K) \times (m(SC) \cdot K)$ correlation matrices $\boldsymbol{R}_s(\boldsymbol{\rho})$ for $s \in S$ (see Sect. 10.3).

Partially modified and fully modified GEE modeling can be extended using the likelihood function $L(SC;\boldsymbol{\theta}) = \exp\left(\ell(SC;\boldsymbol{\theta})\right)$ for individual outcome measurements $y_{sc,u}$ with indexes $sc \in SC$ and $1 \leq u \leq K$ equal to the product over $s \in S$ of the terms $L(O_s;\boldsymbol{\theta})$ where $O_s = \{\boldsymbol{y}_s, \boldsymbol{X}_s, \boldsymbol{V}_s\}$ denotes an observation and

$$\ell(O_s;\boldsymbol{\theta}) = \log L(O_s;\boldsymbol{\theta}) = -\boldsymbol{e}_s^{\mathrm{T}} \cdot \boldsymbol{\Sigma}_s^{-1} \cdot \boldsymbol{e}_s/2 - (\log|\boldsymbol{\Sigma}_s|)/2 - (m(s) \cdot K \cdot \log(2 \cdot \pi))/2$$

for

$$\boldsymbol{\theta} = \begin{pmatrix} \boldsymbol{\beta} \\ \boldsymbol{\gamma} \end{pmatrix},$$

the $(K \cdot r + q) \times 1$ vector composed of the mean and dispersion parameter vectors $\boldsymbol{\beta}$ and $\boldsymbol{\gamma}$ with $K \cdot r$ and q entries, respectively. Maximizing the likelihood involves using Newton's method to solve

$$\boldsymbol{E}(\boldsymbol{\theta}) = \begin{pmatrix} \boldsymbol{E}(\boldsymbol{\beta}) \\ \boldsymbol{E}(\boldsymbol{\gamma}) \end{pmatrix} = \boldsymbol{0}$$

where $\boldsymbol{E}(\boldsymbol{\beta})$ and $\boldsymbol{E}(\boldsymbol{\gamma})$ are, respectively, $(K \cdot r) \times 1$ and $q \times 1$ vectors. $\boldsymbol{E}'(\boldsymbol{\theta})$ has four component matrices $\boldsymbol{E}'(\boldsymbol{\beta}), \boldsymbol{E}'(\boldsymbol{\gamma}), \boldsymbol{E}'(\boldsymbol{\beta},\boldsymbol{\gamma})$, and $\boldsymbol{E}'(\boldsymbol{\gamma},\boldsymbol{\beta}) = \boldsymbol{E}'^{\mathrm{T}}(\boldsymbol{\beta},\boldsymbol{\gamma})$. $\boldsymbol{E}'(\boldsymbol{\beta}), \boldsymbol{E}'(\boldsymbol{\gamma})$, and $\boldsymbol{E}'(\boldsymbol{\beta},\boldsymbol{\gamma})$ are, respectively, $(K \cdot r) \times (K \cdot r)$, $q \times q$, and $(K \cdot r) \times q$ matrices.

Formulation adjustments for partially modified GEE include:

$$\log|\boldsymbol{\Sigma}_s| = \log|\boldsymbol{R}_s(\boldsymbol{\rho})| + \sum_{c \in C(s)} K \cdot \log \varphi_{sc} + \sum_{c \in C(s)} \sum_{u=1}^{K} \log V\left(\mu_{sc,u}\right);$$

$\boldsymbol{E}(\boldsymbol{\gamma})$ is the sum over $s \in S$ of terms $\boldsymbol{E}_s(\boldsymbol{\gamma})$ with entries

$$E_{s,j}(\boldsymbol{\gamma}) = \boldsymbol{vstde}_{s,j}^{\mathrm{T}} \cdot \boldsymbol{R}_s^{-1}(\boldsymbol{\rho}) \cdot \boldsymbol{stde}_s - \sum_{c \in C(s)} K \cdot v_{sc,j}/2,$$

where $\boldsymbol{vstde}_{s,j}$ is the $(m(SC) \cdot K) \times 1$ vector with entries

$$vstde_{sc,u,j} = v_{sc,j} \cdot stde_{sc,u}/2$$

for $sc \in SC$, $1 \le u \le K$, and $1 \le j \le q$; and $\boldsymbol{E}'(\boldsymbol{\gamma})$ is the sum over $s \in S$ of $\boldsymbol{E}'_s(\boldsymbol{\gamma})$ with entries

$$E'_{s,j,j'}(\boldsymbol{\gamma}) = -\boldsymbol{vvstde}_{s,j,j'}^{\mathrm{T}} \cdot \boldsymbol{R}_s^{-1}(\boldsymbol{\rho}) \cdot \boldsymbol{stde}_s - \boldsymbol{vstde}_{s,j}^{\mathrm{T}} \cdot \boldsymbol{R}_s^{-1}(\boldsymbol{\rho}) \cdot \boldsymbol{vstde}_{s,j'}$$

where $\boldsymbol{vvstde}_{s,j,j'}$ is the $(m(SC) \cdot K) \times 1$ vector with entries

$$vvstde_{sc,u,j,j'} = v_{sc,j} \cdot v_{sc,j'} \cdot stde_{sc,u}/4$$

for $sc \in SC$, $1 \le u \le K$, and $1 \le j, j' \le q$. These adjustments apply as well to fully modified GEE modeling. Also, $\boldsymbol{E}'(\boldsymbol{\beta},\boldsymbol{\gamma})$ is the sum over $s \in S$ of $\boldsymbol{E}'_s(\boldsymbol{\beta},\boldsymbol{\gamma})$ with q $(K \cdot r) \times 1$ column vectors

$$\boldsymbol{E'}_{s,j}(\boldsymbol{\beta},\boldsymbol{\gamma}) = -\boldsymbol{D}_s^{\mathrm{T}} \cdot \boldsymbol{DIAG}\left(\boldsymbol{v\sigma inv}_{s,j}\right) \cdot \boldsymbol{R}_s^{-1}(\boldsymbol{\rho}) \cdot \boldsymbol{stde}_s$$
$$-\boldsymbol{D}_s^{\mathrm{T}} \cdot \boldsymbol{DIAG}(\mathbf{1}/\boldsymbol{\sigma}_s) \cdot \boldsymbol{R}_s^{-1}(\boldsymbol{\rho}) \cdot \boldsymbol{vstde}_{s,j}$$

where $\boldsymbol{v\sigma inv}_{s,j}$ is the $(m(SC) \cdot K) \times 1$ vector with entries

$$v\sigma inv_{sc,u,j} = \frac{v_{sc,j}}{2 \cdot \sigma_{sc,u}}$$

for $sc \in SC$, $1 \le u \le K$, and $1 \le j \le q$.

Fully modified GEE also requires formulation adjustments for $\boldsymbol{E}(\boldsymbol{\beta})$, $\boldsymbol{E}'(\boldsymbol{\beta})$, and $\boldsymbol{E}'(\boldsymbol{\beta},\boldsymbol{\gamma})$. $\boldsymbol{E}(\boldsymbol{\beta})$ is the sum over $s \in S$ of $\boldsymbol{E}_s(\boldsymbol{\beta})$ with entries

$$E_{s,w,j}(\boldsymbol{\beta}) = \frac{\partial_0 \ell(O_s;\boldsymbol{\theta})}{\partial_0 \beta_{w,j}} = \boldsymbol{xstde}_{s,w,j}^{\mathrm{T}} \cdot \boldsymbol{R}_s^{-1}(\boldsymbol{\rho}) \cdot \boldsymbol{stde}_s - \sum_{c \in C(s)} \sum_{u=1}^{K} W_{w,j}\left(\mu_{sc,u}\right)/2$$

where

$$W_{w,j}\left(\mu_{sc,u}\right) = \frac{\frac{\partial V\left(\mu_{sc,u}\right)}{\partial \beta_{w,j}}}{V\left(\mu_{sc,u}\right)},$$

for $1 \le u \le K$ and $1 \le j \le r$. The $(m(SC) \cdot K) \times 1$ vector $\boldsymbol{xstde}_{s,w,j}$ has entries $xstde_{sc,u,w,j}$ satisfying

$$xstde_{sc,u,w,j} = x_{sc,j} \cdot \frac{\left(1 - 2 \cdot \mu_{sc,w}\right) \cdot y_{sc,w} + \mu_{sc,w}}{2 \cdot \sigma_{sc,w}}, w = u,$$

$$xstde_{sc,u,w,j} = -x_{sc,j} \cdot \mu_{sc,w} \cdot \frac{\left(1 - 2 \cdot \mu_{sc,u}\right) \cdot y_{sc,u} + \mu_{sc,u}}{2 \cdot \left(1 - \mu_{sc,u}\right) \cdot \sigma_{sc,u}}, w \ne u,$$

while

$$W_{w,j}\left(\mu_{sc,u}\right) = x_{sc,j} \cdot \left(1 - 2 \cdot \mu_{sc,w}\right), w = u,$$

$$W_{w,j}\left(\mu_{sc,u}\right) = -x_{sc,j} \cdot \mu_{sc,w} \cdot \frac{\left(1 - 2 \cdot \mu_{sc,u}\right)}{\left(1 - \mu_{sc,u}\right)}, w \ne u,$$

for $1 \le u$, $w \le K$ and $1 \le j \le r$. As before, the operator notation $\frac{\partial_0}{\partial_0 \beta_{w,j}}$ is used to indicate that this is not a full partial derivative due to not accounting for the effect of $\beta_{w,j}$ on $\boldsymbol{R}_s(\boldsymbol{\rho})$ (see Sect. 10.3). Note that $W_{w,j}(\mu_{sc,u})$ is a standard partial derivative since $V(\mu_{sc,u})$ does not depend on $\boldsymbol{R}_s(\boldsymbol{\rho})$.

$\boldsymbol{E}'(\boldsymbol{\beta})$ is the sum over $s \in S$ of $\boldsymbol{E}'_s(\boldsymbol{\beta})$ with entries

$$E'_{s,w,j,w',j'}(\boldsymbol{\beta}) = \frac{\partial_0 \boldsymbol{E}_{s,w,j}(\boldsymbol{\beta})}{\partial_0 \beta_{w',j'}}$$

$$= -\boldsymbol{xxstde}^{\mathrm{T}}_{s,wj,w',j'} \cdot \boldsymbol{R}_s^{-1}(\rho) \cdot \boldsymbol{stde}_s - \boldsymbol{xxstde}^{\mathrm{T}}_{s,w,j} \cdot \boldsymbol{R}_s^{-1}(\rho) \cdot \boldsymbol{xxstde}_{s,w',j'}$$

$$- \sum_{c \in C(s)} \sum_{u=1}^{K} W_{w,j,w',j'}(\mu_{sc,u})/2$$

where

$$W_{w,j,w',j'}(\mu_{sc,u}) = \frac{\partial W_{w,j}(\mu_{sc,u})}{\partial \beta_{w',j'}}$$

for $1 \le w,\ w' \le K$ and $1 \le j,\ j' \le r$. The following formulation is needed to compute $\boldsymbol{E}'(\boldsymbol{\beta})$ but can be skipped since it is complicated. The $(m(s) \cdot K) \times 1$ vector $\boldsymbol{xxstde}_{s,w,j,w'j'}$ has entries $xxstde_{sc,u,w,j,w'j'}$ for $sc \in SC$, $1 \le u,\ w,\ w' \le K$, and $1 \le j,\ j' \le r$ satisfying

$$xxstde_{sc,u,w,j,w',j'} = x_{sc,j} \cdot x_{sc,j'} \cdot stde_{sc,w}/4,$$

for $w = u$, $w' = u$;

$$xxstde_{sc,u,w,j,w',j'} = -x_{sc,j} \cdot x_{sc,j'} \cdot \mu_{sc,w'} \cdot \frac{stde_{sc,w}}{4 \cdot (1 - \mu_{sc,w})},$$

for $w = u$, $w' \neq u$;

$$xxstde_{sc,u,w,j,w',j'} = -x_{sc,j} \cdot x_{sc,j'} \cdot \mu_{sc,w} \cdot \frac{stde_{sc,w'}}{4 \cdot (1 - \mu_{sc,w'})},$$

for $w \neq u$, $w' = u$;

$$xxstde_{sc,u,w,j,w',j'} = -x_{sc,j} \cdot x_{sc,j'} \cdot \mu_{sc,w} \cdot \mu_{sc,w'} \cdot \frac{(1 - 4 \cdot \mu_{sc,u}) \cdot y_{sc,u} + 3 \cdot \mu_{sc,u}}{4 \cdot (1 - \mu_{sc,u})^2 \cdot \sigma_{sc,u}},$$

for $w \neq u$, $w' \neq u$, $w' \neq w$; and

$$xxstde_{sc,u,w,j,w',j'} = x_{sc,j} \cdot x_{sc,j'} \cdot \mu_{sc,w} \cdot \frac{a_{sc,u,w} \cdot y_{sc,u} + b_{sc,u,w}}{4 \cdot (1 - \mu_{sc,u})^2 \cdot \sigma_{sc,u}},$$

for $w \neq u$, $w' = w$ where

$$a_{sc,u,w} = 2 \cdot (1 - 2 \cdot \mu_{sc,u}) \cdot (1 - \mu_{sc,u}) - (1 - 4 \cdot \mu_{sc,u}) \cdot \mu_{sc,w}$$

and

$$b_{sc,u,w} = (2 \cdot (1 - \mu_{sc,u}) - 3 \cdot \mu_{sc,w}) \cdot \mu_{sc,u}.$$

Also,

$$W_{w,j,w',j'}(\mu_{sc,u}) = -2 \cdot x_{sc,j} \cdot x_{sc,j'} \cdot V(\mu_{sc,w}),$$

for w=u, $w' = u$;

$$W_{w,j,w',j'}(\mu_{sc,u}) = 2 \cdot x_{sc,j} \cdot x_{sc,j'} \cdot \mu_{sc,w} \cdot \mu_{sc,w'},$$

for $w = u$, $w' \neq u$;

$$W_{w,j,w',j'}(\mu_{sc,u}) = 2 \cdot x_{sc,j} \cdot x_{sc,j'} \cdot \mu_{sc,w} \cdot \mu_{sc,w'},$$

for $w \neq u$, $w' = u$;

$$W_{w,j,w',j'}(\mu_{sc,u}) = x_{sc,j} \cdot x_{sc,j'} \cdot \mu_{sc,w} \cdot \mu_{sc,w'} \cdot \frac{1 - 4 \cdot \mu_{sc,u} + 2 \cdot \mu_{sc,u}^2}{(1 - \mu_{sc,u})^2},$$

for $w \neq u$, $w' \neq u$, $w' \neq w$; and

$$W_{w,j,w',j'}(\mu_{sc,u}) = -x_{sc,j} \cdot x_{sc,j'} \cdot \mu_{sc,w} \cdot \frac{c_{sc,u,w}}{(1 - \mu_{sc,u})^2},$$

for $w \neq u$, $w' = w$ where

$$c_{sc,u,w} = (1 - 2 \cdot \mu_{sc,u}) \cdot (1 - \mu_{sc,u}) - (1 - 4 \cdot \mu_{sc,u} + 2 \cdot \mu_{sc,u}^2) \cdot \mu_{sc,w}.$$

$\boldsymbol{E}'(\boldsymbol{\beta}, \boldsymbol{\gamma})$ is the sum over $s \in S$ of $\boldsymbol{E}'_s(\boldsymbol{\beta}, \boldsymbol{\gamma})$ with entries

$$E'_{s,w,j,j'}(\boldsymbol{\beta}, \boldsymbol{\gamma}) = \frac{\partial_0 \boldsymbol{E}_{s,w,j}(\boldsymbol{\beta})}{\partial_0 \gamma_{j'}} = -\boldsymbol{vxstde}_{s,w,j,j'}^{\mathrm{T}} \cdot \boldsymbol{R}_s^{-1}(\rho) \cdot \boldsymbol{stde}_s$$
$$-\boldsymbol{xstde}_{s,w,j}^{\mathrm{T}} \cdot \boldsymbol{R}_s^{-1}(\rho) \cdot \boldsymbol{vstde}_{s,j'}$$

where $\boldsymbol{vxstde}_{s,w,j,j'}$ is the $(m(s) \cdot K) \times 1$ vector with entries

$$vxstde_{sc,u,w,j,j'} = xstde_{sc,u,w,j} \cdot v_{sc,j'}/2$$

and $\boldsymbol{vstde}_{s,j'}$ is the same as for partially modified GEE modeling, for $sc \in SC$, $1 \leq u,\ w \leq K$, $1 \leq j \leq r$, and $1 \leq j' \leq q$.

Model-based and robust empirical estimates of the covariance matrix for the partially and fully modified GEE estimate

$$\boldsymbol{\theta}(SC) = \begin{pmatrix} \boldsymbol{\beta}(SC) \\ \boldsymbol{\gamma}(SC) \end{pmatrix}$$

of the coefficient parameter vector $\boldsymbol{\theta}$ can be computed similarly to those for partially modified GEE modeling given in Sect. 3.4 and fully modified GEE modeling given in Sect. 4.1. These use the partially and fully modified GEE versions of $\boldsymbol{E}'(\boldsymbol{\theta}(SC))$ and $\boldsymbol{G}(\boldsymbol{\theta}(SC))$ for multinomial regression. $\boldsymbol{G}(\boldsymbol{\theta}(SC))$ is defined so that summing the entries of its rows generates $\boldsymbol{E}(\boldsymbol{\theta}(SC))$. A detailed formulation for $\boldsymbol{G}(\boldsymbol{\theta}(SC))$ is not provided for brevity.

10.3 Alternate Correlation Structures

Let $\boldsymbol{R}_{s,c,c'}$ for $c,\ c' \in C(s)$ denote the $m^2(s)\ K \times K$ component matrices of $\boldsymbol{R}_s(\boldsymbol{\rho})$. The special cases $\boldsymbol{R}_{s,c,c}$ with $c' = c$ are the correlation matrices for $\boldsymbol{y}_{sc}$. The individual outcomes $y_{sc,u}$ are multinomially distributed with sum 1 and covariances satisfying

$$\text{Cov}\left(y_{sc,u}, y_{sc,u'}\right) = \mu_{sc,u} \cdot \left(1 - \mu_{sc,u}\right), u = u',$$

$$\text{Cov}\left(y_{sc,u}, y_{sc,u'}\right) = -\mu_{sc,u} \cdot \mu_{sc,u'}, u \neq u'$$

for $sc \in SC$ and $1 \leq u,\ u' \leq K$ (Lipsitz et al., 1994). Consequently, $\boldsymbol{R}_{s,c,c}$ has diagonal entries with value 1 and off-diagonal entries

$$r_{sc,u,u'} = -\left(\frac{\mu_{sc,u}}{1 - \mu_{sc,u}}\right)^{1/2} \cdot \left(\frac{\mu_{sc,u'}}{1 - \mu_{sc,u'}}\right)^{1/2}$$

for $1 \leq u,\ u' \leq K$ with $u \neq u'$. Note that $\boldsymbol{R}_{s,c,c}$ depends on the mean parameters but not on the correlation parameters. Models are needed for the remaining $m(s) \cdot (m(s) - 1)/2$ component matrices $\boldsymbol{R}_{s,c,c'}$ and their transposes $\boldsymbol{R}_{s,c',c} = \boldsymbol{R}^{\mathrm{T}}_{s,c,c'}$ of dimension $K \times K$ for $c < c'$. These depend only on the correlation parameters for the four correlation structures described in Sects. 10.3.1–10.3.4. Estimates of the parameters for these correlation structures for partially and fully modified GEE are provided in those sections. Note that $\boldsymbol{R}_{s,c,c'}$ is the correlation matrix for $\boldsymbol{y}_{sc}$ with $\boldsymbol{y}_{sc'}$ so that its entries satisfy $r_{s,c,c',u,u'} = \text{Corr}(y_{sc,u}, y_{sc',u'})$ and $r_{s,c,c',u',u} = \text{Corr}(y_{sc,u'}, y_{sc',u})$ for $u \neq u'$, which are correlations between two different pairs of indicator variables and so have different values in general, and $\boldsymbol{R}_{s,c,c'}$ is not symmetric in general.

10.3.1 Independent Correlations

Under the IND correlation structure, the component matrices $\boldsymbol{R}_{s,c,c'}$ have all zero entries for c, $c' \in C(s)$ with $c \neq c'$. In this case, the correlation parameter vector $\boldsymbol{\rho}_{\mathrm{IND}}$ is the constant scalar with value 0. There is no need for an estimate of $\boldsymbol{\rho}_{\mathrm{IND}}$.

10.3.2 Exchangeable Correlations

Under the EC correlation structure, the component matrices $\boldsymbol{R}_{s,c,c'}$ for $c,c' \in C(s)$ with $c < c'$ all equal the same $K \times K$ matrix $\boldsymbol{R}$ with entries $r_{\mathrm{EC},u,u'}$ for $1 \leq u$, $u' \leq K$ while $\boldsymbol{R}_{s,c',c} = \boldsymbol{R}^{\mathrm{T}}$. For a given value of the coefficient parameter vector $\boldsymbol{\theta}$, the associated estimate of $\boldsymbol{R}(\boldsymbol{\theta})$ is computed as

$$\boldsymbol{R}(\boldsymbol{\theta}) = \frac{\sum\limits_{cc' \in CC'} \boldsymbol{stde}_{sc}(\boldsymbol{\theta}) \cdot \boldsymbol{stde}_{sc'}^{\mathrm{T}}(\boldsymbol{\theta})}{D}$$

where CC' is the set of $m(CC')$ observed distinct ordered pairs defined in Sect. 2.4.1 and the denominator D is either the bias-adjusted value $D = m(CC') - r > 0$ assuming this is non-zero or the bias-unadjusted value $D = m(CC')$. The correlation parameters $r_{\mathrm{EC},u,u'}(\boldsymbol{\theta})$ are combined over $1 \leq u$, $u' \leq K$ into the $K^2 \times 1$ correlation parameter vector $\boldsymbol{\rho}_{\mathrm{EC}}(\boldsymbol{\theta})$.

10.3.3 Spatial Autoregressive Order 1 Correlations

As in Sect. 2.3.3, under spatial AR1 correlations, there is a function $t(c)$ increasing in the integers $c \in C$ (e.g., increasing measurement times or dosages) while, for the special case of non-spatial AR1, $t(c) = c$ for $c \in C$. Let $\boldsymbol{R}$ denote a $K \times K$ matrix with entries $r_{\mathrm{AR1},u,u'}$ satisfying $-1 < r_{\mathrm{AR1},u,u'} < 1$ for $1 \leq u$, $u' \leq K$. For c, $c' \in C(s)$ with $c < c'$, let

$$\boldsymbol{R}_{s,c,c'} = \mathrm{power}(\boldsymbol{R}, |t(c') - t(c)|)$$

denote the matrices with entries

$$r_{s,c,c',u,u'} = \text{power}(r_{\text{AR1},u,u'}, |t(c') - t(c)|)$$

for an appropriately defined power transform of the possibly negative entries $r_{\text{AR1},u,u'}$ of $\boldsymbol{R}$ for $1 \leq u,\ u' \leq K$.

Results for AR1 correlations are described in Tables 6.1, 7.1, 8.1, and 9.1 for normally, Poisson, Bernoulli, and exponentially distributed data, respectively. Estimated autocorrelations are not reported in those tables, but they are all positive with values larger than 0.5, indicating that how to transform a negative correlation value is not a crucial issue in many cases of these kinds (and they are assumed to be nonnegative in general). However, the matrices $\boldsymbol{R}_s(\boldsymbol{\rho})$ for multinomial regression often have both positive and negative values and signs of the entries of the submatrices $\boldsymbol{R}_{s,c,c'}$ often are the same for $c,\ c' \in C(s)$ (examples are provided in Chap. 13). For this reason, AR1 correlations in the multinomial regression context are based on sign-preserving power transforms. Formally, define

$$\text{power}(r_{\text{AR1},u,u'}, |t(c') - t(c)|) = \text{sign}(r_{\text{AR1},u,u'}) \cdot |r_{\text{AR1},u,u'}|^{|t(c') - t(c)|}.$$

These power transforms are well-defined for all $r_{\text{AR1},u,u'}$ in the interval $(-1, 1)$ and all $c,\ c' \in C$ with $c' \neq c$, and this does not require that the distances $|t(c') - t(c)|$ be all integers for $c,\ c' \in C$. Since $t(c)$ are unique for $c \in C$, $|t(c') - t(c)| > 0$ for $c' \neq c$, so that $|r_{\text{AR1},u,u'}|^{|t(c') - t(c)|}$ | equals 0 when $r_{\text{AR1},u,u'} = 0$.

In the non-spatial AR1 case, for a given value of the coefficient parameter vector $\boldsymbol{\theta}$, an estimate $\boldsymbol{R}(\boldsymbol{\theta})$ of $\boldsymbol{R}$ has entries $r_{\text{AR1},u,u'}(\boldsymbol{\theta})$ satisfying

$$r_{\text{AR1},u,u'}(\boldsymbol{\theta}) = \frac{\sum_{cc' \in CC'(+1)} stde_{sc,u}(\boldsymbol{\theta}) \cdot stde_{sc',u'}(\boldsymbol{\theta})}{D}$$

where $CC'(+1)$ is the set of $m(CC'(+1))$ observed consecutive index pairs defined in Sect. 2.4.1 and the denominator D is either the bias-adjusted value $D = m(CC'(+1)) - r > 0$ assuming this is non-zero or the bias-unadjusted value $D = m(CC'(+1))$. For the spatial AR1 structure, as in Sect. 2.4.1, let $d(i)$ $1 \leq i \leq n_d$ denote the n_d unique positive distances apart for $cc' \in CC'(+1)$ and let $CC'(+1, i)$ be the subset of $CC'(+1)$ satisfying

$$CC'(+1, i) = \{cc' : cc' \in \text{CC}(+1), |t(c') - t(c)| = d(i)\}$$

of size $m(CC'(+1, i))$. For a given value of the coefficient parameter vector $\boldsymbol{\theta}$, define the n_d estimates $r_{\text{AR1},u,u'}(\boldsymbol{\theta}, i)$ of $r_{\text{AR1},u,u'}(\boldsymbol{\theta})$ as

$$r_{\mathrm{AR1},u,u'}(\boldsymbol{\theta},i) = \mathrm{power}\left(\frac{\sum\limits_{cc'\in CC'(+1,i)} stde_{sc,u}(\boldsymbol{\theta})\cdot \mathrm{stde}_{sc',u'}(\boldsymbol{\theta})}{D(i)}, \frac{1}{d(i)}\right)$$

where the denominator $D(i)$ is either the bias-adjusted value $D(i) = m(CC'(+1,i)) - r > 0$ assuming this is non-zero or the bias-unadjusted value $D(i) = m(CC'(+1,i))$. An estimate of the spatial autocorrelation $r_{\mathrm{AR1},u,u'}(\boldsymbol{\theta})$ is given by the average of the n_d estimates $r_{\mathrm{AR1},u,u'}(\boldsymbol{\theta},i)$, that is

$$r_{\mathrm{AR1},u,u'}(\boldsymbol{\theta}) = \frac{\sum\limits_{i=1}^{n_d} r_{\mathrm{AR1},u,u'}(\boldsymbol{\theta},i)}{n_d}.$$

In the non-spatial case, $n_d = 1$ and the spatial estimate is equivalent to the non-spatial estimate and is the same when $d(1) = 1$. The correlation parameter estimates $r_{\mathrm{AR1},u,u'}(\boldsymbol{\theta})$ are combined over $1 \le u,\ u' \le K$ into the $K^2 \times 1$ correlation parameter vector $\rho_{\mathrm{AR1}}(\boldsymbol{\theta})$.

10.3.4 Unstructured Correlations

Under the UN correlation structure, the component matrices $\boldsymbol{R}_{s,c,c'}$ have entries $r_{\mathrm{UN},c,c',u,u'}$ for $c,\ c' \in C(s)$ with $c < c'$ and $1 \le u,\ u' \le K$ while $\boldsymbol{R}_{s,c',c} = \boldsymbol{R}^{\mathrm{T}}_{s,c,c'}$. For a given value of the coefficient parameter vector $\boldsymbol{\theta}$, the estimate $r_{\mathrm{UN},c,c',u,u'}(\boldsymbol{\theta})$ of the UN correlation parameter $r_{\mathrm{UN},c,c',u,u'}$ is computed as

$$r_{\mathrm{UN},c,c',u,u'}(\boldsymbol{\theta}) = \frac{\sum\limits_{s\in S(cc')} stde_{sc,u}(\boldsymbol{\theta})\cdot stde_{sc',u'}(\boldsymbol{\theta})}{D}$$

where $S(cc')$ is the set of $m(S(cc'))$ observed matched set indexes s with observed values for an index pair cc' in the set CC defined in Sect. 2.4.1 and the denominator D is either the bias-adjusted value $D = m(S(cc')) - r > 0$ assuming this is non-zero or the bias-unadjusted value $D = m(S(cc'))$. The correlation parameter vector ρ_{UN} is estimated by combining the estimates $r_{\mathrm{UN},c,c',u,u'}(\boldsymbol{\theta})$ of the UN correlation parameters over $1 \le c,\ c' \le m$ with $c < c'$ and $1 \le u,\ u' \le K$ into the $(K^2 \cdot m \cdot (m - 1)/2) \times 1$ correlation parameter vector $\rho_{\mathrm{UN}}(\boldsymbol{\theta})$.

The number $K^2 \cdot m \cdot (m - 1)/2$ of UN correlation parameters can be quite large even for relatively small values of K and m. For example, the trichotomous outcome defined in Sect. 13.1 has $K = 2$ and $m = 5$ so that there are 40 UN correlation parameters. This increases to 90 UN correlation parameters for $K = 3$ and 160 UN correlation parameters for $K = 4$. These numbers indicate that it can be impractical to consider the UN correlation structure for some correlated polytomous outcomes.

10.3.5 Degeneracy in Correlation Estimates

For the EC, AR1, and UN correlation structures, generated correlation matrices can be degenerate. However, the correlation matrices $\boldsymbol{R}_s(\boldsymbol{\rho})$ depend on $\boldsymbol{\theta}$ and so change with $s \in S$ except in simple cases where $\boldsymbol{\mu}_s$ is the same for all $s \in S$, and so it is not possible to check a single correlation matrix for degeneracy as in Sect. 3.6. Degeneracy in the multinomial case can be checked by computing the eigenvalues of $\boldsymbol{R}_s(\boldsymbol{\rho})$ over $s \in S$. If any one of these has a non-positive smallest eigenvalue, then the model needs to be dropped from consideration in the search for a solution to $\boldsymbol{E}(\boldsymbol{\theta}) = \boldsymbol{0}$.

10.4 Extended Linear Mixed Modeling

As in Chap. 5, full maximum likelihood estimation is possible, maximizing the likelihood in the correlation parameters as well as in the mean and dispersion parameters. In what follows, revised estimating equations are formulated for mean and dispersion parameters as well as for EC, spatial AR1, and UN correlation parameters. There is now just one alternative estimate of the correlation vector and not bias-adjusted and bias-unadjusted alternatives as for standard, partially modified, and fully modified GEE.

10.4.1 Estimating Equations for Means, Dispersions, and Correlations Based on the Likelihood

The definitions of the log-likelihood function $\ell(SC; \boldsymbol{\theta})$ and the likelihood function $L(SC; \boldsymbol{\theta})$ of Sect. 10.2 apply in the ELMM case without change. However, the parameter vector is now

$$\boldsymbol{\theta} = \begin{pmatrix} \boldsymbol{\beta} \\ \boldsymbol{\gamma} \\ \boldsymbol{\rho} \end{pmatrix}$$

with $K \cdot r + q + p$ entries, where p is the number of correlation parameters. The likelihood $L(SC; \boldsymbol{\theta})$ is maximized in the coefficient parameter vector $\boldsymbol{\theta}$. Specifically, use Newton's method to solve the estimating equations

$$\boldsymbol{E}(\boldsymbol{\theta}) = \frac{\partial \ell(SC; \boldsymbol{\theta})}{\partial \boldsymbol{\theta}} = \sum_{s \in S} \boldsymbol{E}_s(\boldsymbol{\theta}) = \sum_{s \in S} \frac{\partial \ell(\boldsymbol{O}_s; \boldsymbol{\theta})}{\partial \boldsymbol{\theta}} = \boldsymbol{0}$$

where the operator notation $\frac{\partial}{\partial \theta}$ is used to indicate that this is a standard partial derivative vector in $\boldsymbol{\theta}$ since $\boldsymbol{\rho}$ is treated as a separate parameter vector. The associated matrix

$$\boldsymbol{E}'(\boldsymbol{\theta}) = \frac{\partial \boldsymbol{E}(\boldsymbol{\theta})}{\partial \boldsymbol{\theta}}.$$

In this case, $\boldsymbol{E}(\boldsymbol{\theta})$ is a true gradient vector and $\boldsymbol{E}'(\boldsymbol{\theta})$ a true Hessian matrix.

The gradient vector satisfies

$$\boldsymbol{E}(\boldsymbol{\theta}) = \begin{pmatrix} \boldsymbol{E}(\boldsymbol{\beta}) \\ \boldsymbol{E}(\boldsymbol{\gamma}) \\ \boldsymbol{E}(\boldsymbol{\rho}) \end{pmatrix}$$

where $\boldsymbol{E}(\boldsymbol{\gamma})$ is computed as in Sect. 10.2 for partially and fully modified GEE modeling since the correlation matrices do not depend on the dispersion parameters, but $\boldsymbol{E}(\boldsymbol{\beta})$ is now different because $\boldsymbol{R}_s(\boldsymbol{\rho})$ depends on the mean parameter vector $\boldsymbol{\beta}$ (see Sect. 10.3). Specifically,

$$\boldsymbol{E}(\boldsymbol{\beta}) = \boldsymbol{E}_0(\boldsymbol{\beta}) + \boldsymbol{E}_1(\boldsymbol{\beta})$$

where $\boldsymbol{E}_0(\boldsymbol{\beta})$ is computed using fully modified GEE formulas for $\boldsymbol{E}(\boldsymbol{\beta})$ given in Sect. 10.2 and $\boldsymbol{E}_1(\boldsymbol{\beta})$ is the extra amount to account for the dependence of $\boldsymbol{R}_s(\boldsymbol{\rho})$ on $\boldsymbol{\beta}$. Details on the computation of $\boldsymbol{E}(\boldsymbol{\theta})$ are given in Sects. 10.4.2–10.4.3.

$\boldsymbol{E}'(\boldsymbol{\theta})$ has nine component matrices: the $(K \cdot r) \times (K \cdot r)$ matrix

$$\boldsymbol{E}'(\boldsymbol{\beta}) = \frac{\partial \boldsymbol{E}(\boldsymbol{\beta})}{\partial \boldsymbol{\beta}}$$

for the $K \cdot r$ mean parameters, the $q \times q$ matrix

$$\boldsymbol{E}'(\boldsymbol{\gamma}) = \frac{\partial \boldsymbol{E}(\boldsymbol{\gamma})}{\partial \boldsymbol{\gamma}}$$

for the q dispersion parameters computed as in Sect. 10.2 for partially and fully modified GEE modeling, the $p \times p$ matrix

$$\boldsymbol{E}'(\boldsymbol{\rho}) = \frac{\partial \boldsymbol{E}(\boldsymbol{\rho})}{\partial \boldsymbol{\rho}}$$

for the p correlation parameters, the $(K \cdot r) \times q$ matrix

$$\boldsymbol{E}'(\boldsymbol{\beta},\boldsymbol{\gamma}) = \frac{\partial \boldsymbol{E}(\boldsymbol{\beta})}{\partial \boldsymbol{\gamma}}$$

and its transpose $\boldsymbol{E}'(\boldsymbol{\gamma},\boldsymbol{\beta}) = \boldsymbol{E}'^{\mathrm{T}}(\boldsymbol{\beta},\boldsymbol{\gamma})$, the $(K \cdot r) \times p$ matrix

$$\boldsymbol{E}'(\boldsymbol{\beta},\boldsymbol{\rho}) = \frac{\partial \boldsymbol{E}(\boldsymbol{\beta})}{\partial \boldsymbol{\rho}}$$

and its transpose $\boldsymbol{E}'(\boldsymbol{\rho},\boldsymbol{\beta}) = \boldsymbol{E}'^{\mathrm{T}}(\boldsymbol{\beta},\boldsymbol{\rho})$, the $q \times p$ matrix

$$\boldsymbol{E}'(\boldsymbol{\gamma},\boldsymbol{\rho}) = \frac{\partial \boldsymbol{E}(\boldsymbol{\gamma})}{\partial \boldsymbol{\rho}}$$

and its transpose $\boldsymbol{E}'(\boldsymbol{\rho},\boldsymbol{\gamma}) = \boldsymbol{E}'^{\mathrm{T}}(\boldsymbol{\gamma},\boldsymbol{\rho})$. Details on the computation of $\boldsymbol{E}'(\boldsymbol{\theta})$ are given in Sects. 10.4.4–10.4.8.

Model-based and robust empirical estimates of the covariance matrix for the ELMM estimate

$$\boldsymbol{\theta}(SC) = \begin{pmatrix} \boldsymbol{\beta}(SC) \\ \boldsymbol{\gamma}(SC) \\ \boldsymbol{\rho}(SC) \end{pmatrix}$$

of the coefficient parameter vector $\boldsymbol{\theta}$ can be computed similarly to those for ELMM given in Sect. 5.1. These use the ELMM versions of $\boldsymbol{E}'(\boldsymbol{\theta}(SC))$ and $\boldsymbol{G}(\boldsymbol{\theta}(SC))$ for multinomial regression. $\boldsymbol{G}(\boldsymbol{\theta}(SC))$ is defined so that summing the entries of its rows generates $\boldsymbol{E}(\boldsymbol{\theta}(SC))$. A detailed formulation for $\boldsymbol{G}(\boldsymbol{\theta}(SC))$ is not provided for brevity.

The first and second partial derivatives of $\ell(SC;\boldsymbol{\theta})$ are sums over $s \in S$ of associated first and second partial derivatives of $\ell(O_s;\boldsymbol{\theta})$. The next seven sections provide formulations for these derivatives except for the cases $\boldsymbol{E}(\boldsymbol{\gamma})$ and $\boldsymbol{E}'(\boldsymbol{\gamma})$, which are formulated in Sect. 10.2. These formulations are needed to compute $\boldsymbol{E}(\boldsymbol{\theta})$ and $\boldsymbol{E}'(\boldsymbol{\theta})$ but can be skipped since they are complicated.

Derivatives involving the correlation matrices $\boldsymbol{R}_s(\boldsymbol{\rho})$ are based on formulations given in Wolfinger et al. (1994). Their formulas are for $-2 \cdot \ell(O_s;\boldsymbol{\theta})$ and so need to be converted to handle $\ell(O_s;\boldsymbol{\theta})$. Formulas for these derivatives are also given in Schott (2005). Specifically, denote the entries of the parameter vector $\boldsymbol{\theta}$ as θ_i for $1 \le i \le K \cdot r + q + p$. First partial derivatives involving $\boldsymbol{R}_s(\boldsymbol{\rho})$ satisfy

$$\frac{\partial \log|\boldsymbol{R}_s(\boldsymbol{\rho})|}{\partial \theta_i} = \mathrm{tr}\left(\boldsymbol{R}_s^{-1}(\boldsymbol{\rho}) \cdot \frac{\partial \boldsymbol{R}_s(\boldsymbol{\rho})}{\partial \theta_i}\right)$$

and

$$\frac{\partial \boldsymbol{R}_s^{-1}(\boldsymbol{\rho})}{\partial \theta_i} = -\boldsymbol{R}_s^{-1}(\boldsymbol{\rho}) \cdot \frac{\partial \boldsymbol{R}_s(\boldsymbol{\rho})}{\partial \theta_i} \cdot \boldsymbol{R}_s^{-1}(\boldsymbol{\rho}).$$

Note that the dependence of the correlation matrices $\boldsymbol{R}_s(\boldsymbol{\rho})$ on the mean parameter vector $\boldsymbol{\beta}$ is suppressed in the notation to reduce its complexity, and so the above derivatives are non-zero when θ_i corresponds to a mean parameter or a correlation parameter, but are zero when θ_i corresponds to a dispersion parameter. Second partial derivatives involving $\boldsymbol{R}_s(\boldsymbol{\rho})$ satisfy

$$\frac{\partial^2 \log|\boldsymbol{R}_s(\boldsymbol{\rho})|}{\partial \theta_{i'} \, \partial \theta_i} = -\operatorname{tr}\left(\boldsymbol{R}_s^{-1}(\boldsymbol{\rho}) \cdot \frac{\partial \boldsymbol{R}_s(\boldsymbol{\rho})}{\partial \theta_{i'}} \cdot \boldsymbol{R}_s^{-1}(\boldsymbol{\rho}) \cdot \frac{\partial \boldsymbol{R}_s(\boldsymbol{\rho})}{\partial \theta_i}\right) + \operatorname{tr}\left(\boldsymbol{R}_s^{-1}(\boldsymbol{\rho}) \cdot \frac{\partial^2 \boldsymbol{R}_s(\boldsymbol{\rho})}{\partial \theta_{i'} \, \partial \theta_i}\right)$$

and

$$\frac{\partial^2 \boldsymbol{R}_s^{-1}(\boldsymbol{\rho})}{\partial \theta_{i'} \, \partial \theta_i} = 2 \cdot \boldsymbol{R}_s^{-1}(\boldsymbol{\rho}) \cdot \frac{\partial \boldsymbol{R}_s(\boldsymbol{\rho})}{\partial \theta_{i'}} \cdot \boldsymbol{R}_s^{-1}(\boldsymbol{\rho}) \cdot \frac{\partial \boldsymbol{R}_s(\boldsymbol{\rho})}{\partial \theta_i} \cdot \boldsymbol{R}_s^{-1}(\boldsymbol{\rho}) - \boldsymbol{R}_s^{-1}(\boldsymbol{\rho}) \cdot \frac{\partial^2 \boldsymbol{R}_s(\boldsymbol{\rho})}{\partial \theta_{i'} \, \partial \theta_i} \cdot \boldsymbol{R}_s^{-1}(\boldsymbol{\rho})$$

for $1 \leq i, i' \leq K \cdot r + q + p$. These are zero when θ_i or $\theta_{i'}$ correspond to a dispersion parameter. The second derivatives $\frac{\partial^2 \boldsymbol{R}_s(\boldsymbol{\rho})}{\partial \theta_{i'} \partial \theta_i}$ can sometimes be zero so that associated terms are dropped from the second partial derivatives of $\log|\boldsymbol{R}_s(\boldsymbol{\rho})|$ and $\boldsymbol{R}_s^{-1}(\boldsymbol{\rho})$. These cases are identified in what follows.

10.4.2 First Partial Derivatives with Respect to Mean Parameters

The gradient vector $\boldsymbol{E}(\boldsymbol{\beta})$ for the mean parameters satisfies

$$\boldsymbol{E}(\boldsymbol{\beta}) = \boldsymbol{E}_0(\boldsymbol{\beta}) + \boldsymbol{E}_1(\boldsymbol{\beta})$$

where $\boldsymbol{E}_0(\boldsymbol{\beta})$ is computed using fully modified GEE formulas for $\boldsymbol{E}(\boldsymbol{\beta})$ given in Sect. 10.2. $\boldsymbol{E}_1(\boldsymbol{\beta})$ is the sum over $s \in S$ of terms $\boldsymbol{E}_{1,\ s}(\boldsymbol{\beta})$ with entries

$$E_{1,s,w,j}(\rho) = -\boldsymbol{stde}_s^{\mathrm{T}} \cdot \frac{\partial \boldsymbol{R}_s^{-1}(\rho)}{\partial \beta_{w,j}} \cdot \boldsymbol{stde}_s/2 - \frac{\partial \log|\boldsymbol{R}_s(\rho)|}{\partial \beta_{w,j}}/2$$

where $\frac{\partial \log|\boldsymbol{R}_s(\rho)|}{\partial \beta_{w,j}}$ and $\frac{\partial \boldsymbol{R}_s^{-1}(\rho)}{\partial \beta_{w,j}}$ for $1 \leq w \leq K$ and $1 \leq j \leq r$ are defined in Sect. 10.4.1. Using the notation of Sect. 10.3, $\frac{\partial \boldsymbol{R}_s(\rho)}{\partial \beta_{w,j}}$ has component matrices $\frac{\partial \boldsymbol{R}_{s,c,c'}}{\partial \beta_{w,j}}$ for $c, c' \in C(s)$. For $c, c' \in C(s)$ with $c \neq c'$, the off-diagonal component matrices $\boldsymbol{R}_{s,\ c,\ c'}$ satisfy

$$\frac{\partial \boldsymbol{R}_{s,c,c'}}{\partial \beta_{w,j}} = \mathbf{0}$$

for each of the four correlation structures of Sect. 10.3 because they do not depend on $\boldsymbol{\beta}$. The diagonal component matrices $\boldsymbol{R}_{s,\ c,\ c}$ have first partial derivatives $\frac{\partial \boldsymbol{R}_{s,c,c}}{\partial \beta_{w,j}}$ with entries $\frac{\partial r_{s,c,c,u,u'}}{\partial \beta_{w,j}}$ satisfying

$$\frac{\partial r_{s,c,c,u,u'}}{\partial \beta_{w,j}} = x_{sc,j} \cdot r_{s,c,c,u,u'} \cdot \left(1 - \frac{\mu_{sc,u}}{1-\mu_{sc,u'}}\right)/2, w = u;$$

$$\frac{\partial r_{s,c,c,u,u'}}{\partial \beta_{w,j}} = x_{sc,j} \cdot r_{s,c,c,u,u'} \cdot \left(1 - \frac{\mu_{sc,u'}}{1-\mu_{sc,u}}\right)/2, w = u';$$

$$\frac{\partial r_{s,c,c,u,u'}}{\partial \beta_{w,j}} = -x_{sc,j} \cdot r_{s,c,c,u,u'} \cdot \mu_{sc,w} \cdot \left(\frac{1}{1-\mu_{sc,u}} + \frac{1}{1-\mu_{sc,u'}}\right)/2, w \neq u, w \neq u'$$

for $1 \leq u, u', w \leq K$ and $1 \leq j \leq r$.

10.4.3 First Partial Derivatives with Respect to Correlation Parameters

With the entries of $\boldsymbol{\rho}$ denoted by ρ_j for $1 \leq j \leq p$,

$$\boldsymbol{E}(\boldsymbol{\rho}) = \frac{\partial \ell(SC;\boldsymbol{\theta})}{\partial \boldsymbol{\rho}}$$

is the sum over $s \in S$ of $\boldsymbol{E}_s(\boldsymbol{\rho})$ with entries

$$E_{s,j}(\rho) = -\boldsymbol{stde}_s^{\mathrm{T}} \cdot \frac{\partial \boldsymbol{R}_s^{-1}(\rho)}{\partial \rho_j} \cdot \boldsymbol{stde}_s/2 - \frac{\partial \log|\boldsymbol{R}_s(\rho)|}{\partial \rho_j}/2$$

where $\frac{\partial \log|\boldsymbol{R}_s(\rho)|}{\partial \rho_j}$ and $\frac{\partial \boldsymbol{R}_s^{-1}(\rho)}{\partial \rho_j}$ are defined in Sect. 10.4.1 for $1 \le j \le p$. For the four correlation structures of Sect. 10.3, the first partial derivative vector $\frac{\partial \boldsymbol{R}_s(\rho)}{\partial \rho_j}$ has diagonal component matrices

$$\frac{\partial \boldsymbol{R}_{s,c,c}}{\partial \rho_j} = \mathbf{0}$$

for $c \in C(s)$ because $\boldsymbol{R}_{s,c,c}$ do not depend on the correlation parameters.

For independent correlations, the off-diagonal component matrices

$$\frac{\partial \boldsymbol{R}_{s,c,c'}}{\partial \rho_j} = \mathbf{0}$$

because $\boldsymbol{R}_{s,c,c'} = \mathbf{0}$ for $c, c' \in C(s)$, $c \neq c'$.

For exchangeable correlations, $\boldsymbol{R}_{s,c,c'} = \boldsymbol{R}$ for $c, c' \in C(s)$ with $c < c'$ and a fixed $K \times K$ matrix $\boldsymbol{R}$ with $p = K^2$ unique entries ρ_j for $1 \le j \le p$ denoted as $r_{\mathrm{EC},u,u'}$ for $1 \le u, u' \le K$ while $\boldsymbol{R}_{s,c',c} = \boldsymbol{R}^{\mathrm{T}}$. In this case,

$$\frac{\partial \boldsymbol{R}_{s,c,c'}}{\partial r_{\mathrm{EC},u,u'}} = \boldsymbol{J}(u, u')$$

for $c, c' \in C(s)$ with $c < c'$ where $\boldsymbol{J}(u, u')$ is the $K \times K$ matrix with entry 1 in the uth row and u'^{th} column and 0 elsewhere while

$$\frac{\partial \boldsymbol{R}_{s,c',c}}{\partial r_{\mathrm{EC},u,u'}} = \boldsymbol{J}^{\mathrm{T}}(u, u').$$

For spatial autoregressive order 1 correlations,

$$\boldsymbol{R}_{s,c,c'} = \mathrm{power}(\boldsymbol{R}, |t(c') - t(c)|)$$

for $c, c' \in C(s)$ with $c < c'$ and a fixed $K \times K$ matrix $\boldsymbol{R}$ with $p = K^2$ unique entries ρ_j for $1 \le j \le p$ denoted as $r_{\mathrm{AR1},u,u'}$ for $1 \le u, u' \le K$ while $\boldsymbol{R}_{s,c',c} = \boldsymbol{R}^T_{s,c,c'}$. In this case, $\boldsymbol{R}_{s,c,c'}$ for $c, c' \in C(s)$ with $c < c'$ has entries

$$\begin{aligned} r_{s,c,c',u,u'} &= \mathrm{power}(r_{\mathrm{AR1},u,u'}, |t(c') - t(c)|) \\ &= \mathrm{sign}(r_{\mathrm{AR1},u,u'}) \cdot (\mathrm{sign}(r_{\mathrm{AR1},u,u'}) \cdot r_{\mathrm{AR1},u,u'})^{|t(c') - t(c)|} \end{aligned}$$

when $|r_{\mathrm{AR1},u,u'}| > 0$ for $1 \le u, u' \le K$ so that

$$\frac{\partial \boldsymbol{R}_{s,c,c'}}{\partial r_{\text{AR1},u,u'}} = \boldsymbol{J}(c, c', u, u')$$

where $\boldsymbol{J}(c, c', u, u')$ is the $K \times K$ matrix with zero entries except for the entry in the uth row and u'^{th} column satisfying

$$\begin{aligned}
&\frac{\partial r_{s,c,c',u,u'}}{\partial r_{\text{AR1},u,u'}} \\
&\quad = (\text{sign}(r_{\text{AR1},u,u'}))^2 \cdot |t(c') - t(c)| \cdot (\text{sign}(r_{\text{AR1},u,u'}) \cdot r_{\text{AR1},u,u'})^{|t(c') - t(c)| - 1} \\
&\quad = |t(c') - t(c)| \cdot |r_{\text{AR1},u,u'}|^{|t(c') - t(c)| - 1}
\end{aligned}$$

with its sign changed when negative while

$$\frac{\partial \boldsymbol{R}_{s,c',c}}{\partial r_{\text{AR1},u,u'}} = \boldsymbol{J}^{\text{T}}(c, c', u, u').$$

When $|t(c') - t(c)| = 1$, the derivative $\frac{\partial r_{s,c,c',u,u'}}{\partial r_{\text{AR1},u,u'}}$ at $r_{\text{AR1},u,u'} = 0$ from above is $+1$ and from below is -1, and so the derivative is not well-defined. This problem can be circumvented in practice by restricting $|r_{\text{AR1},u,u'}|$ to be greater than some small value.

For unstructured correlations, $\boldsymbol{R}_{s,c,c'}$ have $p = K^2 \cdot m(s) \cdot (m(s) - 1)/2$ entries ρ_j for $1 \leq j \leq p$ denoted as $r_{\text{UN},c,c',u,u'}$ for $c, c' \in C(s)$ with $c < c'$ and $1 \leq u, u' \leq K$ while $\boldsymbol{R}_{s,c',c} = \boldsymbol{R}^{\text{T}}{}_{c,c'}$. In this case,

$$\frac{\partial \boldsymbol{R}_{s,c,c'}}{\partial r_{\text{UN},c,c',u,u'}} = \boldsymbol{J}'(c, c', u, u')$$

for $c, c' \in C(s)$ with $c < c'$ where $\boldsymbol{J}'(c, c', u, u')$ is the $K \times K$ matrix with entry 1 in the uth row and u'^{th} column and 0 elsewhere while

$$\frac{\partial \boldsymbol{R}_{s,c',c}}{\partial r_{\text{UN},c,c',u,u'}} = \boldsymbol{J}'^{\text{T}}(c, c', u, u').$$

On the other hand,

$$\frac{\partial \boldsymbol{R}_{s,d,d'}}{\partial r_{\text{UN},c,c',u,u'}} = \boldsymbol{0}$$

for $d, d' \in C(s)$ with $d \neq c$ or $d' \neq c'$.

10.4.4 Second Partial Derivatives with Respect to Mean Parameters

The matrix $\boldsymbol{E}'(\boldsymbol{\beta})$ for the mean parameters satisfies

$$\boldsymbol{E}'(\boldsymbol{\beta}) = \boldsymbol{E}'_0(\boldsymbol{\beta}) + \boldsymbol{E}'_1(\boldsymbol{\beta}) + \boldsymbol{E}'_2(\boldsymbol{\beta})$$

where $\boldsymbol{E}'_0(\boldsymbol{\beta})$ is computed using formulas for $\boldsymbol{E}'(\boldsymbol{\beta})$ given in Sect. 10.2 for fully modified GEE. $\boldsymbol{E}'_1(\boldsymbol{\beta})$ is the sum over $s \in S$ of terms $\boldsymbol{E}'_{1,s}(\boldsymbol{\beta})$ with entries

$$E'_{1,s,w,j,w',j'}(\boldsymbol{\beta}) = -\boldsymbol{stde}_s^{\mathrm{T}} \cdot \frac{\partial^2 \boldsymbol{R}_s^{-1}(\boldsymbol{\rho})}{\partial \beta_{w',j'}\,\partial \beta_{w,j}} \cdot \boldsymbol{stde}_s/2 - \frac{\partial^2 \log|\boldsymbol{R}_s(\boldsymbol{\rho})|}{\partial \beta_{w',j'}\,\partial \beta_{w,j}}/2$$

where $\frac{\partial^2 \log|\boldsymbol{R}_s(\boldsymbol{\rho})|}{\partial \beta_{w',j'}\,\partial \beta_{w,j}}$ and $\frac{\partial^2 \boldsymbol{R}_s^{-1}(\boldsymbol{\rho})}{\partial \beta_{w',j'}\,\partial \beta_{w,j}}$ for $1 \le w, w' \le K$ and $1 \le j, j' \le r$ are defined in Sect. 10.4.1. Using the notation of Sect. 10.3, $\frac{\partial^2 \boldsymbol{R}_s(\boldsymbol{\rho})}{\partial \beta_{w',j'}\,\partial \beta_{w,j}}$ has component matrices $\frac{\partial^2 \boldsymbol{R}_{s,c,c'}}{\partial \beta_{w',j'}\,\partial \beta_{w,j}}$ for $c, c' \in C(s)$. For $c, c' \in C(s)$ with $c \ne c'$,

$$\frac{\partial^2 \boldsymbol{R}_{s,c,c'}}{\partial \beta_{w',j'}\,\partial \beta_{w,j}} = \mathbf{0}$$

for each of the four correlation structures of Sect. 10.3 because

$$\frac{\partial \boldsymbol{R}_{s,c,c'}}{\partial \beta_{w,j}} = \mathbf{0}.$$

The diagonal component matrices $\boldsymbol{R}_{s,c,c}$ have second partial derivatives $\frac{\partial^2 \boldsymbol{R}_{s,c,c}(\boldsymbol{\rho})}{\partial \beta_{w',j'}\,\partial \beta_{w,j}}$ with entries

$$\frac{\partial^2 r_{s,c,c,u,u'}}{\partial \beta_{w',j'}\,\partial \beta_{w,j}} = x_{sc,j} \cdot \frac{\partial r_{s,c,c,u,u'}}{\partial \beta_{w',j'}} \cdot \left(1 - \frac{\mu_{sc,u}}{1-\mu_{sc,u'}}\right)/2 + x_{sc,j} \cdot r_{s,c,c,u,u'} \cdot x_{sc,j'} \cdot a_1/2,$$

for $w = u$, $w' = u$;

$$\frac{\partial^2 r_{s,c,c,u,u'}}{\partial \beta_{w',j'}\,\partial \beta_{w,j}} = x_{sc,j} \cdot \frac{\partial r_{s,c,c,u,u'}}{\partial \beta_{w',j'}} \cdot \left(1 - \frac{\mu_{sc,u'}}{1-\mu_{sc,u}}\right)/2 + x_{sc,j} \cdot r_{s,c,c,u,u'} \cdot x_{sc,j'} \cdot a_2/2,$$

for $w = u$, $w' = u'$;

$$\frac{\partial^2 r_{s,c,c,u,u'}}{\partial\beta_{w',j'}\,\partial\beta_{w,j}} = x_{sc,j} \cdot \frac{\partial r_{s,c,c,u,u'}}{\partial\beta_{w',j'}} \cdot \left(1 - \frac{\mu_{sc,u'}}{1-\mu_{sc,u}}\right)/2 + x_{sc,j} \cdot r_{s,c,c,u,u'} \cdot x_{sc,j'} \cdot a_3/2,$$

for $w = u$, $w' \neq u$, $w' \neq u'$;

$$\frac{\partial^2 r_{s,c,c,u,u'}}{\partial\beta_{w',j'}\,\partial\beta_{w,j}} = x_{sc,j} \cdot \frac{\partial r_{s,c,c,u,u'}}{\partial\beta_{w',j'}} \cdot \left(1 - \frac{\mu_{sc,u}}{1-\mu_{sc,u'}}\right)/2 + x_{sc,j} \cdot r_{s,c,c,u,u'} \cdot x_{sc,j'} \cdot a_4/2,$$

for $w' = u$, $w' = u'$;

$$\frac{\partial^2 r_{s,c,c,u,u'}}{\partial\beta_{w',j'}\,\partial\beta_{w,j}} = x_{sc,j} \cdot \frac{\partial r_{s,c,c,u,u'}}{\partial\beta_{w',j'}} \cdot \left(1 - \frac{\mu_{sc,u}}{1-\mu_{sc,u'}}\right)/2 + x_{sc,j} \cdot r_{s,c,c,u,u'} \cdot x_{sc,j'} \cdot a_5/2,$$

for $w = u'$, $w' = u'$;

$$\frac{\partial^2 r_{s,c,c,u,u'}}{\partial\beta_{w',j'}\,\partial\beta_{w,j}} = x_{sc,j} \cdot \frac{\partial r_{s,c,c,u,u'}}{\partial\beta_{w',j'}} \cdot \left(1 - \frac{\mu_{sc,u}}{1-\mu_{sc,u'}}\right)/2 + x_{sc,j} \cdot r_{s,c,c,u,u'} \cdot x_{sc,j'} \cdot a_6/2,$$

for $w = u'$, $w' \neq u$, $w' \neq u'$;

$$\begin{aligned}\frac{\partial^2 r_{s,c,c,u,u'}}{\partial\beta_{w',j'}\,\partial\beta_{w,j}} &= x_{sc,j} \cdot \frac{\partial r_{s,c,c,u,u'}}{\partial\beta_{w',j'}} \cdot \mu_{sc,w} \cdot \left(\frac{1}{1-\mu_{sc,u}} + \frac{1}{1-\mu_{sc,u'}}\right)/2 \\ &\quad + x_{sc,j} \cdot r_{s,c,c,u,u'} \cdot x_{sc,j'} \cdot a_7/2,\end{aligned}$$

for $w \neq u$, $w \neq u'$, $w' = u$;

$$\begin{aligned}\frac{\partial^2 r_{s,c,c,u,u'}}{\partial\beta_{w',j'}\,\partial\beta_{w,j}} &= x_{sc,j} \cdot \frac{\partial r_{s,c,c,u,u'}}{\partial\beta_{w',j'}} \cdot \mu_{sc,w} \cdot \left(\frac{1}{1-\mu_{sc,u}} + \frac{1}{1-\mu_{sc,u'}}\right)/2 \\ &\quad + x_{sc,j} \cdot r_{s,c,c,u,u'} \cdot x_{sc,j'} \cdot a_8/2,\end{aligned}$$

for $w \neq u$, $w \neq u'$, $w' = u'$;

$$\begin{aligned}\frac{\partial^2 r_{s,c,c,u,u'}}{\partial\beta_{w',j'}\,\partial\beta_{w,j}} &= -x_{sc,j} \cdot \frac{\partial r_{s,c,c,u,u'}}{\partial\beta_{w',j'}} \cdot \mu_{sc,w} \cdot \left(\frac{1}{1-\mu_{sc,u}} + \frac{1}{1-\mu_{sc,u'}}\right)/2 \\ &\quad - x_{sc,j} \cdot r_{s,c,c,u,u'} \cdot x_{sc,j'} \cdot a_9/2,\end{aligned}$$

for $w \neq u$, $w \neq u'$, $w' \neq u$, $w' \neq u'$, $w' = w$; and

$$\frac{\partial^2 r_{s,c,c,u,u'}}{\partial \beta_{w',j'} \partial \beta_{w,j}} = -x_{sc,j} \cdot \frac{\partial r_{s,c,c,u,u'}}{\partial \beta_{w',j'}} \cdot \mu_{sc,w} \cdot \left(\frac{1}{1-\mu_{sc,u}} + \frac{1}{1-\mu_{sc,u'}}\right)/2$$
$$-x_{sc,j} \cdot r_{s,c,c,u,u'} \cdot x_{sc,j'} \cdot a_{10}/2,$$

for $w \neq u$, $w \neq u'$, $w' \neq u$, $w' \neq u'$, $w' \neq w$. The quantities a_1-a_{10} satisfy

$$a_1 = -\frac{\mu_{sc,u}}{1-\mu_{sc,u'}} \cdot \left(1 - \frac{\mu_{sc,u}}{1-\mu_{sc,u'}}\right),$$

$$a_2 = 0,$$

$$a_3 = \mu_{sc,w'} \cdot \frac{\mu_{sc,u}}{\left(1-\mu_{sc,u\prime}\right)^2},$$

$$a_4 = 0,$$

$$a_5 = -\frac{\mu_{sc,u'}}{1-\mu_{sc,u}} \cdot \left(1 - \frac{\mu_{sc,u'}}{1-\mu_{sc,u}}\right),$$

$$a_6 = \mu_{sc,w'} \cdot \frac{\mu_{sc,u'}}{\left(1-\mu_{sc,u}\right)^2},$$

$$a_7 = -\mu_{sc,w} \cdot \frac{\mu_{sc,u}}{\left(1-\mu_{sc,u'}\right)^2},$$

$$a_8 = -\mu_{sc,w} \cdot \frac{\mu_{sc,u'}}{\left(1-\mu_{sc,u}\right)^2},$$

$$a_9 = \mu_{sc,w} \cdot \left(\frac{1}{1-\mu_{sc,u}} + \frac{1}{1-\mu_{sc,u'}} - \mu_{sc,w} \cdot \left(\frac{1}{\left(1-\mu_{sc,u}\right)^2} + \frac{1}{\left(1-\mu_{sc,u\prime}\right)^2}\right)\right),$$

and

$$a_{10} = -\mu_{sc,w} \cdot -\mu_{sc,w'} \cdot \left(\frac{1}{\left(1-\mu_{sc,u}\right)^2} + \frac{1}{\left(1-\mu_{sc,u'}\right)^2}\right).$$

$\boldsymbol{E}'_2(\boldsymbol{\beta})$ is the sum over $s \in S$ of terms $\boldsymbol{E}'_{2,s}(\boldsymbol{\beta})$ with entries

$$E'_{2,s,w,j,w',j'}(\boldsymbol{\beta}) = \boldsymbol{xstde}_{s,w,j}^{\mathrm{T}} \cdot \frac{\partial \boldsymbol{R}_s^{-1}(\boldsymbol{\rho})}{\partial \beta_{w',j'}} \cdot \boldsymbol{stde}_s + \boldsymbol{xstde}_{s,w',j'}^{\mathrm{T}} \cdot \frac{\partial \boldsymbol{R}_s^{-1}(\boldsymbol{\rho})}{\partial \beta_{w,j}} \cdot \boldsymbol{stde}_s,$$

where $\frac{\partial \boldsymbol{R}_s^{-1}(\boldsymbol{\rho})}{\partial \beta_{w',j'}}$ and $\frac{\partial \boldsymbol{R}_s^{-1}(\boldsymbol{\rho})}{\partial \beta_{w,j}}$ for $1 \leq w,\ w' \leq K$ and $1 \leq j,\ j' \leq r$ are defined in Sect. 10.4.1.

10.4.5 Second Partial Derivatives with Respect to Correlation Parameters

With the entries of $\boldsymbol{\rho}$ denoted by ρ_j for $1 \le j \le p$,

$$\boldsymbol{E}'(\boldsymbol{\rho}) = \frac{\partial \boldsymbol{E}(\boldsymbol{\rho})}{\partial \boldsymbol{\rho}}$$

is the sum over $s \in S$ of $\boldsymbol{E}'_s(\boldsymbol{\rho})$ with entries satisfying

$$E'_{s,j,j'}(\boldsymbol{\rho}) = -\boldsymbol{stde}_s^{\mathrm{T}} \cdot \frac{\partial^2 \boldsymbol{R}_s^{-1}(\boldsymbol{\rho})}{\partial \rho_{j'}\,\partial \rho_j} \cdot \boldsymbol{stde}_s/2 - \frac{\partial^2 \log|\boldsymbol{R}_s(\boldsymbol{\rho})|}{\partial \rho_{j'}\,\partial \rho_j}/2$$

where $\frac{\partial^2 \log|\boldsymbol{R}_s(\boldsymbol{\rho})|}{\partial \rho_{j'}\,\partial \rho_j}$ and $\frac{\partial^2 \boldsymbol{R}_s^{-1}(\boldsymbol{\rho})}{\partial \rho_{j'}\,\partial \rho_j}$ for $1 \le j, j' \le p$ are defined in Sect. 10.4.1. For the four correlation structures of Sect. 10.3, the second partial derivatives of the diagonal component matrices $\boldsymbol{R}_{s,c,c}$ for $c \in C(s)$ satisfy

$$\frac{\partial^2 \boldsymbol{R}_{s,c,c}}{\partial \rho_{j'}\,\partial \rho_j} = \boldsymbol{0}$$

because $\boldsymbol{R}_{s,c,c}$ do not depend on the correlation parameters. For independent, exchangeable, and unstructured correlations, the off-diagonal component matrices $\boldsymbol{R}_{s,c,c'}$ satisfy

$$\frac{\partial^2 \boldsymbol{R}_{s,c,c'}}{\partial \rho_{j'}\,\partial \rho_j} = \boldsymbol{0}$$

for $1 \le j, j' \le p$ because $\frac{\partial \boldsymbol{R}_{s,c,c'}}{\partial \rho_j}$ are constant in those parameters for c, $c' \in C(s)$ with $c \ne c'$. For these correlation structures, terms based on $\frac{\partial^2 \boldsymbol{R}_s(\boldsymbol{\rho})}{\partial \rho_{j'}\,\partial \rho_j}$ are dropped from the second partial derivatives of $\log|\boldsymbol{R}_s(\boldsymbol{\rho})|$ and $\boldsymbol{R}_s^{-1}(\boldsymbol{\rho})$.

For spatial autoregressive order 1 correlations with entries ρ_j denoted as $r_{\mathrm{AR1},u,u'}$ for $1 \le u$, $u' \le K$, the off-diagonal component matrices $\boldsymbol{R}_{s,c,c'}$ satisfy

$$\frac{\partial^2 \boldsymbol{R}_{s,c,c'}}{\partial \rho_{j'}\,\partial \rho_j} = \boldsymbol{0}$$

for $j' \ne j$ because $\frac{\partial \boldsymbol{R}_{s,c,c'}}{\partial \rho_j}$ only depends on ρ_j for c, $c' \in C(s)$ with $c \ne c'$ so that then terms based on $\frac{\partial^2 \boldsymbol{R}_s(\boldsymbol{\rho})}{\partial \rho_{j'}\,\partial \rho_j}$ are dropped from associated second partial derivatives of $\log|\boldsymbol{R}_s(\boldsymbol{\rho})|$ and $\boldsymbol{R}_s^{-1}(\boldsymbol{\rho})$. The off-diagonal component matrices

$$\frac{\partial^2 \boldsymbol{R}_{s,c,c'}}{\partial \rho_j^2} = \boldsymbol{J}''(c,c',u,u)$$

for $j' = j$ and c, $c' \in C(s)$ with $c < c'$ when $\rho_j = r_{\mathrm{AR1},u,u'}$ where $\boldsymbol{J}''(c,c',u,u)$ is the $K \times K$ matrix with entry

$$\frac{\partial^2 r_{s,c,c,u,u'}}{\partial r^2_{\mathrm{AR1},u,u'}} = \mathrm{sign}(r_{\mathrm{AR1},u,u'}) \cdot |t(c') - t(c)| \cdot (|t(c') - t(c)| - 1) \cdot |r_{\mathrm{AR1},u,u'}|^{|t(c') - t(c)| - 2}$$

in the uth row and u'^{th} column with the signed changed back if negative and zero elsewhere while

$$\frac{\partial^2 \boldsymbol{R}_{s,c',c}}{\partial \rho_j^2} = \boldsymbol{J}''^{\mathrm{T}}(c,c',u,u),$$

which is guaranteed to hold by restricting $|r_{\mathrm{AR1},u,u'}|$ to be greater than some small value.

10.4.6 Second Partial Derivatives with Respect to Mean and Dispersion Parameters

As indicated in Sect. 10.2, $\boldsymbol{E}(\gamma)$ is the sum over $s \in S$ of terms $\boldsymbol{E}_s(\gamma)$ with entries

$$E_{s,j'}(\gamma) = \boldsymbol{vstde}^{\mathrm{T}}_{s,j'} \cdot \boldsymbol{R}_s^{-1}(\rho) \cdot \boldsymbol{stde}_s - \sum_{c \in C(s)} K \cdot v_{sc,j'}/2,$$

for $1 \le j' \le q$ so that $\boldsymbol{E}'(\gamma, \boldsymbol{\beta})$ is the sum over $s \in S$ of $\boldsymbol{E}'_s(\gamma, \boldsymbol{\beta})$ where

$$\boldsymbol{E}'_s(\gamma, \boldsymbol{\beta}) = \boldsymbol{E}'_{0,s}(\gamma, \boldsymbol{\beta}) + \boldsymbol{E}'_{1,s}(\gamma, \boldsymbol{\beta}).$$

$\boldsymbol{E}'_{0,s}(\gamma, \boldsymbol{\beta})$ has entries

$$\boldsymbol{E}'_{0,s,j',w,j}(\gamma, \boldsymbol{\beta}) = -\boldsymbol{xvstde}^{\mathrm{T}}_{s,j',w,j} \cdot \boldsymbol{R}_s^{-1}(\rho) \cdot \boldsymbol{stde}_s - \boldsymbol{vstde}^{\mathrm{T}}_{s,j'} \cdot \boldsymbol{R}_s^{-1}(\rho) \cdot \boldsymbol{xstde}_{s,w,j}$$

where $\boldsymbol{xstde}_{s,w,j}$ is defined in Sect. 10.2 and $\boldsymbol{xvstde}_{s,j',w,j}$ is the $(m(SC) \cdot K) \times 1$ vector with entries

$$xvstde_{sc,u,j',w,j} = xstde_{sc,u,w,j} \cdot v_{sc,j'}/2.$$

$\mathbf{E}'_{1,s}(\boldsymbol{\gamma},\boldsymbol{\beta})$ has entries

$$\mathbf{E}'_{1,s,j',w,j}(\boldsymbol{\gamma},\boldsymbol{\beta}) = \mathbf{vstde}^{\mathrm{T}}_{s,j'} \cdot \frac{\partial \mathbf{R}_s^{-1}(\boldsymbol{\rho})}{\partial \beta_{w,j}} \cdot \mathbf{stde}_s$$

for $1 \le j' \le q$, $1 \le w \le K$, and $1 \le j \le r$. The formula for $\frac{\partial \mathbf{R}_s^{-1}(\boldsymbol{\rho})}{\partial \beta_{w,j}}$ is given in Sect. 10.4.1 and $\mathbf{E}'(\boldsymbol{\beta},\boldsymbol{\gamma}) = \mathbf{E}'^{\mathrm{T}}(\boldsymbol{\gamma},\boldsymbol{\beta})$.

10.4.7 Second Partial Derivatives with Respect to Mean and Correlation Parameters

As indicated in Sect. 10.4.2,

$$\mathbf{E}(\boldsymbol{\beta}) = \mathbf{E}_0(\boldsymbol{\beta}) + \mathbf{E}_1(\boldsymbol{\beta})$$

so that

$$\mathbf{E}'(\boldsymbol{\beta},\boldsymbol{\rho}) = \mathbf{E}'_0(\boldsymbol{\beta},\boldsymbol{\rho}) + \mathbf{E}'_1(\boldsymbol{\beta},\boldsymbol{\rho})$$

and $\mathbf{E}'(\boldsymbol{\rho},\boldsymbol{\beta}) = \mathbf{E}'^{\mathrm{T}}(\boldsymbol{\beta},\boldsymbol{\rho})$. Also, $\mathbf{E}_0(\boldsymbol{\beta})$ is the sum over $s \in S$ of

$$E_{0,s,w,j}(\boldsymbol{\beta}) = \mathbf{xstde}^{\mathrm{T}}_{s,w,j} \cdot \mathbf{R}_s^{-1}(\boldsymbol{\rho}) \cdot \mathbf{stde}_s - \sum_{c \in C(s)} \sum_{u=1}^{K} W_{w,j}(\mu_{sc,u})/2$$

for $1 \le w \le K$ and $1 \le j \le r$ so that, with the entries of $\boldsymbol{\rho}$ denoted by $\rho_{j'}$ for $1 \le j' \le p$, $\mathbf{E}'_0(\boldsymbol{\beta},\boldsymbol{\rho})$ is the sum over $s \in S$ of $\mathbf{E}'_{0,\,s}(\boldsymbol{\beta},\boldsymbol{\rho})$ with entries

$$E'_{0,s,w,j,j'}(\boldsymbol{\beta},\boldsymbol{\rho}) = \mathbf{xstde}^{\mathrm{T}}_{s,w,j} \cdot \frac{\partial \mathbf{R}_s^{-1}(\boldsymbol{\rho})}{\partial \rho_{j'}} \cdot \mathbf{stde}_s$$

where the formula for $\frac{\partial \mathbf{R}_s^{-1}(\boldsymbol{\rho})}{\partial \rho_{j'}}$ is provided in Sect. 10.4.1. $\mathbf{E}'_1(\boldsymbol{\beta},\boldsymbol{\rho})$ is the sum over $s \in S$ of $\mathbf{E}'_{1,\,s}(\boldsymbol{\beta},\boldsymbol{\rho})$ with entries

$$E'_{1,s,w,j,j'}(\boldsymbol{\beta},\boldsymbol{\rho}) = -\mathbf{stde}^{\mathrm{T}}_s \cdot \frac{\partial^2 \mathbf{R}_s^{-1}(\boldsymbol{\rho})}{\partial \rho_{j'}\,\partial \beta_{w,j}} \cdot \mathbf{stde}_s/2 - \frac{\partial^2 \log|\mathbf{R}_s(\boldsymbol{\rho})|}{\partial \rho_{j'}\,\partial \beta_{w,j}}/2$$

where $\frac{\partial^2 \log|\boldsymbol{R}_s(\boldsymbol{\rho})|}{\partial \rho_{j'}\,\partial \beta_{w,j}}$ and $\frac{\partial^2 \boldsymbol{R}_s^{-1}(\boldsymbol{\rho})}{\partial \rho_{j'}\,\partial \beta_{w,j}}$ for $1 \le w \le K$, $1 \le j \le r$, and $1 \le j' \le p$ are defined in Sect. 10.4.1. Note that the first partial derivatives $\frac{\partial \boldsymbol{R}_s(\boldsymbol{\rho})}{\partial \beta_{K,j}}$ do not depend on $\boldsymbol{\rho}$ (see Sect. 10.4.2) so that

$$\frac{\partial^2 \boldsymbol{R}_s(\boldsymbol{\rho})}{\partial \rho_{j'}\,\partial \beta_{K,j}} = \mathbf{0},$$

and so terms based on $\frac{\partial^2 \boldsymbol{R}_s(\boldsymbol{\rho})}{\partial \rho_{j'}\,\partial \beta_{K,j}}$ are dropped from the second partial derivatives of $\log|\boldsymbol{R}_s(\boldsymbol{\rho})|$ and $\boldsymbol{R}_s^{-1}(\boldsymbol{\rho})$.

10.4.8 Second Partial Derivatives with Respect to Dispersion and Correlation Parameters

As indicated in Sect. 10.2, $\boldsymbol{E}(\boldsymbol{\gamma})$ is the sum over $s \in S$ of terms $\boldsymbol{E}_s(\boldsymbol{\gamma})$ with entries

$$E_{s,j'}(\boldsymbol{\gamma}) = \boldsymbol{vstde}_{s,j'}^{\mathrm{T}} \cdot \boldsymbol{R}_s^{-1}(\boldsymbol{\rho}) \cdot \boldsymbol{stde}_s - \sum_{c \in C(s)} K \cdot v_{sc,j'}/2,$$

for $1 \le j \le q$ so that, with the entries of $\boldsymbol{\rho}$ denoted by $\rho_{j'}$ for $1 \le j' \le p$, $\boldsymbol{E}'_s(\boldsymbol{\gamma},\boldsymbol{\rho})$ has entries

$$\boldsymbol{E}'_{s,j,j'}(\boldsymbol{\gamma},\boldsymbol{\rho}) = \boldsymbol{vstde}_{s,j'}^{\mathrm{T}} \cdot \frac{\partial \boldsymbol{R}_s^{-1}(\boldsymbol{\rho})}{\partial \rho_{j'}} \cdot \boldsymbol{stde}_s/2$$

where the formula for $\frac{\partial \boldsymbol{R}_s^{-1}(\boldsymbol{\rho})}{\partial \rho_{j'}}$ is provided in Sect. 10.4.1 and $\boldsymbol{E}'(\boldsymbol{\rho},\boldsymbol{\gamma}) = \boldsymbol{E}'^{\mathrm{T}}(\boldsymbol{\gamma},\boldsymbol{\rho})$.

References

Lipsitz, S. R., Kim, K., & Zhao, L. (1994). Analysis of repeated categorical data using generalized estimating equations. *Statistics in Medicine, 13*, 1149–1163.

Miller, M. E., Davis, C. S., & Landis, J. R. (1993). The analysis of longitudinal polytomous data: Generalized estimating equations and connections with weighted least squares. *Biometrics, 49*, 1033–1044.

Schott, J. R. (2005). *Matrix analysis for statistics* (2nd ed.). John Wiley & Sons.

Wolfinger, R., Tobias, R., & Sall, J. (1994). Computing gaussian likelihoods and their derivatives for general linear mixed models. *SIAM Journal on Scientific Computing, 6*, 1294–1310.

Chapter 11
Ordinal Regression

Abstract Ordinal regression modeling of correlated sets of polytomous outcomes using the cumulative logit link function based on either individual outcomes or cumulative outcomes is addressed allowing for non-constant dispersions. For both of these two types of outcomes, formulations are provided for standard generalized estimating equations (GEE) modeling, for partially modified GEE modeling, for fully modified GEE modeling, and for extended linear mixed modeling (ELMM). These formulations include estimating equations, gradient vectors, and Hessian matrices. Alternate correlation structures and their estimation are also addressed.

Keywords Correlated polytomous outcomes · Extended linear mixed modeling · Generalized estimating equations · Ordinal regression · Newton's method · Non-constant dispersions

Introduction This chapter addresses ordinal regression modeling of correlated polytomous outcomes (Lipsitz et al. 1994; Miller et al. 1993) based on either individual outcomes (Sect. 11.1) or cumulative outcomes (Sect. 11.2). For both of these two cases, formulations are provided for standard GEE modeling, for partially and fully modified GEE modeling, for alternate correlation structures and their estimation, and for ELMM modeling. Direct variance modeling of Sect. 5.7 can be generalized to ordinal regression, but is not considered for brevity.

11.1 Ordinal Regression Based on Individual Outcomes

This section addresses ordinal regression modeling based on individual outcomes. It provides formulations of standard GEE modeling (Sect. 11.1.1), partially and fully modified GEE modeling (Sect. 11.1.2), alternate correlation structures and their

---

Supplementary Information The online version contains supplementary material available at https://doi.org/10.1007/978-3-031-41988-1_11.

G. J. Knafl, *Modeling Correlated Outcomes Using Extensions of Generalized Estimating Equations and Linear Mixed Modeling*,
https://doi.org/10.1007/978-3-031-41988-1_11

estimation (Sect. 11.1.3), and ELMM (Sect. 11.1.4). The formulation for LCV scores of Sect. 2.6, LCV ratio tests of Sect. 2.6.2, and the adaptive modeling process of Sect. 2.7 generalize to ordinal regression based on individual outcomes. However, since the $m(SC)$ polytomous measurements with $K + 1$ possible values are replaced by $m(SC) \cdot K$ dichotomous measurements, LCV scores are normalized by the number $m(SC) \cdot K$ of effective measurements rather than by $m(SC)$. Extensions for this case are similar to those for multinomial regression of Chap. 10, only now the largest value K is treated as the reference category.

Using the notation of Sect. 2.1, the correlated polytomous outcomes y_{sc} for $sc \in SC$ have values $u = 0, 1, \cdots, K$ and are treated as categorically distributed for a total of $m(SC)$ polytomous measurements. The outcome values u represent ordered categories. For $0 \le u \le K$, define individual outcomes $y_{sc,u}$ to be the indicators for $y_{sc} = u$ so that associated means satisfy

$$\mu_{sc,u} = \mathrm{E}y_{sc,u} = \mathrm{P}\left(y_{sc,u} = 1\right) = \mathrm{P}(y_{sc} = u).$$

For $0 \le u \le K$, define cumulative outcomes $y_{sc,\le u}$ to be the indicators for $y_{sc} \le u$ so that associated means satisfy

$$\mu_{sc,\le u} = \mathrm{E}y_{sc,\le u} = \mathrm{P}\left(y_{sc,\le u} = 1\right) = \mathrm{P}(y_{sc} \le u)$$

and then $\mu_{sc,\le K} = 1$. As for logistic regression, the variance function is

$$V(\mu) = \mu \cdot (1 - \mu)$$

with derivative

$$\frac{dV(\mu)}{d\mu} = 1 - 2 \cdot \mu.$$

For brevity, some formulations are given in what follows without computational details.

As in Sect. 2.2, predictor values for the means are denoted by $x_{sc,j}$ for $1 \le j \le r$ and $sc \in SC$ and combined over $1 \le j \le r$ into $r \times 1$ vectors $\boldsymbol{x}_{sc}$, which are combined over $c \in C(s)$ into $m(s) \times r$ predictor matrices $\boldsymbol{X}_s$ with rows $\boldsymbol{x}_{sc}^{\mathrm{T}}$. As in Sect. 3.1, predictor values for the dispersions are still denoted by $v_{sc,j}$ for $1 \le j \le q$ and $sc \in SC$ and combined over $1 \le j \le q$ into $q \times 1$ vectors $\boldsymbol{v}_{sc}$, which are combined over $c \in C(s)$ into $m(s) \times q$ predictor matrices $\boldsymbol{V}_s$ with rows $\boldsymbol{v}_{sc}^{\mathrm{T}}$.

The link function is cumulative logits with logits computed for lower sets of values relative to higher sets of values (but this can be reversed). Formally, for $0 \le u < K$,

$$g\left(\mu_{sc,\leq u}\right)=\text{logit}\left(\mu_{sc,\leq u}\right)=\log\frac{\mu_{sc,\leq u}}{1-\mu_{sc,\leq u}}=\alpha_u+\boldsymbol{x}_{sc}^{\mathrm{T}}\cdot\boldsymbol{\beta}_K$$

for K intercept parameters α_u and a single $r \times 1$ vector $\boldsymbol{\beta}_K$ of slope parameters $\beta_{K,j}$ for $1 \leq j \leq r$. This is also called proportional odds modeling. This formulation assumes that, for $1 \leq j \leq r$, the predictor values $x_{sc,j}$ are not constant in $sc \in SC$ so that $\boldsymbol{\beta}_K$ does not include a redundant intercept parameter. Combine the intercept parameters α_u over $0 \leq u < K$ into the $K \times 1$ vector $\boldsymbol{\alpha}$. Altogether, there are $K + r$ coefficient parameters for modeling the means, which are combined over $0 \leq u < K$ and $1 \leq j \leq r$ into the $(K + r) \times 1$ vector

$$\boldsymbol{\beta}=\begin{pmatrix}\boldsymbol{\alpha}\\ \boldsymbol{\beta}_K\end{pmatrix}.$$

The cumulative means satisfy

$$\mu_{sc,\leq u}=\frac{\exp\left(\alpha_u+\boldsymbol{x}_{sc}^{\mathrm{T}}\cdot\boldsymbol{\beta}_K\right)}{1+\exp\left(\alpha_u+\boldsymbol{x}_{sc}^{\mathrm{T}}\cdot\boldsymbol{\beta}_K\right)}$$

for $sc \in SC$, $0 \leq u < K$ and $\mu_{sc,\leq K} = 1$. These means represent increasing probabilities, which requires that the intercept parameters α_u are increasing in $0 \leq u < K$. A zero-intercept model corresponds to setting $\alpha_0 = 0$, but α_u for $0 < u < K$ are non-zero. The first partial derivatives of $\mu_{sc,\leq u}$ satisfy

$$\frac{\partial\mu_{sc,\leq u}}{\partial\alpha_w}=V\left(\mu_{sc,\leq w}\right),\ w=u,$$

$$\frac{\partial\mu_{sc,\leq u}}{\partial\alpha_w}=0,\ w\neq u,$$

$$\frac{\partial\mu_{sc,\leq u}}{\partial\beta_{K,j}}=x_{sc,j}\cdot V\left(\mu_{sc,\leq u}\right),$$

for $sc \in SC$, $0 \leq u, w < K$, and $1 \leq j \leq r$. The cumulative probabilities are differenced to compute probabilities for the individual outcomes $y_{sc,u}$, that is, for $sc \in SC$, define $\mu_{sc,\leq -1} = 0$ and then

$$\mu_{sc,u}=\mathrm{E}y_{sc,u}=\mathrm{P}\left(y_{sc,u}=1\right)=\mu_{sc,\leq u}-\mu_{sc,\leq u-1}$$

for $0 \leq u \leq K$.

Combine the individual outcomes $y_{sc,u}$, means $\mu_{sc,u}$, and errors $e_{sc,u} = y_{sc,u} - \mu_{sc,u}$ over $0 \leq u < K$ into the $K \times 1$ vectors $\boldsymbol{y}_{sc}$, $\boldsymbol{\mu}_{sc}$, and $\boldsymbol{e}_{sc} = \boldsymbol{y}_{sc} - \boldsymbol{\mu}_{sc}$. Combine the vectors $\boldsymbol{y}_{sc}$, $\boldsymbol{\mu}_{sc}$, and $\boldsymbol{e}_{sc}$ over $c \in C(s)$ into the $(m(SC) \cdot K) \times 1$ vectors $\boldsymbol{y}_s$, $\boldsymbol{\mu}_s$, and $\boldsymbol{e}_s = \boldsymbol{y}_s - \boldsymbol{\mu}_s$ with $\boldsymbol{y}_{sc}$, $\boldsymbol{\mu}_{sc}$, and $\boldsymbol{e}_{sc}$ ordered by the values $c \in C(s)$. The first partial derivatives of $\mu_{sc,u}$ with respect to the intercepts α_w satisfy

$$\frac{\partial \mu_{sc,u}}{\partial \alpha_w} = V\left(\mu_{sc,\leq w}\right), w = u,$$

$$\frac{\partial \mu_{sc,u}}{\partial \alpha_w} = -V\left(\mu_{sc,\leq w}\right), w = u - 1,$$

$$\frac{\partial \mu_{sc,u}}{\partial \alpha_w} = 0, w \neq u, w \neq u - 1,$$

while the partial derivatives with respect to the slopes $\beta_{K,j}$ satisfy

$$\frac{\partial \mu_{sc,u}}{\partial \beta_{K,j}} = x_{sc,j} \cdot \left(V\left(\mu_{sc,u}\right) - V\left(\mu_{sc,u-1}\right)\right)$$

where $V(\mu_{sc,\leq -1}) = 0$, for $0 \leq u, w < K$ and $1 \leq j \leq r$. Covariances for $y_{sc,u}$ are given in Sect. 11.1.3.

11.1.1 Standard GEE Modeling

Let φ be a constant dispersion parameter so that it is constant in sc,u for $sc \in SC$ and $0 \leq u < K$. Define the extended variances

$$\sigma_{sc,u}^2 = \varphi \cdot V\left(\mu_{sc,u}\right),$$

the standardized residuals

$$stde_{sc,u} = e_{sc,u} / \sigma_{sc,u},$$

and the Pearson residuals

$$Pres_{sc,u} = \frac{e_{sc,u}}{V^{1/2}\left(\mu_{sc,u}\right)}$$

for $sc \in SC$ and $0 \leq u < K$. Combine these values over $0 \leq u < K$ into the $K \times 1$ vectors $\boldsymbol{\sigma}_{sc}$, $\boldsymbol{stde}_{sc}$, and $\boldsymbol{Pres}_{sc}$, and then combine these vectors into the $(m(s) \cdot K) \times 1$ vectors $\boldsymbol{\sigma}_s$, $\boldsymbol{stde}_s$, and $\boldsymbol{Pres}_s$ ordered by their values $c \in C(s)$. Model the $(m(s) \cdot K) \times (m(s) \cdot K)$ covariance matrices $\boldsymbol{\Sigma}_s$ as

$$\boldsymbol{\Sigma}_s = \boldsymbol{DIAG}(\boldsymbol{\sigma}_s) \cdot \boldsymbol{R}_s(\rho) \cdot \boldsymbol{DIAG}(\boldsymbol{\sigma}_s)$$

for appropriate choices of the $(m(s) \cdot K) \times (m(s) \cdot K)$ correlation matrices $\boldsymbol{R}_s(\rho)$ for $s \in S$.

Standard GEE modeling can be extended to ordinal regression based on individual outcomes by providing correlation structures and methods for their estimation (see Sect. 11.1.3). The notation of Sect. 2.4 also extends to ordinal regression based on individual outcomes. Specifically, the generalized estimating equations are given by $\boldsymbol{E}(\boldsymbol{\beta}) = \mathbf{0}$ where the $(K + r) \times 1$ vector $\boldsymbol{E}(\boldsymbol{\beta})$ satisfies

$$\boldsymbol{E}(\boldsymbol{\beta}) = \sum_{s \in S} \boldsymbol{E}_s(\boldsymbol{\beta}) = \sum_{s \in S} \boldsymbol{D}_s^{\mathrm{T}} \cdot \boldsymbol{\Sigma}_s^{-1} \cdot \boldsymbol{e}_s,$$

and the $(m(SC) \cdot K) \times (K + r)$ matrices

$$\boldsymbol{D}_s = \frac{\partial \boldsymbol{\mu}_s}{\partial \boldsymbol{\beta}}$$

for $s \in S$ have entries

$$D_{sc,u,w} = \frac{\partial \mu_{sc,u}}{\partial \alpha_w}$$

and

$$D_{sc,u,K,j} = \frac{\partial \mu_{sc,u}}{\partial \beta_{K,j}}$$

for $sc \in SC$, $0 \leq u, w < K$, and $1 \leq j \leq r$. Let

$$\boldsymbol{E}'(\boldsymbol{\beta}) = -\sum_{s \in S} \boldsymbol{D}_s^{\mathrm{T}} \cdot \boldsymbol{\Sigma}_s^{-1} \cdot \boldsymbol{D}_s.$$

The standard GEE estimation process uses Newton's method to iteratively solve $\boldsymbol{E}(\boldsymbol{\beta}) = \mathbf{0}$ with $\boldsymbol{E}(\boldsymbol{\beta})$ serving in the role of the gradient vector and $\boldsymbol{E}'(\boldsymbol{\beta})$ in the role of the Hessian matrix. The bias-adjusted estimate of the constant dispersion parameter φ for a given value of the coefficient parameter vector $\boldsymbol{\beta}$ is

$$\varphi(\boldsymbol{\beta}) = \frac{\sum_{sc \in SC} \boldsymbol{Pres}_{sc}^{\mathrm{T}}(\boldsymbol{\beta}) \cdot \boldsymbol{Pres}_{sc}(\boldsymbol{\beta})}{m(SC) \cdot K - r}$$

assuming $m(SC) \cdot K - r > 0$. Lipsitz et al. (1994) and Miller et al. (1993) assume unit dispersions and not more general constant dispersions.

The likelihood function $L(SC; \boldsymbol{\theta})$ generalizes to handle ordinal regression modeling using individual outcomes in the standard GEE context. This is a special case of the formulation given in Sect. 11.1.2, and so is not provided here.

Model-based and robust empirical estimates of the covariance matrix for the standard GEE estimate $\boldsymbol{\beta}(SC)$ of the coefficient parameter vector $\boldsymbol{\beta}$ can be computed similarly to those for standard GEE modeling given in Sect. 2.4.2. These use the standard GEE versions of $\boldsymbol{E}'(\boldsymbol{\beta}(SC))$ and $\boldsymbol{G}(\boldsymbol{\beta}(SC))$ for ordinal regression using individual outcomes. $\boldsymbol{G}(\boldsymbol{\beta}(SC))$ is defined so that summing the entries of its rows generates $\boldsymbol{E}(\boldsymbol{\beta}(SC))$. A detailed formulation for $\boldsymbol{G}(\boldsymbol{\beta}(SC))$ is not provided for brevity.

11.1.2 Partially and Fully Modified GEE Modeling

As in Sect. 3.1, predictor values for non-constant dispersions are denoted by $v_{sc,j}$ for $1 \le j \le q$ and $sc \in SC$ and combined over $1 \le j \le q$ into $q \times 1$ vectors $\boldsymbol{v}_{sc}$, which are combined over $c \in C(s)$ into $m(s) \times q$ predictor matrices $\boldsymbol{V}_s$ with rows $\boldsymbol{v}_{sc}^{\mathrm{T}}$. Define $\varphi_{sc} = exp\left(\boldsymbol{v}_{sc}^{\mathrm{T}} \cdot \boldsymbol{\gamma}\right)$ as in Sect. 10.2 so that it is constant in u for $0 \le u < K$. Dispersions are readily generalized to change with u, and so this is not considered for brevity. Treating dispersions as constant in u reduces the complexity of models and their computation time. Let

$$\sigma_{sc,u}^2 = \varphi_{sc} \cdot V\left(\mu_{sc,u}\right),$$

$$stde_{sc,u} = e_{sc,u} / \sigma_{sc,u},$$

and

$$Pres_{sc,u} = \frac{e_{sc,u}}{V^{1/2}\left(\mu_{sc,u}\right)},$$

for $sc \in SC$ and $0 \le u < K$. Combine these over $0 \le u < K$ into the $K \times 1$ vectors $\boldsymbol{\sigma}_{sc}$, $\boldsymbol{stde}_{sc}$, and $\boldsymbol{Pres}_{sc}$, and then combine these vectors, respectively, into the $(m(s) \cdot K) \times 1$ vectors $\boldsymbol{\sigma}_s$, $\boldsymbol{stde}_s$, and $\boldsymbol{Pres}_s$ in the order of the values $c \in C(s)$. Model the $(m(s) \cdot K) \times (m(s) \cdot K)$ covariance matrices $\boldsymbol{\Sigma}_s$ as

$$\boldsymbol{\Sigma}_s = \boldsymbol{DIAG}(\boldsymbol{\sigma}_s) \cdot \boldsymbol{R}_s(\boldsymbol{\rho}) \cdot \boldsymbol{DIAG}(\boldsymbol{\sigma}_s)$$

for appropriate choices of the $(m(s) \cdot K) \times (m(s) \cdot K)$ correlation matrices $\boldsymbol{R}_s(\boldsymbol{\rho})$ for $s \in S$ (see Sect. 11.1.3).

As in Sect. 10.2, partially modified and fully modified GEE modeling can be extended using the likelihood function $L(SC;\boldsymbol{\theta}) = \exp(\ell(SC;\boldsymbol{\theta}))$ for individual outcome measurements $y_{sc,u}$ with indexes $sc \in SC$ and $0 \le u < K$ equal to the product over $s \in S$ of the terms $L(O_s;\boldsymbol{\theta})$ where $O_s = \{\boldsymbol{y}_s, \boldsymbol{X}_s, \boldsymbol{V}_s\}$ denotes an observation and

$$\ell(O_s;\boldsymbol{\theta}) = \log L(O_s;\boldsymbol{\theta}) = -\boldsymbol{e}_s^{\mathrm{T}} \cdot \boldsymbol{\Sigma}_s^{-1} \cdot \boldsymbol{e}_s/2 - (\log|\boldsymbol{\Sigma}_s|)/2 - (m(s) \cdot K \cdot \log(2 \cdot \pi))/2$$

for

$$\boldsymbol{\theta} = \begin{pmatrix} \boldsymbol{\beta} \\ \boldsymbol{\gamma} \end{pmatrix},$$

the $(K + r + q) \times 1$ vector composed of the mean and dispersion parameter vectors $\boldsymbol{\beta}$ and $\boldsymbol{\gamma}$ with $K + r$ and q entries, respectively. Maximizing the likelihood involves using Newton's method to solve

$$\boldsymbol{E}(\boldsymbol{\theta}) = \begin{pmatrix} \boldsymbol{E}(\boldsymbol{\beta}) \\ \boldsymbol{E}(\boldsymbol{\gamma}) \end{pmatrix} = \mathbf{0}$$

where $\boldsymbol{E}(\boldsymbol{\beta})$ and $\boldsymbol{E}(\boldsymbol{\gamma})$ are, respectively, $(K + r) \times 1$ and $q \times 1$ vectors. $\boldsymbol{E}'(\boldsymbol{\theta})$ has four component matrices $\boldsymbol{E}'(\boldsymbol{\beta})$, $\boldsymbol{E}'(\boldsymbol{\gamma})$, $\boldsymbol{E}'(\boldsymbol{\beta},\boldsymbol{\gamma})$, and $\boldsymbol{E}'(\boldsymbol{\gamma},\boldsymbol{\beta}) = \boldsymbol{E}'^{\mathrm{T}}(\boldsymbol{\beta},\boldsymbol{\gamma})$. $\boldsymbol{E}'(\boldsymbol{\beta})$, $\boldsymbol{E}'(\boldsymbol{\gamma})$, and $\boldsymbol{E}'(\boldsymbol{\beta},\boldsymbol{\gamma})$ are, respectively, $(K + r) \times (K + r)$, $q \times q$, and $(K + r) \times q$ matrices.

Formulation adjustments for partially modified GEE include:

$$\log|\boldsymbol{\Sigma}_s| = \log|\boldsymbol{R}_s(\boldsymbol{\rho})| + \sum_{c \in C(s)} K \cdot \log \varphi_{sc} + \sum_{c \in C(s)} \sum_{u=1}^{K} \log V\left(\mu_{sc,u}\right);$$

$\boldsymbol{E}(\boldsymbol{\gamma})$ is the sum over $s \in S$ of terms $\boldsymbol{E}_s(\boldsymbol{\gamma})$ with entries

$$E_{s,j}(\boldsymbol{\gamma}) = \boldsymbol{vstde}_{s,j}^{\mathrm{T}} \cdot \boldsymbol{R}_s^{-1}(\boldsymbol{\rho}) \cdot \boldsymbol{stde}_s - \sum_{c \in C(s)} K \cdot v_{sc,j}/2,$$

where $\boldsymbol{vstde}_{s,j}$ is the $(m(SC) \cdot K) \times 1$ vector with entries

$$vstde_{sc,u,j} = v_{sc,j} \cdot stde_{sc,u}/2$$

for $sc \in SC$, $0 \le u < K$, and $1 \le j \le q$; and $\boldsymbol{E}'(\boldsymbol{\gamma})$ is the sum over $s \in S$ of $\boldsymbol{E}'_s(\boldsymbol{\gamma})$ with entries

$$E'_{s,j,j'}(\boldsymbol{\gamma}) = -\boldsymbol{vvstde}_{s,j,j'}^{\mathrm{T}} \cdot \boldsymbol{R}_s^{-1}(\boldsymbol{\rho}) \cdot \boldsymbol{stde}_s - \boldsymbol{vstde}_{s,j}^{\mathrm{T}} \cdot \boldsymbol{R}_s^{-1}(\boldsymbol{\rho}) \cdot \boldsymbol{vstde}_{s,j'}$$

where $\boldsymbol{vvstde}_{s,j,j'}$ is the $(m(SC) \cdot K) \times 1$ vector with entries

$$vvstde_{sc,u,j,j'} = v_{sc,j} \cdot v_{sc,j'} \cdot stde_{sc,u}/4$$

for $sc \in SC$, $0 \le u < K$, and $1 \le j, j' \le q$. These adjustments apply as well to fully modified GEE modeling. Also, $\boldsymbol{E}'(\boldsymbol{\beta},\boldsymbol{\gamma})$ is the sum over $s \in S$ of $\boldsymbol{E}'_s(\boldsymbol{\beta},\boldsymbol{\gamma})$ with q $(K + r) \times 1$ column vectors

$$\boldsymbol{E'}_{s,j}(\boldsymbol{\beta},\boldsymbol{\gamma}) = -\boldsymbol{D}_s^{\mathrm{T}} \cdot \boldsymbol{DIAG}\left(\boldsymbol{v\sigma inv}_{s,j}\right) \cdot \boldsymbol{R}_s^{-1}(\rho) \cdot \boldsymbol{stde}_s$$
$$-\boldsymbol{D}_s^{\mathrm{T}} \cdot \boldsymbol{DIAG}(\boldsymbol{1}/\boldsymbol{\sigma}_s) \cdot \boldsymbol{R}_s^{-1}(\rho) \cdot \boldsymbol{vstde}_{s,j}$$

where $\boldsymbol{v\sigma inv}_{s,j}$ is the $(m(SC) \cdot K) \times 1$ vector with entries

$$v\sigma inv_{sc,u,j} = \frac{v_{sc,j}}{2 \cdot \sigma_{sc,u}}$$

for $sc \in SC$, $0 \leq u < K$, and $1 \leq j \leq q$.

Fully modified GEE also requires formulation adjustments for $\boldsymbol{E}(\boldsymbol{\beta})$, $\boldsymbol{E'}(\boldsymbol{\beta})$, **and** $\boldsymbol{E}$ $'(\boldsymbol{\beta},\boldsymbol{\gamma})$. $\boldsymbol{E}(\boldsymbol{\beta})$ is the sum over $s \in S$ of $\boldsymbol{E}_s(\boldsymbol{\beta})$ with entries

$$E_{s,w}(\boldsymbol{\beta}) = \frac{\partial_0 \ell(O_s;\boldsymbol{\theta})}{\partial_0 \alpha_w} = \boldsymbol{xstde}_{s,w}^{\mathrm{T}} \cdot \boldsymbol{R}_s^{-1}(\rho) \cdot \boldsymbol{stde}_s - \sum_{c \in C(s)} W_{sc,w}/2,$$

$$E_{s,K,j}(\boldsymbol{\beta}) = \frac{\partial_0 \ell(O_s;\boldsymbol{\theta})}{\partial_0 \beta_{K,j}} = \boldsymbol{xstde}_{s,K,j}^{\mathrm{T}} \cdot \boldsymbol{R}_s^{-1}(\rho) \cdot \boldsymbol{stde}_s - \sum_{c \in C(s)} \sum_{u=0}^{K-1} W_{K,j}\left(\mu_{sc,u}\right)/2$$

where

$$W_{sc,w} = \sum_{u=0}^{K-1} \frac{\frac{\partial V\left(\mu_{sc,u}\right)}{\partial \alpha_w}}{V\left(\mu_{sc,u}\right)},$$

$$W_{K,j}\left(\mu_{sc,u}\right) = \frac{\frac{\partial V\left(\mu_{sc,u}\right)}{\partial \beta_{K,j}}}{V\left(\mu_{sc,u}\right)},$$

for $0 \leq u$, $w < K$ and $1 \leq j \leq r$. The $(m(s) \cdot K) \times 1$ vectors $\boldsymbol{xstde}_{s,w}$ **and** $\boldsymbol{xstde}_{s,K,j}$ have entries $xstde_{sc,u,w}$ and $xstde_{sc,u,K,j}$, respectively, where

$$xstde_{sc,u,w} = \frac{\left(1 - 2 \cdot \mu_{sc,w}\right) \cdot y_{sc,w} + \mu_{sc,w}}{2 \cdot V\left(\mu_{sc,w}\right) \cdot \sigma_{sc,w}} \cdot V\left(\mu_{sc,\leq w}\right),$$

for $w = u$ and $0 \leq u < K$;

$$xstde_{sc,u,w} = -\frac{\left(1 - 2 \cdot \mu_{sc,w+1}\right) \cdot y_{sc,w+1} + \mu_{sc,w+1}}{2 \cdot V\left(\mu_{sc,w+1}\right) \cdot \sigma_{sc,w+1}} \cdot V\left(\mu_{sc,\leq w}\right),$$

for $w = u - 1$ and $0 < u < K$;

$$xstde_{sc,u,w} = 0,$$

for $w \neq u$, $w \neq u - 1$ and $0 \leq u < K$; and

$$xstde_{sc,u,Kj} = x_{sc,j} \cdot \frac{\left(1 - 2 \cdot \mu_{sc,u}\right) \cdot y_{sc,u} + \mu_{sc,u}}{2 \cdot V\left(\mu_{sc,u}\right) \cdot \sigma_{sc,u}} \cdot \left(V\left(\mu_{sc,\leq u}\right) - V\left(\mu_{sc,\leq u-1}\right)\right),$$

for $1 \leq j \leq r$. Also,

$$W_{sc,w} = \frac{1 - 2 \cdot \mu_{sc,w}}{V\left(\mu_{sc,w}\right)} \cdot V\left(\mu_{sc,\leq w}\right) - \frac{1 - 2 \cdot \mu_{sc,w+1}}{V\left(\mu_{sc,w+1}\right)} \cdot V\left(\mu_{sc,\leq w}\right),$$

for $0 \leq w < K - 1$;

$$W_{sc,w} = \frac{1 - 2 \cdot \mu_{sc,w}}{V\left(\mu_{sc,w}\right)} \cdot V\left(\mu_{sc,\leq w}\right),$$

for $w = K - 1$; and

$$W_{Kj}\left(\mu_{sc,u}\right) = x_{sc,j} \cdot \frac{1 - 2 \cdot \mu_{sc,u}}{V\left(\mu_{sc,u}\right)} \cdot \left(V\left(\mu_{sc,\leq u}\right) - V\left(\mu_{sc,\leq u-1}\right)\right),$$

for $1 \leq j \leq r$. As before, the operator notation $\frac{\partial_0}{\partial_0 \alpha_w}$ and $\frac{\partial_0}{\partial_0 \beta_{Kj}}$ is used to indicate that these are not full partial derivatives due to not accounting for the effect of α_w and β_{Kj} on $\boldsymbol{R}_s(\rho)$ (see Sect. 11.1.3). Note that $W_{sc,w}$ and $W_{Kj}(\mu_{sc,u})$ are standard partial derivatives since $V(\mu_{sc,u})$ does not depend on $\boldsymbol{R}_s(\rho)$.

$\boldsymbol{E}'(\boldsymbol{\beta})$ is the sum over $s \in S$ of $\boldsymbol{E}'_s(\boldsymbol{\beta})$ with $(K + r)^2$ entries including the K^2 entries

$$E'_{s,w,w'}(\boldsymbol{\beta}) = \frac{\partial_0 \boldsymbol{E}_{s,w}(\boldsymbol{\beta})}{\partial_0 \alpha_{w'}}$$

$$= -\boldsymbol{xxstde}^{\mathrm{T}}_{s,w,w'} \cdot \boldsymbol{R}_s^{-1}(\rho) \cdot \boldsymbol{stde}_s - \boldsymbol{xstde}^{\mathrm{T}}_{s,w} \cdot \boldsymbol{R}_s^{-1}(\rho) \cdot \boldsymbol{xstde}_{s,w'} - \sum_{c \in C(s)} W_{sc,w,w'}/2$$

for $0 \leq w, w' < K$, the $K \cdot r$ entries

$$E'_{s,Kj,w}(\boldsymbol{\beta}) = \frac{\partial_0 \boldsymbol{E}_{s,Kj}(\boldsymbol{\beta})}{\partial_0 \alpha_w}$$

$$= -\boldsymbol{xxstde}^{\mathrm{T}}_{s,Kj,w} \cdot \boldsymbol{R}_s^{-1}(\rho) \cdot \boldsymbol{stde}_s - \boldsymbol{xstde}^{\mathrm{T}}_{s,Kj} \cdot \boldsymbol{R}_s^{-1}(\rho) \cdot \boldsymbol{xstde}_{s,w} - \sum_{c \in C(s)} W_{sc,Kj,w}/2$$

for $0 \leq w < K$, and $1 \leq j \leq r$, the $K \cdot r$ entries

$$E'_{s,w,K,j}(\boldsymbol{\beta}) = \frac{\partial_0 \boldsymbol{E}_{s,w}(\boldsymbol{\beta})}{\partial_0 \beta_{K,j}}$$

$$= -\boldsymbol{xxstde}^{\mathrm{T}}_{s,w,K,j} \cdot \boldsymbol{R}_s^{-1}(\rho) \cdot \boldsymbol{stde}_s - \boldsymbol{xstde}^{\mathrm{T}}_{s,w} \cdot \boldsymbol{R}_s^{-1}(\rho) \cdot \boldsymbol{xstde}_{s,K,j} - \sum_{c \in C(s)} W_{sc,w,K,j}/2$$

for $0 \leq w < K$, and $1 \leq j \leq r$, and the r^2 entries

$$E'_{s,K,j,j'}(\boldsymbol{\beta}) = \frac{\partial_0 \boldsymbol{E}_{s,K,j}(\boldsymbol{\beta})}{\partial_0 \beta_{K,j'}}$$

$$= -\boldsymbol{xxstde}^{\mathrm{T}}_{s,Kj,j'} \cdot \boldsymbol{R}_s^{-1}(\rho) \cdot \boldsymbol{stde}_s - \boldsymbol{xstde}^{\mathrm{T}}_{s,K,j} \cdot \boldsymbol{R}_s^{-1}(\rho) \cdot \boldsymbol{xstde}_{s,K,j'}$$

$$- \sum_{c \in C(s)} \sum_{u=0}^{K-1} W_{K,j,j'}(\mu_{sc,u})/2$$

for $1 \leq j, j' \leq r$ where

$$W_{sc,w,w'} = \frac{\partial W_{sc,w}}{\partial \alpha_{w'}},$$

$$W_{sc,K,j,w} = \sum_{u=0}^{K-1} \frac{\partial W_{K,j}(\mu_{sc,u})}{\partial \alpha_{w}},$$

$$W_{sc,w,K,j} = \frac{\partial W_{sc,w}}{\partial \beta_{K,j}},$$

$$W_{K,j,j'}(\mu_{sc,u}) = \frac{\partial W_{K,j}(\mu_{sc,u})}{\partial \beta_{K,j'}}.$$

The following formulation is needed to compute $\boldsymbol{E}'(\boldsymbol{\beta})$ but is complex and so can be skipped. For $0 \leq w, w' < K$ and $1 \leq j, j' \leq r$, the $(m(s) \cdot K) \times 1$ vectors $\boldsymbol{xxstde}_{s,w,w'}$, $\boldsymbol{xxstde}_{s,w,K,j}$, $\boldsymbol{xxstde}_{s,K,j,w}$, and $\boldsymbol{xxstde}_{s,K,j,j'}$ have entries $xxstde_{sc,u,w,w'}$, $xxstde_{sc,u,w,K,j}$, $xxstde_{sc,u,K,j,w}$, and $xxstde_{sc,u,K,j,j'}$, respectively, with the following formulations. For $0 \leq u < K$, $w = u$, $w' = u$,

$$xxstde_{sc,u,w,w} = \frac{a_{1,sc,w} \cdot y_{sc,w} + b_{1,sc,w}}{4 \cdot V^2(\mu_{sc,w}) \cdot \sigma_{sc,w}} \cdot V(\mu_{sc,\leq w}),$$

$$a_{1,sc,w} = \left(3 - 8 \cdot \mu_{sc,w} + 8 \cdot \mu^2_{sc,w}\right) \cdot V(\mu_{sc,\leq w})$$
$$- 2 \cdot V(\mu_{sc,w}) \cdot (1 - 2 \cdot \mu_{sc,w}) \cdot (1 - 2 \cdot \mu_{sc,\leq w}),$$

$$b_{1,sc,w} = \mu_{sc,w} \cdot (1 - 4 \cdot \mu_{sc,w}) \cdot V(\mu_{sc,\leq w}) - 2 \cdot V(\mu_{sc,w}) \cdot \mu_{sc,w} \cdot (1 - 2 \cdot \mu_{sc,\leq w});$$

for $0 < u < K$, $w = u$, $w' = u - 1$,

$$xxstde_{sc,u,w,w-1} = -\frac{a_{2,sc,w} \cdot y_{sc,w} + b_{2,sc,w}}{4 \cdot V^2\left(\mu_{sc,w}\right) \cdot \sigma_{sc,w}} \cdot V\left(\mu_{sc,\leq w-1}\right) \cdot V\left(\mu_{sc,\leq w}\right),$$

$$a_{2,sc,w} = 3 - 8 \cdot \mu_{sc,u} + 8 \cdot \mu_{sc,u}^2,$$

$$b_{2,sc,w} = \mu_{sc,w} \cdot \left(1 - 4 \cdot \mu_{sc,w}\right);$$

for $0 < u < K$, $w = u - 1$, $w' = u$,

$$xxstde_{sc,u,w,w+1} = -\frac{a_{2,sc,w+1} \cdot y_{sc,w+1} + b_{2,sc,w+1}}{4 \cdot V^2\left(\mu_{sc,w+1}\right) \cdot \sigma_{sc,w+1}} \cdot V\left(\mu_{sc,\leq w}\right) \cdot V\left(\mu_{sc,\leq w+1}\right);$$

for $0 < u < K$, $w = u - 1$, $w' = u - 1$,

$$xxstde_{sc,u,w,w} = \frac{a_{3,sc,w} \cdot y_{sc,w+1} + b_{3,sc,w}}{4 \cdot V^2\left(\mu_{sc,w+1}\right) \cdot \sigma_{sc,w+1}} \cdot V\left(\mu_{sc,\leq w}\right),$$

$$a_{3,sc,w} = \left(3 - 8 \cdot \mu_{sc,w+1} + 8 \cdot \mu_{sc,w+1}^2\right) \cdot V\left(\mu_{sc,\leq w}\right)$$
$$+2 \cdot V\left(\mu_{sc,w+1}\right) \cdot \left(1 - 2 \cdot \mu_{sc,w+1}\right) \cdot \left(1 - 2 \cdot \mu_{sc,\leq w}\right),$$

$$b_{3,sc,w} = \mu_{sc,w+1} \cdot \left(1 - 4 \cdot \mu_{sc,w+1}\right) \cdot V\left(\mu_{sc,\leq w}\right)$$
$$+ 2 \cdot V\left(\mu_{sc,w+1}\right) \cdot \mu_{sc,w+1} \cdot \left(1 - 2 \cdot \mu_{sc,\leq w}\right);$$

for $0 \leq u < K$, $w \neq u$, $w \neq u - 1$, $w' \neq u$, $w' \neq u - 1$,

$$xxstde_{sc,u,w,w'} = 0;$$

for $1 \leq j, j' \leq r$,

$$xxstde_{sc,u,K,j,j'} = x_{scj} \cdot x_{scj'} \cdot \frac{a_{4,sc,u} \cdot y_{sc,u} + b_{4,sc,u}}{4 \cdot V^2\left(\mu_{sc,u}\right) \cdot \sigma_{sc,u}},$$

$$a_{4,sc,u} = \left(3 - 8 \cdot \mu_{sc,u} + 8 \cdot \mu_{sc,u}^2\right) \cdot \left(V\left(\mu_{sc,\leq u}\right) - V\left(\mu_{sc,\leq u-1}\right)\right)^2$$
$$-2 \cdot V\left(\mu_{sc,u}\right) \cdot \left(1 - 2 \cdot \mu_{sc,u}\right) \cdot \left(V\left(\mu_{sc,\leq u}\right) \cdot \left(1 - 2 \cdot \mu_{sc,\leq u}\right) - V\left(\mu_{sc,\leq u-1}\right)\right.$$
$$\left.\cdot \left(1 - 2 \cdot \mu_{sc,\leq u-1}\right)\right),$$

$$b_{4,sc,u} = \mu_{sc,u} \cdot \left(1 - 4 \cdot \mu_{sc,u}\right) \cdot \left(V\left(\mu_{sc,\leq u}\right) - V\left(\mu_{sc,\leq u-1}\right)\right)^2$$

$$-2 \cdot V\left(\mu_{sc,u}\right) \cdot \mu_{sc,u} \cdot \left(V\left(\mu_{sc,\leq u}\right) \cdot \left(1 - 2 \cdot \mu_{sc,\leq u}\right) - V\left(\mu_{sc,\leq u-1}\right) \cdot \left(1 - 2 \cdot \mu_{sc,\leq u-1}\right)\right);$$

for $0 \leq u < K$, $w = u$, $1 \leq j \leq r$,

$$xxstde_{sc,u,w,K,j} = x_{sc,j} \cdot \frac{a_{5,sc,w} \cdot y_{sc,w} + b_{5,sc,w}}{4 \cdot V^2(\mu_{sc,w}) \cdot \sigma_{sc,w}} \cdot V(\mu_{sc,\le w}),$$

$$a_{5,sc,w} = \left(3 - 8 \cdot \mu_{sc,w} + 8 \cdot \mu_{sc,w}^2\right) \cdot \left(V(\mu_{sc,\le w}) - V(\mu_{sc,\le w-1})\right)$$
$$- 2 \cdot V(\mu_{sc,w}) \cdot (1 - 2 \cdot \mu_{sc,w}) \cdot (1 - 2 \cdot \mu_{sc,\le w})$$

$$b_{5,sc,w} = \mu_{sc,w} \cdot (1 - 4 \cdot \mu_{sc,w}) \cdot \left(V(\mu_{sc,\le w}) - V(\mu_{sc,\le w-1})\right)$$
$$- 2 \cdot V(\mu_{sc,w}) \cdot \mu_{sc,w} \cdot (1 - 2 \cdot \mu_{sc,\le w}),$$

$$xxstde_{sc,u,K,j,w} = xxstde_{sc,u,w,K,j};$$

for $0 < u < K$, $w = u - 1$, $1 \le j \le r$,

$$xxstde_{sc,u,w,K,j} = -x_{sc,j} \cdot \frac{a_{6,sc,w} \cdot y_{sc,w+1} + b_{6,sc,w}}{4 \cdot V^2(\mu_{sc,w+1}) \cdot \sigma_{sc,w+1}} \cdot V(\mu_{sc,\le w}),$$

$$a_{6,sc,w} = \left(3 - 8 \cdot \mu_{sc,w+1} + 8 \cdot \mu_{sc,w+1}^2\right) \cdot \left(V(\mu_{sc,\le w+1}) - V(\mu_{sc,\le w})\right)$$
$$- 2 \cdot V(\mu_{sc,w+1}) \cdot (1 - 2 \cdot \mu_{sc,w+1}) \cdot (1 - 2 \cdot \mu_{sc,\le w})$$

$$b_{6,sc,w} = \mu_{sc,w+1} \cdot (1 - 4 \cdot \mu_{sc,w+1}) \cdot \left(V(\mu_{sc,\le w+1}) - V(\mu_{sc,\le w})\right)$$
$$- 2 \cdot V(\mu_{sc,w+1}) \cdot \mu_{sc,w+1} \cdot (1 - 2 \cdot \mu_{sc,\le w}),$$

$$xxstde_{sc,u,K,j,w} = xxstde_{sc,u,w,K,j};$$

and for $0 \le u < K$, $w \ne u$, $w \ne u - 1$, $1 \le j \le r$,

$$xxstde_{sc,u,w,K,j} = xxstde_{sc,u,K,j,w} = 0.$$

Also, for $0 \le w < K - 1$, $w' = w$,

$$W_{sc,w,w} = -\frac{c_{1,sc,w}}{V^2(\mu_{sc,w})} \cdot V(\mu_{sc,\le w}) - \frac{c_{2,sc,w}}{V^2(\mu_{sc,w+1})} \cdot V(\mu_{sc,\le w})$$

$$c_{1,sc,w} = \left(1 - 2 \cdot \mu_{sc,w} + 2 \cdot \mu_{sc,w}^2\right) \cdot V(\mu_{sc,\le w})$$
$$- (1 - 2 \cdot \mu_{sc,w}) \cdot (1 - 2 \cdot \mu_{sc,\le w}) \cdot V(\mu_{sc,w}),$$

$$c_{2,sc,w} = \left(1 - 2 \cdot \mu_{sc,w+1} + 2 \cdot \mu_{sc,w+1}^2\right) \cdot V(\mu_{sc,\le w})$$
$$+ (1 - 2 \cdot \mu_{sc,w+1}) \cdot (1 - 2 \cdot \mu_{sc,\le w}) \cdot V(\mu_{sc,w+1});$$

for $w = K - 1$, $w' = w$,

$$W_{sc,w,w} = -\frac{c_{1,sc,w}}{V^2(\mu_{sc,w})} \cdot V(\mu_{sc,\leq w});$$

for $0 < w < K$, $w' = w - 1$,

$$W_{sc,w,w-1} = \frac{1 - 2 \cdot \mu_{sc,w} + 2 \cdot \mu_{sc,w}^2}{V^2(\mu_{sc,w})} \cdot V(\mu_{sc,\leq w-1}) \cdot V(\mu_{sc,\leq w});$$

for $0 \leq w < K - 1$, $w' = w + 1$,

$$W_{sc,w,w+1} = \frac{1 - 2 \cdot \mu_{sc,w+1} + 2 \cdot \mu_{sc,w+1}^2}{V^2(\mu_{sc,w+1})} \cdot V(\mu_{sc,\leq w}) \cdot V(\mu_{sc,\leq w+1});$$

for $w' \neq w - 1$, $w' \neq w$, $w' \neq w + 1$,

$$W_{sc,w,w} = 0;$$

for $1 \leq j, j' \leq r$,

$$W_{sc,K,j,j'}(\mu_{sc,u}) = -x_{scj} \cdot x_{scj'} \cdot \frac{c_{3,sc,u}}{V^2(\mu_{sc,u})}$$

$$\begin{aligned} c_{3,sc,u} = {} & (1 - 2 \cdot \mu_{sc,u} + 2 \cdot \mu_{sc,u}^2) \cdot (V(\mu_{sc,\leq u}) - V(\mu_{sc,\leq u-1}))^2 \\ & - (1 - 2 \cdot \mu_{sc,u}) \cdot (1 - 2 \cdot \mu_{sc,\leq u}) \cdot V(\mu_{sc,\leq u}) \cdot V(\mu_{sc,u}) \\ & + (1 - 2 \cdot \mu_{sc,u}) \cdot (1 - 2 \cdot \mu_{sc,\leq u-1}) \cdot V(\mu_{sc,\leq u-1}) \cdot V(\mu_{sc,u}); \end{aligned}$$

for $0 \leq w < K - 1$, $1 \leq j \leq r$,

$$W_{sc,w,K,j} = -x_{scj} \cdot \frac{c_{4,sc,w}}{V^2(\mu_{sc,w})} \cdot V(\mu_{sc,\leq w}) + x_{scj} \cdot \frac{c_{5,sc,w}}{V^2(\mu_{sc,w+1})} \cdot V(\mu_{sc,\leq w}),$$

$$\begin{aligned} c_{4,sc,w} = {} & (1 - 2 \cdot \mu_{sc,w} + 2 \cdot \mu_{sc,w}^2) \cdot (V(\mu_{sc,\leq w}) - V(\mu_{sc,\leq w-1})) \\ & - (1 - 2 \cdot \mu_{sc,w}) \cdot (1 - 2 \cdot \mu_{sc,\leq w}) \cdot V(\mu_{sc,w}), \end{aligned}$$

$$\begin{aligned} c_{5,sc,w} = {} & (1 - 2 \cdot \mu_{sc,w+1} + 2 \cdot \mu_{sc,w+1}^2) \cdot (V(\mu_{sc,\leq w+1}) - V(\mu_{sc,\leq w})) \\ & - (1 - 2 \cdot \mu_{sc,w+1}) \cdot (1 - 2 \cdot \mu_{sc,\leq w}) \cdot V(\mu_{sc,w+1}); \end{aligned}$$

for $w = K - 1$, $1 \leq j \leq r$,

$$W_{sc,w,K,j} = -x_{sc,j} \cdot \frac{c_{4,sc,w}}{V^2\left(\mu_{sc,w}\right)} \cdot V\left(\mu_{sc,\leq w}\right);$$

and for $0 \leq w < K$, $1 \leq j \leq r$.

$$W_{sc,K,j,w} = W_{sc,w,K,j}.$$

$\boldsymbol{E}'(\boldsymbol{\beta},\boldsymbol{\gamma})$ is the sum over $s \in S$ of $\boldsymbol{E}'_s(\boldsymbol{\beta},\boldsymbol{\gamma})$ with entries

$$E'_{s,w,j'}(\boldsymbol{\beta},\boldsymbol{\gamma}) = \frac{\partial_0 \boldsymbol{E}_{s,w}(\boldsymbol{\beta})}{\partial_0 \gamma_{j'}} = -\boldsymbol{vxstde}_{s,w,j'}^{\mathrm{T}} \cdot \boldsymbol{R}_s^{-1}(\rho) \cdot \boldsymbol{stde}_s$$
$$-\boldsymbol{xstde}_{s,w}^{\mathrm{T}} \cdot \boldsymbol{R}_s^{-1}(\rho) \cdot \boldsymbol{vstde}_{s,j'},$$
$$E'_{s,K,j,j'}(\boldsymbol{\beta},\boldsymbol{\gamma}) = \frac{\partial_0 \boldsymbol{E}_{s,K,j}(\boldsymbol{\beta})}{\partial_0 \gamma_{j'}} = -\boldsymbol{vxstde}_{s,K,j,j'}^{\mathrm{T}} \cdot \boldsymbol{R}_s^{-1}(\rho) \cdot \boldsymbol{stde}_s$$
$$-\boldsymbol{xstde}_{s,K,j}^{\mathrm{T}} \cdot \boldsymbol{R}_s^{-1}(\rho) \cdot \boldsymbol{vstde}_{s,j'},$$

where $\boldsymbol{vxstde}_{s,w,j'}$ is the $(m(s) \cdot K) \times 1$ vector with entries

$$vxstde_{sc,u,w,j'} = xstde_{sc,u,w} \cdot v_{sc,j'}/2,$$

$\boldsymbol{vxstde}_{s,K,j,j'}$ is the $(m(s) \cdot K) \times 1$ vector with entries

$$vxstde_{sc,u,K,j,j'} = xstde_{sc,u,K,j} \cdot v_{sc,j'}/2,$$

and $\boldsymbol{vstde}_{s,j'}$ is the same as for partially modified GEE modeling, for $sc \in SC$, $0 \leq u$, $w < K$, $1 \leq j \leq r$, and $1 \leq j' \leq q$.

Model-based and robust empirical estimates of the covariance matrix for the partially and fully modified GEE estimate

$$\boldsymbol{\theta}(SC) = \begin{pmatrix} \boldsymbol{\beta}(SC) \\ \boldsymbol{\gamma}(SC) \end{pmatrix}$$

of the coefficient parameter vector $\boldsymbol{\theta}$ can be computed similarly to those for partially modified GEE modeling given in Sect. 3.4 and fully modified GEE modeling given in Sect. 4.1. These use the partially and fully modified GEE versions of $\boldsymbol{E}'(\boldsymbol{\theta}(SC))$ and $\boldsymbol{G}(\boldsymbol{\theta}(SC))$ for ordinal regression using individual outcomes. $\boldsymbol{G}(\boldsymbol{\theta}(SC))$ is defined so that summing the entries of its rows generates $\boldsymbol{E}(\boldsymbol{\theta}(SC))$. A detailed formulation for $\boldsymbol{G}(\boldsymbol{\theta}(SC))$ is not provided for brevity.

11.1.3 Alternate Correlation Structures

As in Sect. 10.3, let $\boldsymbol{R}_{s,c,c'}$ for c, $c' \in C(s)$ denote the $m^2(s)$ $K \times K$ component matrices of $\boldsymbol{R}_s(\boldsymbol{\rho})$. The special cases $\boldsymbol{R}_{s,c,c}$ with $c' = c$ are the correlation matrices for $\boldsymbol{y}_{sc}$. The individual outcomes $y_{sc,u}$ for $sc \in SC$ and $0 \leq u < K$ are multinomially distributed with sum 1 and covariances satisfying

$$\mathrm{Cov}\left(y_{sc,u}, y_{sc,u'}\right) = \mu_{sc,u} \cdot \left(1 - \mu_{sc,u}\right), u = u',$$
$$\mathrm{Cov}\left(y_{sc,u}, y_{sc,u'}\right) = -\mu_{sc,u} \cdot \mu_{sc,u'}, u \neq u'$$

(Lipsitz et al. 1994). Consequently, $\boldsymbol{R}_{s,c,c}$ has diagonal entries with value 1 and off-diagonal entries

$$r_{sc,u,u'} = -\left(\frac{\mu_{sc,u}}{1 - \mu_{sc,u}}\right)^{½} \cdot \left(\frac{\mu_{sc,u\prime}}{1 - \mu_{sc,u\prime}}\right)^{½}$$

for $0 \leq u$, $u' < K$ with $u \neq u'$. Note that $\boldsymbol{R}_{s,c,c}$ depends on the mean parameters but not on the correlation parameters. Models are needed for the remaining $m(s) \cdot (1 - m(s))/2$ component matrices $\boldsymbol{R}_{s,c,c'}$ and their transposes $\boldsymbol{R}_{s,c',c} = \boldsymbol{R}^{\mathrm{T}}_{s,c,c'}$ of dimension $K \times K$ for $c < c'$. These depend only on the correlation parameters for the four correlation structures described in Sects. 11.1.3.1–11.1.3.4. Estimates of the parameters for these correlation structures for partially and fully modified GEE are provided in those sections. Note that $\boldsymbol{R}_{s,c,c'}$ is the correlation matrix for $\boldsymbol{y}_{sc}$ and $\boldsymbol{y}_{sc'}$ so that its entries satisfy $r_{s,c,c',u,u'} = \mathrm{Corr}(y_{sc,u}, y_{sc',u'})$ and $r_{s,c,c',u',u} = \mathrm{Corr}(y_{sc,u'}, y_{sc',u})$ for $u \neq u'$, which are correlations between two different pairs of indicator variables and so have different values in general, and $\boldsymbol{R}_{s,c,c'}$ is not symmetric in general.

11.1.3.1 Independent Correlations

Under the IND correlation structure, the component matrices $\boldsymbol{R}_{s,c,c'}$ have all zero entries for c, $c' \in C(s)$ with $c \neq c'$. In this case, the correlation parameter vector $\boldsymbol{\rho}_{\mathrm{IND}}$ is the constant scalar with value 0. There is no need for an estimate of $\boldsymbol{\rho}_{\mathrm{IND}}$.

11.1.3.2 Exchangeable Correlations

Under the EC correlation structure, the component matrices $\boldsymbol{R}_{s,c,c'}$ for c, $c' \in C(s)$ with $c < c'$ all equal the same $K \times K$ matrix $\boldsymbol{R}$ with entries $r_{\mathrm{EC},u,u'}$ for $0 \leq u$, $u' < K$ while $\boldsymbol{R}_{s,c',c} = \boldsymbol{R}^{\mathrm{T}}$. For a given value of the coefficient parameter vector $\boldsymbol{\theta}$, the associated estimate of $\boldsymbol{R}(\boldsymbol{\theta})$ is computed as

$$\boldsymbol{R}(\boldsymbol{\theta}) = \frac{\sum\limits_{cc' \in CC'} \boldsymbol{stde}_{sc}(\boldsymbol{\theta}) \cdot \boldsymbol{stde}_{sc'}^{\mathrm{T}}(\boldsymbol{\theta})}{D}$$

where CC' is the set of $m(CC')$ observed distinct ordered pairs defined in Sect. 2.4.1 and the denominator D is either the bias-adjusted value $D = m(CC') - r > 0$ assuming this is non-zero or the bias-unadjusted value $D = m(CC')$. The correlation parameters $r_{\mathrm{EC},u,u'}(\boldsymbol{\theta})$ are combined over $0 \leq u,\ u' < K$ into the $K^2 \times 1$ correlation parameter vector $\boldsymbol{\rho}_{\mathrm{EC}}(\boldsymbol{\theta})$.

11.1.3.3 Autoregressive Correlations

As in Sect. 2.3.3, under spatial AR1 correlations, there is a function $t(c)$ increasing in the integers $c \in C$ (e.g., increasing measurement times or dosages) while, for the special case of non-spatial AR1, $t(c) = c$ for $c \in C$. Let $\boldsymbol{R}$ denote a $K \times K$ matrix with entries $r_{\mathrm{AR1},u,u'}$ satisfying $-1 < r_{\mathrm{AR1},u,u'} < 1$ for $1 \leq u,\ u' \leq K$. For $c,c' \in C(s)$ with $c < c'$, let

$$\boldsymbol{R}_{s,c,c'} = \mathrm{power}(\boldsymbol{R}, |t(c') - t(c)|)$$

denote the matrices with entries

$$r_{s,c,c',u,u'} = \mathrm{power}(r_{\mathrm{AR1},u,u'}, |t(c') - t(c)|)$$

for an appropriately defined power transform of the possibly negative entries $r_{\mathrm{AR1},u,u'}$ of $\boldsymbol{R}$ for $0 \leq u,\ u' < K$.

As justified in Sect. 10.3.3 for multinomial regression, spatial AR1 correlations in the context of ordinal regression with individual outcomes are also based on sign-preserving power transforms. Formally, define

$$\mathrm{power}(r_{\mathrm{AR1},u,u'}, |t(c') - t(c)|) = \mathrm{sign}(r_{\mathrm{AR1},u,u'}) \cdot |r_{\mathrm{AR1},u,u'}|^{|t(c') - t(c)|}.$$

These power transforms are well-defined for all $r_{\mathrm{AR1},u,u'}$ in the interval $(-1, 1)$ and all $c,\ c' \in C$ with $c' \neq c$, and this does not require that the distances $|t(c') - t(c)|$ be all integers for $c,\ c' \in C$. Since $t(c)$ are unique for $c \in C$, $|t(c') - t(c)| > 0$ for $c' \neq c$, so that $|r_{\mathrm{AR1},u,u'}|^{|t(c') - t(c)|}$ | equals 0 when $r_{\mathrm{AR1},u,u'} = 0$.

In the non-spatial AR1 case, for a given value of the coefficient parameter vector $\boldsymbol{\theta}$, an estimate $\boldsymbol{R}(\boldsymbol{\theta})$ of $\boldsymbol{R}$ has entries $r_{\mathrm{AR1},u,u'}(\boldsymbol{\theta})$ satisfying

$$r_{\mathrm{AR1},u,u'}(\boldsymbol{\theta}) = \frac{\sum\limits_{cc' \in CC'(+1)} stde_{sc,u}(\boldsymbol{\theta}) \cdot stde_{sc',u'}(\boldsymbol{\theta})}{D}$$

where $CC'(+1)$ is the set of $m(CC'(+1))$ observed consecutive index pairs defined in Sect. 2.4.1 and the denominator D is either the bias-adjusted value $D = m(CC'(+1)) - r > 0$ assuming this is non-zero or the bias-unadjusted value $D = m(CC'(+1))$. For the spatial AR1 structure, as in Sect. 2.4.1, let $d(i)$ $1 \le i \le n_d$ denote the n_d unique positive distances apart for $cc' \in CC'(+1)$ and let $CC'(+1, i)$ be the subset of $CC'(+1)$ satisfying

$$CC'(+1,i) = \{cc' : cc' \in CC(+1), |t(c') - t(c)| = d(i)\}$$

of size $m(CC'(+1, i))$. For a given value of the coefficient parameter vector $\boldsymbol{\theta}$, define the n_d estimates $r_{\text{AR1},u,u'}(\boldsymbol{\theta}, i)$ of $r_{\text{AR1},u,u'}(\boldsymbol{\theta})$ as

$$r_{\text{AR1},u,u'}(\boldsymbol{\theta}, i) = \text{power}\left(\frac{\sum\limits_{cc' \in CC'(+1,i)} stde_{sc,u}(\boldsymbol{\theta}) \cdot \text{stde}_{sc',u'}(\boldsymbol{\theta})}{D(i)}, \frac{1}{d(i)} \right)$$

where the denominator $D(i)$ is either the bias-adjusted value $D(i) = m(CC'(+1, i)) - r > 0$ assuming this is non-zero or the bias-unadjusted value $D(i) = m(CC'(+1, i))$. An estimate of the spatial autocorrelation $r_{\text{AR1},u,u'}(\boldsymbol{\theta})$ is given by the average of the n_d estimates $r_{\text{AR1},u,u'}(\boldsymbol{\theta}, i)$, that is

$$r_{\text{AR1},u,u'}(\boldsymbol{\theta}) = \frac{\sum\limits_{i=1}^{n_d} r_{\text{AR1},u,u'}(\boldsymbol{\theta}, i)}{n_d}.$$

In the non-spatial case, $n_d = 1$ and the spatial estimate is equivalent to the non-spatial estimate and is the same when $d(1) = 1$. The correlation parameter estimates $r_{\text{AR1},u,u'}(\boldsymbol{\theta})$ are combined over $0 \le u, u' < K$ into the $K^2 \times 1$ correlation parameter vector $\rho_{\text{AR1}}(\boldsymbol{\theta})$.

11.1.3.4 Unstructured Correlations

Under the UN correlation structure, the component matrices $\boldsymbol{R}_{s,c,c'}$ have entries $r_{\text{UN},c,c',u,u'}$ for $c,c' \in C(s)$ with $c < c'$ and $0 \le u, u' < K$ while $\boldsymbol{R}_{s,c',c} = \boldsymbol{R}^{\text{T}}_{s,c,c'}$. For a given value of the coefficient parameter vector $\boldsymbol{\theta}$, the estimate $r_{\text{UN},c,c',u,u'}(\boldsymbol{\theta})$ of the UN correlation parameter $r_{\text{UN},c,c',u,u'}$ is computed as

$$r_{\text{UN},c,c',u,u'}(\boldsymbol{\theta}) = \frac{\sum\limits_{s \in S(cc')} stde_{sc,u}(\boldsymbol{\theta}) \cdot stde_{sc',u'}(\boldsymbol{\theta})}{D}$$

where $S(cc')$ is the set of $m(S(cc'))$ observed matched set indexes for each possible index pair cc' in the set CC defined in Sect. 2.4.1 and the denominator D is either the bias-adjusted value $D = m(S(cc')) - r > 0$ assuming this is non-zero or the bias-unadjusted value $D = m(S(cc'))$. The correlation parameter vector $\boldsymbol{\rho}_{\text{UN}}$ is estimated by combining the estimates $r_{\mathrm{UN},c,c',u,u'}(\boldsymbol{\theta})$ of the UN correlation parameters over $1 \le c, c' \le m$ with $c < c'$ and $1 \le u, u' \le K$ into the $(K^2 \cdot m \cdot (m-1)/2) \times 1$ correlation parameter vector $\boldsymbol{\rho}_{\mathrm{UN}}(\boldsymbol{\theta})$. As in Sect. 10.3, the number $K^2 \cdot m \cdot (m-1)/2$ of UN correlation parameters can be quite large even for relatively small values of K and m so that it can be impractical to consider the UN correlation structure for some correlated polytomous outcomes.

11.1.3.5 Degeneracy in Correlation Estimates

For the EC, spatial AR1, and UN correlation structures, generated correlation matrices can be degenerate. However, the correlation matrices $\boldsymbol{R}_s(\boldsymbol{\rho})$ depend on $\boldsymbol{\theta}$ and so change with $s \in S$ except in simple cases where $\boldsymbol{\mu}_s$ is the same for all $s \in S$, and so it is not possible to check a single correlation matrix for degeneracy as in Sect. 3.6. Degeneracy in the case of ordinal regression based on individual outcomes can be checked by computing the eigenvalues of $\boldsymbol{R}_s(\boldsymbol{\rho})$ over $s \in S$. If any one of these has a non-positive smallest eigenvalue, then the model needs to be dropped from consideration in the search for a solution to $\boldsymbol{E}(\boldsymbol{\theta}) = \boldsymbol{0}$.

11.1.4 *Extended Linear Mixed Modeling*

As in Sect. 10.4, full maximum likelihood estimation is possible, maximizing the likelihood in the correlation parameters as well as in the mean and dispersion parameters. In what follows, revised estimating equations are formulated for mean and dispersion parameters as well as for EC, spatial AR1, and UN correlation parameters. There is now just one alternative estimate of the correlation vector and not bias-adjusted and bias-unadjusted alternatives as for standard, partially modified, and fully modified GEE.

11.1.4.1 Estimating Equations for Means, Dispersions, and Correlations Based on the Likelihood

The definitions of the log-likelihood $\ell(SC;\boldsymbol{\theta})$ and the likelihood function $L(SC;\boldsymbol{\theta})$ of Sect. 11.1.2 apply in this case without change. However, the parameter vector is now

$$\boldsymbol{\theta} = \begin{pmatrix} \boldsymbol{\beta} \\ \boldsymbol{\gamma} \\ \boldsymbol{\rho} \end{pmatrix}$$

with $K + r + q + p$ entries, where p is the number of correlation parameters. The likelihood function $L(SC;\boldsymbol{\theta})$ is maximized in the coefficient parameter vector $\boldsymbol{\theta}$. Specifically, use Newton's method to solve the estimating equations

$$\boldsymbol{E}(\boldsymbol{\theta}) = \frac{\partial \ell(SC;\boldsymbol{\theta})}{\partial \boldsymbol{\theta}} = \sum_{s \in S} \boldsymbol{E}_s(\boldsymbol{\theta}) = \sum_{s \in S} \frac{\partial \ell(O_s;\boldsymbol{\theta})}{\partial \boldsymbol{\theta}} = \mathbf{0}$$

where the operator notation $\frac{\partial}{\partial \boldsymbol{\theta}}$ is used to indicate that this is a standard partial derivative vector in $\boldsymbol{\theta}$ since $\boldsymbol{\rho}$ is treated as a separate parameter vector. The associated matrix

$$\boldsymbol{E}'(\boldsymbol{\theta}) = \frac{\partial \boldsymbol{E}(\boldsymbol{\theta})}{\partial \boldsymbol{\theta}}.$$

In this case, $\boldsymbol{E}(\boldsymbol{\theta})$ is a true gradient vector and $\boldsymbol{E}'(\boldsymbol{\theta})$ a true Hessian matrix.

The gradient vector satisfies

$$\boldsymbol{E}(\boldsymbol{\theta}) = \begin{pmatrix} \boldsymbol{E}(\boldsymbol{\beta}) \\ \boldsymbol{E}(\boldsymbol{\gamma}) \\ \boldsymbol{E}(\boldsymbol{\rho}) \end{pmatrix}$$

where $\boldsymbol{E}(\boldsymbol{\gamma})$ is computed as in Sect. 11.1.2 for partially and fully modified GEE modeling since the correlation matrices do not depend on the dispersion parameters, but $\boldsymbol{E}(\boldsymbol{\beta})$ is now different because $\boldsymbol{R}_s(\boldsymbol{\rho})$ depends on the mean parameter vector $\boldsymbol{\beta}$ (see Sect. 11.1.3). Specifically,

$$\boldsymbol{E}(\boldsymbol{\beta}) = \boldsymbol{E}_0(\boldsymbol{\beta}) + \boldsymbol{E}_1(\boldsymbol{\beta})$$

where $\boldsymbol{E}_0(\boldsymbol{\beta})$ is computed using fully modified GEE formulas for $\boldsymbol{E}(\boldsymbol{\beta})$ given in Sect. 11.1.2 and $\boldsymbol{E}_1(\boldsymbol{\beta})$ is the extra amount to account for the dependence of $\boldsymbol{R}_s(\boldsymbol{\rho})$ on $\boldsymbol{\beta}$. Details on the computation of $\boldsymbol{E}(\boldsymbol{\theta})$ are given in Sects. 11.1.4.2–11.1.4.3.

The Hessian matrix $\boldsymbol{E}'(\boldsymbol{\theta})$ has nine component matrices: the $(K + r) \times (K + r)$ matrix

$$\boldsymbol{E}'(\boldsymbol{\beta}) = \frac{\partial \boldsymbol{E}(\boldsymbol{\beta})}{\partial \boldsymbol{\beta}}$$

for the $K + r$ mean parameters, the $q \times q$ matrix

$$\boldsymbol{E}'(\boldsymbol{\gamma}) = \frac{\partial \boldsymbol{E}(\boldsymbol{\gamma})}{\partial \boldsymbol{\gamma}}$$

for the q dispersion parameters computed as in Sect. 11.1.2 for partially and fully modified GEE modeling, the p×p matrix

$$\boldsymbol{E}'(\boldsymbol{\rho}) = \frac{\partial \boldsymbol{E}(\boldsymbol{\rho})}{\partial \boldsymbol{\rho}}$$

for the p correlation parameters, the $(K + r) \times q$ matrix

$$\boldsymbol{E}'(\boldsymbol{\beta}, \boldsymbol{\gamma}) = \frac{\partial \boldsymbol{E}(\boldsymbol{\beta})}{\partial \boldsymbol{\gamma}}$$

and its transpose $\boldsymbol{E}'(\boldsymbol{\gamma}, \boldsymbol{\beta}) = \boldsymbol{E}'^{\mathrm{T}}(\boldsymbol{\beta}, \boldsymbol{\gamma})$, the $(K + r) \times p$ matrix

$$\boldsymbol{E}'(\boldsymbol{\beta}, \boldsymbol{\rho}) = \frac{\partial \boldsymbol{E}(\boldsymbol{\beta})}{\partial \boldsymbol{\rho}}$$

and its transpose $\boldsymbol{E}'(\boldsymbol{\rho}, \boldsymbol{\beta}) = \boldsymbol{E}'^{\mathrm{T}}(\boldsymbol{\gamma}, \boldsymbol{\rho})$, the $q \times p$ matrix

$$\boldsymbol{E}'(\boldsymbol{\gamma}, \boldsymbol{\rho}) = \frac{\partial \boldsymbol{E}(\boldsymbol{\gamma})}{\partial \boldsymbol{\rho}}$$

and its transpose $\boldsymbol{E}'(\boldsymbol{\rho}, \boldsymbol{\gamma}) = \boldsymbol{E}'^{\mathrm{T}}(\boldsymbol{\gamma}, \boldsymbol{\rho})$. Details on the computation of $\boldsymbol{E}'(\boldsymbol{\theta})$ are given in Sects. 11.1.4.4–11.1.4.8.

Model-based and robust empirical estimates of the covariance matrix for the ELMM estimate

$$\boldsymbol{\theta}(SC) = \begin{pmatrix} \beta(SC) \\ \gamma(SC) \\ \rho(SC) \end{pmatrix}$$

of the coefficient parameter vector $\boldsymbol{\theta}$ can be computed similarly to those for ELMM given in Sect. 5.1. These use the ELMM versions of $\boldsymbol{E}'(\boldsymbol{\theta}(SC))$ and $\boldsymbol{G}(\boldsymbol{\theta}(SC))$ for ordinal regression using individual outcomes. $\boldsymbol{G}(\boldsymbol{\theta}(SC))$ is defined so that summing the entries of its rows generates $\boldsymbol{E}(\boldsymbol{\theta}(SC))$. A detailed formulation for $\boldsymbol{G}(\boldsymbol{\theta}(SC))$ is not provided for brevity.

The first and second partial derivatives of $\ell(SC;\boldsymbol{\theta})$ are sums over $s \in S$ of associated first and second partial derivatives of $\ell(O_s;\boldsymbol{\theta})$. The next seven sections provide formulations for these derivatives except for the cases $\boldsymbol{E}(\boldsymbol{\gamma})$ and $\boldsymbol{E}'(\boldsymbol{\gamma})$, which are formulated in Sect. 11.1.2. These formulations are needed to compute $\boldsymbol{E}(\boldsymbol{\theta})$ and $\boldsymbol{E}'(\boldsymbol{\theta})$ but are complex and so can be skipped.

Derivatives involving the correlation matrices $\boldsymbol{R}_s(\boldsymbol{\rho})$ are based on formulations given in Wolfinger et al. (1994). Their formulas are for $-2 \cdot \ell(O_s;\boldsymbol{\theta})$ and so need to be converted to handle $\ell(O_s;\boldsymbol{\theta})$. Formulas for these derivatives are also given in Schott (2005). Specifically, denote the entries of the parameter vector $\boldsymbol{\theta}$ as θ_i for $1 \leq i \leq K + r + q + p$. First partial derivatives involving $\boldsymbol{R}_s(\boldsymbol{\rho})$ satisfy

$$\frac{\partial \log|\boldsymbol{R}_s(\rho)|}{\partial \theta_i} = \mathrm{tr}\left(\boldsymbol{R}_s^{-1}(\rho) \cdot \frac{\partial \boldsymbol{R}_s(\rho)}{\partial \theta_i}\right)$$

and

$$\frac{\partial \boldsymbol{R}_s^{-1}(\rho)}{\partial \theta_i} = -\boldsymbol{R}_s^{-1}(\rho) \cdot \frac{\partial \boldsymbol{R}_s(\rho)}{\partial \theta_i} \cdot \boldsymbol{R}_s^{-1}(\rho).$$

Note that the dependence of the correlation matrices $\boldsymbol{R}_s(\rho)$ on the mean parameters $\boldsymbol{\beta}$ is suppressed in the notation to reduce its complexity, and so the above derivatives are non-zero when θ_i corresponds to a mean parameter or a correlation parameter, but are zero when θ_i corresponds to a dispersion parameter. Second partial derivatives involving $\boldsymbol{R}_s(\rho)$ satisfy

$$\frac{\partial^2 \log|\boldsymbol{R}_s(\rho)|}{\partial \theta_{i'}\,\partial \theta_i} = -\,\mathrm{tr}\left(\boldsymbol{R}_s^{-1}(\rho) \cdot \frac{\partial \boldsymbol{R}_s(\rho)}{\partial \theta_{i'}} \cdot \boldsymbol{R}_s^{-1}(\rho) \cdot \frac{\partial \boldsymbol{R}_s(\rho)}{\partial \theta_i}\right)$$
$$+\,\mathrm{tr}\left(\boldsymbol{R}_s^{-1}(\rho) \cdot \frac{\partial^2 \boldsymbol{R}_s(\rho)}{\partial \theta_{i'}\,\partial \theta_i}\right)$$

and

$$\frac{\partial^2 \boldsymbol{R}_s^{-1}(\rho)}{\partial \theta_{i'}\,\partial \theta_i} = 2 \cdot \boldsymbol{R}_s^{-1}(\rho) \cdot \frac{\partial \boldsymbol{R}_s(\rho)}{\partial \theta_{i'}} \cdot \boldsymbol{R}_s^{-1}(\rho) \cdot \frac{\partial \boldsymbol{R}_s(\rho)}{\partial \theta_i} \cdot \boldsymbol{R}_s^{-1}(\rho)$$
$$-\boldsymbol{R}_s^{-1}(\rho) \cdot \frac{\partial^2 \boldsymbol{R}_s(\rho)}{\partial \theta_{i'}\,\partial \theta_i} \cdot \boldsymbol{R}_s^{-1}(\rho)$$

for $1 \le i, i' \le K + r + q + p$. These are zero when θ_i or $\theta_{i'}$ correspond to a dispersion parameter. The second partial derivatives $\frac{\partial^2 \boldsymbol{R}_s(\rho)}{\partial \theta_{i'}\,\partial \theta_i}$ can sometimes be zero so that associated terms are dropped from the second partial derivatives of $\log|\boldsymbol{R}_s(\rho)|$ and $\boldsymbol{R}_s^{-1}(\rho)$. These cases are identified in what follows.

11.1.4.2 First Partial Derivatives with Respect to Mean Parameters

The gradient vector $\boldsymbol{E}(\boldsymbol{\beta})$ for the mean parameters satisfies

$$\boldsymbol{E}(\boldsymbol{\beta}) = \boldsymbol{E}_0(\boldsymbol{\beta}) + \boldsymbol{E}_1(\boldsymbol{\beta})$$

where $\boldsymbol{E}_0(\boldsymbol{\beta})$ is computed using fully modified GEE formulas for $\boldsymbol{E}(\boldsymbol{\beta})$ given in Sect. 11.1.2. $\boldsymbol{E}_1(\boldsymbol{\beta})$ is the sum over $s \in S$ of terms $\boldsymbol{E}_{1,s}(\boldsymbol{\beta})$ with entries

$$E_{1,s,w}(\boldsymbol{\rho}) = -\boldsymbol{stde}_s^{\mathrm{T}} \cdot \frac{\partial \boldsymbol{R}_s^{-1}(\boldsymbol{\rho})}{\partial \alpha_w} \cdot \boldsymbol{stde}_s/2 - \frac{\partial \log|\boldsymbol{R}_s(\boldsymbol{\rho})|}{\partial \alpha_w}/2,$$

$$E_{1,s,K,j}(\boldsymbol{\rho}) = -\boldsymbol{stde}_s^{\mathrm{T}} \cdot \frac{\partial \boldsymbol{R}_s^{-1}(\boldsymbol{\rho})}{\partial \beta_{K,j}} \cdot \boldsymbol{stde}_s/2 - \frac{\partial \log|\boldsymbol{R}_s(\boldsymbol{\rho})|}{\partial \beta_{K,j}}/2$$

where the above first partial derivatives of $\log|\boldsymbol{R}_s(\boldsymbol{\rho})|$ and $\boldsymbol{R}_s^{-1}(\boldsymbol{\rho})$ are defined in Sect. 11.1.4.1 for $0 \leq w < K$ and $1 \leq j \leq r$. Using the notation of Sect. 11.1.3, $\frac{\partial \boldsymbol{R}_s(\boldsymbol{\rho})}{\partial \alpha_w}$ and $\frac{\partial \boldsymbol{R}_s(\boldsymbol{\rho})}{\partial \beta_{w,j}}$ have component matrices $\frac{\partial \boldsymbol{R}_{s,c,c'}}{\partial \alpha_w}$ and $\frac{\partial \boldsymbol{R}_{s,c,c'}}{\partial \beta_{w,j}}$ for c, $c' \in C(s)$. For c, $c' \in C(s)$ with $c \neq c'$, the off-diagonal component matrices $\boldsymbol{R}_{s,c,c'}$ satisfy

$$\frac{\partial \boldsymbol{R}_{s,c,c'}}{\partial \alpha_w} = \frac{\partial \boldsymbol{R}_{s,c,c'}}{\partial \beta_{K,j}} = \mathbf{0}$$

for each of the four correlation structures of Sect. 11.1.3 because they do not depend on $\boldsymbol{\beta}$. The diagonal component matrices $\boldsymbol{R}_{s,c,c}$ have first partial derivatives $\frac{\partial \boldsymbol{R}_{s,c,c}}{\partial \alpha_w}$ and $\frac{\partial \boldsymbol{R}_{s,c,c}}{\partial \beta_{w,j}}$ with entries $\frac{\partial r_{s,c,c,u,u'}}{\partial \alpha_w}$ and $\frac{\partial r_{s,c,c,u,u'}}{\partial \beta_{w,j}}$, respectively, satisfying

$$\frac{\partial r_{s,c,c,u,u'}}{\partial \alpha_w} = r_{s,c,c,u,u'} \cdot \left(\frac{1}{V(\mu_{sc,u})} - \frac{1}{V(\mu_{sc,u+1})}\right) \cdot V(\mu_{sc,\leq u})/2, w = u, u' = u + 1;$$

$$\frac{\partial r_{s,c,c,u,u'}}{\partial \alpha_w} = r_{s,c,c,u,u'} \cdot \frac{V(\mu_{sc,\leq u})}{V(\mu_{sc,u})}/2, w = u, u' > u + 1;$$

$$\frac{\partial r_{s,c,c,u,u'}}{\partial \alpha_w} = -r_{s,c,c,u,u'} \cdot \frac{V(\mu_{sc,\leq u-1})}{V(\mu_{sc,u})}/2, w = u - 1;$$

$$\frac{\partial r_{s,c,c,u,u'}}{\partial \alpha_w} = r_{s,c,c,u,u'} \cdot \frac{V(\mu_{sc,\leq u'})}{V(\mu_{sc,u'})}/2, w = u';$$

$$\frac{\partial r_{s,c,c,u,u'}}{\partial \alpha_w} = -r_{s,c,c,u,u'} \cdot \frac{V(\mu_{sc,\leq u'-1})}{V(\mu_{sc,u'})}/2, w = u' - 1, u' > u + 1;$$

$$\frac{\partial r_{s,c,c,u,u'}}{\partial \alpha_w} = 0, w \neq u, w \neq u - 1, w \neq u', w \neq u' - 1;$$

$$\frac{\partial r_{s,c,c,u,u'}}{\partial \beta_{K,j}}$$

$$= x_{sc,j} \cdot r_{s,c,c,u,u'} \cdot \left(\frac{V(\mu_{sc,\le u}) - V(\mu_{sc,\le u-1})}{V(\mu_{sc,u})} + \frac{V(\mu_{sc,\le u'}) - V(\mu_{sc,\le u'-1})}{V(\mu_{sc,u'})} \right) /2,$$

for $0 \le u, u', w < K$ and $1 \le j \le r$. Note that the case $w = u' - 1$, $u = u' - 1$ is covered by the case $w = u$, $u' = u + 1$ while the cases $w < u' - 1$ and $w > u'$ are covered by the case $w \ne u$, $w \ne u - 1$, $w \ne u'$, $w \ne u' - 1$.

11.1.4.3 First Partial Derivatives with Respect to Correlation Parameters

With the entries of $\boldsymbol{\rho}$ denoted by ρ_j for $1 \le j \le p$,

$$\boldsymbol{E}(\boldsymbol{\rho}) = \frac{\partial \ell(SC;\boldsymbol{\theta})}{\partial \boldsymbol{\rho}}$$

is the sum over $s \in S$ of $\boldsymbol{E}_s(\boldsymbol{\rho})$ with entries

$$E_{s,j}(\boldsymbol{\rho}) = -\boldsymbol{stde}_s^{\mathrm{T}} \cdot \frac{\partial \boldsymbol{R}_s^{-1}(\boldsymbol{\rho})}{\partial \rho_j} \cdot \boldsymbol{stde}_s/2 - \frac{\partial \log|\boldsymbol{R}_s(\boldsymbol{\rho})|}{\partial \rho_j}/2$$

where the above first partial derivatives of $\log|\boldsymbol{R}_s(\boldsymbol{\rho})|$ and $\boldsymbol{R}_s^{-1}(\boldsymbol{\rho})$ are defined in Sect. 11.1.4.1 for $1 \le j \le p$. For the four correlation structures of Sect. 11.1.3, the first partial derivative vector $\frac{\partial \boldsymbol{R}_s(\boldsymbol{\rho})}{\partial \rho_j}$ has diagonal component matrices

$$\frac{\partial \boldsymbol{R}_{s,c,c}}{\partial \rho_j} = \boldsymbol{0}$$

for $c \in C(s)$ because $\boldsymbol{R}_{s,c,c}$ do not depend on the correlation parameters.

For independent correlations, the off-diagonal component matrices

$$\frac{\partial \boldsymbol{R}_{s,c,c'}}{\partial \rho_j} = \boldsymbol{0}$$

because $\boldsymbol{R}_{s,c,c'} = \boldsymbol{0}$ for $c, c' \in C(s)$, $c \ne c'$.

For exchangeable correlations, $\boldsymbol{R}_{s,c,c'} = \boldsymbol{R}$ for $c,c' \in C(s)$ with $c < c'$ and a fixed $K \times K$ matrix $\boldsymbol{R}$ with $p = K^2$ unique entries ρ_j for $1 \le j \le p$ denoted as $r_{\mathrm{EC},u,u'}$ for $0 \le u, u' < K$ while $\boldsymbol{R}_{s,c',c} = \boldsymbol{R}^{\mathrm{T}}$. In this case,

$$\frac{\partial \boldsymbol{R}_{s,c,c'}}{\partial r_{\mathrm{EC},u,u'}} = \boldsymbol{J}(u,u')$$

for $c, c' \in C(s)$ with $c < c'$ where $\boldsymbol{J}(u, u')$ is the $K \times K$ matrix with entry 1 in the uth row and u'^{th} column and 0 elsewhere while

$$\frac{\partial \boldsymbol{R}_{s,c',c}}{\partial r_{\mathrm{EC},u,u'}} = \boldsymbol{J}^{\mathrm{T}}(u,u').$$

For spatial autoregressive order 1 correlations,

$$\boldsymbol{R}_{s,c,c'} = \mathrm{power}(\boldsymbol{R}, |t(c') - t(c)|)$$

for $c, c' \in C(s)$ with $c < c'$ and a fixed $K \times K$ matrix $\boldsymbol{R}$ with $p = K^2$ unique entries ρ_j for $1 \leq j \leq p$ denoted as $r_{\mathrm{AR1},u,u'}$ for $0 \leq u,u' < K$ while $\boldsymbol{R}_{s,c',c} = \boldsymbol{R}^T_{s,c,c'}$. In this case, $\boldsymbol{R}_{s,c,c'}$ for $c, c' \in C(s)$ with $c < c'$ has entries

$$\begin{aligned} r_{s,c,c',u,u'} &= \mathrm{power}(r_{\mathrm{AR1},u,u'}, |t(c') - t(c)|) \\ &= \mathrm{sign}(r_{\mathrm{AR1},u,u'}) \cdot (\mathrm{sign}(r_{\mathrm{AR1},u,u'}) \cdot r_{\mathrm{AR1},u,u'})^{|t(c') - t(c)|} \end{aligned}$$

when $|r_{\mathrm{AR1},u,u'}| > 0$ for $0 \leq u,\ u' < K$ so that

$$\frac{\partial \boldsymbol{R}_{s,c,c'}}{\partial r_{\mathrm{AR1},u,u'}} = \boldsymbol{J}(c,c',u,u')$$

where $\boldsymbol{J}(c, c', u, u')$ is the $K \times K$ matrix with zero entries except for the entry in the uth row and u'^{th} column satisfying

$$\begin{aligned} &\frac{\partial r_{s,c,c',u,u'}}{\partial r_{\mathrm{AR1},u,u'}} \\ &\quad = (\mathrm{sign}(r_{\mathrm{AR1},u,u'}))^2 \cdot |t(c') - t(c)| \cdot (\mathrm{sign}(r_{\mathrm{AR1},u,u'}) \cdot r_{\mathrm{AR1},u,u'})^{|t(c') - t(c)| - 1} \\ &\quad = |t(c') - t(c)| \cdot |r_{\mathrm{AR1},u,u'}|^{|t(c') - t(c)| - 1} \end{aligned}$$

with its sign changed when negative while

$$\frac{\partial \boldsymbol{R}_{s,c',c}}{\partial r_{\mathrm{AR1},u,u'}} = \boldsymbol{J}^{\mathrm{T}}(c,c',u,u').$$

When $|t(c') - t(c)| = 1$, the derivative $\frac{\partial r_{s,c,c',u,u'}}{\partial r_{\mathrm{AR1},u,u'}}$ at $r_{\mathrm{AR1},u,u'} = 0$ from above is $+1$ and from below is -1, and so the derivative is not well-defined. This problem can be circumvented in practice by restricting $|r_{\mathrm{AR1},u,u'}|$ to be greater than some small value.

For unstructured correlations, $\boldsymbol{R}_{s,c,c'}$ have $p = K^2 \cdot m(s) \cdot (m(s) - 1)/2$ entries ρ_j for $1 \le j \le p$ denoted as $r_{\mathrm{UN},c,c',u,u'}$ for c, $c' \in C(s)$ with $c < c'$ and $0 \le u$, $u' < K$ while $\boldsymbol{R}_{s,c',c} = \boldsymbol{R}^{\mathrm{T}}$. In this case,

$$\frac{\partial \boldsymbol{R}_{s,c,c'}}{\partial r_{\mathrm{UN},c,c',u,u'}} = \boldsymbol{J}'(c, c', u, u')$$

for c, $c' \in C(s)$ with $c < c'$ where $\boldsymbol{J}'(c, c', u, u')$ is the $K \times K$ matrix with entry 1 in the uth row and u'^{th} column and 0 elsewhere while

$$\frac{\partial \boldsymbol{R}_{s,c',c}}{\partial r_{\mathrm{UN},c,c',u,u'}} = \boldsymbol{J}'^{\mathrm{T}}(c, c', u, u').$$

On the other hand, for d, $d' \in C(s)$ with $d < d'$

$$\frac{\partial \boldsymbol{R}_{s,d,d'}}{\partial r_{\mathrm{UN},c,c',u,u'}} = \boldsymbol{0}$$

when $d \neq c$ or $d' \neq c'$.

11.1.4.4 Second Partial Derivatives with Respect to Mean Parameters

The matrix $\boldsymbol{E}'(\boldsymbol{\beta})$ for the mean parameters satisfies

$$\boldsymbol{E}'(\boldsymbol{\beta}) = \boldsymbol{E}'_0(\boldsymbol{\beta}) + \boldsymbol{E}'_1(\boldsymbol{\beta}) + \boldsymbol{E}'_2(\boldsymbol{\beta})$$

where $\boldsymbol{E}'_0(\boldsymbol{\beta})$ is computed using formulas for $\boldsymbol{E}'(\boldsymbol{\beta})$ given in Sect. 11.1.2 for fully modified GEE. $\boldsymbol{E}'_1(\boldsymbol{\beta})$ is the sum over $s \in S$ of terms $\boldsymbol{E}'_{1,s}(\boldsymbol{\beta})$ with entries

$$E'_{1,s,w,w'}(\boldsymbol{\beta}) = -\,\boldsymbol{stde}_s^{\mathrm{T}} \cdot \frac{\partial^2 \boldsymbol{R}_s^{-1}(\boldsymbol{\rho})}{\partial \alpha_{w'}\,\partial \alpha_w} \cdot \boldsymbol{stde}_s/2 - \frac{\partial^2 \log|\boldsymbol{R}_s(\boldsymbol{\rho})|}{\partial \alpha_{w'}\,\partial \alpha_w}/2,$$

$$E'_{1,s,w,Kj}(\boldsymbol{\beta}) = -\,\boldsymbol{stde}_s^{\mathrm{T}} \cdot \frac{\partial^2 \boldsymbol{R}_s^{-1}(\boldsymbol{\rho})}{\partial \beta_{Kj}\,\partial \alpha_w} \cdot \boldsymbol{stde}_s/2 - \frac{\partial^2 \log|\boldsymbol{R}_s(\boldsymbol{\rho})|}{\partial \beta_{Kj}\alpha_w}/2,$$

$$E'_{1,s,Kj,w}(\boldsymbol{\beta}) = -\,\boldsymbol{stde}_s^{\mathrm{T}} \cdot \frac{\partial^2 \boldsymbol{R}_s^{-1}(\boldsymbol{\rho})}{\partial \alpha_w\,\partial \beta_{Kj}} \cdot \boldsymbol{stde}_s/2 - \frac{\partial^2 \log|\boldsymbol{R}_s(\boldsymbol{\rho})|}{\partial \alpha_w\,\partial \beta_{Kj}}/2,$$

$$E'_{1,s,Kj,j'}(\boldsymbol{\beta}) = -\,\boldsymbol{stde}_s^{\mathrm{T}} \cdot \frac{\partial^2 \boldsymbol{R}_s^{-1}(\boldsymbol{\rho})}{\partial \beta_{Kj'}\,\partial \beta_{Kj}} \cdot \boldsymbol{stde}_s/2 - \frac{\partial^2 \log|\boldsymbol{R}_s(\boldsymbol{\rho})|}{\partial \beta_{Kj'}\,\partial \beta_{Kj}}/2$$

where the above second partial derivatives of $\log|\boldsymbol{R}_s(\boldsymbol{\rho})|$ and $\boldsymbol{R}_s^{-1}(\boldsymbol{\rho})$ are defined in Sect. 11.1.4.1 for $0 \le w$, $w' < K$ and $1 \le j, j' \le r$. Using the notation of Sect. 11.1.3, second partial derivatives of component matrices $\boldsymbol{R}_{s,c,c'}$ for c, $c' \in C(s)$ with $c \neq c'$, are all zero matrices for each of the four correlation structures of Sect. 11.1.3 because they depend only on the correlation parameters and not on the mean parameters. The diagonal component matrices $\boldsymbol{R}_{s,c,c}$ have second partial derivatives with entries satisfying the following for the first partial derivatives $\frac{\partial r_{s,c,c,u,u'}}{\partial \alpha_w}$ and $\frac{\partial r_{s,c,c,u,u'}}{\partial \beta_{K,j}}$ defined in Sect. 11.1.4.3. For $w = u$ and $u' = u + 1$,

$$\frac{\partial^2 r_{s,c,c,u,u'}}{\partial \alpha_{w'}\,\partial \alpha_w} = \frac{\partial r_{s,c,c,u,u'}}{\partial \alpha_{w'}} \cdot \left(\frac{1}{V\left(\mu_{sc,u}\right)} - \frac{1}{V\left(\mu_{sc,u+1}\right)}\right) \cdot V\left(\mu_{sc,\le u}\right)/2 + r_{s,c,c,u,u'} \cdot a_1/2$$

where

$$a_1 = \left(\frac{1}{\mu_{sc,u}} - \frac{1}{1-\mu_{sc,u}}\right) \cdot \frac{V\left(\mu_{sc,\le u}\right) \cdot V\left(\mu_{sc,\le u-1}\right)}{V\left(\mu_{sc,u}\right)}$$

when $w' = u - 1$;

$$\begin{aligned} a_1 = {} & \left(1 - 2 \cdot \mu_{sc,\le u}\right) \cdot \left(\frac{1}{V\left(\mu_{sc,u}\right)} - \frac{1}{V\left(\mu_{sc,u+1}\right)}\right) \cdot V\left(\mu_{sc,\le u}\right) \\ & - \left(\frac{1}{\mu_{sc,u}} - \frac{1}{1-\mu_{sc,u}}\right) \cdot \frac{V^2\left(\mu_{sc,\le u}\right)}{V\left(\mu_{sc,u}\right)} \\ & + \left(\frac{1}{\mu_{sc,u+1}} - \frac{1}{1-\mu_{sc,u+1}}\right) \cdot \frac{1}{V\left(\mu_{sc,u+1}\right)} \end{aligned}$$

when $w' = u$;

$$a_1 = \left(\frac{1}{\mu_{sc,u+1}} - \frac{1}{1-\mu_{sc,u+1}}\right) \cdot \frac{V\left(\mu_{sc,\le u}\right) \cdot V\left(\mu_{sc,\le u+1}\right)}{V\left(\mu_{sc,u+1}\right)}$$

when $w' = u'$;

$$a_1 = 0$$

when $w' \neq u$, $w' \neq u - 1$, $w' \neq u'$, $w' \neq u' - 1$; and

$$\frac{\partial^2 r_{s,c,c,u,u'}}{\partial\beta_{K,j}\partial\alpha_w} = \frac{\partial r_{s,c,c,u,u'}}{\partial\beta_{K,j}} \cdot \left(\frac{1}{V(\mu_{sc,u})} - \frac{1}{V(\mu_{sc,u+1})}\right) \cdot V(\mu_{sc,\le u})/2$$
$$+ r_{s,c,c,u,u'} \cdot x_{sc,j} \cdot b_1/2$$

where

$$b_1 = (1 - 2\cdot\mu_{sc,\le u}) \cdot \left(\frac{1}{V(\mu_{sc,u})} - \frac{1}{V(\mu_{sc,u+1})}\right) \cdot V(\mu_{sc,\le u})$$
$$- \left(\frac{1}{\mu_{sc,u}} - \frac{1}{1-\mu_{sc,u}}\right) \cdot \frac{V(\mu_{sc,\le u}) - V(\mu_{sc,\le u-1})}{V(\mu_{sc,u})} \cdot V(\mu_{sc,\le u})$$
$$+ \left(\frac{1}{\mu_{sc,u+1}} - \frac{1}{1-\mu_{sc,u+1}}\right) \cdot \frac{V(\mu_{sc,\le u+1}) - V(\mu_{sc,\le u})}{V(\mu_{sc,u+1})} \cdot V(\mu_{sc,\le u}).$$

For $w = u$ and $u' > u + 1$,

$$\frac{\partial^2 r_{s,c,c,u,u'}}{\partial\alpha_{w'}\partial\alpha_w} = \frac{\partial r_{s,c,c,u,u'}}{\partial\alpha_{w'}} \cdot \frac{V(\mu_{sc,\le u})}{V(\mu_{sc,u})}/2 + r_{s,c,c,u,u'} \cdot a_2/2$$

where

$$a_2 = \left(\frac{1}{\mu_{sc,u}} - \frac{1}{1-\mu_{sc,u}}\right) \cdot \frac{V(\mu_{sc,\le u}) \cdot V(\mu_{sc,\le u-1})}{V(\mu_{sc,u})}$$

when $w' = u - 1$;

$$a_2 = \left(1 - 2\cdot\mu_{sc,\le u} - V(\mu_{sc,\le u}) \cdot \left(\frac{1}{\mu_{sc,u}} - \frac{1}{1-\mu_{sc,u}}\right)\right) \cdot \frac{V(\mu_{sc,\le u})}{V(\mu_{sc,u})}$$

when $w' = u$, $u' > u + 1$;

$$a_2 = 0$$

when $w' = u'$ or when $w' = u' - 1$ or when $w \ne u$, $w \ne u'$, $w' \ne u$, $w' \ne u'$; and

$$\frac{\partial^2 r_{s,c,c,u,u'}}{\partial\beta_{K,j}\partial\alpha_w} = \frac{\partial r_{s,c,c,u,u'}}{\partial\beta_{K,j}} \cdot \frac{V(\mu_{sc,\le u})}{V(\mu_{sc,u})}/2 + r_{s,c,c,u,u'} \cdot x_{sc,j} \cdot b_2/2$$

where

$$b_2 = \left(1 - 2 \cdot \mu_{sc, \leq u}\right) \cdot \frac{V\left(\mu_{sc, \leq u}\right)}{V\left(\mu_{sc,u}\right)} - \left(\frac{1}{\mu_{sc,u}} - \frac{1}{1 - \mu_{sc,u}}\right) \cdot \frac{V\left(\mu_{sc, \leq u}\right) - V\left(\mu_{sc, \leq u-1}\right)}{V\left(\mu_{sc,u}\right)}.$$

For $w = u - 1$,

$$\frac{\partial^2 r_{s,c,c,u,u'}}{\partial \alpha_{w'} \partial \alpha_w} = -\frac{\partial r_{s,c,c,u,u'}}{\partial \alpha_{w'}} \cdot \frac{V\left(\mu_{sc, \leq u-1}\right)}{V\left(\mu_{sc,u}\right)} /2 - r_{s,c,c,u,u'} \cdot a_3/2$$

where

$$a_3 = \left(1 - 2 \cdot \mu_{sc, \leq u-1} + V\left(\mu_{sc, \leq u-1}\right) \cdot \left(\frac{1}{\mu_{sc,u}} - \frac{1}{1 - \mu_{sc,u}}\right)\right) \cdot \frac{V\left(\mu_{sc, \leq u-1}\right)}{V\left(\mu_{sc,u}\right)}$$

when $w' = u - 1$;

$$a_3 = -\left(\frac{1}{\mu_{sc,u}} - \frac{1}{1 - \mu_{sc,u}}\right) \cdot \frac{V\left(\mu_{sc, \leq u}\right) \cdot V\left(\mu_{sc, \leq u-1}\right)}{V\left(\mu_{sc,u}\right)}$$

when $w' = u$, $u' \geq u + 1$;

$$a_3 = 0$$

when $w' = u'$ or when $w' = u' - 1$ with $u' > u + 1$ or when $w \neq u$, $w \neq u'$, $w' \neq u$, $w' \neq u'$; and

$$\frac{\partial^2 r_{s,c,c,u,u'}}{\partial \beta_{Kj} \partial \alpha_w} = -\frac{\partial r_{s,c,c,u,u'}}{\partial \beta_{Kj}} \cdot \frac{V\left(\mu_{sc, \leq u-1}\right)}{V\left(\mu_{sc,u}\right)} /2 - r_{s,c,c,u,u'} \cdot x_{scj} \cdot b_3/2$$

where

$$b_3 = \left(1 - 2 \cdot \mu_{sc, \leq u-1} - \left(V\left(\mu_{sc, \leq u}\right) - V\left(\mu_{sc, \leq u-1}\right)\right) \cdot \left(\frac{1}{\mu_{sc,u}} - \frac{1}{1 - \mu_{sc,u}}\right)\right) \cdot \frac{V\left(\mu_{sc, \leq u-1}\right)}{V\left(\mu_{sc,u}\right)}.$$

For $w = u'$,

$$\frac{\partial^2 r_{s,c,c,u,u'}}{\partial \alpha_{w'} \partial \alpha_w} = \frac{\partial r_{s,c,c,u,u'}}{\partial \alpha_{w'}} \cdot \frac{V\left(\mu_{sc, \leq u'}\right)}{V\left(\mu_{sc,u'}\right)} /2 + r_{s,c,c,u,u'} \cdot a_4/2$$

where

$$a_4 = \left(\frac{1}{\mu_{sc,u+1}} - \frac{1}{1-\mu_{sc,u+1}}\right) \cdot \frac{V(\mu_{sc,\le u}) \cdot V(\mu_{sc,\le u+1})}{V(\mu_{sc,u+1})}$$

when $w' = u$, $u' = u + 1$;

$$a_4 = \left(1 - 2 \cdot \mu_{sc,\le u'} - V(\mu_{sc,\le u'}) \cdot \left(\frac{1}{\mu_{sc,u'}} - \frac{1}{1-\mu_{sc,u'}}\right)\right) \cdot \frac{V(\mu_{sc,\le u'})}{V(\mu_{sc,u'})}$$

when $w' = u'$;

$$a_4 = \left(\frac{1}{\mu_{sc,u'}} - \frac{1}{1-\mu_{sc,u'}}\right) \cdot \frac{V(\mu_{sc,\le u'}) \cdot V(\mu_{sc,\le u'-1})}{V(\mu_{sc,u'})}$$

when $w' = u' - 1$, $u' > u + 1$;

$$a_4 = 0$$

when $w' = u$, $u' > u + 1$ or when $w' = u - 1$ or when $w \ne u$, $w \ne u'$, $w' \ne u$, $w' \ne u'$; and

$$\frac{\partial^2 r_{s,c,c,u,u'}}{\partial \beta_{K,j} \partial \alpha_w} = \frac{\partial r_{s,c,c,u,u'}}{\partial \beta_{K,j}} \cdot \frac{V(\mu_{sc,\le u'})}{V(\mu_{sc,u'})} / 2 + r_{s,c,c,u,u'} \cdot x_{sc,j} \cdot b_4/2$$

where

$$b_4 = \left(1 - 2 \cdot \mu_{sc,\le u'} - \left(V(\mu_{sc,\le u'}) - V(\mu_{sc,\le u'-1})\right)\right) \cdot \left(\frac{1}{\mu_{sc,u'}} - \frac{1}{1-\mu_{sc,u'}}\right)\Bigg) \cdot \frac{V(\mu_{sc,\le u'})}{V(\mu_{sc,u'})}.$$

For $w = u' - 1$ and $u' >$ u + 1,

$$\frac{\partial^2 r_{s,c,c,u,u'}}{\partial \alpha_{w'} \partial \alpha_w} = - \frac{\partial r_{s,c,c,u,u'}}{\partial \alpha_{w'}} \cdot \frac{V(\mu_{sc,\le u'-1})}{V(\mu_{sc,u'})} / 2 - r_{s,c,c,u,u'} \cdot a_5/2$$

where

$$a_5 = -\left(\frac{1}{\mu_{sc,u'}} - \frac{1}{1-\mu_{sc,u'}}\right) \cdot \frac{V(\mu_{sc,\le u'}) \cdot V(\mu_{sc,\le u'-1})}{V(\mu_{sc,u'})}$$

when $w' = u'$;

$$a_5 = \left(1 - 2 \cdot \mu_{sc, \le u' - 1} + V\left(\mu_{sc, \le u' - 1}\right) \cdot \left(\frac{1}{\mu_{sc,u'}} - \frac{1}{1 - \mu_{sc,u'}}\right)\right) \cdot \frac{V\left(\mu_{sc, \le u' - 1}\right)}{V\left(\mu_{sc,u'}\right)}$$

when $w' = u' - 1$, $u' > u + 1$;

$$a_5 = 0$$

when $w' = u$ or when $w' = u - 1$ or when $w \neq u$, $w \neq u'$, $w' \neq u$, $w' \neq u'$; and

$$\frac{\partial^2 r_{s,c,c,u,u'}}{\partial \beta_{K,j} \partial \alpha_w} = -\frac{\partial r_{s,c,c,u,u'}}{\partial \beta_{K,j}} \cdot \frac{V\left(\mu_{sc, \le u' - 1}\right)}{V\left(\mu_{sc,u'}\right)} /2 - r_{s,c,c,u,u'} \cdot x_{sc,j} \cdot b_5/2$$

where

$$b_5 = \begin{array}{l} \left(1 - 2 \cdot \mu_{sc, \le u' - 1} - \left(V\left(\mu_{sc, \le u'}\right) - V\left(\mu_{sc, \le u' - 1}\right)\right) \cdot \left(\frac{1}{\mu_{sc,u'}} - \frac{1}{1 - \mu_{sc,u'}}\right)\right) \\ \cdot \frac{V\left(\mu_{sc, \le u' - 1}\right)}{V\left(\mu_{sc,u'}\right)}. \end{array}$$

For $w \neq u$, $w \neq u - 1$, $w \neq u'$, and $w \neq u' - 1$ as well as for $w' \neq u$, $w' \neq u - 1$, $w' \neq u'$, and $w' \neq u' - 1$,

$$\frac{\partial^2 r_{s,c,c,u,u'}}{\partial \alpha_{w'} \partial \alpha_w} = \frac{\partial^2 r_{s,c,c,u,u'}}{\partial \alpha_w \partial \beta_{K,j}} = 0.$$

Also, the diagonal component matrices $\boldsymbol{R}_{s,c,c}$ have second partial derivatives with entries satisfying the following for first partial derivatives $\frac{\partial r_{s,c,c,u,u'}}{\partial \beta_{K,j}}$

$$\begin{aligned} &\frac{\partial^2 r_{s,c,c,u,u'}}{\partial \alpha_w \partial \beta_{K,j}} \\ &= x_{sc,j} \cdot \frac{\partial r_{s,c,c,u,u'}}{\partial \alpha_w} \cdot \left(\frac{V\left(\mu_{sc,\le u}\right) - V\left(\mu_{sc,\le u-1}\right)}{V\left(\mu_{sc,u}\right)} + \frac{V\left(\mu_{sc,\le u'}\right) - V\left(\mu_{sc,\le u'-1}\right)}{V\left(\mu_{sc,u'}\right)}\right)/2 \\ &\qquad + x_{sc,j} \cdot r_{s,c,c,u,u'} \cdot a_6/2 \end{aligned}$$

where

$$a_6 = \left(1 - 2 \cdot \mu_{sc,\le u} - \left(V\left(\mu_{sc,\le u}\right) - V\left(\mu_{sc,\le u-1}\right)\right) \cdot \left(\frac{1}{\mu_{sc,u}} - \frac{1}{1 - \mu_{sc,u}}\right)\right) \cdot \frac{V\left(\mu_{sc,\le u}\right)}{V\left(\mu_{sc,u}\right)}$$

$$-\left(1-2\cdot\mu_{sc,\le u'-1}-\left(V\left(\mu_{sc,\le u'}\right)-V\left(\mu_{sc,\le u'-1}\right)\right)\cdot\left(\frac{1}{\mu_{sc,u'}}-\frac{1}{1-\mu_{sc,u'}}\right)\right)\cdot\frac{V\left(\mu_{sc,\le u'-1}\right)}{V\left(\mu_{sc,u'}\right)}$$

when $w = u$, $u' = u + 1$;

$$a_6=\left(1-2\cdot\mu_{sc,\le u}-\left(V\left(\mu_{sc,\le u}\right)-V\left(\mu_{sc,\le u-1}\right)\right)\cdot\left(\frac{1}{\mu_{sc,u}}-\frac{1}{1-\mu_{sc,u}}\right)\right)\cdot\frac{V\left(\mu_{sc,\le u}\right)}{V\left(\mu_{sc,u}\right)}$$

when $w = u$, $u' > u + 1$;

$$a_6=-\left(1-2\cdot\mu_{sc,\le u-1}-\left(V\left(\mu_{sc,\le u}\right)-V\left(\mu_{sc,\le u-1}\right)\right)\cdot\left(\frac{1}{\mu_{sc,u}}-\frac{1}{1-\mu_{sc,u}}\right)\right)\cdot\frac{V\left(\mu_{sc,\le u-1}\right)}{V\left(\mu_{sc,u}\right)}$$

when $w = u - 1$;

$$a_6=\left(1-2\cdot\mu_{sc,\le u'}-\left(V\left(\mu_{sc,\le u'}\right)-V\left(\mu_{sc,\le u'-1}\right)\right)\cdot\left(\frac{1}{\mu_{sc,u'}}-\frac{1}{1-\mu_{sc,u'}}\right)\right)\cdot\frac{V\left(\mu_{sc,\le u'}\right)}{V\left(\mu_{sc,u'}\right)}$$

when $w = u'$;

$$a_6=-\left(1-2\cdot\mu_{sc,\le u'-1}-\left(V\left(\mu_{sc,\le u'}\right)-V\left(\mu_{sc,\le u'-1}\right)\right)\cdot\left(\frac{1}{\mu_{sc,u'}}-\frac{1}{1-\mu_{sc,u'}}\right)\right)\cdot\frac{V\left(\mu_{sc,\le u'-1}\right)}{V\left(\mu_{sc,u'}\right)}$$

when $w = u' - 1$, $u' >$ u + 1;

$$a_6=0$$

when $w \ne u$, $w \ne u'$, $w' \ne u$, $w' \ne u'$; and

$$\frac{\partial^2 r_{s,c,c,u,u'}}{\partial\beta_{K,j'}\partial\beta_{K,j}}$$

$$= x_{sc,j}\cdot\frac{\partial r_{s,c,c,u,u'}}{\beta_{K,j'}}\cdot\left(\frac{V(\mu_{sc,\leq u}) - V(\mu_{sc,\leq u-1})}{V(\mu_{sc,u})} + \frac{V(\mu_{sc,\leq u'}) - V(\mu_{sc,\leq u'-1})}{V(\mu_{sc,u'})}\right)/2$$

$$+ x_{sc,j}\cdot x_{sc,j'}\cdot r_{s,c,c,u,u'}\cdot b_6/2$$

where

$$b_6 = -\frac{\left(V(\mu_{sc,\leq u}) - V(\mu_{sc,\leq u-1})\right)^2}{V(\mu_{sc,u})}\cdot\left(\frac{1}{\mu_{sc,u}} - \frac{1}{1-\mu_{sc,u}}\right)$$

$$+ \frac{(1-2\cdot\mu_{sc,\leq u})\cdot V(\mu_{sc,\leq u}) - (1-2\cdot\mu_{sc,\leq u-1})\cdot V(\mu_{sc,\leq u-1})}{V(\mu_{sc,u})}$$

$$-\frac{\left(V(\mu_{sc,\leq u'}) - V(\mu_{sc,\leq u'-1})\right)^2}{V(\mu_{sc,u'})}\cdot\left(\frac{1}{\mu_{sc,u'}} - \frac{1}{1-\mu_{sc,u'}}\right)$$

$$+ \frac{(1-2\cdot\mu_{sc,\leq u'})\cdot V(\mu_{sc,\leq u'}) - (1-2\cdot\mu_{sc,\leq u'-1})\cdot V(\mu_{sc,\leq u'-1})}{V(\mu_{sc,u'})}.$$

Cases not listed are not possible; for example, for $w = u$, $u' = u + 1$, cases for w' with $u' > u + 1$ are not possible.

$\boldsymbol{E}'_2(\boldsymbol{\beta})$ is the sum over $s \in S$ of terms $\boldsymbol{E}'_{2,s}(\boldsymbol{\beta})$ with entries

$$E'_{2,s,w,w'}(\boldsymbol{\beta}) = \boldsymbol{xstde}_{s,w}^{\mathrm{T}}\cdot\frac{\partial\boldsymbol{R}_s^{-1}(\boldsymbol{\rho})}{\partial\alpha_{w'}}\cdot\boldsymbol{stde}_s + \boldsymbol{xstde}_{s,w'}^{\mathrm{T}}\cdot\frac{\partial\boldsymbol{R}_s^{-1}(\boldsymbol{\rho})}{\partial\alpha_w}\cdot\boldsymbol{stde}_s,$$

$$E'_{2,s,K,j,w}(\boldsymbol{\beta}) = \boldsymbol{xstde}_{s,K,j}^{\mathrm{T}}\cdot\frac{\partial\boldsymbol{R}_s^{-1}(\boldsymbol{\rho})}{\partial\alpha_w}\cdot\boldsymbol{stde}_s + \boldsymbol{xstde}_{s,w}^{\mathrm{T}}\cdot\frac{\partial\boldsymbol{R}_s^{-1}(\boldsymbol{\rho})}{\partial\beta_{K,j}}\cdot\boldsymbol{stde}_s,$$

$$E'_{2,s,w,K,j}(\boldsymbol{\beta}) = \boldsymbol{xstde}_{s,w}^{\mathrm{T}}\cdot\frac{\partial\boldsymbol{R}_s^{-1}(\boldsymbol{\rho})}{\partial\beta_{K,j}}\cdot\boldsymbol{stde}_s + \boldsymbol{xstde}_{s,K,j}^{\mathrm{T}}\cdot\frac{\partial\boldsymbol{R}_s^{-1}(\boldsymbol{\rho})}{\partial\alpha_w}\cdot\boldsymbol{stde}_s,$$

$$E'_{2,s,K,j,j'}(\boldsymbol{\beta}) = \boldsymbol{xstde}_{s,K,j}^{\mathrm{T}}\cdot\frac{\partial\boldsymbol{R}_s^{-1}(\boldsymbol{\rho})}{\partial\beta_{K,j'}}\cdot\boldsymbol{stde}_s + \boldsymbol{xstde}_{s,K,j'}^{\mathrm{T}}\cdot\frac{\partial\boldsymbol{R}_s^{-1}(\boldsymbol{\rho})}{\partial\beta_{K,j}}\cdot\boldsymbol{stde}_s,$$

where $\boldsymbol{xstde}_{s,w}$ and $\boldsymbol{xstde}_{s,K,j}$ are defined in Sect. 11.1.2 and the first partial derivatives of $\boldsymbol{R}_s^{-1}(\boldsymbol{\rho})$ are defined in Sect. 11.1.4.1, for $0 \leq w, w' < K$ and $1 \leq j, j' \leq r$.

11.1.4.5 Second Partial Derivatives with Respect to Correlation Parameters

With the entries of $\boldsymbol{\rho}$ denoted by ρ_j for $1 \leq j \leq p$,

$$\boldsymbol{E}'(\boldsymbol{\rho}) = \frac{\partial \boldsymbol{E}(\boldsymbol{\rho})}{\partial \boldsymbol{\rho}}$$

is the sum over $s \in S$ of $\boldsymbol{E}'_s(\boldsymbol{\rho})$ with entries satisfying

$$E'_{s,j,j'}(\boldsymbol{\rho}) = -\,\boldsymbol{stde}_s^{\mathrm{T}} \cdot \frac{\partial^2 \boldsymbol{R}_s^{-1}(\boldsymbol{\rho})}{\partial \rho_{j'}\, \partial \rho_j} \cdot \boldsymbol{stde}_s/2 - \frac{\partial^2 \log|\boldsymbol{R}_s(\boldsymbol{\rho})|}{\partial \rho_{j'}\, \partial \rho_j}/2$$

where the above second partial derivatives of $\log|\boldsymbol{R}_s(\boldsymbol{\rho})|$ and $\boldsymbol{R}_s^{-1}(\boldsymbol{\rho})$ are defined in Sect. 11.1.4.1 for $1 \leq j, j' \leq p$. For the four correlation structures of Sect. 11.1.3, the second partial derivatives of the diagonal component matrices $\boldsymbol{R}_{s,c,c}$ for $c \in C(s)$ satisfy

$$\frac{\partial^2 \boldsymbol{R}_{s,c,c}}{\partial \rho_{j'}\, \partial \rho_j} = \boldsymbol{0}$$

because $\boldsymbol{R}_{s,c,c}$ do not depend on the correlation parameters. For independent, exchangeable, and unstructured correlations, the off-diagonal component matrices $\boldsymbol{R}_{s,c,c'}$ satisfy

$$\frac{\partial^2 \boldsymbol{R}_{s,c,c'}}{\partial \rho_{j'}\, \partial \rho_j} = \boldsymbol{0}$$

for $1 \leq j, j' \leq p$ because $\frac{\partial \boldsymbol{R}_{s,c,c'}}{\partial \rho_j}$ are constant in those parameters for c, $c' \in C(s)$ with $c \neq c'$. For these correlation structures, terms based on $\frac{\partial^2 \boldsymbol{R}_s(\boldsymbol{\rho})}{\partial \rho_{j'}\, \partial \rho_j}$ are dropped from the second partial derivatives of $\log|\boldsymbol{R}_s(\boldsymbol{\rho})|$ and $\boldsymbol{R}_s^{-1}(\boldsymbol{\rho})$.

For spatial autoregressive order 1 correlations with entries ρ_j denoted as $r_{\mathrm{AR1},u,u'}$ for $0 \leq u$, $u' < K$, the off-diagonal component matrices $\boldsymbol{R}_{s,c,c'}$ satisfy

$$\frac{\partial^2 \boldsymbol{R}_{s,c,c'}}{\partial \rho_{j'}\, \partial \rho_j} = \boldsymbol{0}$$

for $j' \neq j$ because $\frac{\partial \boldsymbol{R}_{s,c,c'}}{\partial \rho_j}$ only depends on ρ_j for $c,c' \in C(s)$ with $c \neq c'$, so that then terms based on $\frac{\partial^2 \boldsymbol{R}_s(\boldsymbol{\rho})}{\partial \rho_{j'}\, \partial \rho_j}$ are dropped from associated second partial derivatives of $\log|\boldsymbol{R}_s(\boldsymbol{\rho})|$ and $\boldsymbol{R}_s^{-1}(\boldsymbol{\rho})$. The off-diagonal component matrices

$$\frac{\partial^2 \boldsymbol{R}_{s,c,c'}}{\partial \rho_j^2} = \boldsymbol{J}''(c, c', u, u)$$

for $j' = j$ and $c, c' \in C(s)$ with $c < c'$ when $\rho_j = r_{\mathrm{AR1},u,u'}$ where $\boldsymbol{J}''(c, c', u, u)$ is the $K \times K$ matrix with entry

$$\frac{\partial^2 r_{s,c,c,u,u'}}{\partial r^2_{\mathrm{AR1},u,u'}} = \mathrm{sign}(r_{\mathrm{AR1},u,u'}) \cdot |t(c') - t(c)| \cdot (|t(c') - t(c)| - 1) \cdot |r_{\mathrm{AR1},u,u'}|^{|t(c') - t(c)| - 2}$$

in the uth row and u'^{th} column with the signed changed back if negative and zero elsewhere while

$$\frac{\partial^2 \boldsymbol{R}_{s,c',c}}{\partial \rho_j^2} = \boldsymbol{J}''^{\mathrm{T}}(c, c', u, u),$$

which is guaranteed to hold by restricting $|r_{\mathrm{AR1},u,u'}|$ to be greater than some small value.

11.1.4.6 Second Partial Derivatives with Respect to Mean and Dispersion Parameters

As indicated in Sect. 11.1.2, $\boldsymbol{E}(\boldsymbol{\gamma})$ is the sum over $s \in S$ of terms $\boldsymbol{E}_s(\boldsymbol{\gamma})$ with entries

$$E_{s,j'}(\boldsymbol{\gamma}) = \boldsymbol{vstde}^{\mathrm{T}}_{s,j'} \cdot \boldsymbol{R}_s^{-1}(\boldsymbol{\rho}) \cdot \boldsymbol{stde}_s - \sum_{c \in C(s)} K \cdot v_{sc,j'}/2,$$

for $1 \leq j' \leq q$ so that $\boldsymbol{E}'(\boldsymbol{\gamma}, \boldsymbol{\beta})$ is the sum over $s \in S$ of $\boldsymbol{E}'_s(\boldsymbol{\gamma}, \boldsymbol{\beta})$ where

$$\boldsymbol{E}'_s(\boldsymbol{\gamma}, \boldsymbol{\beta}) = \boldsymbol{E}'_{0,s}(\boldsymbol{\gamma}, \boldsymbol{\beta}) + \boldsymbol{E}'_{1,s}(\boldsymbol{\gamma}, \boldsymbol{\beta}).$$

$\boldsymbol{E}'_{0,s}(\boldsymbol{\gamma}, \boldsymbol{\beta})$ has entries

$$\boldsymbol{E}'_{0,s,j',w}(\boldsymbol{\gamma}, \boldsymbol{\beta}) = -\boldsymbol{xvstde}^{\mathrm{T}}_{s,j',w} \cdot \boldsymbol{R}_s^{-1}(\boldsymbol{\rho}) \cdot \boldsymbol{stde}_s - \boldsymbol{vstde}^{\mathrm{T}}_{s,j'} \cdot \boldsymbol{R}_s^{-1}(\boldsymbol{\rho}) \cdot \boldsymbol{xstde}_{s,w},$$

$$\boldsymbol{E}'_{0,s,j',Kj}(\boldsymbol{\gamma}, \boldsymbol{\beta}) = -\boldsymbol{xvstde}^{\mathrm{T}}_{s,j',Kj} \cdot \boldsymbol{R}_s^{-1}(\boldsymbol{\rho}) \cdot \boldsymbol{stde}_s - \boldsymbol{vstde}^{\mathrm{T}}_{s,j'} \cdot \boldsymbol{R}_s^{-1}(\boldsymbol{\rho}) \cdot \boldsymbol{xstde}_{s,Kj}$$

where $\boldsymbol{xstde}_{s,w}$ and $\boldsymbol{xstde}_{s,Kj}$ are defined in Sect. 11.1.2 and $\boldsymbol{xvstde}_{s,j',\mathrm{w}}$, and $\boldsymbol{xvstde}_{s,j',Kj}$ are the $(m(SC) \cdot K) \times 1$ vectors with entries

$$xvstde_{sc,u,j',w} = xstde_{sc,u,w} \cdot v_{sc,j'}/2,$$

$$xvstde_{sc,u,j',Kj} = xstde_{sc,u,Kj} \cdot v_{sc,j'}/2.$$

$\boldsymbol{E}'_{1,s}(\boldsymbol{\gamma},\boldsymbol{\beta})$ has entries

$$\boldsymbol{E}'_{1,s,j',w}(\boldsymbol{\gamma},\boldsymbol{\beta}) = \boldsymbol{vstde}_{s,j'}^{\mathrm{T}} \cdot \frac{\partial \boldsymbol{R}_s^{-1}(\boldsymbol{\rho})}{\partial \alpha_w} \cdot \boldsymbol{stde}_s,$$

$$\boldsymbol{E}'_{1,s,j',Kj}(\boldsymbol{\gamma},\boldsymbol{\beta}) = \boldsymbol{vstde}_{s,j'}^{\mathrm{T}} \cdot \frac{\partial \boldsymbol{R}_s^{-1}(\boldsymbol{\rho})}{\partial \beta_{Kj}} \cdot \boldsymbol{stde}_s$$

for $1 \le j' \le q$, $1 \le w \le K$, and $1 \le j \le r$. The formulas for the above first partial derivatives of $\boldsymbol{R}_s^{-1}(\boldsymbol{\rho})$ are defined in Sect. 11.1.4.1 and $\boldsymbol{E}'(\boldsymbol{\beta},\boldsymbol{\gamma}) = \boldsymbol{E}'^{\mathrm{T}}(\boldsymbol{\gamma},\boldsymbol{\beta})$.

11.1.4.7 Second Partial Derivatives with Respect to Mean and Correlation Parameters

As indicated in Sect. 11.1.4.2,

$$\boldsymbol{E}(\boldsymbol{\beta}) = \boldsymbol{E}_0(\boldsymbol{\beta}) + \boldsymbol{E}_1(\boldsymbol{\beta})$$

so that

$$\boldsymbol{E}'(\boldsymbol{\beta},\boldsymbol{\rho}) = \boldsymbol{E}'_0(\boldsymbol{\beta},\boldsymbol{\rho}) + \boldsymbol{E}'_1(\boldsymbol{\beta},\boldsymbol{\rho})$$

and $\boldsymbol{E}'(\boldsymbol{\rho},\boldsymbol{\beta}) = \boldsymbol{E}'^{\mathrm{T}}(\boldsymbol{\beta},\boldsymbol{\rho})$. Also, $\boldsymbol{E}_0(\boldsymbol{\beta})$ is the sum over $s \in S$ of $\boldsymbol{E}_{0,s}(\boldsymbol{\beta})$ with entries

$$E_{0,s,w}(\boldsymbol{\beta}) = \boldsymbol{xstde}_{s,w}^{\mathrm{T}} \cdot \boldsymbol{R}_s^{-1}(\boldsymbol{\rho}) \cdot \boldsymbol{stde}_s - \sum_{c \in C(s)} W_{sc,w}/2,$$

$$E_{0,s,Kj}(\boldsymbol{\beta}) = \boldsymbol{xstde}_{s,Kj}^{\mathrm{T}} \cdot \boldsymbol{R}_s^{-1}(\boldsymbol{\rho}) \cdot \boldsymbol{stde}_s - \sum_{c \in C(s)} \sum_{u=0}^{K-1} W_{Kj}(\mu_{sc,u})/2$$

for $0 \le w < K$ and $1 \le j \le r$ so that, with the entries of $\boldsymbol{\rho}$ denoted by $\rho_{j'}$ for $1 \le j' \le p$, $\boldsymbol{E}'_0(\boldsymbol{\beta},\boldsymbol{\rho})$ is the sum over $s \in S$ of $\boldsymbol{E}'_{0,s}(\boldsymbol{\beta},\boldsymbol{\rho})$ with entries

$$E'_{0,s,w,j'}(\boldsymbol{\beta},\boldsymbol{\rho}) = \boldsymbol{xstde}_{s,w}^{\mathrm{T}} \cdot \frac{\partial \boldsymbol{R}_s^{-1}(\boldsymbol{\rho})}{\partial \rho_{j'}} \cdot \boldsymbol{stde}_s,$$

$$E'_{0,s,K,j,j'}(\boldsymbol{\beta},\boldsymbol{\rho}) = \boldsymbol{xstde}^{\mathrm{T}}_{s,K,j} \cdot \frac{\partial \boldsymbol{R}_s^{-1}(\boldsymbol{\rho})}{\partial \rho_{j'}} \cdot \boldsymbol{stde}_s$$

where the above first partial derivatives of $\boldsymbol{R}_s^{-1}(\boldsymbol{\rho})$ are defined in Sect. 11.1.4.1. $\boldsymbol{E}'_1(\boldsymbol{\beta},\boldsymbol{\rho})$ is the sum over $s \in S$ of $\boldsymbol{E}'_{1,s}(\boldsymbol{\beta},\boldsymbol{\rho})$ with entries

$$E'_{1,s,w,j'}(\boldsymbol{\beta},\boldsymbol{\rho}) = -\boldsymbol{stde}_s^{\mathrm{T}} \cdot \frac{\partial^2 \boldsymbol{R}_s^{-1}(\boldsymbol{\rho})}{\partial \rho_{j'}\,\partial \alpha_w} \cdot \boldsymbol{stde}_s/2 - \frac{\partial^2 \log|\boldsymbol{R}_s(\boldsymbol{\rho})|}{\partial \rho_{j'}\,\partial \alpha_w}/2,$$

$$E'_{1,s,K,j,j'}(\boldsymbol{\beta},\boldsymbol{\rho}) = -\boldsymbol{stde}_s^{\mathrm{T}} \cdot \frac{\partial^2 \boldsymbol{R}_s^{-1}(\boldsymbol{\rho})}{\partial \rho_{j'}\,\partial \beta_{K,j}} \cdot \boldsymbol{stde}_s/2 - \frac{\partial^2 \log|\boldsymbol{R}_s(\boldsymbol{\rho})|}{\partial \rho_{j'}\,\partial \beta_{K,j}}/2$$

where the above second partial derivatives of $\log|\boldsymbol{R}_s(\boldsymbol{\rho})|$ and $\boldsymbol{R}_s^{-1}(\boldsymbol{\rho})$ are defined in Sect. 11.1.4.1 for $0 \le w < K$, $1 \le j \le r$, and $1 \le j' \le q$. Note that the first partial derivatives $\frac{\partial \boldsymbol{R}_s(\boldsymbol{\rho})}{\partial \alpha_w}$ and $\frac{\partial \boldsymbol{R}_s(\boldsymbol{\rho})}{\partial \beta_{K,j}}$ do not depend on $\boldsymbol{\rho}$ (see Sect. 11.1.4.2), so that

$$\frac{\partial^2 \boldsymbol{R}_s(\boldsymbol{\rho})}{\partial \rho_{j'}\,\partial \alpha_w} = \frac{\partial^2 \boldsymbol{R}_s(\boldsymbol{\rho})}{\partial \rho_{j'}\,\partial \beta_{K,j}} = \boldsymbol{0},$$

and so terms based on these second partial derivatives are dropped from the second partial derivatives of $\log|\boldsymbol{R}_s(\boldsymbol{\rho})|$ and $\boldsymbol{R}_s^{-1}(\boldsymbol{\rho})$.

11.1.4.8 Second Partial Derivatives with Respect to Dispersion and Correlation Parameters

As indicated in Sect. 11.1.2, $\boldsymbol{E}(\boldsymbol{\gamma})$ is the sum over $s \in S$ of terms $\boldsymbol{E}_s(\boldsymbol{\gamma})$ with entries

$$E_{s,j'}(\boldsymbol{\gamma}) = \boldsymbol{vstde}^{\mathrm{T}}_{s,j'} \cdot \boldsymbol{R}_s^{-1}(\boldsymbol{\rho}) \cdot \boldsymbol{stde}_s - \sum_{c \in C(s)} K \cdot v_{sc,j'}/2,$$

for $1 \le j \le q$ so that, with the entries of $\boldsymbol{\rho}$ denoted by $\rho_{j'}$ for $1 \le j' \le p$, $\boldsymbol{E}'_s(\boldsymbol{\gamma},\boldsymbol{\rho})$ has entries

$$\boldsymbol{E}'_{s,j,j'}(\boldsymbol{\gamma},\boldsymbol{\rho}) = \boldsymbol{vstde}^{\mathrm{T}}_{s,j'} \cdot \frac{\partial \boldsymbol{R}_s^{-1}(\boldsymbol{\rho})}{\partial \rho_{j'}} \cdot \boldsymbol{stde}_s/2$$

where the above first partial derivatives of $\boldsymbol{R}_s^{-1}(\boldsymbol{\rho})$ are defined in Sect. 11.1.4.1 and $\boldsymbol{E}'(\boldsymbol{\rho},\boldsymbol{\gamma}) = \boldsymbol{E}'^{\mathrm{T}}(\boldsymbol{\gamma},\boldsymbol{\rho})$.

11.2 Ordinal Regression Based on Cumulative Outcomes

This section addresses ordinal regression modeling based on cumulative outcomes. It provides formulations of standard GEE modeling (Sect. 11.2.1), partially and fully modified GEE modeling (Sect. 11.2.2), alternate correlation structures and their estimation (Sect. 11.2.3), and ELMM (Sect. 11.2.4). The formulation for LCV scores of Sect. 2.6, LCV ratio tests of Sect. 2.6.2, and the adaptive modeling process of Sect. 2.7 generalize to ordinal regression based on cumulative outcomes. However, since the $m(SC)$ polytomous measurements with $K + 1$ possible values are replaced by $m(SC) \cdot K$ dichotomous measurements, LCV scores are normalized by the number $m(SC) \cdot K$ of effective measurements rather than by $m(SC)$.

Using the notation of Sect. 11.1, for $sc \in SC$, combine the cumulative outcomes $y_{sc,\le u}$, means $\mu_{sc,\le u}$, and errors $e_{sc,\le u} = y_{sc,\le u} - \mu_{sc,\le u}$ over $0 \le u < K$ into the $K \times 1$ vectors $\mathbf{y}_{sc}$, $\boldsymbol{\mu}_{sc}$, and $\mathbf{e}_{sc} = \mathbf{y}_{sc} - \boldsymbol{\mu}_{sc}$. Combine the vectors $\mathbf{y}_{sc}$, $\boldsymbol{\mu}_{sc}$, and $\mathbf{e}_{sc}$ over $c \in C(s)$ into the $(m(SC) \cdot K) \times 1$ vectors $\mathbf{y}_s$, $\boldsymbol{\mu}_s$, and $\mathbf{e}_s = \mathbf{y}_s - \boldsymbol{\mu}_s$ with $\mathbf{y}_{sc}$, $\boldsymbol{\mu}_{sc}$, and $\mathbf{e}_{sc}$ ordered by the values $c \in C(s)$. Note that the same notation is used for these vectors in Sect. 11.1, but they are computed there using the individual outcomes $y_{sc,u}$ rather than the cumulative outcomes $y_{sc,\le u}$. The means $\mu_{sc,\le u}$ have the same definitions in terms of the parameter vector

$$\boldsymbol{\beta} = \begin{pmatrix} \boldsymbol{\alpha} \\ \boldsymbol{\beta}_K \end{pmatrix}$$

and have the same derivatives based on the variance function $V(\mu_{sc,\le u})$. The individual outcomes $y_{sc,u}$, their means, and associated residuals are not used in the formulations of this section.

11.2.1 Standard GEE Modeling

Let φ be a constant dispersion parameter so that it is constant in $sc,\le u$ for $sc \in SC$ and $0 \le u < K$. Define the extended variances

$$\sigma^2_{sc,\le u} = \varphi \cdot V(\mu_{sc,\le u}),$$

the standardized residuals

$$stde_{sc,\le u} = e_{sc,\le u} / \sigma_{sc,\le u},$$

and the Pearson residuals

$$Pres_{sc,\leq u} = \frac{e_{sc,\leq u}}{V^{1/2}\left(\mu_{sc,\leq u}\right)}$$

for $sc \in SC$ and $0 \leq u < K$. Combine these values over $0 \leq u < K$ into the $K \times 1$ vectors $\boldsymbol{\sigma}_{sc}$, $\boldsymbol{stde}_{sc}$, and $\boldsymbol{Pres}_{sc}$, and then combine these vectors into the $(m(SC) \cdot K) \times 1$ vectors $\boldsymbol{\sigma}_s$, $\boldsymbol{stde}_s$, and $\boldsymbol{Pres}_s$ ordered by their values $c \in C(s)$. Model the $(m(SC) \cdot K) \times (m(SC) \cdot K)$ covariance matrices $\boldsymbol{\Sigma}_s$ as

$$\boldsymbol{\Sigma}_s = \boldsymbol{DIAG}(\boldsymbol{\sigma}_s) \cdot \boldsymbol{R}_s(\boldsymbol{\rho}) \cdot \boldsymbol{DIAG}(\boldsymbol{\sigma}_s)$$

for appropriate choices of the $(m(SC) \cdot K) \times (m(SC) \cdot K)$ correlation matrices $\boldsymbol{R}_s(\boldsymbol{\rho})$ for $s \in S$.

Standard GEE modeling can be extended to ordinal regression based on cumulative outcomes by providing correlation structures and methods for their estimation (see Sect. 11.2.3). The notation of Sect. 2.4 also extends to ordinal regression using cumulative outcomes. Specifically, the generalized estimating equations are given by $\boldsymbol{E}(\boldsymbol{\beta}) = \boldsymbol{0}$ where the $(K + r) \times 1$ vector $\boldsymbol{E}(\boldsymbol{\beta})$ satisfies

$$\boldsymbol{E}(\boldsymbol{\beta}) = \sum_{s \in S} \boldsymbol{E}_s(\boldsymbol{\beta}) = \sum_{s \in S} \boldsymbol{D}_s^{\mathrm{T}} \cdot \boldsymbol{\Sigma}_s^{-1} \cdot \boldsymbol{e}_s,$$

and the $(m(SC) \cdot K) \times (K + r)$ matrices

$$\boldsymbol{D}_s = \frac{\partial \boldsymbol{\mu}_s}{\partial \boldsymbol{\beta}}$$

for $s \in S$ have entries

$$D_{sc,\leq u,w} = \frac{\partial \mu_{sc,\leq u}}{\partial \alpha_w}$$

and

$$D_{sc,\leq u,K,j} = \frac{\partial \mu_{sc,\leq u}}{\partial \beta_{K,j}}$$

based on derivatives as defined in Sect. 11.1 for $sc \in SC$, $0 \leq u$, $w < K$, and $1 \leq j \leq r$. Let

$$\boldsymbol{E}'(\boldsymbol{\beta}) = -\sum_{s \in S} \boldsymbol{D}_s^{\mathrm{T}} \cdot \boldsymbol{\Sigma}_s^{-1} \cdot \boldsymbol{D}_s.$$

The standard GEE estimation process uses Newton's method to iteratively solve $\boldsymbol{E}(\boldsymbol{\beta}) = \boldsymbol{0}$ with $\boldsymbol{E}(\boldsymbol{\beta})$ serving in the role of the gradient vector and $\boldsymbol{E}'(\boldsymbol{\beta})$ in the role of the Hessian matrix. The bias-adjusted estimate of the constant dispersion parameter φ for a given value of the coefficient parameter vector $\boldsymbol{\beta}$ is

$$\varphi(\boldsymbol{\beta}) = \frac{\sum\limits_{sc\in SC} \boldsymbol{Pres}_{sc}^{\mathrm{T}}(\boldsymbol{\beta}) \cdot \boldsymbol{Pres}_{sc}(\boldsymbol{\beta})}{m(SC) \cdot K - r}$$

assuming $m(SC) \cdot K - r > 0$. Lipsitz et al. (1994) and Miller et al. (1993) assume unit dispersions and not more general constant dispersions. For the ordinal regression case based on cumulative logits, models in those references are expressed in terms of individual outcomes $y_{sc,u}$ computed from cumulative outcomes $y_{sc,\leq u}$ as in Sect. 11.1 and not in terms of cumulative outcomes directly as addressed in Sect. 11.2.

The likelihood function $L(SC;\boldsymbol{\theta})$ generalizes to handle ordinal regression modeling using cumulative outcomes in the standard GEE context. This is a special case of the formulation given in Sect. 11.2.2, and so is not provided here.

Model-based and robust empirical estimates of the covariance matrix for the standard GEE estimate $\boldsymbol{\beta}(SC)$ of the coefficient parameter vector $\boldsymbol{\beta}$ can be computed similarly to those for standard GEE modeling given in Sect. 2.4.2. These use the standard GEE versions of $\boldsymbol{E}'(\boldsymbol{\beta}(SC))$ and $\boldsymbol{G}(\boldsymbol{\beta}(SC))$ for ordinal regression using cumulative outcomes. $\boldsymbol{G}(\boldsymbol{\beta}(SC))$ is defined so that summing the entries of its rows generates $\boldsymbol{E}(\boldsymbol{\beta}(SC))$. A detailed formulation for $\boldsymbol{G}(\boldsymbol{\beta}(SC))$ is not provided for brevity.

11.2.2 Partially and Fully Modified GEE Modeling

Define non-constant dispersions $\varphi_{sc} = exp\left(\boldsymbol{v}_{sc}^{\mathrm{T}} \cdot \boldsymbol{\gamma}\right)$ as in Sect. 11.1.2 so that they are constant in u for $0 \leq u < K$. Dispersions are readily generalized to change with u, and so this is not considered for brevity. Treating dispersions as constant in u reduces the complexity of models and their computation time. Let

$$\sigma_{sc,\leq u}^2 = \varphi_{sc} \cdot V\left(\mu_{sc,\leq u}\right),$$

$$stde_{sc,\leq u} = e_{sc,\leq u} / \sigma_{sc,\leq u},$$

and

$$Pres_{sc,\leq u} = \frac{e_{sc,\leq u}}{V^{½}\left(\mu_{sc,\leq u}\right)},$$

for $sc \in SC$ and $0 \leq u < K$. Combine these over $0 \leq u < K$ into the $K \times 1$ vectors $\boldsymbol{\sigma}_{sc}$, $\boldsymbol{stde}_{sc}$, and $\boldsymbol{Pres}_{sc}$, and then combine these vectors, respectively, into the $(m(SC) \cdot K) \times 1$ vectors $\boldsymbol{\sigma}_s$, $\boldsymbol{stde}_s$, and $\boldsymbol{Pres}_s$ in the order of the values $c \in C(s)$. Model the $(m(SC) \cdot K) \times (m(SC) \cdot K)$ covariance matrices $\boldsymbol{\Sigma}_s$ as

$$\boldsymbol{\Sigma}_s = \boldsymbol{DIAG}(\boldsymbol{\sigma}_s) \cdot \boldsymbol{R}_s(\rho) \cdot \boldsymbol{DIAG}(\boldsymbol{\sigma}_s)$$

for appropriate choices of the $(m(SC) \cdot K) \times (m(SC) \cdot K)$ correlation matrices $\boldsymbol{R}_s(\rho)$ for $s \in S$ (see Sect. 11.2.3).

As in Sects. 10.2 and 11.1.2, partially modified and fully modified GEE modeling can be extended using the likelihood function $L(SC;\boldsymbol{\theta}) = \exp(\ell(SC;\boldsymbol{\theta}))$ for cumulative outcome measurements $y_{sc,\le u}$ with indexes $sc \in SC$ and $0 \le u < K$ equal to the product over $s \in S$ of the terms $L(O_s;\boldsymbol{\theta})$ where $O_s = \{\boldsymbol{y}_s, \boldsymbol{X}_s, \boldsymbol{V}_s\}$ denotes an observation and

$$\ell(O_s;\boldsymbol{\theta}) = \log L(O_s;\boldsymbol{\theta}) = -\boldsymbol{e}_s^{\mathrm{T}} \cdot \boldsymbol{\Sigma}_s^{-1} \cdot \boldsymbol{e}_s/2 - (\log|\boldsymbol{\Sigma}_s|)/2 - (m(s) \cdot K \cdot \log(2 \cdot \pi))/2$$

for

$$\boldsymbol{\theta} = \begin{pmatrix} \beta \\ \gamma \end{pmatrix},$$

the $(K + r + q) \times 1$ vector composed of the mean and dispersion parameter vectors $\boldsymbol{\beta}$ and $\boldsymbol{\gamma}$ with $K + r$ and q entries, respectively. Maximizing the likelihood involves using Newton's method to solve

$$\boldsymbol{E}(\boldsymbol{\theta}) = \begin{pmatrix} E(\beta) \\ E(\gamma) \end{pmatrix} = \boldsymbol{0}$$

where $\boldsymbol{E}(\boldsymbol{\beta})$ and $\boldsymbol{E}(\boldsymbol{\gamma})$ are, respectively, $(K + r) \times 1$ and $q \times 1$ vectors. $\boldsymbol{E}'(\boldsymbol{\theta})$ has four component matrices $\boldsymbol{E}'(\boldsymbol{\beta})$, $\boldsymbol{E}'(\boldsymbol{\gamma})$, $\boldsymbol{E}'(\boldsymbol{\beta},\boldsymbol{\gamma})$, and $\boldsymbol{E}'(\boldsymbol{\gamma},\boldsymbol{\beta}) = \boldsymbol{E}'^{\mathrm{T}}(\boldsymbol{\beta},\boldsymbol{\gamma})$. $\boldsymbol{E}'(\boldsymbol{\beta})$, $\boldsymbol{E}'(\boldsymbol{\gamma})$, and $\boldsymbol{E}'(\boldsymbol{\beta},\boldsymbol{\gamma})$ are, respectively, $(K + r) \times (K + r)$, $q \times q$, and $(K + r) \times q$ matrices.

Formulation adjustments for partially modified GEE include:

$$\log|\boldsymbol{\Sigma}_s| = \log|\boldsymbol{R}_s(\boldsymbol{\rho})| + \sum_{c \in C(s)} K \cdot \log \varphi_{sc} + \sum_{c \in C(s)} \sum_{u=1}^{K} \log V(\mu_{sc,\le u});$$

$\boldsymbol{E}(\boldsymbol{\gamma})$ is the sum over $s \in S$ of terms $\boldsymbol{E}_s(\boldsymbol{\gamma})$ with entries

$$E_{s,j}(\gamma) = \boldsymbol{vstde}_{s,j}^{\mathrm{T}} \cdot \boldsymbol{R}_s^{-1}(\rho) \cdot \boldsymbol{stde}_s - \sum_{c \in C(s)} K \cdot v_{sc,j}/2,$$

where $\boldsymbol{vstde}_{s,j}$ is the $(m(SC) \cdot K) \times 1$ vector with entries

$$vstde_{sc,\le u,j} = v_{sc,j} \cdot stde_{sc,\le u}/2$$

for $sc \in SC$, $0 \le u < K$, and $1 \le j \le q$; and $\boldsymbol{E}'(\boldsymbol{\gamma})$ is the sum over $s \in S$ of $\boldsymbol{E}'_s(\gamma)$ with entries

$$E'_{s,j,j'}(\gamma) = -\boldsymbol{vvstde}^{\mathrm{T}}_{s,j,j'} \cdot \boldsymbol{R}_s^{-1}(\rho) \cdot \boldsymbol{stde}_s - \boldsymbol{vstde}^{\mathrm{T}}_{s,j} \cdot \boldsymbol{R}_s^{-1}(\rho) \cdot \boldsymbol{vstde}_{s,j'}$$

where $\boldsymbol{vvstde}_{s,j,j'}$ is the $(m(SC) \cdot K) \times 1$ vector with entries

$$vvstde_{sc,\leq u,j,j'} = v_{sc,j} \cdot v_{sc,j'} \cdot stde_{sc,\leq u}/4$$

for $sc \in SC$, $0 \leq u < K$, and $1 \leq j, j' \leq q$. These adjustments apply as well to fully modified GEE modeling. Also, $\boldsymbol{E}'(\boldsymbol{\beta},\boldsymbol{\gamma})$ is the sum over $s \in S$ of $\boldsymbol{E}'_s(\boldsymbol{\beta},\boldsymbol{\gamma})$ with q $(K + r) \times 1$ column vectors

$$\begin{aligned}\boldsymbol{E}'_{s,j}(\boldsymbol{\beta},\boldsymbol{\gamma}) = &-\boldsymbol{D}_s^{\mathrm{T}} \cdot \boldsymbol{DIAG}\left(\boldsymbol{v\sigma inv}_{s,j}\right) \cdot \boldsymbol{R}_s^{-1}(\rho) \cdot \boldsymbol{stde}_s \\ &- \boldsymbol{D}_s^{\mathrm{T}} \cdot \boldsymbol{DIAG}(\boldsymbol{1}/\boldsymbol{\sigma}_s) \cdot \boldsymbol{R}_s^{-1}(\rho) \cdot \boldsymbol{vstde}_{s,j}\end{aligned}$$

where $\boldsymbol{v\sigma inv}_{s,j}$ is the $(m(SC) \cdot K) \times 1$ vector with entries

$$v\sigma inv_{sc,\leq u,j} = \frac{v_{sc,j}}{2 \cdot \sigma_{sc,\leq u}}$$

for $sc \in SC$, $0 \leq u < K$, and $1 \leq j \leq q$.

Fully modified GEE also requires formulation adjustments for $\boldsymbol{E}(\boldsymbol{\beta})$, $\boldsymbol{E}'(\boldsymbol{\beta})$, **and** $\boldsymbol{E}'(\boldsymbol{\beta},\boldsymbol{\gamma})$. $\boldsymbol{E}(\boldsymbol{\beta})$ is the sum over $s \in S$ of $\boldsymbol{E}_s(\boldsymbol{\beta})$ with entries

$$E_{s,w}(\boldsymbol{\beta}) = \frac{\partial_0 \ell(O_s;\boldsymbol{\theta})}{\partial_0 \alpha_w} = \boldsymbol{xstde}^{\mathrm{T}}_{s,w} \cdot \boldsymbol{R}_s^{-1}(\rho) \cdot \boldsymbol{stde}_s - \sum_{c \in C(s)} W_{sc,w}/2,$$

$$E_{s,K,j}(\boldsymbol{\beta}) = \frac{\partial_0 \ell(O_s;\boldsymbol{\theta})}{\partial_0 \beta_{K,j}} = \boldsymbol{xstde}^{\mathrm{T}}_{s,K,j} \cdot \boldsymbol{R}_s^{-1}(\rho) \cdot \boldsymbol{stde}_s - \sum_{c \in C(s)} \sum_{u=0}^{K-1} W_{K,j}\left(\mu_{sc,\leq u}\right)/2$$

where

$$W_{sc,w} = \sum_{u=0}^{K-1} \frac{\frac{\partial V\left(\mu_{sc,\leq u}\right)}{\partial \alpha_w}}{V\left(\mu_{sc,\leq u}\right)},$$

$$W_{K,j}\left(\mu_{sc,\leq u}\right) = \frac{\frac{\partial V\left(\mu_{sc,\leq u}\right)}{\partial \beta_{K,j}}}{V\left(\mu_{sc,\leq u}\right)},$$

for $0 \leq u$, $w < K$ and $1 \leq j \leq r$. The $(m(SC) \cdot K) \times 1$ vectors $\boldsymbol{xstde}_{s,w}$ **and** $\boldsymbol{xstde}_{s,K,j}$ have entries $xstde_{sc,\leq u,w}$ and $xstde_{sc,\leq u,K,j}$, respectively, where for $0 \leq u$, $w < K$,

$$xstde_{sc,\leq u,w} = \frac{\left(1-2\cdot\mu_{sc,\leq w}\right)\cdot y_{sc,\leq w}+\mu_{sc,\leq w}}{2\cdot\sigma_{sc,\leq w}},$$

for $w = u$;

$$xstde_{sc,\leq u,w} = 0,$$

for $w \neq u$; and

$$xstde_{sc,\leq u,Kj} = x_{scj}\cdot\frac{\left(1-2\cdot\mu_{sc,\leq u}\right)\cdot y_{sc,\leq u}+\mu_{sc,\leq u}}{2\cdot\sigma_{sc,\leq u}},$$

for $1 \leq j \leq r$;

$$W_{sc,w} = 1-2\cdot\mu_{sc,\leq w},$$

for $w = u$;

$$W_{sc,w} = 0,$$

for $w \neq u$; and

$$W_{Kj}\left(\mu_{sc,\leq u}\right) = x_{scj}\cdot 1-2\cdot\mu_{sc,\leq u},$$

for $1 \leq j \leq r$. As before, the operator notation $\frac{\partial_0}{\partial_0\alpha_w}$ and $\frac{\partial_0}{\partial_0\beta_{Kj}}$ is used to indicate that these are not full partial derivatives due to not accounting for the effect of α_w and β_{Kj} on $\boldsymbol{R}_s(\boldsymbol{\rho})$ (see Sect. 11.2.3). Note that $W_{sc,w}$ and $W_{Kj}(\mu_{sc,\leq u})$ are standard partial derivatives since $V(\mu_{sc,\leq u})$ does not depend on $\boldsymbol{R}_s(\boldsymbol{\rho})$.

$\boldsymbol{E}'(\boldsymbol{\beta})$ is the sum over $s \in S$ of $\boldsymbol{E}'_s(\boldsymbol{\beta})$ with $(K + r)^2$ entries including the K^2 entries

$$E'_{s,w,w'}(\boldsymbol{\beta}) = \frac{\partial_0\boldsymbol{E}_{s,w}(\boldsymbol{\beta})}{\partial_0\alpha_{w'}}$$

$$= -\boldsymbol{xxstde}^{\mathrm{T}}_{s,w,w'}\cdot\boldsymbol{R}_s^{-1}(\boldsymbol{\rho})\cdot\boldsymbol{stde}_s - \boldsymbol{xstde}^{\mathrm{T}}_{s,w}\cdot\boldsymbol{R}_s^{-1}(\boldsymbol{\rho})\cdot\boldsymbol{xstde}_{s,w'} - \sum_{c\in C(s)} W_{sc,w,w'}/2$$

for $0 \leq w, w' < K$, the $K \cdot r$ entries

$$E'_{s,Kj,w}(\boldsymbol{\beta}) = \frac{\partial_0\boldsymbol{E}_{s,Kj}(\boldsymbol{\beta})}{\partial_0\alpha_w}$$

$$= -\boldsymbol{xxstde}_{s,K,j,w}^{\mathrm{T}} \cdot \boldsymbol{R}_s^{-1}(\boldsymbol{\rho}) \cdot \boldsymbol{stde}_s - \boldsymbol{xstde}_{s,K,j}^{\mathrm{T}} \cdot \boldsymbol{R}_s^{-1}(\boldsymbol{\rho}) \cdot \boldsymbol{xstde}_{s,w} - \sum_{c\in C(s)} W_{sc,K,j,w}/2$$

for $0 \leq w < K$, and $1 \leq j \leq r$, the $K \cdot r$ entries

$$E'_{s,w,K,j}(\boldsymbol{\beta}) = \frac{\partial_0 \boldsymbol{E}_{s,w}(\boldsymbol{\beta})}{\partial_0 \beta_{K,j}}$$

$$= -\boldsymbol{xxstde}_{s,w,K,j}^{\mathrm{T}} \cdot \boldsymbol{R}_s^{-1}(\boldsymbol{\rho}) \cdot \boldsymbol{stde}_s - \boldsymbol{xstde}_{s,w}^{\mathrm{T}} \cdot \boldsymbol{R}_s^{-1}(\boldsymbol{\rho}) \cdot \boldsymbol{xstde}_{s,K,j} - \sum_{c\in C(s)} W_{sc,w,K,j}/2$$

for $0 \leq w < K$, and $1 \leq j \leq r$, and the r^2 entries

$$E'_{s,K,j,j'}(\boldsymbol{\beta}) = \frac{\partial_0 \boldsymbol{E}_{s,K,j}(\boldsymbol{\beta})}{\partial_0 \beta_{K,j'}}$$

$$= -\boldsymbol{xxstde}_{s,Kj,j'}^{\mathrm{T}} \cdot \boldsymbol{R}_s^{-1}(\boldsymbol{\rho}) \cdot \boldsymbol{stde}_s - \boldsymbol{xstde}_{s,K,j}^{\mathrm{T}} \cdot \boldsymbol{R}_s^{-1}(\boldsymbol{\rho}) \cdot \boldsymbol{xstde}_{s,K,j'}$$
$$- \sum_{c\in C(s)} \sum_{u=0}^{K-1} W_{K,j,j'}\left(\mu_{sc,\leq u}\right)/2$$

for $1 \leq j, j' \leq r$ where

$$W_{sc,w,w'} = \frac{\partial W_{sc,w}}{\partial \alpha_{w'}},$$

$$W_{sc,K,j,w} = \sum_{u=0}^{K-1} \frac{\partial W_{K,j}\left(\mu_{sc,\leq u}\right)}{\partial \alpha_{w}},$$

$$W_{sc,w,K,j} = \frac{\partial W_{sc,w}}{\partial \beta_{K,j}},$$

$$W_{K,j,j'}\left(\mu_{sc,\leq u}\right) = \frac{\partial W_{K,j}\left(\mu_{sc,\leq u}\right)}{\partial \beta_{K,j'}}.$$

For $0 \leq w, w' < K$ and $1 \leq j, j' \leq r$, the $(m(SC) \cdot K) \times 1$ vectors $\boldsymbol{xxstde}_{s,w,w'}$, $\boldsymbol{xxstde}_{s,w,K,j}$, $\boldsymbol{xxstde}_{s,K,j,w}$, and $\boldsymbol{xxstde}_{s,K,j,j'}$ have entries $xxstde_{sc,\leq u,w,w'}$, $xxstde_{sc,\leq u,w,K,j}$, $xxstde_{sc,\leq u,K,j,w}$, and $xxstde_{sc,\leq u,K,j,j'}$, respectively, with the following formulations. For $0 \leq u < K$, $w = u$, $w' = u'$,

$$xxstde_{sc,\leq u,w,w} = stde_{sc,\leq w}/4, w = u, w = u';$$

$$xxstde_{sc,\leq u,w,w'} = 0, w \neq u \text{ or } w \neq u';$$

$$xxstde_{sc,\leq u,w,K,j} = xxstde_{sc,\leq u,K,j,w} = x_{sc,j} \cdot stde_{sc,\leq w}/4, w = u;$$
$$xxstde_{sc,\leq u,w,K,j} = xxstde_{sc,\leq u,K,j,w} = 0, w \neq u;$$
$$xxstde_{sc,\leq u,K,j,j'} = x_{sc,j} \cdot x_{sc,j'} \cdot stde_{sc,\leq w}/4$$

while

$$W_{sc,w,w} = -2 \cdot V\left(\mu_{sc,\leq w}\right), w' = w;$$
$$W_{sc,w,w'} = 0, w' \neq w;$$
$$W_{sc,w,K,j} = W_{sc,K,j,w} = -2 \cdot x_{sc,j} \cdot V\left(\mu_{sc,\leq u}\right);$$
$$W_{K,j,j'}\left(\mu_{sc,\leq u}\right) = -2 \cdot x_{sc,j} \cdot x_{sc,j'} \cdot V\left(\mu_{sc,\leq u}\right)$$

for $0 \leq u$, w, $w' < K$ and $1 \leq j, j' \leq r$.

$\boldsymbol{E}'(\boldsymbol{\beta}, \boldsymbol{\gamma})$ is the sum over $s \in S$ of $\boldsymbol{E}'_s(\boldsymbol{\beta}, \boldsymbol{\gamma})$ with entries

$$E'_{s,w,j'}(\boldsymbol{\beta}, \boldsymbol{\gamma}) = \frac{\partial \boldsymbol{E}_{s,w}(\boldsymbol{\beta})}{\partial \gamma_{j'}} = -\boldsymbol{vxstde}^{\mathrm{T}}_{s,w,j'} \cdot \boldsymbol{R}_s^{-1}(\rho) \cdot \boldsymbol{stde}_s$$
$$-\boldsymbol{xstde}^{\mathrm{T}}_{s,w} \cdot \boldsymbol{R}_s^{-1}(\rho) \cdot \boldsymbol{vstde}_{s,j'},$$
$$E'_{s,K,j,j'}(\boldsymbol{\beta}, \boldsymbol{\gamma}) = \frac{\partial \boldsymbol{E}_{s,K,j}(\boldsymbol{\beta})}{\partial \gamma_{j'}} = -\boldsymbol{vxstde}^{\mathrm{T}}_{s,K,j,j'} \cdot \boldsymbol{R}_s^{-1}(\rho) \cdot \boldsymbol{stde}_s$$
$$-\boldsymbol{xstde}^{\mathrm{T}}_{s,K,j} \cdot \boldsymbol{R}_s^{-1}(\rho) \cdot \boldsymbol{vstde}_{s,j'},$$

where $\boldsymbol{vxstde}_{s,w,j'}$ is the $(m(SC) \cdot K) \times 1$ vector with entries

$$vxstde_{sc,\leq u,w,j'} = xstde_{sc,\leq u,w} \cdot v_{sc,j'}/2,$$

$\boldsymbol{vxstde}_{s,K,j,j'}$ is the $(m(SC) \cdot K) \times 1$ vector with entries

$$vxstde_{sc,\leq u,K,j,j'} = xstde_{sc,u,K,j} \cdot v_{sc,j'}/2,$$

and $\boldsymbol{vstde}_{s,j'}$ is the same as for partially modified GEE modeling, for $sc \in SC$, $0 \leq u$, $w < K$, $1 \leq j \leq r$, and $1 \leq j' \leq q$.

Model-based and robust empirical estimates of the covariance matrix for the partially and fully modified GEE estimate

$$\boldsymbol{\theta}(SC) = \begin{pmatrix} \beta(SC) \\ \gamma(SC) \end{pmatrix}$$

of the coefficient parameter vector $\boldsymbol{\theta}$ can be computed similarly to those for partially modified GEE modeling given in Sect. 3.4 and fully modified GEE modeling given in Sect. 4.1. These use the partially and fully modified GEE versions of $\boldsymbol{E}'(\boldsymbol{\theta}(SC))$ and $\boldsymbol{G}(\boldsymbol{\theta}(SC))$ for ordinal regression using cumulative outcomes. $\boldsymbol{G}(\boldsymbol{\theta}(SC))$ is defined so that summing the entries of its rows generates $\boldsymbol{E}(\boldsymbol{\theta}(SC))$. A detailed formulation for $\boldsymbol{G}(\boldsymbol{\theta}(SC))$ is not provided for brevity.

11.2.3 Alternate Correlation Structures

As in Sects. 10.3 and 11.1.3, let $\boldsymbol{R}_{s,c,c'}$ for $c,c' \in C(s)$ denote the $m^2(s)$ $K \times K$ component matrices of $\boldsymbol{R}_s(\boldsymbol{\rho})$. The special cases $\boldsymbol{R}_{s,c,c}$ with $c' = c$ are the correlation matrices for $\boldsymbol{y}_{sc}$. The cumulative outcomes $y_{sc,\le u}$ for $sc \in SC$ have covariances for $0 \le u \le w < K$ satisfying

$$\begin{aligned}
\mathrm{Cov}\left(y_{sc,\le u}, y_{sc,\le w}\right) &= \mathrm{Cov}\left(\sum_{u'=0}^{u} y_{sc,u'}, \sum_{u''=0}^{w} y_{sc,u''}\right) \\
&= \sum_{u'=0}^{u}\sum_{u''=0}^{w} \mathrm{Cov}\left(y_{sc,u'}, y_{sc,u''}\right) \\
&= \sum_{u'=0}^{u}\left(\mathrm{Cov}\left(y_{sc,u'}, y_{sc,u'}\right) + \sum_{u''=0}^{u'-1}\mathrm{Cov}\left(y_{sc,u'}, y_{sc,u''}\right) + \sum_{u''=u'+1}^{w}\mathrm{Cov}\left(y_{sc,u'}, y_{sc,u''}\right)\right) \\
&= \sum_{u'=0}^{u}\left(\mu_{sc,u'}\cdot\left(1-\mu_{sc,u'}\right) - \sum_{u''=0}^{u'-1}\mu_{sc,u'}\cdot\mu_{sc,u''} - \sum_{u''=u'+1}^{w}\mu_{sc,u'}\cdot\mu_{sc,u''}\right) \\
&= \sum_{u'=0}^{u}\mu_{sc,u'}\cdot\left(1-\mu_{sc,u'} - \sum_{u''=0}^{u'-1}\mu_{sc,u''} - \sum_{u''=u'+1}^{w}\mu_{sc,u''}\right) = \sum_{u'=0}^{u}\mu_{sc,u'}\cdot\left(1-\mu_{sc,\le w}\right) \\
&= \mu_{sc,\le u}\cdot\left(1-\mu_{sc,\le w}\right)
\end{aligned}$$

Consequently, $\boldsymbol{R}_{s,c,c}$ has diagonal entries with value 1 and off-diagonal entries

$$r_{sc,u,u'} = \left(\frac{\mu_{sc,\le u}}{1-\mu_{sc,\le u}}\right)^{½}\cdot\left(\frac{\mu_{sc,\le u\prime}}{1-\mu_{sc,\le u\prime}}\right)^{-½} = r_{sc,u',u}$$

for $0 \le u,\ u' < K$ with $u < u'$. Note that $\boldsymbol{R}_{s,c,c}$ depends on the mean parameters but not on the correlation parameters. The dependence of the correlation matrices $\boldsymbol{R}_s(\boldsymbol{\rho})$ on the mean parameters $\boldsymbol{\beta}$ is suppressed in the notation to reduce the complexity of the notation. Models are needed for the remaining $m(s)\cdot(m(s) - 1)/2$ component matrices $\boldsymbol{R}_{s,c,c'}$ and their transposes $\boldsymbol{R}_{s,c',c} = \boldsymbol{R}^{\mathrm{T}}_{s,c,c'}$ of dimension $K \times K$ for $c < c'$. These are based on either IND, EC, spatial AR1, or UN correlation structures. Formulations, estimates, and degeneracy issues for $\boldsymbol{R}_{s,c,c'}$ with $c < c'$ are the same as for ordinal regression with individual outcomes as given in Sect. 11.1.3 except that these represent correlations between cumulative outcomes and so computed using $stde_{sc,\le u}$ rather than $stde_{sc,u}$.

11.2.4 Extended Linear Mixed Modeling

As in Sect. 11.1.4, full maximum likelihood estimation is possible, maximizing the likelihood in the correlation parameters as well as in the mean and dispersion parameters. In what follows, revised estimating equations are formulated for mean and dispersion parameters as well as for EC, spatial AR1, and UN correlation parameters. There is now just one alternative estimate of the correlation vector and not bias-adjusted and bias-unadjusted alternatives as for standard, partially modified, and fully modified GEE.

11.2.4.1 Estimating Equations for Means, Dispersions, and Correlations Based on the Likelihood

As for the fully modified GEE case, the definitions of the log-likelihood function $\ell(SC;\boldsymbol{\theta})$ and the likelihood function $L(SC;\boldsymbol{\theta})$ of Sect. 11.2.2 apply in this case without change. However, the parameter vector is now

$$\boldsymbol{\theta} = \begin{pmatrix} \beta \\ \gamma \\ \rho \end{pmatrix}$$

with $K + r + q + p$ entries, where p is the number of correlation parameters. The likelihood $L(SC;\boldsymbol{\theta})$ is maximized in the coefficient parameter vector $\boldsymbol{\theta}$. Specifically, use Newton's method to solve the estimating equations

$$\boldsymbol{E}(\boldsymbol{\theta}) = \frac{\partial \ell(SC;\boldsymbol{\theta})}{\partial \boldsymbol{\theta}} = \sum_{s \in S} \boldsymbol{E}_s(\boldsymbol{\theta}) = \sum_{s \in S} \frac{\partial \ell(O_s;\boldsymbol{\theta})}{\partial \boldsymbol{\theta}} = \mathbf{0}$$

where the operator notation $\frac{\partial}{\partial \boldsymbol{\theta}}$ is used to indicate that this is a standard partial derivative vector in $\boldsymbol{\theta}$ since $\boldsymbol{\rho}$ is treated as a separate parameter vector. The associated matrix

$$\boldsymbol{E}'(\boldsymbol{\theta}) = \frac{\partial \boldsymbol{E}(\boldsymbol{\theta})}{\partial \boldsymbol{\theta}}.$$

In this case, $\boldsymbol{E}(\boldsymbol{\theta})$ is a true gradient vector and $\boldsymbol{E}'(\boldsymbol{\theta})$ a true Hessian matrix.

The gradient vector satisfies

$$\boldsymbol{E}(\boldsymbol{\theta}) = \begin{pmatrix} E(\beta) \\ E(\gamma) \\ E(\rho) \end{pmatrix}$$

where $\boldsymbol{E}(\gamma)$ is computed as in Sect. 11.2.2 for partially and fully modified GEE modeling since the correlation matrices do not depend on the dispersion parameters, but $\boldsymbol{E}(\boldsymbol{\beta})$ is now different because $\boldsymbol{R}_s(\boldsymbol{\rho})$ depends on the mean parameter vector $\boldsymbol{\beta}$ (see Sect. 11.2.3). Specifically,

$$\boldsymbol{E}(\boldsymbol{\beta}) = \boldsymbol{E}_0(\boldsymbol{\beta}) + \boldsymbol{E}_1(\boldsymbol{\beta})$$

where $\boldsymbol{E}_0(\boldsymbol{\beta})$ is computed using fully modified GEE formulas for $\boldsymbol{E}(\boldsymbol{\beta})$ given in Sect. 11.2.2 and $\boldsymbol{E}_1(\boldsymbol{\beta})$ is the extra amount to account for the dependence of $\boldsymbol{R}_s(\boldsymbol{\rho})$ on $\boldsymbol{\beta}$. Details on the computation of $\boldsymbol{E}(\boldsymbol{\theta})$ are given in Sects. 11.2.4.2–11.2.4.3.

The Hessian matrix $\boldsymbol{E}'(\boldsymbol{\theta})$ has nine component matrices: the $(K + r) \times (K + r)$ matrix

$$\boldsymbol{E}'(\boldsymbol{\beta}) = \frac{\partial \boldsymbol{E}(\boldsymbol{\beta})}{\partial \boldsymbol{\beta}}$$

for the $K + r$ mean parameters, the $q \times q$ matrix

$$\boldsymbol{E}'(\gamma) = \frac{\partial \boldsymbol{E}(\gamma)}{\partial \gamma}$$

for the q dispersion parameters computed as in Sect. 11.2.2 for partially and fully modified GEE modeling, the $p \times p$ matrix

$$\boldsymbol{E}'(\boldsymbol{\rho}) = \frac{\partial \boldsymbol{E}(\boldsymbol{\rho})}{\partial \boldsymbol{\rho}}$$

for the p correlation parameters, the $(K + r) \times q$ matrix

$$\boldsymbol{E}'(\boldsymbol{\beta}, \gamma) = \frac{\partial \boldsymbol{E}(\boldsymbol{\beta})}{\partial \gamma}$$

and its transpose $\boldsymbol{E}'(\gamma, \boldsymbol{\beta}) = \boldsymbol{E}'^{\mathrm{T}}(\boldsymbol{\beta}, \gamma)$, the $(K + r) \times p$ matrix

$$\boldsymbol{E}'(\boldsymbol{\beta}, \boldsymbol{\rho}) = \frac{\partial \boldsymbol{E}(\boldsymbol{\beta})}{\partial \boldsymbol{\rho}}$$

and its transpose $\boldsymbol{E}'(\boldsymbol{\rho}, \boldsymbol{\beta}) = \boldsymbol{E}'^{\mathrm{T}}(\gamma, \boldsymbol{\rho})$, the $q \times p$ matrix

$$\boldsymbol{E}'(\gamma, \boldsymbol{\rho}) = \frac{\partial \boldsymbol{E}(\gamma)}{\partial \boldsymbol{\rho}}$$

and its transpose $\boldsymbol{E}'(\boldsymbol{\rho}, \gamma) = \boldsymbol{E}'^{\mathrm{T}}(\gamma, \boldsymbol{\rho})$. Details on the computation of $\boldsymbol{E}'(\boldsymbol{\theta})$ are given in Sects. 11.2.4.4–11.2.4.8.

Model-based and robust empirical estimates of the covariance matrix for the ELMM estimate

$$\boldsymbol{\theta}(SC) = \begin{pmatrix} \beta(SC) \\ \gamma(SC) \\ \rho(SC) \end{pmatrix}$$

of the coefficient parameter vector $\boldsymbol{\theta}$ can be computed similarly to those for ELMM given in Sect. 5.1. These use the ELMM versions of $\boldsymbol{E}'(\boldsymbol{\theta}(SC))$ and $\boldsymbol{G}(\boldsymbol{\theta}(SC))$ for ordinal regression using cumulative outcomes. $\boldsymbol{G}(\boldsymbol{\theta}(SC))$ is defined so that summing the entries of its rows generates $\boldsymbol{E}(\boldsymbol{\theta}(SC))$. A detailed formulation for $\boldsymbol{G}(\boldsymbol{\theta}(SC))$ is not provided for brevity.

The first and second partial derivatives of $\ell(SC;\boldsymbol{\theta})$ are sums over $s \in S$ of associated first and second partial derivatives of $\ell(O_s;\boldsymbol{\theta})$. The next seven sections provide formulations for these derivatives except for the cases $\boldsymbol{E}(\boldsymbol{\gamma})$ and $\boldsymbol{E}'(\boldsymbol{\gamma})$, which are formulated in Sect. 11.2.2. These formulations are needed to compute $\boldsymbol{E}(\boldsymbol{\theta})$ and $\boldsymbol{E}'(\boldsymbol{\theta})$ but are complex and so can be skipped. Formulas for first and second partial derivatives of $\log|\boldsymbol{R}_s(\boldsymbol{\rho})|$ and of $\boldsymbol{R}_s^{-1}(\boldsymbol{\rho})$ are the same as those provided in Sect. 11.1.4.1.

11.2.4.2 First Partial Derivatives with Respect to Mean Parameters

Formulas for this case are the same as provided in Sect. 11.1.4.2, but using the correlation matrices $\boldsymbol{R}_s(\boldsymbol{\rho})$ for ordinal regression based on cumulative outcomes, rather than based on individual outcomes, and the partial derivative formulations of Sect. 11.2.4.1 only now the first partial derivatives of $\boldsymbol{R}_{s,c,c}$ have entries $\frac{\partial r_{s,c,c,u,u'}}{\partial \alpha_w}$ and $\frac{\partial r_{s,c,c,u,u'}}{\partial \beta_{w,j}}$, respectively, satisfying

$$\frac{\partial r_{s,c,c,u,u'}}{\partial \alpha_w} = r_{s,c,c,u,u'}/2, w = u,$$

$$\frac{\partial r_{s,c,c,u,u'}}{\partial \alpha_w} = -r_{s,c,c,u,u'}/2, w = u',$$

$$\frac{\partial r_{s,c,c,u,u'}}{\partial \alpha_w} = 0, w \neq u, w \neq u',$$

$$\frac{\partial r_{s,c,c,u,u'}}{\partial \beta_{K,j}} = 0,$$

for $0 \leq u, u', \mathrm{w} < K$ and $1 \leq j \leq r$. Note that $E_{1,s,K,j}(\boldsymbol{\rho}) = 0$ for $1 \leq j \leq r$.

11.2.4.3 First Partial Derivatives with Respect to Correlation Parameters

Formulas for this case are the same as provided in Sect. 11.1.4.3, but using the correlation matrices $\boldsymbol{R}_s(\boldsymbol{\rho})$ for ordinal regression based on cumulative outcomes, rather than based on individual outcomes, and the partial derivative formulations of Sect. 11.2.4.1. For IND, EC, spatial AR1, and UN correlations, the partial derivatives $\frac{\partial \boldsymbol{R}_{s,c,c'}}{\partial \rho_j}$ for the off-diagonal component matrices $\boldsymbol{R}_{s,c,c'}$ are the same as those provided in Sect. 11.1.4.3.

11.2.4.4 Second Partial Derivatives with Respect to Mean Parameters

Formulas for this case are the same as provided in Sect. 11.1.4.4, but using the correlation matrices $\boldsymbol{R}_s(\boldsymbol{\rho})$ for ordinal regression based on cumulative outcomes, rather than based on individual outcomes, and the partial derivative formulations of Sect. 11.2.4.1 only now the second partial derivatives of $\boldsymbol{R}_{s,c,c}$ have entries satisfying the following. For $w = u$, $w' = u$ or $w = u'$, $w' = u'$,

$$\frac{\partial^2 r_{s,c,c,u,u'}}{\partial \alpha_{w'}\,\partial \alpha_w} = r_{s,c,c,u,u'}/4;$$

for $w = u$, $w' = u'$ or $w = u'$, $w' = u$,

$$\frac{\partial^2 r_{s,c,c,u,u'}}{\partial \alpha_{w'}\,\partial \alpha_w} = -\,r_{s,c,c,u,u'}/4;$$

for $w \neq u$, $w \neq u'$, $w' \neq u$, $w' \neq u'$,

$$\frac{\partial^2 r_{s,c,c,u,u'}}{\partial \alpha_{w'}\,\partial \alpha_w} = 0;$$

and

$$\frac{\partial^2 r_{s,c,c,u,u'}}{\partial \alpha_w \partial \beta_{Kj}} = \frac{\partial^2 r_{s,c,c,u,u'}}{\partial \beta_{Kj} \partial \alpha_w} = \frac{\partial^2 r_{s,c,c,u,u'}}{\partial \beta_{Kj'}\,\partial \beta_{Kj}} = 0.$$

Note that

$$E'_{1,s,w,Kj}(\boldsymbol{\beta}) = E'_{1,s,Kj,w}(\boldsymbol{\beta}) = E'_{1,s,Kj,j'}(\boldsymbol{\beta}) = 0$$

for $0 \leq w < K$ and $1 \leq j, j' \leq r$. Since $\frac{\partial \boldsymbol{R}_s^{-1}(\boldsymbol{\rho})}{\partial \beta_{Kj}} = \boldsymbol{0}$, three of the four formulas for the entries of $\boldsymbol{E'}_{2,s}(\boldsymbol{\beta})$ simplify to

$$E'_{2,s,K,j,w}(\boldsymbol{\beta}) = E'_{2,s,w,K,j}(\boldsymbol{\beta}) = \boldsymbol{xstde}^{\mathrm{T}}_{s,K,j} \cdot \frac{\partial \boldsymbol{R}_s^{-1}(\boldsymbol{\rho})}{\partial \alpha_w} \cdot \boldsymbol{stde}_s,$$

$$E'_{2,s,K,j,K,j'}(\boldsymbol{\beta}) = 0.$$

11.2.4.5 Second Partial Derivatives with Respect to Correlation Parameters

Formulas for this case are the same as provided in Sect. 11.1.4.5, but using the correlation matrices $\boldsymbol{R}_s(\boldsymbol{\rho})$ for ordinal regression based on cumulative outcomes, rather than based on individual outcomes, and the partial derivative formulations of Sect. 11.2.4.1.

11.2.4.6 Second Partial Derivatives with Respect to Mean and Dispersion Parameters

Formulas for this case are the same as provided in Sect. 11.1.4.6, but using the correlation matrices $\boldsymbol{R}_s(\boldsymbol{\rho})$ for ordinal regression based on cumulative outcomes, rather than based on individual outcomes, and the partial derivative formulations of Sect. 11.2.4.1 with $\boldsymbol{xstde}_{s,w}$, $\boldsymbol{xstde}_{s,K,j}$, $\boldsymbol{xvstde}_{s,j',w}$, and $\boldsymbol{xvstde}_{s,j',K,j}$ as formulated in Sect. 11.2.2 for $1 \le j' \le q$, $1 \le w \le K$, and $1 \le j \le r$. Moreover, since $\frac{\partial \boldsymbol{R}_s^{-1}(\boldsymbol{\rho})}{\partial \beta_{K,j}} = \boldsymbol{0}$,

$$E'_{1,s,j',K,j}(\boldsymbol{\gamma},\boldsymbol{\beta}) = \boldsymbol{0}.$$

11.2.4.7 Second Partial Derivatives with Respect to Mean and Correlation Parameters

Formulas for this case are the same as provided in Sect. 11.1.4.7, but using the correlation matrices $\boldsymbol{R}_s(\boldsymbol{\rho})$ for ordinal regression based on cumulative outcomes, rather than based on individual outcomes, and the partial derivative formulations of Sect. 11.2.4.1 with $\boldsymbol{xstde}_{s,w}$ and $\boldsymbol{xstde}_{s,K,j}$ as formulated in Sect. 11.2.2 for $1 \le w \le K$ and $1 \le j \le r$. However, in this case $\frac{\partial \boldsymbol{R}_s(\boldsymbol{\rho})}{\partial \beta_{K,j}} = \boldsymbol{0}$, and so $E'_{0,s,K,j,j'}(\boldsymbol{\beta},\boldsymbol{\rho}) = 0$, for $1 \le j \le r$.

11.2.4.8 Second Partial Derivatives with Respect to Dispersion and Correlation Parameters

Formulas for this case are the same as provided in Sect. 11.1.4.8, but using the correlation matrices $\boldsymbol{R}_s(\boldsymbol{\rho})$ for ordinal regression based on cumulative outcomes, rather than based on individual outcomes, and the partial derivative formulations of Sect. 11.2.4.1 with $\boldsymbol{vstde}_{s,j'}$ as formulated in Sect. 11.2.2 for $1 \le j' \le q$.

References

Lipsitz, S. R., Kim, K., & Zhao, L. (1994). Analysis of repeated categorical data using generalized estimating equations. *Statistics in Medicine, 13*, 1149–1163.

Miller, M. E., Davis, C. S., & Landis, J. R. (1993). The analysis of longitudinal polytomous data: Generalized estimating equations and connections with weighted least squares. *Biometrics, 49*, 1033–1044.

Schott, J. R. (2005). *Matrix analysis for statistics* (2nd ed.). John Wiley & Sons.

Wolfinger, R., Tobias, R., & Sall, J. (1994). Computing gaussian likelihoods and their derivatives for general linear mixed models. *SIAM Journal on Scientific Computing, 6*, 1294–1310.

Chapter 12
Discrete Regression

Abstract Discrete regression of outcomes with a discrete number of possible numeric values is addressed, as an alternative to multinomial and ordinal regression. The outcome values can represent categories, but should be truly numeric, as for ordinal categories, and not nominal numeric codes for nonnumeric categories. The outcome values can also be actual numbers, as for pain level ratings. Formulations are provided for standard generalized estimating equations (GEE) modeling, partially modified GEE modeling, fully modified GEE modeling, and extended linear mixed modeling (ELMM) of correlated sets of univariate discrete outcomes. Formulations are also provided for estimation for singleton univariate discrete outcomes as needed to generate initial estimates for parameter estimation of models for correlated sets of univariate discrete outcomes. Distributions for discrete outcomes are modeled using multinomial, ordinal, and censored Poisson probabilities. Non-constant dispersions are addressed using both extended and direct variance modeling.

Keywords Correlated discrete outcomes · Direct variance modeling · Discrete regression · Extended linear mixed modeling · Generalized estimating equations · Non-constant dispersions

Introduction This chapter addresses discrete regression of outcomes with a discrete number of numeric values treated as univariate outcomes without considering indicators for that outcome's values (as in Chaps. 10–11). Section 12.1 formulates the case of singleton univariate discrete outcomes while Sect. 12.2 addresses correlated sets of univariate discrete outcomes. The formulations for likelihood functions, LCV scores, LCV ratio tests, and the adaptive modeling process of Part 1 apply to both singleton univariate discrete outcomes and correlated sets of univariate discrete outcomes. Some details for the following formulations are not provided for brevity.

Supplementary Information The online version contains supplementary material available at https://doi.org/10.1007/978-3-031-41988-1_12.

G. J. Knafl, *Modeling Correlated Outcomes Using Extensions of Generalized Estimating Equations and Linear Mixed Modeling*,
https://doi.org/10.1007/978-3-031-41988-1_12

12.1 Singleton Univariate Discrete Outcomes

Let y_s for $s \in S$ be univariate discrete outcomes with a finite number of increasing values d_u for $0 \le u \le K$ and associated probabilities $p_{s,u} = \mathrm{P}(y_s = d_u)$ for $0 \le u \le K$. The means of such univariate discrete outcomes satisfy

$$\mu_s = \mathrm{E}y_s = \sum_{u=0}^{K} d_u \cdot p_{s,u}$$

while their variances satisfy

$$\mathrm{Var}(y_s) = \sum_{u=0}^{K} (d_u - \mu_s)^2 \cdot p_{s,u} = \left(\sum_{u=0}^{K} d_u^2 \cdot p_{s,u} \right) - \mu_s^2 = \mathrm{E}y_s^2 - \mu_s^2.$$

This variance is not a direct function $V(\mu_s)$ of the means as in generalized linear modeling, and so the use of a deviance function based on integrating $2 \cdot (y_s - t)/V(t)$ as in Sect. 4.4 is not a practical option. Consequently, dispersion parameter estimation based on extended generalized linear modeling is not feasible for univariate discrete outcomes, but extended linear modeling (Sect. 4.4) can be used instead. The variances, though, can be considered a function $V(\boldsymbol{p}_s)$ of the vector $\boldsymbol{p}_s$ of probabilities $p_{s,u}$ for the outcome y_s, but this distinction is not utilized in formulations that follow. Models are expressed in terms of $\mathrm{Var}(y_s)$ instead. Define the residuals as $e_s = y_s - \mu_s$. Means and variances can be computed for outcomes with values corresponding to nominal categories, but that seems inappropriate because means and variances are inherently numeric except in the case of outcomes with two nominal categories coded as 0 and 1 (Sect. 2.2.3).

Count outcome variables are discrete and are usually treated as infinite taking on every possible nonnegative integer value. These outcomes can be modeled using Poisson regression (Sects. 2.2.2 and 4.2.2). However, in practice count outcomes take on a bounded set of observed nonnegative integer values, and so could be modeled as finite-valued discrete outcomes instead. Also, count outcomes are sometimes finite because they are censored so that the largest outcome value represents that integer value as well as all larger integer values.

Probabilities for finite-valued singleton discrete outcomes can be multinomial as addressed in Sect. 12.1.1, ordinal as addressed in Sect. 12.1.2, or censored Poisson as addressed in Sect. 12.1.3. Section 12.1.4 addresses direct variance modeling of singleton univariate discrete outcomes.

12.1.1 Multinomial Probabilities

For predictor values $x_{s,j}$, combine them over $1 \leq j \leq r$ into the $r \times 1$ vectors $\boldsymbol{x}_s$ for $s \in S$. The probabilities $p_{s,u}$ are modeled multinomially using generalized logits with the smallest value d_0 as the reference category (but any other value can be used instead) as follows:

$$g(p_{s,u}) = \log \frac{p_{s,u}}{p_{s,0}} = \boldsymbol{x}_s^{\mathrm{T}} \cdot \boldsymbol{\beta}_u$$

for K $r \times 1$ vectors $\boldsymbol{\beta}_u$ of coefficient parameters $\beta_{u,j}$ for $1 \leq u \leq K$ and $1 \leq j \leq r$. Combine the vectors $\boldsymbol{\beta}_u$ over $1 \leq u \leq K$ into the composite $(K \cdot r) \times 1$ vector $\boldsymbol{\beta}$. For $s \in S$, the probabilities satisfy

$$p_{s,u} = \frac{\exp\left(\boldsymbol{x}_s^{\mathrm{T}} \cdot \boldsymbol{\beta}_u\right)}{1 + \sum_{u'=1}^{K} \exp\left(\boldsymbol{x}_s^{\mathrm{T}} \cdot \boldsymbol{\beta}_{u'}\right)}$$

for $1 \leq u \leq K$ and

$$p_{s,0} = \frac{1}{1 + \sum_{u'=1}^{K} \exp\left(\boldsymbol{x}_s^{\mathrm{T}} \cdot \boldsymbol{\beta}_{u'}\right)}.$$

Their partial derivatives $\frac{\partial p_{s,u}}{\partial \beta_{w,j}}$ satisfy

$$\frac{\partial p_{s,u}}{\partial \beta_{w,j}} = x_{s,j} \cdot p_{s,w} \cdot \left(1 - p_{s,w}\right), w = u,$$

$$\frac{\partial p_{s,u}}{\partial \beta_{w,j}} = -x_{s,j} \cdot p_{s,u} \cdot p_{s,w}, w \neq u,$$

and

$$\frac{\partial p_{s,0}}{\partial \beta_{w,j}} = -x_{s,j} \cdot p_{s,0} \cdot p_{s,w},$$

for $1 \leq u$, $w \leq K$, $1 \leq j \leq r$, and $s \in S$.

For predictor values $v_{s,j}$, combine them over $1 \leq j \leq q$ into the $q \times 1$ vectors $\boldsymbol{v}_s$ for $s \in S$. Model the natural log of the non-constant dispersions in terms of these predictor values, that is,

$$\log \varphi_s = \boldsymbol{v}_s^{\mathrm{T}} \cdot \boldsymbol{\gamma}$$

where $\boldsymbol{\gamma}$ is a $q \times 1$ vector of coefficient parameters. Define the extended variances as

$$\sigma_s^2 = \varphi_s \cdot \mathrm{Var}(y_s),$$

and the standardized residuals as

$$stde_s = e_s / \sigma_s.$$

Denote an observation by $O_s = \{y_s, \boldsymbol{x}_s, \boldsymbol{v}_s\}$ and the likelihood function $L(S;\boldsymbol{\theta})$ as the product of terms $L(O_s;\boldsymbol{\theta})$ for $s \in S$ satisfying

$$\begin{aligned}\ell(O_s;\boldsymbol{\theta}) = \log L(O_s;\boldsymbol{\theta}) &= -\,stde_s^2/2 - \left(\log \sigma_s^2\right)/2 - (\log(2\cdot\pi))/2 \\ &= stde_s^2/2 - (\log \varphi_s)/2 - (\log \mathrm{Var}(y_s))/2 - (\log(2\cdot\pi))/2\end{aligned}$$

where

$$\boldsymbol{\theta} = \begin{pmatrix} \boldsymbol{\beta} \\ \boldsymbol{\gamma} \end{pmatrix}.$$

For a discrete univariate outcome with unit dispersions, it is possible to utilize instead the true likelihood based on the probabilities $p_{s,u}$. The function $L(S;\boldsymbol{\theta})$ is not an exact likelihood, but has the advantages of accounting for the variances along with non-unit dispersions and of being readily generalized to handle correlated univariate outcomes (Sect. 12.2).

The likelihood $L(S;\boldsymbol{\theta})$ can be maximized using Newton's method to generate estimates

$$\boldsymbol{\theta}(S) = \begin{pmatrix} \boldsymbol{\beta}(S) \\ \boldsymbol{\gamma}(S) \end{pmatrix}$$

by solving

$$\boldsymbol{E}(\boldsymbol{\theta}) = \frac{\partial \ell(S;\boldsymbol{\theta})}{\partial \boldsymbol{\theta}} = \begin{pmatrix} \boldsymbol{E}(\boldsymbol{\beta}) \\ \boldsymbol{E}(\boldsymbol{\gamma}) \end{pmatrix} = \begin{pmatrix} \dfrac{\partial \ell(S;\boldsymbol{\theta})}{\partial \boldsymbol{\beta}} \\ \dfrac{\partial \ell(S;\boldsymbol{\theta})}{\partial \boldsymbol{\gamma}} \end{pmatrix} = \boldsymbol{0}$$

where $\boldsymbol{E}(\boldsymbol{\beta})$ and $\boldsymbol{E}(\boldsymbol{\gamma})$ are, respectively, $(K \cdot r) \times 1$ and $q \times 1$ vectors. $\boldsymbol{E}(\boldsymbol{\beta})$ is the sum over $s \in S$ of $\boldsymbol{E}_s(\boldsymbol{\beta})$ with $K \cdot r$ entries

$$E_{s,w,j}(\boldsymbol{\beta}) = xstde_{s,w,j} \cdot stde_s - W_{s,w,j}/2$$

where

$$xstde_{s,w,j} = \frac{\partial \mu_s}{\partial \beta_{w,j}} / \sigma_s + stde_s \cdot W_{s,w,j}/2,$$

$$\frac{\partial \mu_s}{\partial \beta_{w,j}} = x_{s,j} \cdot p_{s,w} \cdot (d_w - \mu_s),$$

$$W_{s,w,j} = \frac{\frac{\partial \mathrm{Var}(y_s)}{\partial \beta_{w,j}}}{\mathrm{Var}(y_s)},$$

$$\frac{\partial \mathrm{Var}(y_s)}{\partial \beta_{w,j}} = x_{s,j} \cdot p_{s,w} \cdot \left(d_w^2 - \mathrm{E}y_s^2 - 2 \cdot \mu_s \cdot (d_w - \mu_s)\right),$$

for $1 \le w \le K$, $1 \le j \le r$. $\boldsymbol{E}(\boldsymbol{\gamma})$ is the sum over $s \in S$ of $\boldsymbol{E}_s(\boldsymbol{\gamma})$ with q entries

$$E_{s,j}(\boldsymbol{\gamma}) = vstde_{s,j} \cdot stde_s - v_{s,j}/2$$

where

$$vstde_{s,j} = v_{s,j} \cdot stde_s/2$$

for $1 \le j \le q$.

$\boldsymbol{E}'(\boldsymbol{\theta})$ has four component matrices: the $(K \cdot r) \times (K \cdot r)$ matrix

$$\boldsymbol{E}'(\boldsymbol{\beta}) = \frac{\partial \boldsymbol{E}(\boldsymbol{\beta})}{\partial \boldsymbol{\beta}}$$

for the $K \cdot r$ mean coefficients, the $q \times q$ matrix

$$\boldsymbol{E}'(\boldsymbol{\gamma}) = \frac{\partial \boldsymbol{E}(\boldsymbol{\gamma})}{\partial \boldsymbol{\gamma}}$$

for the q dispersion coefficients, the $(K \cdot r) \times q$ matrix

$$\boldsymbol{E}'(\boldsymbol{\beta}, \boldsymbol{\gamma}) = \frac{\partial \boldsymbol{E}(\boldsymbol{\beta})}{\partial \boldsymbol{\gamma}},$$

and its transpose $\boldsymbol{E}'(\boldsymbol{\gamma}, \boldsymbol{\beta}) = \boldsymbol{E}'^{\mathrm{T}}(\boldsymbol{\beta}, \boldsymbol{\gamma})$. $\boldsymbol{E}'(\boldsymbol{\beta})$ is the sum over $s \in S$ of $\boldsymbol{E}'_s(\boldsymbol{\beta})$ with entries

$$E'_{s,w,j,w',j'}(\boldsymbol{\beta}) = -xxstde_{s,w,j,w',j'} \cdot stde_s - xstde_{s,w,j} \cdot xstde_{s,w',j'} - W_{s,w,j,w',j'}/2$$

where

$$xxstde_{s,w,j,w',j'} = -\frac{\frac{\partial^2 \mu_s}{\partial \beta_{w',j'} \partial \beta_{w,j}}}{\sigma_s} + \frac{\partial \mu_s}{\partial \beta_{w,j}} \cdot \frac{W_{s,w',j'}}{2 \cdot \sigma_s} + xstde_{s,w',j'} \cdot \frac{W_{s,w,j}}{2}$$

$$- stde_s \cdot \frac{W_{s,w,j,w',j'}}{2},$$

$$\frac{\partial^2 \mu_s}{\partial \beta_{w',j'} \partial \beta_{w,j}} = x_{s,j} \cdot x_{s,j'} \cdot p_{s,w} \cdot \left(1 - 2 \cdot p_{s,w}\right) \cdot (d_w - \mu_s), w' = w,$$

$$\frac{\partial^2 \mu_s}{\partial \beta_{w',j'} \partial \beta_{w,j}} = -x_{s,j} \cdot x_{s,j'} \cdot p_{s,w} \cdot p_{s,w'} \cdot (d_w + d_{w'} - 2 \cdot \mu_s), w' \neq w,$$

$$W_{s,w,j,w',j'} = \frac{\partial W_{s,w,j}}{\partial \beta_{w',j'}} = \frac{\frac{\partial^2 \mathrm{Var}(y_s)}{\partial \beta_{w',j'} \partial \beta_{w,j}}}{\mathrm{Var}(y_s)} - \frac{\frac{\partial \mathrm{Var}(y_s)}{\partial \beta_{w',j'}} \cdot \frac{\partial \mathrm{Var}(y_s)}{\partial \beta_{w,j}}}{\mathrm{Var}^2(y_s)},$$

$$\frac{\partial^2 \mathrm{Var}(y_s)}{\partial \beta_{w',j'} \partial \beta_{w,j}} = x_{s,j} \cdot x_{s,j'} \cdot p_{s,w} \cdot \left(1 - p_{s,w}\right) \cdot \left(d_w^2 - \mathrm{Ey}_s^2 - 2 \cdot \mu_s \cdot (d_w - \mu_s)\right)$$

$$+ x_{s,j} \cdot x_{s,j'} \cdot p_{s,w}^2 \cdot \left(\mathrm{Ey}_s^2 - d_w^2 + 2 \cdot (2 \cdot \mu_s - d_w) \cdot (d_w - \mu_s)\right), w' = w,$$

$$\frac{\partial^2 \mathrm{Var}(y_s)}{\partial \beta_{w',j'} \partial \beta_{w,j}} = -x_{s,j} \cdot x_{s,j'} \cdot p_{s,w} \cdot p_{s,w'} \cdot \left(d_w^2 - \mathrm{Ey}_s^2 - 2 \cdot \mu_s \cdot (d_w - \mu_s)\right)$$

$$+ x_{s,j} \cdot x_{s,j'} \cdot p_{s,w} \cdot p_{s,w'} \cdot \left(\mathrm{Ey}_s^2 - d_{w'}^2 + 2 \cdot (2 \cdot \mu_s - d_{w'}) \cdot (d_{w'} - \mu_s)\right), w' \neq w,$$

for $1 \leq w, w' \leq K$ and $1 \leq j, j' \leq r$. $\boldsymbol{E}'(\boldsymbol{\gamma})$ is the sum over $s \in S$ of $\boldsymbol{E}'_s(\gamma)$ with entries

$$E'_{s,j,j'}(\boldsymbol{\gamma}) = -vvstde_{s,j,j'} \cdot stde_s - vstde_{s,j} \cdot vstde_{s,j'}$$

where

$$vvstde_{s,j,j'} = v_{s,j} \cdot v_{s,j'} \cdot stde_s/4$$

for $1 \leq j, j' \leq q$. $\boldsymbol{E}'(\boldsymbol{\beta}, \boldsymbol{\gamma})$ is the sum over $s \in S$ of $\boldsymbol{E}'_s(\boldsymbol{\beta}, \boldsymbol{\gamma})$ with entries

$$E'_{s,w,j,j'}(\boldsymbol{\beta}, \boldsymbol{\gamma}) = -vxstde_{s,w,j,j'} \cdot stde_s - xstde_{s,w,j} \cdot vstde_{s,j'}$$

and

$$vxstde_{s,w,j,j'} = xstde_{s,w,j} \cdot v_{s,j'} \cdot /2$$

for $1 \le w \le K$, $1 \le j \le r$, and $1 \le j' \le q$.

Model-based and robust empirical estimates of the covariance matrix for the estimate $\boldsymbol{\theta}(SC)$ of the parameter vector $\boldsymbol{\theta}$ can be computed using $\mathbf{E}'(\boldsymbol{\theta}(SC))$ and $\mathbf{G}(\boldsymbol{\theta}(SC))$ for multinomial probabilities. $\mathbf{G}(\boldsymbol{\theta}(SC))$ is defined so that summing the entries of its rows generates $\mathbf{E}(\boldsymbol{\theta}(SC))$. A detailed formulation for $\mathbf{G}(\boldsymbol{\theta}(SC))$ is not provided for brevity.

12.1.2 Ordinal Probabilities

For predictor values $x_{s,j}$, combine them over $1 \le j \le r$ into the $r \times 1$ vectors $\mathbf{x}_s$ for $s \in S$. For $s \in S$, define cumulative probabilities

$$p_{s,\le u} = \mathrm{P}(y_s \le d_u), 0 \le u < K,$$
$$p_{s,\le K} = \mathrm{P}(y_s \le d_K) = 1.$$

The link function is cumulative logits computed for lower sets of values relative to higher sets of values (but this can be reversed). This assumes that outcome values are in increasing order. Formally, for $0 \le u < K$,

$$g(p_{s,\le u}) = \mathrm{logit}(p_{s,\le u}) = \log \frac{p_{s,\le u}}{1 - p_{s,\le u}} = \alpha_u + \mathbf{x}_s^{\mathrm{T}} \cdot \boldsymbol{\beta}_K$$

for K intercept parameters α_u and a single $r \times 1$ vector $\boldsymbol{\beta}_K$ of slope parameters $\beta_{K,j}$ for $1 \le j \le r$. This formulation assumes that, for $1 \le j \le r$, the predictor values $x_{s,j}$ are not constant in $s \in S$ so that $\boldsymbol{\beta}_K$ does not include a redundant intercept parameter. Combine the intercept parameters α_u over $0 \le u < K$ into the $K \times 1$ vector $\boldsymbol{\alpha}$. Altogether, there are $K + r$ coefficient parameters for modeling the probabilities, which are combined over $0 \le u < K$ and $1 \le j \le r$ into the $(K + r) \times 1$ vector

$$\boldsymbol{\beta} = \begin{pmatrix} \boldsymbol{\alpha} \\ \boldsymbol{\beta}_K \end{pmatrix}.$$

A zero-intercept model corresponds to setting $\alpha_0 = 0$, but α_u for $0 < u < K$ are non-zero.

The cumulative probabilities satisfy

$$p_{s,\le u} = \frac{\exp(\alpha_u + \mathbf{x}_s^{\mathrm{T}} \cdot \boldsymbol{\beta}_K)}{1 + \exp(\alpha_u + \mathbf{x}_s^{\mathrm{T}} \cdot \boldsymbol{\beta}_K)}$$

for $0 \leq u < K$ and $s \in S$. For $0 \leq u$, $w < K$, $1 \leq j \leq r$, and $s \in S$, the first partial derivatives of $p_{s,\leq u}$ satisfy

$$\frac{\partial p_{s,\leq u}}{\partial \alpha_w} = p_{s,\leq w} \cdot \left(1 - p_{s,\leq w}\right), w = u,$$

$$\frac{\partial p_{s,\leq u}}{\partial \alpha_w} = 0, w \neq u,$$

$$\frac{\partial p_{s,\leq u}}{\partial \beta_{K,j}} = x_{s,j} \cdot p_{s,\leq u} \cdot \left(1 - p_{s,\leq u}\right).$$

The cumulative probabilities are differenced to compute probabilities $p_{s,u} = \mathrm{P}(y_s = d_u)$, that is, for $s \in S$, define $p_{s,\leq -1} = 0$ and then $p_{s,u} = p_{s,\leq u} - p_{s,\leq u-1}$ for $0 \leq u \leq K$.

For predictor values $v_{s,j}$, combine them over $1 \leq j \leq q$ into the $q \times 1$ vectors $\boldsymbol{v}_s$ for $s \in S$. Model the natural log of the non-constant dispersions in terms of these predictor values, that is,

$$\log \varphi_s = \boldsymbol{v}_s^{\mathrm{T}} \cdot \boldsymbol{\gamma}$$

where $\boldsymbol{\gamma}$ is a $q \times 1$ vector of coefficient parameters. Define the extended variances as

$$\sigma_s^2 = \varphi_s \cdot \mathrm{Var}(y_s),$$

and the standardized residuals as

$$stde_s = e_s / \sigma_s.$$

Denote an observation by $O_s = \{y_s, \boldsymbol{x}_s, \boldsymbol{v}_s\}$ and the likelihood function $L(S;\boldsymbol{\theta})$ as the product of terms $L(O_s;\boldsymbol{\theta})$ for $s \in S$ satisfying

$$\begin{aligned}\ell(O_s;\boldsymbol{\theta}) = \log L(O_s;\boldsymbol{\theta}) &= -\,stde_s^2/2 - \left(\log \sigma_s^2\right)/2 - (\log(2 \cdot \pi))/2 \\ &= stde_s^2/2 - (\log \varphi_s)/2 - (\log \mathrm{Var}(y_s))/2 - (\log(2 \cdot \pi))/2\end{aligned}$$

where

$$\boldsymbol{\theta} = \begin{pmatrix} \beta \\ \gamma \end{pmatrix}.$$

For a discrete univariate outcome with unit dispersions, it is possible to utilize instead the true likelihood based on the probabilities $p_{s,u}$. The function $L(S;\boldsymbol{\theta})$ is not an exact likelihood, but has the advantages of directly accounting for the variances along with non-unit dispersions and of being readily generalized to handle correlated univariate outcomes (Sect. 12.2).

The likelihood $L(S;\boldsymbol{\theta})$ can be maximized using Newton's method to generate estimates

$$\boldsymbol{\theta}(S) = \begin{pmatrix} \beta(S) \\ \gamma(S) \end{pmatrix}$$

by solving

$$\boldsymbol{E}(\boldsymbol{\theta}) = \frac{\partial \ell(S;\boldsymbol{\theta})}{\partial \boldsymbol{\theta}} = \begin{pmatrix} \boldsymbol{E}(\boldsymbol{\beta}) \\ \boldsymbol{E}(\boldsymbol{\gamma}) \end{pmatrix} = \begin{pmatrix} \dfrac{\partial \ell(S;\boldsymbol{\theta})}{\partial \boldsymbol{\beta}} \\ \dfrac{\partial \ell(S;\boldsymbol{\theta})}{\partial \boldsymbol{\gamma}} \end{pmatrix} = \mathbf{0}$$

where $\boldsymbol{E}(\boldsymbol{\beta})$ and $\boldsymbol{E}(\boldsymbol{\gamma})$ are, respectively, $(K + r) \times 1$ and $q \times 1$ vectors. $\boldsymbol{E}(\boldsymbol{\beta})$ is the sum over $s \in S$ of $\boldsymbol{E}_s(\boldsymbol{\beta})$ with $K + r$ entries

$$E_{s,w}(\boldsymbol{\beta}) = xstde_{s,w} \cdot stde_s - W_{s,w}/2,$$
$$E_{s,K,j}(\boldsymbol{\beta}) = xstde_{s,K,j} \cdot stde_s - W_{s,K,j}/2,$$

where

$$xstde_{s,w} = \frac{\partial \mu_s}{\partial \alpha_w} / \sigma_s + stde_s \cdot W_{s,w}/2,$$
$$\frac{\partial \mu_s}{\partial \alpha_w} = p_{s,\leq w} \cdot \left(1 - p_{s,\leq w}\right) \cdot \left(d_w - d_{w-1}\right),$$
$$xstde_{s,K,j} = \frac{\partial \mu_s}{\partial \beta_{K,j}} / \sigma_s + stde_s \cdot W_{s,K,j}/2,$$
$$\frac{\partial \mu_s}{\partial \beta_{K,j}} = x_{s,j} \cdot \sum_{u=0}^{K-1} \left(p_{s,\leq u} \cdot \left(1 - p_{s,\leq u}\right) \cdot \left(d_u - d_{u-1}\right)\right),$$
$$W_{s,w} = \frac{\frac{\partial \mathrm{Var}(y_s)}{\partial \alpha_w}}{\mathrm{Var}(y_s)},$$
$$\frac{\partial \mathrm{Var}(y_s)}{\partial \alpha_w} = p_{s,\leq w} \cdot \left(1 - p_{s,\leq w}\right) \cdot \left(d_w - d_{w+1}\right) \cdot \left(d_w + d_{w+1} - 2 \cdot \mu_s\right),$$
$$W_{s,K,j} = \frac{\frac{\partial \mathrm{Var}(y_s)}{\partial \beta_{K,j}}}{\mathrm{Var}(y_s)},$$

$$\frac{\partial \mathrm{Var}(y_s)}{\partial \beta_{K,j}} = x_{s,j} \cdot \sum_{u=0}^{K-1} \left(p_{s,\le u} \cdot \left(1 - p_{s,\le u}\right) \cdot (d_u - d_{u+1}) \cdot (d_u + d_{u+1} - 2 \cdot \mu_s)\right),$$

for $0 \le w < K$ and $1 \le j \le r$. $\boldsymbol{E}(\gamma)$ is the sum over $s \in S$ of $\boldsymbol{E}_s(\gamma)$ with q entries

$$E_{s,j}(\boldsymbol{\gamma}) = vstde_{s,j} \cdot stde_s - v_{s,j}/2$$

where

$$vstde_{s,j} = v_{s,j} \cdot stde_s/2$$

for $1 \le j \le q$.

$\boldsymbol{E}'(\boldsymbol{\theta})$ has four component matrices: the $(K + r) \times (K + r)$ matrix

$$\boldsymbol{E}'(\boldsymbol{\beta}) = \frac{\partial \boldsymbol{E}(\boldsymbol{\beta})}{\partial \boldsymbol{\beta}}$$

for the $K + r$ mean coefficients, the $q \times q$ matrix

$$\boldsymbol{E}'(\boldsymbol{\gamma}) = \frac{\partial \boldsymbol{E}(\boldsymbol{\gamma})}{\partial \boldsymbol{\gamma}}$$

for the q dispersion coefficients, the $(K + r) \times q$ matrix

$$\boldsymbol{E}'(\boldsymbol{\beta}, \boldsymbol{\gamma}) = \frac{\partial \boldsymbol{E}(\boldsymbol{\beta})}{\partial \boldsymbol{\gamma}},$$

and its transpose $\boldsymbol{E}'(\boldsymbol{\gamma}, \boldsymbol{\beta}) = \boldsymbol{E}'^{\mathrm{T}}(\boldsymbol{\beta}, \boldsymbol{\gamma})$. $\boldsymbol{E}'(\boldsymbol{\beta})$ is the sum over $s \in S$ of $\boldsymbol{E}'_s(\boldsymbol{\beta})$ with entries

$$\begin{aligned}
E'_{s,w,w'}(\boldsymbol{\beta}) &= -xxstde_{s,w,w'} \cdot stde_s - xstde_{s,w} \cdot xstde_{s,w'} - W_{s,w,w'}/2, \\
E'_{s,w,K,j}(\boldsymbol{\beta}) &= -xxstde_{s,w,K,j} \cdot stde_s - xstde_{s,w} \cdot xstde_{s,K,j} - W_{s,w,K,j}/2, \\
E'_{s,K,j,w'}(\boldsymbol{\beta}) &= -xxstde_{s,K,j,w'} \cdot stde_s - xstde_{s,K,j} \cdot xstde_{s,w'} - W_{s,K,j,w'}/2, \\
E'_{s,K,j,j'}(\boldsymbol{\beta}) &= -xxstde_{s,K,j,j'} \cdot stde_s - xstde_{s,K,j} \cdot xstde_{s,K,j'} - W_{s,K,j,j'}/2,
\end{aligned}$$

where

$$xxstde_{s,w,w'} = -\frac{\frac{\partial^2 \mu_s}{\partial \alpha_{w'} \partial \alpha_w}}{\sigma_s} + \frac{\partial \mu_s}{\partial \alpha_w} \cdot \frac{W_{s,w'}}{2 \cdot \sigma_s} + xstde_{s,w'} \cdot \frac{W_{s,w}}{2} - stde_s \cdot \frac{W_{s,w,w'}}{2},$$

$$\frac{\partial^2 \mu_s}{\partial \alpha_{w'} \partial \alpha_w} = p_{s,\le w} \cdot \left(1 - p_{s,\le w}\right) \cdot \left(1 - 2 \cdot p_{s,\le w}\right) \cdot \left(d_w - d_{w+1}\right), w' = w,$$

$$\frac{\partial^2 \mu_s}{\partial \alpha_{w'} \partial \alpha_w} = 0, w' \ne w;$$

$$xxstde_{s,w,Kj} = -\frac{\frac{\partial^2 \mu_s}{\partial \beta_{Kj} \partial \alpha_w}}{\sigma_s} + \frac{\partial \mu_s}{\partial \alpha_w} \cdot \frac{W_{s,Kj}}{2 \cdot \sigma_s} + xstde_{s,Kj} \cdot \frac{W_{s,w}}{2} - stde_s \cdot \frac{W_{s,w,Kj}}{2},$$

$$\frac{\partial^2 \mu_s}{\partial \beta_{Kj} \partial \alpha_w} = x_{s,j} \cdot p_{s,\le w} \cdot \left(1 - p_{s,\le w}\right) \cdot \left(1 - 2 \cdot p_{s,\le w}\right) \cdot \left(d_w - d_{w+1}\right);$$

$$xxstde_{s,Kj,w'} = -\frac{\frac{\partial^2 \mu_s}{\partial \alpha_{w'} \partial \beta_{Kj}}}{\sigma_s} + \frac{\partial \mu_s}{\partial \beta_{Kj}} \cdot \frac{W_{s,w'}}{2 \cdot \sigma_s} + xstde_{s,w'} \cdot \frac{W_{s,Kj}}{2} - stde_s \cdot \frac{W_{s,Kj,w'}}{2},$$

$$\frac{\partial^2 \mu_s}{\partial \alpha_{w'} \partial \beta_{Kj}} = x_{s,j} \cdot p_{s,\le w'} \cdot \left(1 - p_{s,\le w'}\right) \cdot \left(1 - 2 \cdot p_{s,\le w'}\right) \cdot \left(d_{w'} - d_{w'+1}\right);$$

$$xxstde_{s,Kjj'} = -\frac{\frac{\partial^2 \mu_s}{\partial \beta_{Kj'} \partial \beta_{Kj}}}{\sigma_s} + \frac{\partial \mu_s}{\partial \beta_{Kj}} \cdot \frac{W_{s,Kj'}}{2 \cdot \sigma_s} + xstde_{s,Kj'} \cdot \frac{W_{s,Kj}}{2} - stde_s \cdot \frac{W_{s,Kjj'}}{2},$$

$$\frac{\partial^2 \mu_s}{\partial \beta_{Kj'} \partial \beta_{Kj}} = x_{s,j} \cdot x_{s,j'} \cdot \sum_{u=0}^{K-1} \left(p_{s,\le u} \cdot \left(1 - p_{s,\le u}\right) \cdot \left(1 - 2 \cdot p_{s,\le u}\right) \cdot \left(d_u - d_{u+1}\right)\right);$$

$$W_{s,w,w'} = \frac{\partial W_{s,w}}{\partial \alpha_{w'}} = \frac{\frac{\partial^2 \mathrm{Var}(y_s)}{\partial \alpha_{w'} \partial \alpha_w}}{\mathrm{Var}(y_s)} - \frac{\frac{\partial \mathrm{Var}(y_s)}{\partial \alpha_{w'}} \cdot \frac{\partial \mathrm{Var}(y_s)}{\partial \alpha_w}}{\mathrm{Var}^2(y_s)},$$

$$\frac{\partial^2 \mathrm{Var}(y_s)}{\partial \alpha_{w'} \partial \alpha_w} = p_{s,\le w} \cdot \left(1 - p_{s,\le w}\right) \cdot \left(d_w - d_{w+1}\right) \cdot$$
$$\left(\left(1 - 2 \cdot p_{s,\le w}\right) \cdot \left(d_w + d_{w+1} - 2 \cdot \mu_s\right) - 2 \cdot p_{s,\le w} \cdot \left(1 - p_{s,\le w}\right)\right), w' = w,$$

$$\frac{\partial^2 \mathrm{Var}(y_s)}{\partial \alpha_{w'} \partial \alpha_w} =$$
$$-2 \cdot p_{s,\le w} \cdot \left(1 - p_{s,\le w}\right) \cdot p_{s,\le w'} \cdot \left(1 - p_{s,\le w'}\right) \cdot \left(d_w - d_{w+1}\right) \cdot \left(d_{w'} - d_{w'+1}\right), w' \ne w;$$

$$W_{s,w,Kj} = \frac{\partial W_{s,w}}{\partial \beta_{Kj}} = \frac{\frac{\partial^2 \mathrm{Var}(y_s)}{\partial \beta_{Kj} \partial \alpha_w}}{\mathrm{Var}(y_s)} - \frac{\frac{\partial \mathrm{Var}(y_s)}{\partial \beta_{Kj}} \cdot \frac{\partial \mathrm{Var}(y_s)}{\partial \alpha_w}}{\mathrm{Var}^2(y_s)},$$

$$\frac{\partial^2 \mathrm{Var}(y_s)}{\partial \beta_{Kj} \partial \alpha_w} = x_{s,j} \cdot p_{s,\le w} \cdot \left(1 - p_{s,\le w}\right) \cdot \left(d_w - d_{w+1}\right) \cdot$$

$$\left(\left(1-2\cdot p_{s,\leq w}\right)\cdot\left(d_w+d_{w+1}-2\cdot\mu_s\right)-2\cdot\sum_{u=0}^{K-1}\left(p_{s,\leq u}\cdot\left(1-p_{s,\leq u}\right)\cdot\left(d_u-d_{u+1}\right)\right)\right);$$

$$W_{s,K,j,w'}=\frac{\partial W_{s,K,j}}{\partial\alpha_{w'}}=\frac{\frac{\partial^2\text{Var}(y_s)}{\partial\alpha_{w'}\partial\beta_{K,j}}}{\text{Var}(y_s)}-\frac{\frac{\partial\text{Var}(y_s)}{\partial\alpha_{w'}}\cdot\frac{\partial\text{Var}(y_s)}{\partial\beta_{K,j}}}{\text{Var}^2(y_s)},$$

$$\frac{\partial^2\text{Var}(y_s)}{\partial\alpha_{w'}\partial\beta_{K,j}}=x_{s,j}\cdot p_{s,\leq w'}\cdot\left(1-p_{s,\leq w'}\right)\cdot\left(d_{w'}-d_{w'+1}\right)\cdot$$
$$\left(\left(1-2\cdot p_{s,\leq w'}\right)\cdot\left(d_{w'}+d_{w'+1}-2\cdot\mu_s\right)-2\right.$$
$$\left.\cdot\sum_{u=0}^{K-1}\left(p_{s,\leq u}\cdot\left(1-p_{s,\leq u}\right)\cdot\left(d_u-d_{u+1}\right)\right)\right);$$

$$W_{s,K,j,j'}=\frac{\partial W_{s,K,j}}{\partial\beta_{K,j'}}=\frac{\frac{\partial^2\text{Var}(y_s)}{\partial\beta_{K,j'}\partial\beta_{K,j}}}{\text{Var}(y_s)}-\frac{\frac{\partial\text{Var}(y_s)}{\partial\beta_{K,j'}}\cdot\frac{\partial\text{Var}(y_s)}{\partial\beta_{K,j}}}{\text{Var}^2(y_s)},$$

$$\frac{\partial^2\text{Var}(y_s)}{\partial\beta_{K,j'}\partial\beta_{K,j}}=x_{s,j}\cdot x_{s,j'}\cdot\sum_{u=0}^{K-1}$$
$$\times\left(p_{s,\leq u}\cdot\left(1-p_{s,\leq u}\right)\cdot\left(1-2\cdot p_{s,\leq u}\right)\cdot\left(d_u-d_{u+1}\right)\cdot\left(d_u+d_{u+1}-2\cdot\mu_s\right)\right)$$
$$-2\cdot x_{s,j}\cdot x_{s,j'}\cdot\left(\sum_{u=0}^{K-1}\left(p_{s,\leq u}\cdot\left(1-p_{s,\leq u}\right)\cdot\left(d_u-d_{u+1}\right)\right)\right)^2$$

for $0\leq w, w' < K$ and $1\leq j, j'\leq r$. $\boldsymbol{E}'(\boldsymbol{\gamma})$ is the sum over $s\in S$ of $\boldsymbol{E}'_s(\boldsymbol{\gamma})$ with entries

$$E'_{s,j,j'}(\boldsymbol{\gamma})=-vvstde_{s,j,j'}\cdot stde_s-vstde_{s,j}\cdot vstde_{s,j'}$$

where

$$vvstde_{s,j,j'}=v_{s,j}\cdot v_{s,j'}\cdot stde_s/4$$

for $1\leq j, j'\leq q$. $\boldsymbol{E}'(\boldsymbol{\beta},\boldsymbol{\gamma})$ is the sum over $s\in S$ of $\boldsymbol{E}'_s(\boldsymbol{\beta},\boldsymbol{\gamma})$ with entries

$$E'_{s,w,j'}(\boldsymbol{\beta},\boldsymbol{\gamma})=-vxstde_{s,w,j'}\cdot stde_s-xstde_{s,w}\cdot vstde_{s,j'},$$
$$E'_{s,K,j,j'}(\boldsymbol{\beta},\boldsymbol{\gamma})=-vxstde_{s,K,j,j'}\cdot stde_s-xstde_{s,K,j}\cdot vstde_{s,j'}$$

and

$$vxstde_{s,w,j'}=xstde_{s,w}\cdot v_{s,j'}/2,$$

$$vxstde_{s,K,j,j'} = xstde_{s,K,j} \cdot v_{s,j'}/2$$

for $0 \leq w < K$, $1 \leq j \leq r$, and $1 \leq j' \leq q$.

Model-based and robust empirical estimates of the covariance matrix for the estimate $\boldsymbol{\theta}(SC)$ of the parameter vector $\boldsymbol{\theta}$ can be computed using $\boldsymbol{E}'(\boldsymbol{\theta}(SC))$ and $\boldsymbol{G}(\boldsymbol{\theta}(SC))$ for ordinal probabilities. $\boldsymbol{G}(\boldsymbol{\theta}(SC))$ is defined so that summing the entries of its rows generates $\boldsymbol{E}(\boldsymbol{\theta}(SC))$. A detailed formulation for $\boldsymbol{G}(\boldsymbol{\theta}(SC))$ is not provided for brevity.

12.1.3 Censored Poisson Probabilities

For predictor values $x_{s,j}$, combine them over $1 \leq j \leq r$ into the $r \times 1$ vectors $\boldsymbol{x}_s$ for $s \in S$. Censored Poisson probabilities $p_{s,u} = \mathrm{P}(y_s = d_u)$ are modeled using the natural log link function as follows

$$p_{s,u} = \exp(-\lambda_s) \cdot \frac{\lambda_s^u}{u!}, 0 \leq u < K,$$

$$p_{s,K} = 1 - \sum_{u=0}^{K-1} p_{s,u},$$

$$\log \lambda_s = \boldsymbol{x}_s^{\mathrm{T}} \cdot \boldsymbol{\beta},$$

for a $r \times 1$ vector $\boldsymbol{\beta}$ of coefficient parameters β_j for $1 \leq j \leq r$. The first partial derivatives $\frac{\partial \lambda_s}{\partial \beta_j}$ and $\frac{\partial p_{s,u}}{\partial \beta_j}$ satisfy

$$\frac{\partial \lambda_s}{\partial \beta_j} = x_{s,j} \cdot \lambda_s,$$

$$\frac{\partial p_{s,u}}{\partial \beta_j} = x_{s,j} \cdot p_{s,u} \cdot (u - \lambda_s), 0 \leq u < K,$$

$$\frac{\partial p_{s,K}}{\partial \beta_j} = - \sum_{u=0}^{K-1} \frac{\partial p_{s,u}}{\partial \beta_j},$$

for $1 \leq j \leq r$ and $s \in S$. The associated second partial derivatives satisfy

$$\frac{\partial^2 \lambda_s}{\partial \beta_{j'} \partial \beta_j} = x_{s,j} \cdot x_{s,j'} \cdot \lambda_s,$$

$$\frac{\partial^2 p_{s,u}}{\partial \beta_{j'} \partial \beta_j} = x_{s,j} \cdot x_{s,j'} \cdot p_{s,u} \cdot \left((u - \lambda_s)^2 - \lambda_s \right), 0 \leq u < K,$$

$$\frac{\partial^2 p_{s,K}}{\partial \beta_{j'} \partial \beta_j} = - \sum_{u=0}^{K-1} \frac{\partial^2 p_{s,u}}{\partial \beta_{j'} \partial \beta_j},$$

for $1 \leq j, j' \leq r$ and $s \in S$.

For predictor values $v_{s,j}$, combine them over $1 \leq j \leq q$ into the $q \times 1$ vectors $\boldsymbol{v}_s$ for $s \in S$. Model the natural log of the non-constant dispersions in terms of these predictor values, that is,

$$\log \varphi_s = \boldsymbol{v}_s^{\mathrm{T}} \cdot \boldsymbol{\gamma}$$

where $\boldsymbol{\gamma}$ is a $q \times 1$ vector of coefficient parameters. Define the extended variances as

$$\sigma_s^2 = \varphi_s \cdot \mathrm{Var}(y_s),$$

and the standardized residuals as

$$stde_s = e_s / \sigma_s.$$

Denote an observation by $O_s = \{y_s, \boldsymbol{x}_s, \boldsymbol{v}_s\}$ and the likelihood function $L(S;\boldsymbol{\theta})$ as the product of terms $L(O_s;\boldsymbol{\theta})$ for $s \in S$ satisfying

$$\begin{aligned} \ell(O_s;\boldsymbol{\theta}) &= \log L(O_s;\boldsymbol{\theta}) = - stde_s^2/2 - \left(\log \sigma_s^2\right)/2 - (\log(2 \cdot \pi))/2 \\ &= stde_s^2/2 - (\log \varphi_s)/2 - (\log \mathrm{Var}(y_s))/2 - (\log(2 \cdot \pi))/2 \end{aligned}$$

where

$$\boldsymbol{\theta} = \begin{pmatrix} \beta \\ \gamma \end{pmatrix}.$$

For a discrete univariate outcome with unit dispersions, it is possible to utilize instead the true likelihood based on the probabilities $p_{s,u}$. The function $L(S;\boldsymbol{\theta})$ is not an exact likelihood, but has the advantages of accounting for the variances along with non-unit dispersions and of being readily generalized to handle correlated univariate outcomes (Sect. 12.2).

The likelihood $L(S;\boldsymbol{\theta})$ can be maximized using Newton's method to generate estimates

$$\boldsymbol{\theta}(S) = \begin{pmatrix} \boldsymbol{\beta}(S) \\ \boldsymbol{\gamma}(S) \end{pmatrix}$$

by solving

$$\boldsymbol{E}(\boldsymbol{\theta}) = \frac{\partial \ell(S;\boldsymbol{\theta})}{\partial \boldsymbol{\theta}} = \begin{pmatrix} \boldsymbol{E}(\boldsymbol{\beta}) \\ \boldsymbol{E}(\boldsymbol{\gamma}) \end{pmatrix} = \begin{pmatrix} \dfrac{\partial \ell(S;\boldsymbol{\theta})}{\partial \boldsymbol{\beta}} \\ \dfrac{\partial \ell(S;\boldsymbol{\theta})}{\partial \boldsymbol{\gamma}} \end{pmatrix} = \mathbf{0}$$

where $\boldsymbol{E}(\boldsymbol{\beta})$ and $\boldsymbol{E}(\boldsymbol{\gamma})$ are, respectively, $r \times 1$ and $q \times 1$ vectors. $\boldsymbol{E}(\boldsymbol{\beta})$ is the sum over $s \in S$ of $\boldsymbol{E}_s(\boldsymbol{\beta})$ with r entries

$$E_{s,j}(\boldsymbol{\beta}) = xstde_{s,j} \cdot stde_s - W_{s,j}/2$$

where

$$xstde_{s,j} = \frac{\partial \mu_s}{\partial \beta_j} / \sigma_s + stde_s \cdot W_{s,j}/2,$$

$$\frac{\partial \mu_s}{\partial \beta_j} = \sum_{u=0}^{K-1} (d_u - d_K) \cdot \frac{\partial p_{s,u}}{\partial \beta_j},$$

$$W_{s,j} = \frac{\frac{\partial \mathrm{Var}(y_s)}{\partial \beta_j}}{\mathrm{Var}(y_s)},$$

$$\frac{\partial \mathrm{Var}(y_s)}{\partial \beta_j} = \sum_{u=0}^{K-1} \left((d_u - d_K) \cdot (d_u + d_K - 2 \cdot \mu_s) \cdot \frac{\partial p_{s,u}}{\partial \beta_j} \right),$$

for $1 \leq j \leq r$. $\boldsymbol{E}(\boldsymbol{\gamma})$ is the sum over $s \in S$ of $\boldsymbol{E}_s(\boldsymbol{\gamma})$ with q entries

$$E_{s,j}(\boldsymbol{\gamma}) = vstde_{s,j} \cdot stde_s - v_{s,j}/2$$

where

$$vstde_{s,j} = v_{s,j} \cdot stde_s/2$$

for $1 \leq j \leq q$.

$\boldsymbol{E}'(\boldsymbol{\theta})$ has four component matrices: the $r \times r$ matrix

$$\boldsymbol{E}'(\boldsymbol{\beta}) = \frac{\partial \boldsymbol{E}(\boldsymbol{\beta})}{\partial \boldsymbol{\beta}}$$

for the r mean coefficients, the $q \times q$ matrix

$$\boldsymbol{E}'(\boldsymbol{\gamma}) = \frac{\partial \boldsymbol{E}(\boldsymbol{\gamma})}{\partial \boldsymbol{\gamma}}$$

for the q dispersion coefficients, the $r \times q$ matrix

$$\boldsymbol{E}'(\boldsymbol{\beta},\boldsymbol{\gamma}) = \frac{\partial \boldsymbol{E}(\boldsymbol{\beta})}{\partial \boldsymbol{\gamma}},$$

and its transpose $\boldsymbol{E}'(\boldsymbol{\gamma},\boldsymbol{\beta}) = \boldsymbol{E}'^{\mathrm{T}}(\boldsymbol{\beta},\boldsymbol{\gamma})$. $\boldsymbol{E}'(\boldsymbol{\beta})$ is the sum over $s \in S$ of $\boldsymbol{E}'_s(\boldsymbol{\beta})$ with entries

$$E'_{s,j,j'}(\boldsymbol{\beta}) = -xxstde_{s,j,j'} \cdot stde_s - xstde_{s,j} \cdot xstde_{s,j'} - W_{s,j,j'}/2$$

where

$$xxstde_{s,j,j'} = -\frac{\frac{\partial^2 \mu_s}{\partial \beta_{j'}\,\partial \beta_j}}{\sigma_s} + \frac{\partial \mu_s}{\partial \beta_j} \cdot \frac{W_{s,j'}}{2 \cdot \sigma_s} + xstde_{s,j'} \cdot \frac{W_{s,j}}{2} - stde_s \cdot \frac{W_{s,j,j'}}{2},$$

$$\frac{\partial^2 \mu_s}{\partial \beta_{j'}\,\partial \beta_j} = \sum_{u=0}^{K-1} (d_u - d_K) \cdot \frac{\partial^2 p_{s,u}}{\partial \beta_{j'}\,\partial \beta_j},$$

$$W_{s,j,j'} = \frac{\partial W_{s,j}}{\partial \beta_{j'}} = \frac{\frac{\partial^2 \mathrm{Var}(y_s)}{\partial \beta_{j'}\,\partial \beta_j}}{\mathrm{Var}(y_s)} - \frac{\frac{\partial \mathrm{Var}(y_s)}{\partial \beta_{j'}} \cdot \frac{\partial \mathrm{Var}(y_s)}{\partial \beta_j}}{\mathrm{Var}^2(y_s)},$$

$$\frac{\partial^2 \mathrm{Var}(y_s)}{\partial \beta_{j'}\,\partial \beta_j} = \sum_{u=0}^{K-1} \left((d_u - d_K) \cdot (d_u + d_K - 2 \cdot \mu_s) \cdot \frac{\partial^2 p_{s,u}}{\partial \beta_{j'}\,\partial \beta_j} - 2 \cdot \frac{\partial \mu_s}{\partial \beta_j} \cdot \frac{\partial p_{s,u}}{\partial \beta_{j'}} \right),$$

for $1 \leq j, j' \leq r$. $\boldsymbol{E}'(\boldsymbol{\gamma})$ is the sum over $s \in S$ of $\boldsymbol{E}'_s(\boldsymbol{\gamma})$ with entries

$$E'_{s,j,j'}(\boldsymbol{\gamma}) = -vvstde_{s,j,j'} \cdot stde_s - vstde_{s,j} \cdot vstde_{s,j'}$$

where

$$vvstde_{s,j,j'} = v_{s,j} \cdot v_{s,j'} \cdot stde_s/4$$

for $1 \leq j, j' \leq q$. $\boldsymbol{E}'(\boldsymbol{\beta},\boldsymbol{\gamma})$ is the sum over $s \in S$ of $\boldsymbol{E}'_s(\boldsymbol{\beta},\boldsymbol{\gamma})$ with entries

$$E'_{s,j,j'}(\boldsymbol{\beta},\boldsymbol{\gamma}) = -vxstde_{s,j,j'} \cdot stde_s - xstde_{s,j} \cdot vstde_{s,j'}$$

and

$$vxstde_{s,j,j'} = xstde_{s,j} \cdot v_{s,j'}/2$$

for $1 \le j \le r$ and $1 \le j' \le q$.

Model-based and robust empirical estimates of the covariance matrix for the estimate $\boldsymbol{\theta}(SC)$ of the parameter vector $\boldsymbol{\theta}$ can be computed using $\mathbf{E}'(\boldsymbol{\theta}(SC))$ and $\mathbf{G}(\boldsymbol{\theta}(SC))$ for censored Poisson probabilities. $\mathbf{G}(\boldsymbol{\theta}(SC))$ is defined so that summing the entries of its rows generates $\mathbf{E}(\boldsymbol{\theta}(SC))$. A detailed formulation for $\mathbf{G}(\boldsymbol{\theta}(SC))$ is not provided for brevity.

12.1.4 Direct Variance Modeling

This section provides the formulation for direct variance modeling, as first addressed in Sect. 5.7, of singleton univariate discrete outcomes. Section 12.1.4.1 addresses direct variance modeling using multinomial probabilities, Sect. 12.1.4.2 ordinal probabilities, and Sect. 12.1.4.3 censored Poisson probabilities. As in Sect. 5.7, formulations are provided only for the ELMM case.

The variances are $\sigma_s^2 = \varphi_s$ and the standardized residuals $stde_s = e_s/\sigma_s$. The likelihood $L(S;\boldsymbol{\theta})$ is the product of terms $L(O_s;\boldsymbol{\theta})$ for $s \in S$ satisfying

$$\begin{aligned}\ell(O_s;\boldsymbol{\theta}) &= \log L(O_s;\boldsymbol{\theta}) = -\,stde_s^2/2 - \left(\log\sigma_s^2\right)/2 - (\log(2\cdot\pi))/2 \\ &= stde_s^2/2 - (\log\varphi_s)/2 - (\log(2\cdot\pi))/2\end{aligned}$$

where

$$\boldsymbol{\theta} = \begin{pmatrix}\boldsymbol{\beta}\\ \boldsymbol{\gamma}\end{pmatrix}.$$

To maximize $L(S;\boldsymbol{\theta})$, solve

$$\mathbf{E}(\boldsymbol{\theta}) = \frac{\partial\ell(S;\boldsymbol{\theta})}{\partial\boldsymbol{\theta}} = \begin{pmatrix}\mathbf{E}(\boldsymbol{\beta})\\ \mathbf{E}(\boldsymbol{\gamma})\end{pmatrix} = \begin{pmatrix}\dfrac{\partial\ell(S;\boldsymbol{\theta})}{\partial\boldsymbol{\beta}}\\ \dfrac{\partial\ell(S;\boldsymbol{\theta})}{\partial\boldsymbol{\gamma}}\end{pmatrix} = \mathbf{0}.$$

12.1.4.1 Multinomial Probabilities

$\mathbf{E}(\boldsymbol{\beta})$ is the $(K \cdot r) \times 1$ vector equaling the sum over $s \in S$ of $\mathbf{E}_s(\boldsymbol{\beta})$ with entries

$$E_{s,w,j}(\boldsymbol{\beta}) = xstde_{s,w,j} \cdot stde_s$$

where

$$xstde_{s,w,j} = \frac{\partial \mu_s}{\partial \beta_{w,j}} / \sigma_s,$$

$$\frac{\partial \mu_s}{\partial \beta_{w,j}} = x_{s,j} \cdot p_{s,w} \cdot (d_w - \mu_s),$$

for $1 \leq w \leq K$ and $1 \leq j \leq r$. $\boldsymbol{E}(\boldsymbol{\gamma})$ has the same formulation as in Sect. 12.1.1. $\boldsymbol{E}'(\boldsymbol{\theta})$ has four component matrices: the $(K \cdot r) \times (K \cdot r)$ matrix

$$\boldsymbol{E}'(\boldsymbol{\beta}) = \frac{\partial \boldsymbol{E}(\boldsymbol{\beta})}{\partial \boldsymbol{\beta}}$$

for the $K \cdot r$ mean coefficients, the $q \times q$ matrix

$$\boldsymbol{E}'(\boldsymbol{\gamma}) = \frac{\partial \boldsymbol{E}(\boldsymbol{\gamma})}{\partial \boldsymbol{\gamma}}$$

for the q dispersion coefficients, the $(K \cdot r) \times q$ matrix

$$\boldsymbol{E}'(\boldsymbol{\beta},\boldsymbol{\gamma}) = \frac{\partial \boldsymbol{E}(\boldsymbol{\beta})}{\partial \boldsymbol{\gamma}},$$

and its transpose $\boldsymbol{E}'(\boldsymbol{\gamma},\boldsymbol{\beta}) = \boldsymbol{E}'^{\mathrm{T}}(\boldsymbol{\beta},\boldsymbol{\gamma})$. $\boldsymbol{E}'(\boldsymbol{\beta})$ is the sum over $s \in S$ of $\boldsymbol{E}'_s(\boldsymbol{\beta})$ with entries

$$E'_{s,w,j,w',j'}(\boldsymbol{\beta}) = -xxstde_{s,w,j,w',j'} \cdot stde_s - xstde_{s,w,j} \cdot xstde_{s,w',j'}$$

where

$$xxstde_{s,w,j,w',j'} = -\frac{\partial^2 \mu_s}{\partial \beta_{w',j'} \partial \beta_{w,j}} / \sigma_s,$$

$$\frac{\partial^2 \mu_s}{\partial \beta_{w',j'} \partial \beta_{w,j}} = x_{s,j} \cdot x_{s,j'} \cdot p_{s,w} \cdot \left(1 - 2 \cdot p_{s,w}\right) \cdot (d_w - \mu_s), w' = w,$$

$$\frac{\partial^2 \mu_s}{\partial \beta_{w',j'} \partial \beta_{w,j}} = -x_{s,j} \cdot x_{s,j'} \cdot p_{s,w} \cdot p_{s,w'} \cdot (d_w + d_{w'} - 2 \cdot \mu_s), w' \neq w,$$

for $1 \leq w, w' \leq K$ and $1 \leq j, j' \leq r$. $\boldsymbol{E}'(\boldsymbol{\gamma})$ has the same formulation as in Sect. 12.1.1 as does $\boldsymbol{E}'(\boldsymbol{\beta},\boldsymbol{\gamma})$, but using the revised $xstde_{s,w,j}$.

12.1.4.2 Ordinal Probabilities

$\boldsymbol{E}(\boldsymbol{\beta})$ is the $(K + r) \times 1$ vector equaling the sum over $s \in S$ of $\boldsymbol{E}_s(\boldsymbol{\beta})$ with entries

$$E_{s,w}(\boldsymbol{\beta}) = xstde_{s,w} \cdot stde_s,$$
$$E_{s,K,j}(\boldsymbol{\beta}) = xstde_{s,K,j} \cdot stde_s,$$

where

$$xstde_{s,w} = \frac{\partial \mu_s}{\partial \alpha_w} / \sigma_s,$$
$$\frac{\partial \mu_s}{\partial \alpha_w} = p_{s,\leq w} \cdot \left(1 - p_{s,\leq w}\right) \cdot \left(d_w - d_{w-1}\right),$$
$$xstde_{s,K,j} = \frac{\partial \mu_s}{\partial \beta_{K,j}} / \sigma_s,$$
$$\frac{\partial \mu_s}{\partial \beta_{K,j}} = x_{s,j} \cdot \sum_{u=0}^{K-1} \left(p_{s,\leq u} \cdot \left(1 - p_{s,\leq u}\right) \cdot \left(d_u - d_{u-1}\right)\right),$$

for $0 \leq w < K$ and $1 \leq j \leq r$. $\boldsymbol{E}(\boldsymbol{\gamma})$ has the same formulation as in Sect. 12.1.2. $\boldsymbol{E}'(\boldsymbol{\theta})$ has four component matrices: the $(K + r) \times (K + r)$ matrix

$$\boldsymbol{E}'(\boldsymbol{\beta}) = \frac{\partial \boldsymbol{E}(\boldsymbol{\beta})}{\partial \boldsymbol{\beta}}$$

for the $K + r$ mean coefficients, the $q \times q$ matrix

$$\boldsymbol{E}'(\boldsymbol{\gamma}) = \frac{\partial \boldsymbol{E}(\boldsymbol{\gamma})}{\partial \boldsymbol{\gamma}}$$

for the q dispersion coefficients, the $(K + r) \times q$ matrix

$$\boldsymbol{E}'(\boldsymbol{\beta}, \boldsymbol{\gamma}) = \frac{\partial \boldsymbol{E}(\boldsymbol{\beta})}{\partial \boldsymbol{\gamma}},$$

and its transpose $\boldsymbol{E}'(\boldsymbol{\gamma}, \boldsymbol{\beta}) = \boldsymbol{E}'^{\mathrm{T}}(\boldsymbol{\beta}, \boldsymbol{\gamma})$. $\boldsymbol{E}'(\boldsymbol{\beta})$ is the sum over $s \in S$ of $\boldsymbol{E}'_s(\boldsymbol{\beta})$ with entries

$$E'_{s,w,w'}(\boldsymbol{\beta}) = -xxstde_{s,w,w'} \cdot stde_s - xstde_{s,w} \cdot xstde_{s,w'},$$
$$E'_{s,w,K,j}(\boldsymbol{\beta}) = -xxstde_{s,w,K,j} \cdot stde_s - xstde_{s,w} \cdot xstde_{s,K,j},$$

$$E'_{s,K\,j,w'}(\boldsymbol{\beta}) = -\,xxstde_{s,K\,j,w'} \cdot stde_s - xstde_{s,K\,j} \cdot xstde_{s,w'}/2,$$

$$E'_{s,K\,j,j'}(\boldsymbol{\beta}) = -\,xxstde_{s,K\,j,j'} \cdot stde_s - xstde_{s,K\,j} \cdot xstde_{s,K\,j'}/2,$$

where

$$xxstde_{s,w,w'} = -\frac{\partial^2 \mu_s}{\partial \alpha_{w'}\,\partial \alpha_w}/\sigma_s,$$

$$\frac{\partial^2 \mu_s}{\partial \alpha_{w'}\,\partial \alpha_w} = p_{s,\le w} \cdot \left(1 - p_{s,\le w}\right) \cdot \left(1 - 2 \cdot p_{s,\le w}\right) \cdot (d_w - d_{w+1}),\ w' = w,$$

$$\frac{\partial^2 \mu_s}{\partial \alpha_{w'}\,\partial \alpha_w} = 0,\ w' \ne w;$$

$$xxstde_{s,w,K\,j} = -\frac{\partial^2 \mu_s}{\partial \beta_{K\,j}\,\partial \alpha_w}/\sigma_s,$$

$$\frac{\partial^2 \mu_s}{\partial \beta_{K\,j}\,\partial \alpha_w} = x_{s,j} \cdot p_{s,\le w} \cdot \left(1 - p_{s,\le w}\right) \cdot \left(1 - 2 \cdot p_{s,\le w}\right) \cdot (d_w - d_{w+1});$$

$$xxstde_{s,K\,j,w'} = -\frac{\partial^2 \mu_s}{\partial \alpha_{w'}\,\partial \beta_{K\,j}}/\sigma_s,$$

$$\frac{\partial^2 \mu_s}{\partial \alpha_{w'}\,\partial \beta_{K\,j}} = x_{s,j} \cdot p_{s,\le w'} \cdot \left(1 - p_{s,\le w'}\right) \cdot \left(1 - 2 \cdot p_{s,\le w'}\right) \cdot (d_{w'} - d_{w'+1});$$

$$xxstde_{s,K\,j,j'} = -\frac{\partial^2 \mu_s}{\partial \beta_{K\,j'}\,\partial \beta_{K\,j}}/\sigma_s,$$

$$\frac{\partial^2 \mu_s}{\partial \beta_{K\,j'}\,\partial \beta_{K\,j}} = x_{s,j} \cdot x_{s,j'} \cdot \sum_{u=0}^{K-1} \left(p_{s,\le u} \cdot \left(1 - p_{s,\le u}\right) \cdot \left(1 - 2 \cdot p_{s,\le u}\right) \cdot (d_u - d_{u+1})\right),$$

for $1 \le w, w' < K$ and $1 \le j, j' \le r$. $\boldsymbol{E}'(\boldsymbol{\gamma})$ has the same formulation as in Sect. 12.1.1 as does $\boldsymbol{E}'(\boldsymbol{\beta}, \boldsymbol{\gamma})$, but using the revised $xstde_{s,w,j}$.

12.1.4.3 Censored Poisson Probabilities

$\boldsymbol{E}(\boldsymbol{\beta})$ is the $r \times 1$ vector equaling the sum over $s \in S$ of $\boldsymbol{E}_s(\boldsymbol{\beta})$ with entries

$$E_{s,j}(\boldsymbol{\beta}) = xstde_{s,j} \cdot stde_s$$

where

$$xstde_{s,j} = \frac{\partial \mu_s}{\partial \beta_j} / \sigma_s,$$

$$\frac{\partial \mu_s}{\partial \beta_j} = \sum_{u=0}^{K-1} (d_u - d_K) \cdot \frac{\partial p_{s,u}}{\partial \beta_j},$$

for $1 \le j \le r$ where $\frac{\partial p_{s,u}}{\partial \beta_j}$ for $0 \le u \le K$ are defined in Sect. 12.1.3. $\boldsymbol{E}(\boldsymbol{\gamma})$ has the same formulation as in Sect. 12.1.3. $\boldsymbol{E}'(\boldsymbol{\theta})$ has four component matrices: the $r \times r$ matrix

$$\boldsymbol{E}'(\boldsymbol{\beta}) = \frac{\partial \boldsymbol{E}(\boldsymbol{\beta})}{\partial \boldsymbol{\beta}}$$

for the r mean coefficients, the $q \times q$ matrix

$$\boldsymbol{E}'(\boldsymbol{\gamma}) = \frac{\partial \boldsymbol{E}(\boldsymbol{\gamma})}{\partial \boldsymbol{\gamma}}$$

for the q dispersion coefficients, the $r \times q$ matrix

$$\boldsymbol{E}'(\boldsymbol{\beta}, \boldsymbol{\gamma}) = \frac{\partial \boldsymbol{E}(\boldsymbol{\beta})}{\partial \boldsymbol{\gamma}},$$

and its transpose $\boldsymbol{E}'(\boldsymbol{\gamma}, \boldsymbol{\beta}) = \boldsymbol{E}'^{\mathrm{T}}(\boldsymbol{\beta}, \boldsymbol{\gamma})$. $\boldsymbol{E}'(\boldsymbol{\beta})$ is the sum over $s \in S$ of $\boldsymbol{E}'_s(\boldsymbol{\beta})$ with entries

$$E'_{s,j,j'}(\boldsymbol{\beta}) = -xxstde_{s,j,j'} \cdot stde_s - xstde_{s,j} \cdot xstde_{s,j'}$$

where

$$xxstde_{s,j,j'} = -\frac{\partial^2 \mu_s}{\partial \beta_{j'} \partial \beta_j} / \sigma_s,$$

$$\frac{\partial^2 \mu_s}{\partial \beta_{j'} \partial \beta_j} = \sum_{u=0}^{K-1} (d_u - d_K) \cdot \frac{\partial^2 p_{s,u}}{\partial \beta_{j'} \partial \beta_j},$$

for $1 \le j, j' \le r$ where $\frac{\partial^2 p_{s,u}}{\partial \beta_{j'} \partial \beta_j}$ is defined in Sect. 12.1.3. $\boldsymbol{E}'(\boldsymbol{\gamma})$ has the same formulation as in Sect. 12.1.1 as does $\boldsymbol{E}'(\boldsymbol{\beta}, \boldsymbol{\gamma})$, but using the revised $xstde_{s,w,j}$.

12.2 Correlated Univariate Discrete Outcomes

Using the notation of Sect. 2.1, let y_{sc} for $sc \in SC$ be discrete outcomes with a finite number of increasing values d_u for $0 \leq u \leq K$ and associated probabilities $p_{sc,u} = \mathrm{P}(y_{sc} = d_u)$ for $0 \leq u \leq K$. The means of such univariate discrete outcomes satisfy

$$\mu_{sc} = \mathrm{E}y_{sc} = \sum_{u=0}^{K} d_u \cdot p_{sc,u}$$

while their variances satisfy

$$\mathrm{Var}(y_{sc}) = \sum_{u=0}^{K} (d_u - \mu_{sc})^2 \cdot p_{sc,u} = \left(\sum_{u=0}^{K} d_u^2 \cdot p_{sc,u}\right) - \mu_{sc}^2 = \mathrm{E}y_{sc}^2 - \mu_{sc}^2.$$

This variance is not a direct function $V(\mu_{sc})$ of the means as in generalized linear modeling, but it can be considered a function $V(\boldsymbol{p}_{sc})$ of the vector $\boldsymbol{p}_{sc}$ of probabilities $p_{sc,u}$ for the outcome y_{sc}. This distinction is not utilized in formulations that follow. Models are expressed instead in terms of $\mathrm{Var}(y_{sc})$. Define the residuals as $e_{sc} = y_{sc} - \mu_{sc}$. Combine y_{sc}, μ_{sc}, and e_{sc} over $c \in C(s)$ into the $m(s) \times 1$ vectors $\boldsymbol{y}_s$, $\boldsymbol{\mu}_s$, and $\boldsymbol{e}_s = \boldsymbol{y}_s - \boldsymbol{\mu}_s$. Probabilities for these correlated discrete outcomes can be multinomial as addressed in Sect. 12.2.1, ordinal as addressed in Sect. 12.2.2, or censored Poisson as addressed in Sect. 12.2.3. Section 12.2.4 addresses direct variance modeling of correlated univariate discrete outcomes.

Standard GEE, partially modified GEE, fully modified GEE, and ELMM extend to correlated discrete outcomes similarly to formulations provided in Chaps. 2–5, respectively. Details are provided in what follows. The likelihood function $L(SC;\boldsymbol{\theta})$ of Sect. 2.5, LCV scores of Sect. 2.6, and the adaptive modeling process of Sect. 2.7 apply to modeling of discrete outcomes using multinomial, ordinal, and censored Poisson probabilities.

12.2.1 Multinomial Probabilities

For predictor values $x_{sc,j}$, combine them over $1 \leq j \leq r$ into the $r \times 1$ vectors $\boldsymbol{x}_{sc}$ for $sc \in SC$. Let $\boldsymbol{X}_s$ denote the $m(s) \times r$ predictor matrix with rows $\boldsymbol{x}_{sc}^{\mathrm{T}}$. The probabilities $p_{sc,u}$ are modeled multinomially using generalized logits with the smallest value d_0 as the reference category (but any other value can be used instead) as follows:

$$g(p_{sc,u}) = \log \frac{p_{sc,u}}{p_{sc,0}} = \boldsymbol{x}_{sc}^{\mathrm{T}} \cdot \boldsymbol{\beta}_u$$

for K $r \times 1$ vectors $\boldsymbol{\beta}_u$ of coefficient parameters $\beta_{u,j}$ for $1 \leq u \leq K$ and $1 \leq j \leq r$. Combine the vectors $\boldsymbol{\beta}_u$ over $1 \leq u \leq K$ into the composite $(K \cdot r) \times 1$ vector $\boldsymbol{\beta}$. For $sc \in SC$, the probabilities satisfy

$$p_{sc,u} = \frac{\exp\left(\boldsymbol{x}_{sc}^{\mathrm{T}} \cdot \boldsymbol{\beta}_u\right)}{1 + \sum_{u'=1}^{K} \exp\left(\boldsymbol{x}_{sc}^{\mathrm{T}} \cdot \boldsymbol{\beta}_{u'}\right)}$$

for $1 \leq u \leq K$ and

$$p_{sc,0} = \frac{1}{1 + \sum_{u'=1}^{K} \exp\left(\boldsymbol{x}_{sc}^{\mathrm{T}} \cdot \boldsymbol{\beta}_{u'}\right)}.$$

Their first partial derivatives satisfy

$$\frac{\partial p_{sc,u}}{\partial \beta_{w,j}} = x_{sc,j} \cdot p_{sc,w} \cdot \left(1 - p_{sc,w}\right), w = u,$$

$$\frac{\partial p_{sc,u}}{\partial \beta_{w,j}} = -x_{sc,j} \cdot p_{sc,u} \cdot p_{sc,w}, w \neq u,$$

and

$$\frac{\partial p_{sc,0}}{\partial \beta_{w,j}} = -x_{sc,j} \cdot p_{sc,0} \cdot p_{sc,w},$$

for $1 \leq u, w \leq K$, $1 \leq j \leq r$, and $sc \in SC$. In what follows, extensions are provided for standard GEE modeling (Sect. 12.2.1.1), partially modified GEE modeling (Sect. 12.2.1.2), fully modified GEE modeling (Sect. 12.2.1.3), and extended linear mixed modeling (Sect. 12.2.1.4).

12.2.1.1 Standard GEE Modeling

The formulations of Chap. 2 apply except that $\mathrm{Var}(y_{sc})$ is no longer a simple function of the means μ_{sc}. The constant dispersions are still based on a constant parameter φ as in Sect. 2.2 . Define the extended variances

$$\sigma_{sc}^2 = \varphi \cdot \mathrm{Var}(y_{sc}),$$

the standardized residuals

$$stde_{sc} = e_{sc}/\sigma_{sc},$$

and the Pearson residuals

$$Pres_{sc} = \frac{e_{sc}}{\mathrm{Var}^{1/2}(y_{sc})}$$

for $sc \in SC$. Combine these, respectively, into the $m(s) \times 1$ vectors $\boldsymbol{\sigma}_s$, $\boldsymbol{stde}_s$, and $\boldsymbol{Pres}_s$ ordered by their values $c \in C(s)$. Model the $m(s) \times m(s)$ covariance matrices $\boldsymbol{\Sigma}_s$ as

$$\boldsymbol{\Sigma}_s = \boldsymbol{DIAG}(\boldsymbol{\sigma}_s) \cdot \boldsymbol{R}_s(\boldsymbol{\rho}) \cdot \boldsymbol{DIAG}(\boldsymbol{\sigma}_s)$$

for appropriate choices of the $m(s) \times m(s)$ correlation matrices $\boldsymbol{R}_s(\boldsymbol{\rho})$ for $s \in S$. The estimating equations for the mean parameters

$$\boldsymbol{E}(\boldsymbol{\beta}) = \sum_{s \in S} \boldsymbol{E}_s(\boldsymbol{\beta}) = \sum_{s \in S} \boldsymbol{D}_s^{\mathrm{T}} \cdot \boldsymbol{\Sigma}_s^{-1} \cdot \boldsymbol{e}_s,$$

are based on the $m(s) \times (K \cdot r)$ matrices

$$\boldsymbol{D}_s = \frac{\partial \boldsymbol{\mu}_s}{\partial \boldsymbol{\beta}}$$

for $s \in S$ with entries

$$D_{sc,w,j} = \frac{\partial \mu_{sc}}{\partial \beta_{w,j}} = x_{sc,j} \cdot p_{sc,w} \cdot (d_w - \mu_{sc})$$

for $sc \in SC$, $1 \le w \le K$, and $1 \le j \le r$ while

$$\boldsymbol{E}'(\boldsymbol{\beta}) = -\sum_{s \in S} \boldsymbol{D}_s^{\mathrm{T}} \cdot \boldsymbol{\Sigma}_s^{-1} \cdot \boldsymbol{D}_s.$$

The bias-adjusted estimate of the constant dispersion parameter φ for a given value of the coefficient parameter vector $\boldsymbol{\beta}$ is

$$\varphi(\boldsymbol{\beta}) = \frac{\sum_{s \in S} \boldsymbol{Pres}_s^{\mathrm{T}}(\boldsymbol{\beta}) \cdot \boldsymbol{Pres}_s(\boldsymbol{\beta})}{m(SC) - r}$$

assuming $m(SC) - r > 0$. Compute correlation estimates for the correlation structures of Sect. 2.3 using the formulas of Sect. 2.4.1. Model-based and robust empirical estimates of the covariance matrix for the standard GEE estimate $\boldsymbol{\beta}(SC)$ of the mean coefficient parameter vector $\boldsymbol{\beta}$ can be computed as in Sect. 2.4.2.

12.2.1.2 Partially Modified GEE Modeling

The formulation of Chap. 3 applies with $V(\mu_{sc})$ replaced by $\mathrm{Var}(y_{sc})$. For predictor values $v_{sc,j}$, combine them over $1 \le j \le q$ into the $q \times 1$ vectors $\boldsymbol{v}_{sc}$ for $sc \in SC$, and model the natural log of the non-constant dispersions in terms of these predictor values, that is,

$$\log \varphi_{sc} = \boldsymbol{v}_{sc}^{\mathrm{T}} \cdot \boldsymbol{\gamma}$$

where $\boldsymbol{\gamma}$ is a $q \times 1$ vector of coefficient parameters. Let $\boldsymbol{V}_s$ denote the $m(s) \times q$ predictor matrix with rows $\boldsymbol{v}_{sc}^{\mathrm{T}}$. Define the extended variances as

$$\sigma_{sc}^2 = \varphi_{sc} \cdot V(\mu_{sc})$$

and the standardized residuals as

$$stde_{sc} = e_{sc}/\sigma_{sc}.$$

Combine the extended standard deviations and standardized residuals over $c \in C(s)$ into the $m(s) \times 1$ vectors $\boldsymbol{\sigma}_s$ and $\boldsymbol{stde}_s$ for $s \in S$.

Denote an observation by $O_s = \{\boldsymbol{y}_s, \boldsymbol{X}_s, \boldsymbol{V}_s\}$ and define the likelihood function $L(SC;\boldsymbol{\theta})$ to be the product of terms $L(O_s;\boldsymbol{\theta})$ for $s \in S$ satisfying

$$\ell(O_s;\boldsymbol{\theta}) = \log L(O_s;\boldsymbol{\theta}) = -\boldsymbol{e}_s^{\mathrm{T}} \cdot \boldsymbol{\Sigma}_s^{-1} \cdot \boldsymbol{e}_s/2 - (\log|\boldsymbol{\Sigma}_s|)/2 - (m(s) \cdot \log(2 \cdot \pi))/2$$

where

$$\boldsymbol{\theta} = \begin{pmatrix} \boldsymbol{\beta} \\ \boldsymbol{\gamma} \end{pmatrix}$$

and the $m(s) \times m(s)$ covariance matrix $\boldsymbol{\Sigma}_s$ of $\boldsymbol{y}_s$ satisfies

$$\boldsymbol{\Sigma}_s = \boldsymbol{DIAG}(\boldsymbol{\sigma}_s) \cdot \boldsymbol{R}_s(\rho) \cdot \boldsymbol{DIAG}(\boldsymbol{\sigma}_s)$$

for appropriate choices of the $m(s) \times m(s)$ correlation matrices $\boldsymbol{R}_s(\rho)$ for $s \in S$. Estimating equations $\boldsymbol{E}(\boldsymbol{\gamma}) = \boldsymbol{0}$ for the dispersion parameters can be generated by maximizing the likelihood $L(SC;\boldsymbol{\theta})$ in $\boldsymbol{\gamma}$, that is,

$$\boldsymbol{E}(\boldsymbol{\gamma}) = \frac{\partial_0 \ell(SC;\boldsymbol{\theta})}{\partial_0 \boldsymbol{\gamma}}$$

where the operator notation $\frac{\partial_0}{\partial_0 \gamma}$ is used to indicate that this is not the full partial derivative vector for $\ell(SC;\boldsymbol{\theta})$ in $\boldsymbol{\gamma}$ due to not accounting for the effect of $\boldsymbol{\gamma}$ on $\boldsymbol{R}_s(\boldsymbol{\rho})$. $\boldsymbol{E}(\boldsymbol{\gamma})$ is the sum over $s \in S$ of $\boldsymbol{E}_s(\boldsymbol{\gamma})$ with entries

$$E_{s,j}(\boldsymbol{\gamma}) = \boldsymbol{vstde}_{s,j}^{\mathrm{T}} \cdot \boldsymbol{R}_s^{-1}(\boldsymbol{\rho}) \cdot \boldsymbol{stde}_s - \sum_{c \in C(s)} v_{sc,j}/2$$

where $\boldsymbol{vstde}_{s,j}$ is the $m(s) \times 1$ vector with entries

$$vstde_{sc,j} = v_{sc,j} \cdot stde_{sc}/2$$

for $sc \in SC$ and $1 \le j \le q$. Now, combine these with the $K \cdot r$ standard GEE mean estimating equations $\boldsymbol{E}(\boldsymbol{\beta}) = \boldsymbol{0}$ to solve for joint estimates of $\boldsymbol{\beta}$ and $\boldsymbol{\gamma}$. Then, use Newton's method to iteratively solve for

$$\boldsymbol{E}(\boldsymbol{\theta}) = \begin{pmatrix} \boldsymbol{E}(\boldsymbol{\beta}) \\ \boldsymbol{E}(\boldsymbol{\gamma}) \end{pmatrix} = \boldsymbol{0}$$

with $\boldsymbol{E}(\boldsymbol{\theta})$ in the role of the gradient vector and the $(K \cdot r + q) \times (K \cdot r + q)$ matrix $\boldsymbol{E}'(\boldsymbol{\theta})$ in the role of the Hessian matrix.

$\boldsymbol{E}'(\boldsymbol{\theta})$ has four component matrices: the $(K \cdot r) \times (K \cdot r)$ matrix $\boldsymbol{E}'(\boldsymbol{\beta})$ for the $K \cdot r$ mean coefficients as used in standard GEE modeling, the $q \times q$ matrix

$$\boldsymbol{E}'(\boldsymbol{\gamma}) = \frac{\partial_0 \boldsymbol{E}(\boldsymbol{\gamma})}{\partial_0 \boldsymbol{\gamma}}$$

for the q dispersion coefficients, the $(K \cdot r) \times q$ matrix

$$\boldsymbol{E}'(\boldsymbol{\beta}, \boldsymbol{\gamma}) = \frac{\partial_0 \boldsymbol{E}(\boldsymbol{\beta})}{\partial_0 \boldsymbol{\gamma}},$$

and its transpose $\boldsymbol{E}'(\boldsymbol{\gamma}, \boldsymbol{\beta}) = \boldsymbol{E}'^{\mathrm{T}}(\boldsymbol{\beta}, \boldsymbol{\gamma})$. $\boldsymbol{E}'(\boldsymbol{\gamma})$ is the sum over $s \in S$ of $\boldsymbol{E}'_s(\boldsymbol{\gamma})$ with entries

$$E'_{s,j,j'}(\boldsymbol{\gamma}) = -\boldsymbol{vvstde}_{s,j,j'}^{\mathrm{T}} \cdot \boldsymbol{R}_s^{-1}(\boldsymbol{\rho}) \cdot \boldsymbol{stde}_s - \boldsymbol{vstde}_{s,j}^{\mathrm{T}} \cdot \boldsymbol{R}_s^{-1}(\boldsymbol{\rho}) \cdot \boldsymbol{vstde}_{s,j'}$$

where $\boldsymbol{vvstde}_{s,j,j'}$ is the $m(s) \times 1$ vector with entries

$$vvstde_{sc,j,j'} = v_{sc,j} \cdot v_{sc,j'} \cdot stde_{sc}/4$$

for $sc \in SC$ and $1 \le j, j' \le q$. $\boldsymbol{E}'(\boldsymbol{\beta}, \boldsymbol{\gamma})$ is the sum over $s \in S$ of $\boldsymbol{E}'_s(\boldsymbol{\beta}, \boldsymbol{\gamma})$ with q $(K \cdot r) \times 1$ column vectors

$$\begin{aligned}\boldsymbol{E}'_{s,j}(\boldsymbol{\beta},\boldsymbol{\gamma}) &= -\boldsymbol{D}_s^{\mathrm{T}}\cdot\boldsymbol{DIAG}(\boldsymbol{v\sigma inv}_{s,j})\cdot\boldsymbol{R}_s^{-1}(\boldsymbol{\rho})\cdot\boldsymbol{stde}_s\\ &-\boldsymbol{D}_s^{\mathrm{T}}\cdot\boldsymbol{DIAG}(\mathbf{1}/\boldsymbol{\sigma}_s)\cdot\boldsymbol{R}_s^{-1}(\boldsymbol{\rho})\cdot\boldsymbol{vstde}_{s,j}\end{aligned}$$

where $\boldsymbol{v\sigma inv}_{s,j}$ is the $m(s)\times 1$ vector with entries

$$v\sigma inv_{sc,j}=\frac{v_{sc,j}}{2\cdot\sigma_{sc}}$$

for $sc\in SC$ and $1\le j\le q$. Model-based and robust empirical estimates of the covariance matrix for the partially modified GEE estimate $\boldsymbol{\theta}(SC)$ of the mean coefficient parameter vector $\boldsymbol{\theta}$ can be computed as in Sect. 3.4.

Given a value for the vector $\boldsymbol{\theta}$ of all coefficient parameters, an estimate of the correlation parameter vector $\boldsymbol{\rho}$ can be based on the associated standardized residuals $stde_{sc}(\boldsymbol{\theta})$ determined by non-constant dispersions $\varphi_{sc}(\boldsymbol{\gamma})$ computed with the current value for $\boldsymbol{\gamma}$. Calculate the revised correlation estimates for the correlation structures of Sect. 2.3 using the formulas of Sect. 2.4.1 evaluated with the revised standardized residuals $stde_{sc}(\boldsymbol{\theta})$.

12.2.1.3 Fully Modified GEE Modeling

The formulation of Chap. 4 applies with $V(\mu_{sc})$ replaced by $\mathrm{Var}(y_{sc})$ extending the formulation of Sect. 12.2.1.2 using the same likelihood function $L(SC;\boldsymbol{\theta})$ and

$$\boldsymbol{E}(\boldsymbol{\theta})=\begin{pmatrix}\boldsymbol{E}(\boldsymbol{\beta})\\ \boldsymbol{E}(\boldsymbol{\gamma})\end{pmatrix}$$

with $\boldsymbol{E}(\boldsymbol{\gamma})$ computed as in Sect. 12.2.1.2.

$$\boldsymbol{E}(\boldsymbol{\beta})=\frac{\partial_0\ell(SC;\boldsymbol{\theta})}{\partial_0\boldsymbol{\beta}}$$

is the sum over $s\in S$ of $\boldsymbol{E}_s(\boldsymbol{\beta})$ with entries

$$E_{s,w,j}(\boldsymbol{\beta})=\boldsymbol{xstde}_{s,w,j}^{\mathrm{T}}\cdot\boldsymbol{R}_s^{-1}(\boldsymbol{\rho})\cdot\boldsymbol{stde}_s-\sum_{c\in C(s)}W_{sc,w,j}/2$$

where $\boldsymbol{xstde}_{s,w,j}$ is the $m(s)\times 1$ vector with entries

$$xstde_{sc,w,j}=\frac{\partial\mu_{sc}}{\partial\beta_{w,j}}/\sigma_{sc}+stde_{sc}\cdot W_{sc,w,j}/2,$$

$$W_{sc,w,j} = \frac{\frac{\partial \mathrm{Var}(y_{sc})}{\partial \beta_{w,j}}}{\mathrm{Var}(y_{sc})},$$

$$\frac{\partial \mathrm{Var}(y_{sc})}{\partial \beta_{w,j}} = x_{sc,j} \cdot p_{sc,w} \cdot \left(d_w^2 - \mathrm{E}y_{sc}^2 - 2 \cdot \mu_{sc} \cdot (d_w - \mu_{sc})\right),$$

and $\frac{\partial \mu_{sc}}{\partial \beta_{w,j}}$ is defined in Sect. 12.2.1.1, for $1 \le w \le K$, $1 \le j \le r$, and $sc \in SC$. As before, use Newton's method to iteratively solve $\boldsymbol{E}(\boldsymbol{\theta}) = \boldsymbol{0}$. The correlation estimates are the same as those in Sect. 12.2.1.2.

$\boldsymbol{E}'(\boldsymbol{\theta})$ has four component matrices: the $(K \cdot r) \times (K \cdot r)$ matrix

$$\boldsymbol{E}'(\boldsymbol{\beta}) = \frac{\partial_0 \boldsymbol{E}(\boldsymbol{\beta})}{\partial_0 \boldsymbol{\beta}}$$

for the $K \cdot r$ mean coefficients, the $q \times q$ matrix

$$\boldsymbol{E}'(\boldsymbol{\gamma}) = \frac{\partial_0 \boldsymbol{E}(\boldsymbol{\gamma})}{\partial_0 \boldsymbol{\gamma}}$$

for the q dispersion coefficients as computed in Sect. 12.2.1.2, the $(K \cdot r) \times q$ matrix

$$\boldsymbol{E}'(\boldsymbol{\beta}, \boldsymbol{\gamma}) = \frac{\partial_0 \boldsymbol{E}(\boldsymbol{\beta})}{\partial_0 \boldsymbol{\gamma}},$$

and its transpose $\boldsymbol{E}'(\boldsymbol{\gamma}, \boldsymbol{\beta}) = \boldsymbol{E}'^{\mathrm{T}}(\boldsymbol{\beta}, \boldsymbol{\gamma})$. $\boldsymbol{E}'(\boldsymbol{\beta})$ is the sum over $s \in S$ of $\boldsymbol{E}'_s(\boldsymbol{\beta})$ with entries

$$E'_{s,w,j,w',j'}(\boldsymbol{\beta}) = -\boldsymbol{xxstde}^{\mathrm{T}}_{s,wj,w',j'} \cdot \boldsymbol{R}_s^{-1}(\boldsymbol{\rho}) \cdot \boldsymbol{stde}_s$$
$$- \boldsymbol{xstde}^{\mathrm{T}}_{s,w,j} \cdot \boldsymbol{R}_s^{-1}(\boldsymbol{\rho}) \cdot \boldsymbol{xstde}_{s,w',j'} - \sum_{c \in C(s)} W_{sc,w,j,w',j'}/2$$

where $\boldsymbol{xxstde}_{s,w,j,w',j'}$ is the $m(s) \times 1$ vector with entries

$$xxstde_{sc,w,j,w',j'} = -\frac{\frac{\partial^2 \mu_{sc}}{\partial \beta_{w',j'} \partial \beta_{w,j}}}{\sigma_{sc}} + \frac{\partial \mu_{sc}}{\partial \beta_{w,j}} \cdot \frac{W_{sc,w',j'}}{2 \cdot \sigma_{sc}} + xstde_{sc,w',j'} \cdot \frac{W_{sc,w,j}}{2}$$
$$- stde_{sc} \cdot \frac{W_{sc,w,j,w',j'}}{2},$$

$$\frac{\partial^2 \mu_{sc}}{\partial \beta_{w',j'} \partial \beta_{w,j}} = x_{sc,j} \cdot x_{sc,j'} \cdot p_{sc,w} \cdot \left(1 - 2 \cdot p_{sc,w}\right) \cdot (d_w - \mu_{sc}), w' = w,$$

$$\frac{\partial^2 \mu_{sc}}{\partial \beta_{w',j'}\,\partial \beta_{w,j}} = -x_{sc,j} \cdot x_{sc,j'} \cdot p_{sc,w} \cdot p_{sc,w'} \cdot (d_w + d_{w'} - 2 \cdot \mu_{sc}), w' \neq w,$$

$$W_{sc,w,j,w',j'} = \frac{\partial W_{sc,w,j}}{\partial \beta_{w',j'}} = \frac{\frac{\partial^2 \mathrm{Var}(y_{sc})}{\partial \beta_{w',j'}\,\partial \beta_{w,j}}}{\mathrm{Var}(y_{sc})} - \frac{\frac{\partial \mathrm{Var}(y_{sc})}{\partial \beta_{w',j'}} \cdot \frac{\partial \mathrm{Var}(y_{sc})}{\partial \beta_{w,j}}}{\mathrm{Var}^2(y_{sc})},$$

$$\frac{\partial^2 \mathrm{Var}(y_{sc})}{\partial \beta_{w',j'}\,\partial \beta_{w,j}} = x_{sc,j} \cdot x_{sc,j'} \cdot p_{sc,w} \cdot (1 - p_{sc,w}) \cdot (d_w^2 - \mathrm{E}y_{sc}^2 - 2 \cdot \mu_{sc} \cdot (d_w - \mu_{sc}))$$

$$+x_{sc,j} \cdot x_{sc,j'} \cdot p_{sc,w}^2 \cdot (\mathrm{E}y_{sc}^2 - d_w^2 + 2 \cdot (2 \cdot \mu_{sc} - d_w) \cdot (d_w - \mu_{sc})), w' = w,$$

$$\frac{\partial^2 \mathrm{Var}(y_{sc})}{\partial \beta_{w',j'}\,\partial \beta_{w,j}} = -x_{sc,j} \cdot x_{sc,j'} \cdot p_{sc,w} \cdot p_{sc,w'} \cdot (d_w^2 - \mathrm{E}y_{sc}^2 - 2 \cdot \mu_{sc} \cdot (d_w - \mu_{sc}))$$

$$+x_{sc,j} \cdot x_{sc,j'} \cdot p_{sc,w} \cdot p_{sc,w'} \cdot (\mathrm{E}y_{sc}^2 - d_{w'}^2 + 2 \cdot (2 \cdot \mu_{sc} - d_{w'}) \cdot (d_{w'} - \mu_{sc})), w' \neq w,$$

for $1 \leq w, w' \leq K$ and $1 \leq j, j' \leq r$. $\boldsymbol{E}'(\boldsymbol{\beta},\boldsymbol{\gamma})$ is the sum over $s \in S$ of $\boldsymbol{E}'_s(\boldsymbol{\beta},\boldsymbol{\gamma})$ with entries

$$E'_{s,w,j,j'}(\boldsymbol{\beta},\boldsymbol{\gamma}) = -\boldsymbol{vxstde}_{s,w,j,j'}^{\mathrm{T}} \cdot \boldsymbol{R}_s^{-1}(\boldsymbol{\rho}) \cdot \boldsymbol{stde}_s - \boldsymbol{xstde}_{s,w,j}^{\mathrm{T}} \cdot \boldsymbol{R}_s^{-1}(\boldsymbol{\rho}) \cdot \boldsymbol{vstde}_{s,j'}$$

where $\boldsymbol{vxstde}_{s,w,j,j'}$ is the $m(s) \times 1$ vector with entries

$$vxstde_{sc,w,j,j'} = xstde_{sc,w,j} \cdot v_{sc,j'}/2$$

and $\boldsymbol{vstde}_{s,j'}$ is defined in Sect. 12.2.1.2 for $sc \in SC$, $1 \leq w \leq K$, $1 \leq j \leq r$, and $1 \leq j' \leq q$. Model-based and robust empirical estimates of the covariance matrix for the fully modified GEE estimate $\boldsymbol{\theta}(SC)$ of the mean coefficient parameter vector $\boldsymbol{\theta}$ can be computed as in Sect. 4.1.

12.2.1.4 Extended Linear Mixed Modeling

The formulation of Chap. 5 applies with $V(\mu_{sc})$ replaced by $\mathrm{Var}(y_{sc})$ extending the formulation of Sect. 12.2.1.3. The likelihood function $L(SC;\boldsymbol{\theta})$ is the same as defined in Sect. 12.2.1.2 except that the parameter vector is now

$$\boldsymbol{\theta} = \begin{pmatrix} \boldsymbol{\beta} \\ \boldsymbol{\gamma} \\ \boldsymbol{\rho} \end{pmatrix}$$

with $K \cdot r + q + p$ entries where p is the number of correlation parameters. The likelihood $L(SC;\boldsymbol{\theta})$ is maximized in the coefficient parameter vector $\boldsymbol{\theta}$. Specifically, use Newton's method to solve the estimating equations

$$\boldsymbol{E}(\boldsymbol{\theta}) = \frac{\partial \ell(SC;\boldsymbol{\theta})}{\partial \boldsymbol{\theta}} = \sum_{s \in S} \boldsymbol{E}_s(\boldsymbol{\theta}) = \sum_{s \in S} \frac{\partial \ell(O_s;\boldsymbol{\theta})}{\partial \boldsymbol{\theta}} = \mathbf{0}$$

where the operator notation $\frac{\partial}{\partial \theta}$ is used to indicate that this is a standard partial derivative vector in $\boldsymbol{\theta}$ since $\boldsymbol{\rho}$ is treated as a separate parameter vector. The associated matrix

$$\boldsymbol{E}'(\boldsymbol{\theta}) = \frac{\partial \boldsymbol{E}(\boldsymbol{\theta})}{\partial \boldsymbol{\theta}}.$$

In this case, $\boldsymbol{E}(\boldsymbol{\theta})$ is a true gradient vector and $\boldsymbol{E}'(\boldsymbol{\theta})$ a true Hessian matrix. The four correlation structures of Sect. 2.3 can still be considered. In all cases, there is just one alternative estimate of the correlation vector and not bias-adjusted and bias-unadjusted alternatives as for standard, partially modified, and fully modified GEE. The EC and spatial AR1 cases can be handled without storing associated correlation matrices (Sects. 5.3–5.4), providing efficient computation of associated estimates for data with relatively large numbers m of conditions.

The gradient vector satisfies

$$\boldsymbol{E}(\boldsymbol{\theta}) = \begin{pmatrix} \boldsymbol{E}(\boldsymbol{\beta}) \\ \boldsymbol{E}(\boldsymbol{\gamma}) \\ \boldsymbol{E}(\boldsymbol{\rho}) \end{pmatrix}$$

where $\boldsymbol{E}(\boldsymbol{\gamma})$ is computed as in Sect. 12.2.1.2 for partially modified GEE modeling and $\boldsymbol{E}(\boldsymbol{\beta})$ is computed as in Sect. 12.2.1.3 for fully modified GEE modeling since the correlation matrices do not depend on the dispersion parameters. With the entries of $\boldsymbol{\rho}$ denoted by ρ_j for $1 \le j \le p$,

$$\boldsymbol{E}(\boldsymbol{\rho}) = \frac{\partial \ell(SC;\boldsymbol{\theta})}{\partial \boldsymbol{\rho}}$$

is the sum over $s \in S$ of $\boldsymbol{E}_s(\boldsymbol{\rho})$ with entries

$$E_{s,j}(\boldsymbol{\rho}) = -\,\boldsymbol{stde}_s^{\mathrm{T}} \cdot \frac{\partial \boldsymbol{R}_s^{-1}(\boldsymbol{\rho})}{\partial \rho_j} \cdot \boldsymbol{stde}_s/2 - \frac{\partial \log|\boldsymbol{R}_s(\boldsymbol{\rho})|}{\partial \rho_j}/2$$

where $\boldsymbol{R}_s(\boldsymbol{\rho})$ changes with the correlation structure but does not depend on the mean and dispersion parameters.

$\boldsymbol{E}'(\boldsymbol{\theta})$ has nine component matrices: the $(K \cdot r) \times (K \cdot r)$ matrix

$$\boldsymbol{E}'(\boldsymbol{\beta}) = \frac{\partial \boldsymbol{E}(\boldsymbol{\beta})}{\partial \boldsymbol{\beta}}$$

for the $K \cdot r$ mean parameters computed as in Sect. 12.2.1.3 for fully modified GEE modeling, the $q \times q$ matrix

$$\boldsymbol{E}'(\boldsymbol{\gamma}) = \frac{\partial \boldsymbol{E}(\boldsymbol{\gamma})}{\partial \boldsymbol{\gamma}}$$

for the q dispersion parameters computed as in Sect. 12.2.1.2 for partially modified GEE modeling, the $p \times p$ matrix

$$\boldsymbol{E}'(\boldsymbol{\rho}) = \frac{\partial \boldsymbol{E}(\boldsymbol{\rho})}{\partial \boldsymbol{\rho}}$$

for the p correlation parameters, the $(K \cdot r) \times q$ matrix

$$\boldsymbol{E}'(\boldsymbol{\beta}, \boldsymbol{\gamma}) = \frac{\partial \boldsymbol{E}(\boldsymbol{\beta})}{\partial \boldsymbol{\gamma}}$$

and its transpose $\boldsymbol{E}'(\boldsymbol{\gamma}, \boldsymbol{\beta}) = \boldsymbol{E}'^{\mathrm{T}}(\boldsymbol{\beta}, \boldsymbol{\gamma})$ computed as in Sect. 12.2.1.3 for fully modified GEE modeling, the $(K \cdot r) \times p$ matrix

$$\boldsymbol{E}'(\boldsymbol{\beta}, \boldsymbol{\rho}) = \frac{\partial \boldsymbol{E}(\boldsymbol{\beta})}{\partial \boldsymbol{\rho}}$$

and its transpose $\boldsymbol{E}'(\boldsymbol{\rho}, \boldsymbol{\beta}) = \boldsymbol{E}'^{\mathrm{T}}(\boldsymbol{\beta}, \boldsymbol{\rho})$, the $q \times p$ matrix

$$\boldsymbol{E}'(\boldsymbol{\gamma}, \boldsymbol{\rho}) = \frac{\partial \boldsymbol{E}(\boldsymbol{\gamma})}{\partial \boldsymbol{\rho}}$$

and its transpose $\boldsymbol{E}'(\boldsymbol{\rho}, \boldsymbol{\gamma}) = \boldsymbol{E}'^{\mathrm{T}}(\boldsymbol{\gamma}, \boldsymbol{\rho})$. $\boldsymbol{E}'(\boldsymbol{\rho})$ is the sum over $s \in S$ of $\boldsymbol{E}'_s(\boldsymbol{\rho})$ with entries satisfying

$$E'_{s,j,j'}(\boldsymbol{\rho}) = -\boldsymbol{stde}_s^{\mathrm{T}} \cdot \frac{\partial^2 \boldsymbol{R}_s^{-1}(\boldsymbol{\rho})}{\partial \rho_{j'}\, \partial \rho_j} \cdot \boldsymbol{stde}_s/2 - \frac{\partial^2 \log|\boldsymbol{R}_s(\boldsymbol{\rho})|}{\partial \rho_{j'}\, \partial \rho_j}/2.$$

$\boldsymbol{E}'(\boldsymbol{\beta}, \boldsymbol{\rho})$ is the sum over $s \in S$ of $\boldsymbol{E}'_s(\boldsymbol{\beta}, \boldsymbol{\rho})$ with entries

$$E'_{s,w,j,j'}(\boldsymbol{\beta}, \boldsymbol{\rho}) = \boldsymbol{xstde}_{s,w,j}^{\mathrm{T}} \cdot \frac{\partial \boldsymbol{R}_s^{-1}(\boldsymbol{\rho})}{\partial \rho_{j'}} \cdot \boldsymbol{stde}_s$$

for $1 \le w \le K$, $1 \le j \le r$, and $1 \le j' \le p$ where $\boldsymbol{xstde}_{s,w,j}$ is defined in Sect. 12.2.1.3. $\boldsymbol{E}'(\boldsymbol{\gamma}, \boldsymbol{\rho})$ is the sum over $s \in S$ of $\boldsymbol{E}'_s(\boldsymbol{\gamma}, \boldsymbol{\rho})$ with entries

$$E'_{s,j,j'}(\gamma,\rho) = \boldsymbol{vstde}^{\mathrm{T}}_{s,w,j} \cdot \frac{\partial \boldsymbol{R}_s^{-1}(\rho)}{\partial \rho_{j'}} \cdot \boldsymbol{stde}_s$$

for $1 \le j \le q$ and $1 \le j' \le p$ where $\boldsymbol{vstde}_{s,w,j}$ is defined in Sect. 12.2.1.2. Formulations for first and second partial derivatives of $\log|\boldsymbol{R}_s(\boldsymbol{\rho})|$ and $\boldsymbol{R}_s^{-1}(\boldsymbol{\rho})$ with respect to $\boldsymbol{\rho}$ needed to compute $\boldsymbol{E}(\boldsymbol{\rho})$, $\boldsymbol{E}'(\boldsymbol{\rho})$, $\boldsymbol{E}'(\boldsymbol{\beta},\boldsymbol{\rho})$, and $\boldsymbol{E}'(\gamma,\boldsymbol{\rho})$ are provided in Sects. 5.3–5.5 for the EC, spatial AR1, and UN structures, respectively. These partial derivatives are dropped for the IND correlation structure. Model-based and robust empirical estimates of the covariance matrix for the ELMM estimate $\boldsymbol{\theta}(SC)$ of the parameter vector $\boldsymbol{\theta}$ can be computed as in Sect. 5.1.

12.2.2 Ordinal Probabilities

For $sc \in SC$, define cumulative probabilities

$$p_{sc,\le u} = \mathrm{P}(y_{sc} \le d_u), 0 \le u < K,$$
$$p_{sc,\le K} = \mathrm{P}(y_{sc} \le d_K) = 1.$$

The link function is cumulative logits computed for lower sets of values relative to higher sets of values (but this can be reversed). This assumes that outcome values are in increasing order. Formally, for predictor values $x_{sc,j}$, combine them over $1 \le j \le r$ into the $r \times 1$ vectors $\boldsymbol{x}_{sc}$ for $sc \in SC$. Let $\boldsymbol{X}_s$ denote the $m(s) \times r$ predictor matrix with rows $\boldsymbol{x}^{\mathrm{T}}_{sc}$. Model the probabilities $p_{sc,\le u}$ for $0 \le u < K$ and $sc \in SC$ ordinally as

$$g(p_{sc,\le u}) = \mathrm{logit}(p_{sc,\le u}) = \log \frac{p_{sc,\le u}}{1 - p_{sc,\le u}} = \alpha_u + \boldsymbol{x}^{\mathrm{T}}_{sc} \cdot \boldsymbol{\beta}_K$$

for K intercept parameters α_u and a single $r \times 1$ vector $\boldsymbol{\beta}_K$ of slope parameters $\beta_{K,j}$ for $1 \le j \le r$. This formulation assumes that, for $1 \le j \le r$, the predictor values $x_{sc,j}$ are not constant in $sc \in SC$ so that $\boldsymbol{\beta}_K$ does not include a redundant intercept parameter. Combine the intercept parameters α_u over $0 \le u < K$ into the $K \times 1$ vector $\boldsymbol{\alpha}$. Altogether, there are $K + r$ coefficient parameters for modeling the probabilities, which are combined over $0 \le u < K$ and $1 \le j \le r$ into the $(K + r) \times 1$ vector

$$\boldsymbol{\beta} = \begin{pmatrix} \boldsymbol{\alpha} \\ \boldsymbol{\beta}_K \end{pmatrix}.$$

A zero-intercept model corresponds to setting $\alpha_0 = 0$, but α_u for $0 < u < K$ are non-zero.

The cumulative probabilities satisfy

$$p_{sc,\leq u} = \frac{\exp(\alpha_u + \boldsymbol{x}_{sc}^{\mathrm{T}} \cdot \boldsymbol{\beta}_K)}{1 + \exp(\alpha_u + \boldsymbol{x}_{sc}^{\mathrm{T}} \cdot \boldsymbol{\beta}_K)}$$

for $0 \leq u < K$ and $sc \in SC$. For $0 \leq u, w < K$, $1 \leq j \leq r$, and $sc \in SC$, the first partial derivatives of $p_{sc,\leq u}$ satisfy

$$\frac{\partial p_{sc,\leq u}}{\partial \alpha_w} = p_{sc,\leq w} \cdot (1 - p_{sc,\leq w}), w = u,$$

$$\frac{\partial p_{sc,\leq u}}{\partial \alpha_w} = 0, w \neq u,$$

$$\frac{\partial p_{sc,\leq u}}{\partial \beta_{K,j}} = x_{sc,j} \cdot p_{sc,\leq u} \cdot (1 - p_{sc,\leq u}).$$

The cumulative probabilities are differenced to compute probabilities $p_{sc,u} = \mathrm{P}(y_{sc} = d_u)$, that is, for $sc \in SC$, define $p_{sc,\leq -1} = 0$ and then $p_{sc,u} = p_{sc,\leq u} - p_{sc,\leq u-1}$ for $0 \leq u \leq K$. In what follows, extensions are provided for standard GEE modeling (Sect. 12.2.2.1), partially modified GEE modeling (Sect. 12.2.2.2), fully modified GEE modeling (Sect. 12.2.2.3), and extended linear mixed modeling (Sect. 12.2.2.4).

12.2.2.1 Standard GEE Modeling

The formulations of Chap. 2 apply except that $\mathrm{Var}(y_{sc})$ is no longer a simple function of the means μ_{sc}. The constant dispersions are still based on a constant parameter φ as in Sect. 2.2 . Define the extended variances

$$\sigma_{sc}^2 = \varphi \cdot \mathrm{Var}(y_{sc}),$$

the standardized residuals

$$stde_{sc} = e_{sc}/\sigma_{sc},$$

and the Pearson residuals

$$Pres_{sc} = \frac{e_{sc}}{\mathrm{Var}^{1/2}(y_{sc})}$$

for $sc \in SC$. Combine these, respectively, into the $m(s) \times 1$ vectors $\boldsymbol{\sigma}_s$, $\boldsymbol{stde}_s$, and $\boldsymbol{Pres}_s$ ordered by their values $c \in C(s)$. Model the $m(s) \times m(s)$ covariance matrices $\boldsymbol{\Sigma}_s$ as

$$\boldsymbol{\Sigma}_s = \boldsymbol{DIAG}(\boldsymbol{\sigma}_s) \cdot \boldsymbol{R}_s(\boldsymbol{\rho}) \cdot \boldsymbol{DIAG}(\boldsymbol{\sigma}_s)$$

for appropriate choices of the $m(s) \times m(s)$ correlation matrices $\boldsymbol{R}_s(\boldsymbol{\rho})$ for $s \in S$. The estimating equations for the mean parameters

$$\boldsymbol{E}(\boldsymbol{\beta}) = \sum_{s\in S} \boldsymbol{E}_s(\boldsymbol{\beta}) = \sum_{s\in S} \boldsymbol{D}_s^{\mathrm{T}} \cdot \boldsymbol{\Sigma}_s^{-1} \cdot \boldsymbol{e}_s,$$

are based on the $m(s) \times (K + r)$ matrices

$$\boldsymbol{D}_s = \frac{\partial \boldsymbol{\mu}_s}{\partial \boldsymbol{\beta}}$$

for $s \in S$ with entries

$$D_{sc,w} = \frac{\partial \mu_{sc}}{\partial \alpha_w} = p_{sc,\leq w} \cdot \left(1 - p_{sc,\leq w}\right) \cdot (d_w - d_{w+1}),$$

$$D_{sc,K,j} = \frac{\partial \mu_{sc}}{\partial \beta_{K,j}} = x_{sc,j} \cdot \sum_{u=0}^{K-1} \left(p_{sc,\leq u} \cdot \left(1 - p_{sc,\leq u}\right) \cdot (d_u - d_{u-1})\right)$$

for $sc \in SC$, $0 \leq w < K$, and $1 \leq j \leq r$ while

$$\boldsymbol{E}'(\boldsymbol{\beta}) = -\sum_{s\in S} \boldsymbol{D}_s^{\mathrm{T}} \cdot \boldsymbol{\Sigma}_s^{-1} \cdot \boldsymbol{D}_s.$$

The bias-adjusted estimate of the constant dispersion parameter φ for a given value of the coefficient parameter vector $\boldsymbol{\beta}$ is

$$\varphi(\boldsymbol{\beta}) = \frac{\sum_{s\in S} \boldsymbol{Pres}_s^{\mathrm{T}}(\boldsymbol{\beta}) \cdot \boldsymbol{Pres}_s(\boldsymbol{\beta})}{m(SC) - r}$$

assuming $m(SC) - r > 0$. Compute correlation estimates for the correlation structures of Sect. 2.3 using the formulas of Sect. 2.4.1. Model-based and robust empirical estimates of the covariance matrix for the standard GEE estimate $\boldsymbol{\beta}(SC)$ of the mean coefficient parameter vector $\boldsymbol{\beta}$ can be computed as in Sect. 2.4.2.

12.2.2.2 Partially Modified GEE Modeling

The formulation of Chap. 3 applies with $V(\mu_{sc})$ replaced by $\mathrm{Var}(y_{sc})$. For predictor values $v_{sc,j}$, combine them over $1 \leq j \leq q$ into the $q \times 1$ vectors $\boldsymbol{v}_{sc}$ for $sc \in SC$, and model the natural log of the non-constant dispersions in terms of these predictor values, that is,

$$\log \varphi_{sc} = \boldsymbol{v}_{sc}^{\mathrm{T}} \cdot \boldsymbol{\gamma}$$

where $\boldsymbol{\gamma}$ is a $q \times 1$ vector of coefficient parameters. Let $\boldsymbol{V}_s$ denote the $m(s) \times q$ predictor matrix with rows $\boldsymbol{v}_{sc}^{\mathrm{T}}$. Define the extended variances as

$$\sigma_{sc}^2 = \varphi_{sc} \cdot V(\mu_{sc})$$

and the standardized residuals as

$$stde_{sc} = e_{sc}/\sigma_{sc}.$$

Combine the extended standard deviations and standardized residuals over $c \in C(s)$ into the $m(s) \times 1$ vectors $\boldsymbol{\sigma}_s$ and $\boldsymbol{stde}_s$ for $s \in S$.

Denote an observation by $O_s = \{\boldsymbol{y}_s, \boldsymbol{X}_s, \boldsymbol{V}_s\}$ and define the likelihood function $L(SC;\boldsymbol{\theta})$ to be the product of terms $L(O_s;\boldsymbol{\theta})$ for $s \in S$ satisfying

$$\ell(O_s;\boldsymbol{\theta}) = \log L(O_s;\boldsymbol{\theta}) = -\boldsymbol{e}_s^{\mathrm{T}} \cdot \boldsymbol{\Sigma}_s^{-1} \cdot \boldsymbol{e}_s/2 - (\log|\boldsymbol{\Sigma}_s|)/2 - (m(s) \cdot \log(2 \cdot \pi))/2$$

where

$$\boldsymbol{\theta} = \begin{pmatrix} \boldsymbol{\beta} \\ \boldsymbol{\gamma} \end{pmatrix}$$

and the $m(s) \times m(s)$ covariance matrix $\boldsymbol{\Sigma}_s$ of $\boldsymbol{y}_s$ satisfies

$$\boldsymbol{\Sigma}_s = \boldsymbol{DIAG}(\boldsymbol{\sigma}_s) \cdot \boldsymbol{R}_s(\boldsymbol{\rho}) \cdot \boldsymbol{DIAG}(\boldsymbol{\sigma}_s)$$

for appropriate choices of the $m(s) \times m(s)$ correlation matrices $\boldsymbol{R}_s(\boldsymbol{\rho})$ for $s \in S$. Estimating equations $\boldsymbol{E}(\boldsymbol{\gamma}) = \boldsymbol{0}$ for the dispersion parameters can be generated by maximizing the likelihood $L(SC;\boldsymbol{\theta})$ in $\boldsymbol{\gamma}$, that is,

$$\boldsymbol{E}(\boldsymbol{\gamma}) = \frac{\partial_0 \ell(SC;\boldsymbol{\theta})}{\partial_0 \boldsymbol{\gamma}}$$

where the operator notation $\frac{\partial_0}{\partial_0 \boldsymbol{\gamma}}$ is used to indicate that this is not the full partial derivative vector for $\ell(SC;\boldsymbol{\theta})$ in $\boldsymbol{\gamma}$ due to not accounting for the effect of $\boldsymbol{\gamma}$ on $\boldsymbol{R}_s(\boldsymbol{\rho})$. $\boldsymbol{E}(\boldsymbol{\gamma})$ is the sum over $s \in S$ of $\boldsymbol{E}_s(\boldsymbol{\gamma})$ with entries

$$E_{s,j}(\gamma) = \boldsymbol{vstde}_{s,j}^{\mathrm{T}} \cdot \boldsymbol{R}_s^{-1}(\rho) \cdot \boldsymbol{stde}_s - \sum_{c \in C(s)} v_{sc,j}/2$$

where $\boldsymbol{vstde}_{s,j}$ is the $m(s) \times 1$ vector with entries

$$vstde_{sc,j} = v_{sc,j} \cdot stde_{sc}/2$$

for $sc \in SC$ and $1 \leq j \leq q$. Now, combine these with the $K + r$ standard GEE mean estimating equations $\boldsymbol{E}(\boldsymbol{\beta}) = \boldsymbol{0}$ to use Newton's method to solve for joint estimates of $\boldsymbol{\beta}$ and $\boldsymbol{\gamma}$. Then, iteratively solve for

$$\boldsymbol{E}(\boldsymbol{\theta}) = \begin{pmatrix} \boldsymbol{E}(\boldsymbol{\beta}) \\ \boldsymbol{E}(\boldsymbol{\gamma}) \end{pmatrix} = \boldsymbol{0}$$

with $\boldsymbol{E}(\boldsymbol{\theta})$ in the role of the gradient vector and the $(K + r + q) \times (K + r + q)$ matrix $\boldsymbol{E}'(\boldsymbol{\theta})$ in the role of the Hessian matrix.

$\boldsymbol{E}'(\boldsymbol{\theta})$ has four component matrices: the $(K + r) \times (K + r)$ matrix

$$\boldsymbol{E}'(\boldsymbol{\beta}) = \frac{\partial_0 \boldsymbol{E}(\boldsymbol{\beta})}{\partial_0 \boldsymbol{\beta}}$$

for $K + r$ the mean coefficients as used in standard GEE modeling, the $q \times q$ matrix

$$\boldsymbol{E}'(\boldsymbol{\gamma}) = \frac{\partial_0 \boldsymbol{E}(\boldsymbol{\gamma})}{\partial_0 \boldsymbol{\gamma}}$$

for the q dispersion coefficients, the $(K + r) \times q$ matrix

$$\boldsymbol{E}'(\boldsymbol{\beta}, \boldsymbol{\gamma}) = \frac{\partial_0 \boldsymbol{E}(\boldsymbol{\beta})}{\partial_0 \boldsymbol{\gamma}},$$

and its transpose $\boldsymbol{E}'(\boldsymbol{\gamma}, \boldsymbol{\beta}) = \boldsymbol{E}'^{\mathrm{T}}(\boldsymbol{\beta}, \boldsymbol{\gamma})$. $\boldsymbol{E}'(\boldsymbol{\gamma})$ is the sum over $s \in S$ of $\boldsymbol{E}'_s(\boldsymbol{\gamma})$ with entries

$$E'_{s,j,j'}(\gamma) = -\boldsymbol{vvstde}_{s,j,j'}^{\mathrm{T}} \cdot \boldsymbol{R}_s^{-1}(\rho) \cdot \boldsymbol{stde}_s - \boldsymbol{vstde}_{s,j}^{\mathrm{T}} \cdot \boldsymbol{R}_s^{-1}(\rho) \cdot \boldsymbol{vstde}_{s,j'}$$

where $\boldsymbol{vvstde}_{s,j,j'}$ is the $m(s) \times 1$ vector with entries

$$vvstde_{sc,j,j'} = v_{sc,j} \cdot v_{sc,j'} \cdot stde_{sc}/4$$

for $sc \in SC$ and $1 \leq j, j' \leq q$. $\boldsymbol{E}'(\boldsymbol{\beta}, \boldsymbol{\gamma})$ is the sum over $s \in S$ of $\boldsymbol{E}'_s(\boldsymbol{\beta}, \boldsymbol{\gamma})$ with q $(K + r) \times 1$ column vectors

$$\begin{aligned}\mathbf{E}'_{s,j}(\boldsymbol{\beta},\boldsymbol{\gamma}) &= -\mathbf{D}_s^{\mathrm{T}}\cdot \mathbf{DIAG}\left(\boldsymbol{v\sigma inv}_{s,j}\right)\cdot \mathbf{R}_s^{-1}(\boldsymbol{\rho})\cdot \mathbf{stde}_s\\ &\quad -\mathbf{D}_s^{\mathrm{T}}\cdot \mathbf{DIAG}(\mathbf{1}/\boldsymbol{\sigma}_s)\cdot \mathbf{R}_s^{-1}(\boldsymbol{\rho})\cdot \mathbf{vstde}_{s,j}\end{aligned}$$

where $\boldsymbol{v\sigma inv}_{s,j}$ is the $m(s) \times 1$ vector with entries

$$v\sigma inv_{sc,j} = \frac{v_{sc,j}}{2\cdot\sigma_{sc}}$$

for $sc \in SC$ and $1 \leq j \leq q$. Model-based and robust empirical estimates of the covariance matrix for the partially modified GEE estimate $\boldsymbol{\theta}(SC)$ of the mean coefficient parameter vector $\boldsymbol{\theta}$ can be computed as in Sect. 3.4.

Given a value for the vector $\boldsymbol{\theta}$ of all coefficient parameters, an estimate of the correlation parameter vector $\boldsymbol{\rho}$ can be based on the associated standardized residuals $stde_{sc}(\boldsymbol{\theta})$ determined by non-constant dispersions $\varphi_{sc}(\boldsymbol{\gamma})$ computed with the current value for $\boldsymbol{\gamma}$. Calculate the revised correlation estimates for the correlation structures of Sect. 2.3 using the formulas of Sect. 2.4.1 evaluated with the revised standardized residuals $stde_{sc}(\boldsymbol{\theta})$.

12.2.2.3 Fully Modified GEE Modeling

The formulation of Chap. 4 applies with $V(\mu_{sc})$ replaced by $\mathrm{Var}(y_{sc})$ extending the formulation of Sect. 12.2.2.2 using the same likelihood function $L(SC;\boldsymbol{\theta})$ and

$$\mathbf{E}(\boldsymbol{\theta}) = \begin{pmatrix}\mathbf{E}(\boldsymbol{\beta})\\ \mathbf{E}(\boldsymbol{\gamma})\end{pmatrix}$$

with $\mathbf{E}(\boldsymbol{\gamma})$ computed as in Sect. 12.2.2.2.

$$\mathbf{E}(\boldsymbol{\beta}) = \frac{\partial_0 \ell(SC;\boldsymbol{\theta})}{\partial_0 \boldsymbol{\beta}}$$

is the sum over $s \in S$ of $\mathbf{E}_s(\boldsymbol{\beta})$ with entries

$$E_{s,w}(\boldsymbol{\beta}) = \mathbf{xstde}_{s,w}^{\mathrm{T}}\cdot \mathbf{R}_s^{-1}(\boldsymbol{\rho})\cdot \mathbf{stde}_s - \sum_{c\in C(s)} W_{sc,w}/2,$$

$$E_{s,K,j}(\boldsymbol{\beta}) = \mathbf{xstde}_{s,K,j}^{\mathrm{T}}\cdot \mathbf{R}_s^{-1}(\boldsymbol{\rho})\cdot \mathbf{stde}_s - \sum_{c\in C(s)} W_{sc,K,j}/2$$

where $\mathbf{xstde}_{s,w}$ and $\mathbf{xstde}_{s,K,j}$ are the $m(s) \times 1$ vector with respective entries

$$xstde_{sc,w} = \frac{\partial \mu_{sc}}{\partial \alpha_w} / \sigma_{sc} + stde_{sc} \cdot W_{sc,w}/2,$$

$$xstde_{sc,Kj} = \frac{\partial \mu_{sc}}{\partial \beta_{Kj}} / \sigma_{sc} + stde_{sc} \cdot W_{sc,Kj}/2,$$

$$W_{sc,w} = \frac{\frac{\partial \mathrm{Var}(y_{sc})}{\partial \alpha_w}}{\mathrm{Var}(y_{sc})},$$

$$\frac{\partial \mathrm{Var}(y_{sc})}{\partial \alpha_w} = p_{sc,\leq w} \cdot \left(1 - p_{sc,\leq w}\right) \cdot (d_w - d_{w+1}) \cdot (d_w + d_{w+1} - 2 \cdot \mu_{sc}),$$

$$W_{sc,Kj} = \frac{\frac{\partial \mathrm{Var}(y_{sc})}{\partial \beta_{Kj}}}{\mathrm{Var}(y_{sc})},$$

$$\frac{\partial \mathrm{Var}(y_{sc})}{\partial \beta_{Kj}} = x_{scj} \cdot \sum_{u=0}^{K-1} \left(p_{sc,\leq u} \cdot \left(1 - p_{sc,\leq u}\right) \cdot (d_u - d_{u+1}) \cdot (d_u + d_{u+1} - 2 \cdot \mu_{sc})\right),$$

and the first partial derivatives $\frac{\partial \mu_{sc}}{\partial \alpha_w}$ and $\frac{\partial \mu_{sc}}{\partial \beta_{Kj}}$ are defined in Sect. 12.2.2.1, for $0 \leq w < K$, $1 \leq j \leq r$, and $sc \in SC$. As before, use Newton's method to iteratively solve $\boldsymbol{E}(\boldsymbol{\theta}) = \boldsymbol{0}$. The correlation estimates are the same as those in Sect. 12.2.2.2.

$\boldsymbol{E}'(\boldsymbol{\theta})$ has four component matrices: the $(K + r) \times (K + r)$ matrix

$$\boldsymbol{E}'(\boldsymbol{\beta}) = \frac{\partial_0 \boldsymbol{E}(\boldsymbol{\beta})}{\partial_0 \boldsymbol{\beta}}$$

for the $K + r$ mean coefficients, the $q \times q$ matrix

$$\boldsymbol{E}'(\boldsymbol{\gamma}) = \frac{\partial_0 \boldsymbol{E}(\boldsymbol{\gamma})}{\partial_0 \boldsymbol{\gamma}}$$

for the q dispersion coefficients as computed in Sect. 12.2.2.2, the $(K + r) \times q$ matrix

$$\boldsymbol{E}'(\boldsymbol{\beta}, \boldsymbol{\gamma}) = \frac{\partial_0 \boldsymbol{E}(\boldsymbol{\beta})}{\partial_0 \boldsymbol{\gamma}},$$

and its transpose $\boldsymbol{E}'(\boldsymbol{\gamma}, \boldsymbol{\beta}) = \boldsymbol{E}'^{\mathrm{T}}(\boldsymbol{\beta}, \boldsymbol{\gamma})$. $\boldsymbol{E}'(\boldsymbol{\beta})$ is the sum over $s \in S$ of $\boldsymbol{E}'_s(\boldsymbol{\beta})$ with entries

$$E'_{s,w,w'}(\boldsymbol{\beta}) = -\boldsymbol{xxstde}^{\mathrm{T}}_{s,w,w'} \cdot \boldsymbol{R}_s^{-1}(\boldsymbol{\rho}) \cdot \boldsymbol{stde}_s - \boldsymbol{xstde}^{\mathrm{T}}_{s,w} \cdot \boldsymbol{R}_s^{-1}(\boldsymbol{\rho}) \cdot \boldsymbol{xstde}_{s,w'}$$
$$- \sum_{c \in C(s)} W_{sc,w,w'}/2,$$

$$E'_{s,w,K,j}(\boldsymbol{\beta}) = -\boldsymbol{xxstde}^{\mathrm{T}}_{s,w,K,j} \cdot \boldsymbol{R}_s^{-1}(\boldsymbol{\rho}) \cdot \boldsymbol{stde}_s - \boldsymbol{xstde}^{\mathrm{T}}_{s,w} \cdot \boldsymbol{R}_s^{-1}(\boldsymbol{\rho}) \cdot \boldsymbol{xstde}_{s,K,j}$$
$$- \sum_{c \in C(s)} W_{sc,w,K,j}/2,$$

$$E'_{s,K,j,w'}(\boldsymbol{\beta}) = -\boldsymbol{xxstde}^{\mathrm{T}}_{s,Kj,w'} \cdot \boldsymbol{R}_s^{-1}(\boldsymbol{\rho}) \cdot \boldsymbol{stde}_s - \boldsymbol{xstde}^{\mathrm{T}}_{s,K,j} \cdot \boldsymbol{R}_s^{-1}(\boldsymbol{\rho}) \cdot \boldsymbol{xstde}_{s,w'}$$
$$- \sum_{c \in C(s)} W_{sc,K,j,w'}/2,$$

$$E'_{s,K,j,j'}(\boldsymbol{\beta}) = -\boldsymbol{xxstde}^{\mathrm{T}}_{s,Kj,j'} \cdot \boldsymbol{R}_s^{-1}(\boldsymbol{\rho}) \cdot \boldsymbol{stde}_s - \boldsymbol{xstde}^{\mathrm{T}}_{s,K,j} \cdot \boldsymbol{R}_s^{-1}(\boldsymbol{\rho}) \cdot \boldsymbol{xstde}_{s,K,j'}$$
$$- \sum_{c \in C(s)} W_{sc,K,j,j'}/2,$$

where $\boldsymbol{xxstde}_{s,w,w'}$, $\boldsymbol{xxstde}_{s,w,K,j}$, $\boldsymbol{xxstde}_{s,K,j,w'}$, and $\boldsymbol{xxstde}_{s,K,j,j'}$ are the $m(s) \times 1$ vectors with respective entries

$$xxstde_{sc,w,w'} = -\frac{\frac{\partial^2 \mu_{sc}}{\partial \alpha_{w'}\,\partial \alpha_w}}{\sigma_{sc}} + \frac{\partial \mu_{sc}}{\partial \alpha_w} \cdot \frac{W_{sc,w'}}{2 \cdot \sigma_{sc}} + xstde_{sc,w'} \cdot \frac{W_{sc,w}}{2} - stde_{sc} \cdot \frac{W_{sc,w,w'}}{2},$$

$$\frac{\partial^2 \mu_{sc}}{\partial \alpha_{w'}\,\partial \alpha_w} = p_{sc,\le w} \cdot \left(1 - p_{sc,\le w}\right) \cdot \left(1 - 2 \cdot p_{sc,\le w}\right) \cdot \left(d_w - d_{w+1}\right), w' = w,$$

$$\frac{\partial^2 \mu_{sc}}{\partial \alpha_{w'}\,\partial \alpha_{w'}} = 0, w' \ne w;$$

$$xxstde_{sc,w,K,j} = -\frac{\frac{\partial^2 \mu_{sc}}{\partial \beta_{K,j}\partial \alpha_w}}{\sigma_{sc}} + \frac{\partial \mu_{sc}}{\partial \alpha_w} \cdot \frac{W_{sc,K,j}}{2 \cdot \sigma_{sc}} + xstde_{sc,K,j} \cdot \frac{W_{sc,w}}{2} - stde_{sc} \cdot \frac{W_{sc,w,K,j}}{2},$$

$$\frac{\partial^2 \mu_{sc}}{\partial \beta_{K,j}\partial \alpha_w} = x_{sc,j} \cdot p_{sc,\le w} \cdot \left(1 - p_{sc,\le w}\right) \cdot \left(1 - 2 \cdot p_{sc,\le w}\right) \cdot \left(d_w - d_{w+1}\right);$$

$$xxstde_{sc,K,j,w'} = -\frac{\frac{\partial^2 \mu_{sc}}{\partial \alpha_{w'}\,\partial \beta_{K,j}}}{\sigma_{sc}} + \frac{\partial \mu_{sc}}{\partial \beta_{K,j}} \cdot \frac{W_{sc,w'}}{2 \cdot \sigma_{sc}} + xstde_{sc,w'} \cdot \frac{W_{sc,K,j}}{2}$$
$$- stde_{sc} \cdot \frac{W_{sc,K,j,w'}}{2},$$

$$\frac{\partial^2 \mu_{sc}}{\partial \alpha_{w'}\,\partial \beta_{K,j}} = x_{sc,j} \cdot p_{sc,\le w'} \cdot \left(1 - p_{sc,\le w'}\right) \cdot \left(1 - 2 \cdot p_{sc,\le w'}\right) \cdot \left(d_{w'} - d_{w'+1}\right);$$

$$xxstde_{sc,K,j,j'} = -\frac{\frac{\partial^2 \mu_{sc}}{\partial \beta_{K,j'}\partial \beta_{K,j}}}{\sigma_{sc}} + \frac{\partial \mu_{sc}}{\partial \beta_{K,j}} \cdot \frac{W_{sc,K,j'}}{2 \cdot \sigma_{sc}} + xstde_{sc,K,j'} \cdot \frac{W_{sc,K,j}}{2}$$
$$- stde_{sc} \cdot \frac{W_{sc,K,j,j'}}{2},$$

$$\frac{\partial^2 \mu_{sc}}{\partial \beta_{K,j'}\partial \beta_{K,j}} = x_{sc,j} \cdot x_{sc,j'} \cdot \sum_{u=0}^{K-1} \left(p_{sc,\le u} \cdot \left(1 - p_{sc,\le u}\right) \cdot \left(1 - 2 \cdot p_{sc,\le u}\right) \cdot (d_u - d_{u+1})\right);$$

$$W_{sc,w,w'} = \frac{\partial W_{sc,w}}{\partial \alpha_{w'}} = \frac{\frac{\partial^2 \mathrm{Var}(y_{sc})}{\partial \alpha_{w'}\partial \alpha_w}}{\mathrm{Var}(y_{sc})} - \frac{\frac{\partial \mathrm{Var}(y_{sc})}{\partial \alpha_{w'}} \cdot \frac{\partial \mathrm{Var}(y_{sc})}{\partial \alpha_w}}{\mathrm{Var}^2(y_{sc})},$$

$$\frac{\partial^2 \mathrm{Var}(y_{sc})}{\partial \alpha_{w'}\partial \alpha_w} = p_{sc,\le w} \cdot \left(1 - p_{sc,\le w}\right) \cdot (d_w - d_{w+1}) \cdot$$
$$\left(\left(1 - 2 \cdot p_{sc,\le w}\right) \cdot (d_w + d_{w+1} - 2 \cdot \mu_{sc}) - 2 \cdot p_{sc,\le w} \cdot \left(1 - p_{s,\le w}\right) \cdot (d_w - d_{w+1})\right), w' = w,$$

$$\frac{\partial^2 \mathrm{Var}(y_{sc})}{\partial \alpha_{w'}\partial \alpha_w} =$$
$$-2 \cdot p_{sc,\le w} \cdot \left(1 - p_{sc,\le w}\right) \cdot p_{sc,\le w'} \cdot \left(1 - p_{sc,\le w'}\right) \cdot (d_w - d_{w+1}) \cdot (d_{w'} - d_{w'+1}), w' \ne w;$$

$$W_{sc,w,K,j} = \frac{\partial W_{sc,w}}{\partial \beta_{K,j}} = \frac{\frac{\partial^2 \mathrm{Var}(y_{sc})}{\partial \beta_{K,j}\partial \alpha_w}}{\mathrm{Var}(y_{sc})} - \frac{\frac{\partial \mathrm{Var}(y_{sc})}{\partial \beta_{K,j}} \cdot \frac{\partial \mathrm{Var}(y_{sc})}{\partial \alpha_w}}{\mathrm{Var}^2(y_{sc})},$$

$$\frac{\partial^2 \mathrm{Var}(y_{sc})}{\partial \beta_{K,j}\partial \alpha_w} = x_{sc,j} \cdot p_{sc,\le w} \cdot \left(1 - p_{sc,\le w}\right) \cdot (d_w - d_{w+1}) \cdot$$
$$\left(\left(1 - 2 \cdot p_{sc,\le w}\right) \cdot (d_w + d_{w+1} - 2 \cdot \mu_{sc}) - 2 \cdot \sum_{u=0}^{K-1} \left(p_{sc,\le u} \cdot \left(1 - p_{sc,\le u}\right) \cdot (d_u - d_{u+1})\right)\right);$$

$$W_{sc,K,j,w'} = \frac{\partial W_{sc,K,j}}{\partial \alpha_{w'}} = \frac{\frac{\partial^2 \mathrm{Var}(y_{sc})}{\partial \alpha_{w'}\partial \beta_{K,j}}}{\mathrm{Var}(y_{sc})} - \frac{\frac{\partial \mathrm{Var}(y_{sc})}{\partial \alpha_{w'}} \cdot \frac{\partial \mathrm{Var}(y_{sc})}{\partial \beta_{K,j}}}{\mathrm{Var}^2(y_{sc})},$$

$$\frac{\partial^2 \mathrm{Var}(y_{sc})}{\partial \alpha_{w'}\partial \beta_{K,j}} = x_{sc,j} \cdot p_{sc,\le w'} \cdot \left(1 - p_{sc,\le w'}\right) \cdot (d_{w'} - d_{w'+1}) \cdot$$
$$\left(\left(1 - 2 \cdot p_{sc,\le w'}\right) \cdot (d_{w'} + d_{w'+1} - 2 \cdot \mu_{sc}) - 2\right.$$
$$\left. \cdot \sum_{u=0}^{K-1} \left(p_{sc,\le u} \cdot \left(1 - p_{sc,\le u}\right) \cdot (d_u - d_{u+1})\right)\right);$$

$$W_{sc,Kjj'} = \frac{\partial W_{sc,Kj}}{\partial \beta_{Kj'}} = \frac{\frac{\partial^2 \text{Var}(y_{sc})}{\partial \beta_{Kj'} \partial \beta_{Kj}}}{\text{Var}(y_{sc})} - \frac{\frac{\partial \text{Var}(y_{sc})}{\partial \beta_{Kj'}} \cdot \frac{\partial \text{Var}(y_{sc})}{\partial \beta_{Kj}}}{\text{Var}^2(y_{sc})},$$

$$\frac{\partial^2 \text{Var}(y_{sc})}{\partial \beta_{Kj'} \partial \beta_{Kj}} = x_{scj} \cdot x_{scj'} \cdot$$

$$\sum_{u=0}^{K-1} (p_{sc,\le u} \cdot (1 - p_{sc,\le u}) \cdot (1 - 2 \cdot p_{sc,\le u}) \cdot (d_u - d_{u+1}) \cdot (d_u + d_{u+1} - 2 \cdot \mu_{sc}))$$

$$-2 \cdot x_{scj} \cdot x_{scj'} \cdot \left(\sum_{u=0}^{K-1} (p_{sc,\le u} \cdot (1 - p_{sc,\le u}) \cdot (d_u - d_{u+1})) \right)^2,$$

for $1 \le w, w' < K$ and $1 \le j, j' \le r$. $\boldsymbol{E}'(\boldsymbol{\gamma})$ is the sum over $s \in S$ of $\boldsymbol{E}'_s(\boldsymbol{\gamma})$ with entries

$$E_{s,jj'}(\boldsymbol{\gamma}) = -vvstde_{s,jj'} \cdot stde_s - vstde_{s,j} \cdot vstde_{s,j'}$$

where

$$vvstde_{sc,jj'} = v_{scj} \cdot v_{scj'} \cdot stde_s/4$$

for $1 \le j, j' \le q$. $\boldsymbol{E}'(\boldsymbol{\beta}, \boldsymbol{\gamma})$ is the sum over $s \in S$ of $\boldsymbol{E}'_s(\boldsymbol{\beta}, \boldsymbol{\gamma})$ with entries

$$E'_{s,wj'}(\boldsymbol{\beta}, \boldsymbol{\gamma}) = -vxstde_{s,wj'} \cdot stde_s - xstde_{s,w} \cdot vstde_{s,j'},$$
$$E'_{s,Kjj'}(\boldsymbol{\beta}, \boldsymbol{\gamma}) = -vxstde_{s,Kjj'} \cdot stde_s - xstde_{s,Kj} \cdot vstde_{s,j'}$$

and

$$vxstde_{sc,wj'} = xstde_{sc,w} \cdot v_{scj'}/2,$$
$$vxstde_{s,Kjj'} = xstde_{sc,Kj} \cdot v_{scj'}/2$$

for $0 \le w < K$, $1 \le j \le r$, and $1 \le j' \le q$. Model-based and robust empirical estimates of the covariance matrix for the GEE estimate $\boldsymbol{\theta}(SC)$ of the parameter vector $\boldsymbol{\theta}$ can be computed as in Sect. 4.1.

12.2.2.4 Extended Linear Mixed Modeling

The formulation of Chap. 5 applies with $V(\mu_{sc})$ replaced by $\text{Var}(y_{sc})$ extending the formulation of Sect. 12.2.2.3. The likelihood function $L(SC; \boldsymbol{\theta})$ is the same as defined in Sect. 12.2.1.2 except that the parameter vector is now

$$\boldsymbol{\theta} = \begin{pmatrix} \boldsymbol{\beta} \\ \boldsymbol{\gamma} \\ \boldsymbol{\rho} \end{pmatrix}$$

with $K + r + q + p$ entries where p is the number of correlation parameters. The likelihood $L(SC;\boldsymbol{\theta})$ is maximized in the coefficient parameter vector $\boldsymbol{\theta}$. Specifically, use Newton's method to solve the estimating equations

$$\mathbf{E}(\boldsymbol{\theta}) = \frac{\partial \ell(SC;\boldsymbol{\theta})}{\partial \boldsymbol{\theta}} = \sum_{s \in S} \mathbf{E}_s(\boldsymbol{\theta}) = \sum_{s \in S} \frac{\partial \ell(O_s;\boldsymbol{\theta})}{\partial \boldsymbol{\theta}} = \mathbf{0}$$

where the operator notation $\frac{\partial}{\partial \boldsymbol{\theta}}$ is used to indicate that this is a standard partial derivative vector in $\boldsymbol{\theta}$ since $\boldsymbol{\rho}$ is treated as a separate parameter vector. The associated matrix

$$\mathbf{E}'(\boldsymbol{\theta}) = \frac{\partial \mathbf{E}(\boldsymbol{\theta})}{\partial \boldsymbol{\theta}}.$$

In this case, $\mathbf{E}(\boldsymbol{\theta})$ is a true gradient vector and $\mathbf{E}'(\boldsymbol{\theta})$ a true Hessian matrix. The four correlation structures of Sect. 2.3 can still be considered. In all cases, there is just one alternative estimate of the correlation vector and not bias-adjusted and bias-unadjusted alternatives as for standard, partially modified, and fully modified GEE. The EC and spatial AR1 cases can be handled without storing associated correlation matrices (Sects. 5.3–5.4), providing efficient computation of associated estimates for data with relatively large numbers m of conditions.

The gradient vector satisfies

$$\mathbf{E}(\boldsymbol{\theta}) = \begin{pmatrix} \mathbf{E}(\boldsymbol{\beta}) \\ \mathbf{E}(\boldsymbol{\gamma}) \\ \mathbf{E}(\boldsymbol{\rho}) \end{pmatrix}$$

where $\mathbf{E}(\boldsymbol{\gamma})$ is computed as in Sect. 12.2.2.2 for partially modified GEE modeling and $\mathbf{E}(\boldsymbol{\beta})$ is computed as in Sect. 12.2.2.3 for fully modified GEE modeling since the correlation matrices do not depend on the dispersion parameters. With the entries of $\boldsymbol{\rho}$ denoted by ρ_j for $1 \le j \le p$,

$$\mathbf{E}(\boldsymbol{\rho}) = \frac{\partial \ell(SC;\boldsymbol{\theta})}{\partial \boldsymbol{\rho}}$$

is the sum over $s \in S$ of $\mathbf{E}_s(\boldsymbol{\rho})$ with entries

$$E_{s,j}(\boldsymbol{\rho}) = -\boldsymbol{stde}_s^{\mathrm{T}} \cdot \frac{\partial \boldsymbol{R}_s^{-1}(\boldsymbol{\rho})}{\partial \rho_j} \cdot \boldsymbol{stde}_s/2 - \frac{\partial \log|\boldsymbol{R}_s(\boldsymbol{\rho})|}{\partial \rho_j}/2$$

where $\boldsymbol{R}_s(\boldsymbol{\rho})$ changes with the correlation structure but does not depend on the mean and dispersion parameters.

$\boldsymbol{E}'(\boldsymbol{\theta})$ has nine component matrices: the $(K + r) \times (K + r)$ matrix

$$\boldsymbol{E}'(\boldsymbol{\beta}) = \frac{\partial \boldsymbol{E}(\boldsymbol{\beta})}{\partial \boldsymbol{\beta}}$$

for the $K + r$ mean parameters computed as in Sect. 12.2.2.3 for fully modified GEE modeling, the $q \times q$ matrix

$$\boldsymbol{E}'(\boldsymbol{\gamma}) = \frac{\partial \boldsymbol{E}(\boldsymbol{\gamma})}{\partial \boldsymbol{\gamma}}$$

for the q dispersion parameters computed as in Sect. 12.2.2.2 for partially modified GEE modeling, the $p \times p$ matrix

$$\boldsymbol{E}'(\boldsymbol{\rho}) = \frac{\partial \boldsymbol{E}(\boldsymbol{\rho})}{\partial \boldsymbol{\rho}}$$

for the p correlation parameters, the $(K + r) \times q$ matrix

$$\boldsymbol{E}'(\boldsymbol{\beta}, \boldsymbol{\gamma}) = \frac{\partial \boldsymbol{E}(\boldsymbol{\beta})}{\partial \boldsymbol{\gamma}}$$

and its transpose $\boldsymbol{E}'(\boldsymbol{\gamma}, \boldsymbol{\beta}) = \boldsymbol{E}'^{\mathrm{T}}(\boldsymbol{\beta}, \boldsymbol{\gamma})$ computed as in Sect. 12.2.2.3 for fully modified GEE modeling, the $(K + r) \times p$ matrix

$$\boldsymbol{E}'(\boldsymbol{\beta}, \boldsymbol{\rho}) = \frac{\partial \boldsymbol{E}(\boldsymbol{\beta})}{\partial \boldsymbol{\rho}}$$

and its transpose $\boldsymbol{E}'(\boldsymbol{\rho}, \boldsymbol{\beta}) = \boldsymbol{E}'^{\mathrm{T}}(\boldsymbol{\beta}, \boldsymbol{\rho})$, the $q \times p$ matrix

$$\boldsymbol{E}'(\boldsymbol{\gamma}, \boldsymbol{\rho}) = \frac{\partial \boldsymbol{E}(\boldsymbol{\gamma})}{\partial \boldsymbol{\rho}}$$

and its transpose $\boldsymbol{E}'(\boldsymbol{\rho}, \boldsymbol{\gamma}) = \boldsymbol{E}'^{\mathrm{T}}(\boldsymbol{\gamma}, \boldsymbol{\rho})$. $\boldsymbol{E}'(\boldsymbol{\rho})$ is the sum over $s \in S$ of $\boldsymbol{E}'_s(\boldsymbol{\rho})$ with entries satisfying

$$E'_{s,j,j'}(\boldsymbol{\rho}) = -\boldsymbol{stde}_s^{\mathrm{T}} \cdot \frac{\partial^2 \boldsymbol{R}_s^{-1}(\boldsymbol{\rho})}{\partial \rho_{j'}\, \partial \rho_j} \cdot \boldsymbol{stde}_s/2 - \frac{\partial^2 \log|\boldsymbol{R}_s(\boldsymbol{\rho})|}{\partial \rho_{j'}\, \partial \rho_j}/2.$$

$\boldsymbol{E}'(\boldsymbol{\beta},\boldsymbol{\rho})$ is the sum over $s \in S$ of $\boldsymbol{E}'_s(\boldsymbol{\beta},\boldsymbol{\rho})$ with entries

$$E'_{s,w,j'}(\boldsymbol{\beta},\boldsymbol{\rho}) = \boldsymbol{xstde}_{s,w}^{\mathrm{T}} \cdot \frac{\partial \boldsymbol{R}_s^{-1}(\boldsymbol{\rho})}{\partial \rho_{j'}} \cdot \boldsymbol{stde}_s,$$

$$E'_{s,K,j,j'}(\boldsymbol{\beta},\boldsymbol{\rho}) = \boldsymbol{xstde}_{s,K,j}^{\mathrm{T}} \cdot \frac{\partial \boldsymbol{R}_s^{-1}(\boldsymbol{\rho})}{\partial \rho_{j'}} \cdot \boldsymbol{stde}_s$$

for $1 \le w < K$, $1 \le j \le r$, and $1 \le j' \le p$ where $\boldsymbol{xstde}_{s,w,j}$ and $\boldsymbol{xstde}_{s,K,j}$ is defined in Sect. 12.2.2.3. $\boldsymbol{E}'(\boldsymbol{\gamma},\boldsymbol{\rho})$ is the sum over $s \in S$ of $\boldsymbol{E}'_s(\boldsymbol{\gamma},\boldsymbol{\rho})$ with entries

$$E'_{s,j,j'}(\boldsymbol{\gamma},\boldsymbol{\rho}) = \boldsymbol{vstde}_{s,w,j}^{\mathrm{T}} \cdot \frac{\partial \boldsymbol{R}_s^{-1}(\boldsymbol{\rho})}{\partial \rho_{j'}} \cdot \boldsymbol{stde}_s$$

for $1 \le j \le q$ and $1 \le j' \le p$ where $\boldsymbol{vstde}_{s,w,j}$ is defined in Sect. 12.2.2.2. Formulations for first and second partial derivatives of $\log|\boldsymbol{R}_s(\boldsymbol{\rho})|$ and $\boldsymbol{R}_s^{-1}(\boldsymbol{\rho})$ with respect to $\boldsymbol{\rho}$ needed to compute $\boldsymbol{E}(\boldsymbol{\rho})$, $\boldsymbol{E}'(\boldsymbol{\rho})$, $\boldsymbol{E}'(\boldsymbol{\beta},\boldsymbol{\rho})$, and $\boldsymbol{E}'(\gamma,\boldsymbol{\rho})$ are provided in Sects. 5.3–5.5 for the EC, spatial AR1, and UN structures. These partial derivatives are dropped for the IND correlation structure. Model-based and robust empirical estimates of the covariance matrix for the ELMM estimate $\boldsymbol{\theta}(SC)$ of the parameter vector $\boldsymbol{\theta}$ can be computed as in Sect. 5.1.

12.2.3 Censored Poisson Probabilities

For predictor values $x_{sc,j}$, combine them over $1 \le j \le r$ into the $r \times 1$ vectors $\boldsymbol{x}_{sc}$ for $sc \in SC$. Let $\boldsymbol{X}_s$ denote the $m(s) \times r$ predictor matrix with rows $\boldsymbol{x}_{sc}^{\mathrm{T}}$. Model the censored Poisson probabilities $p_{sc,u} = \mathrm{P}(y_{sc} = d_u)$ using the natural log link function as follows:

$$p_{sc,u} = \exp(-\lambda_{sc}) \cdot \frac{\lambda_{sc}^u}{u!}, 0 \le u < K,$$

$$p_{sc,K} = 1 - \sum_{u=0}^{K-1} p_{sc,u},$$

$$\log \lambda_{sc} = \boldsymbol{x}_{sc}^{\mathrm{T}} \cdot \boldsymbol{\beta},$$

for an $r \times 1$ vector $\boldsymbol{\beta}$ of coefficient parameters β_j for $1 \le j \le r$. The first partial derivatives $\frac{\partial \lambda_{sc}}{\partial \beta_j}$ and $\frac{\partial p_{sc,u}}{\partial \beta_j}$ satisfy

$$\frac{\partial \lambda_{sc}}{\partial \beta_j} = x_{sc,j} \cdot \lambda_{sc},$$

$$\frac{\partial p_{sc,u}}{\partial \beta_j} = x_{sc,j} \cdot p_{sc,u} \cdot (u - \lambda_{sc}), 0 \le u < K,$$

$$\frac{\partial p_{sc,K}}{\partial \beta_j} = -\sum_{u=0}^{K-1} \frac{\partial p_{sc,u}}{\partial \beta_j},$$

for $1 \le j \le r$ and $sc \in SC$. The associated second partial derivatives satisfy

$$\frac{\partial^2 \lambda_{sc}}{\partial \beta_{j'} \partial \beta_j} = x_{sc,j} \cdot x_{sc,j'} \cdot \lambda_{sc}, 0 \le u < K,$$

$$\frac{\partial^2 p_{sc,u}}{\partial \beta_{j'} \partial \beta_j} = x_{sc,j} \cdot x_{sc,j'} \cdot p_{sc,u} \cdot \left((u - \lambda_{sc})^2 - \lambda_{sc} \right), 0 \le u < K,$$

$$\frac{\partial^2 p_{sc,K}}{\partial \beta_{j'} \partial \beta_j} = -\sum_{u=0}^{K-1} \frac{\partial^2 p_{sc,u}}{\partial \beta_{j'} \partial \beta_j},$$

for $1 \le j, j' \le r$ and $sc \in SC$. In what follows, extensions are provided for standard GEE modeling (Sect. 12.2.3.1), partially modified GEE modeling (Sect. 12.2.3.2), fully modified GEE modeling (Sect. 12.2.3.3), and extended linear mixed modeling (Sect. 12.2.3.4).

12.2.3.1 Standard GEE Modeling

The formulations of Chap. 2 apply except that $\mathrm{Var}(y_{sc})$ is no longer a simple function of the means μ_{sc}. The constant dispersions still equal a constant parameter φ as in Sect. 2.2 . Define the extended variances

$$\sigma_{sc}^2 = \varphi \cdot \mathrm{Var}(y_{sc}),$$

the standardized residuals

$$stde_{sc} = e_{sc} / \sigma_{sc},$$

and the Pearson residuals

$$Pres_{sc} = \frac{e_{sc}}{\mathrm{Var}^{1/2}(y_{sc})}$$

for $sc \in SC$. Combine these, respectively, into the $m(s) \times 1$ vectors $\boldsymbol{\sigma}_s$, $\boldsymbol{stde}_s$, and $\boldsymbol{Pres}_s$ ordered by their values $c \in C(s)$. Model the $m(s) \times m(s)$ covariance matrices $\boldsymbol{\Sigma}_s$ as

$$\boldsymbol{\Sigma}_s = \boldsymbol{DIAG}(\boldsymbol{\sigma}_s) \cdot \boldsymbol{R}_s(\rho) \cdot \boldsymbol{DIAG}(\boldsymbol{\sigma}_s)$$

for appropriate choices of the $m(s) \times m(s)$ correlation matrices $\boldsymbol{R}_s(\rho)$ for $s \in S$. The estimating equations for the mean parameters

$$\boldsymbol{E}(\boldsymbol{\beta}) = \sum_{s \in S} \boldsymbol{E}_s(\boldsymbol{\beta}) = \sum_{s \in S} \boldsymbol{D}_s^{\mathrm{T}} \cdot \boldsymbol{\Sigma}_s^{-1} \cdot \boldsymbol{e}_s,$$

are based on the $m(s) \times r$ matrices

$$\boldsymbol{D}_s = \frac{\partial \boldsymbol{\mu}_s}{\partial \boldsymbol{\beta}}$$

for $s \in S$ with entries

$$D_{sc,j} = \frac{\partial \mu_{sc}}{\partial \beta_j} = \sum_{u=0}^{K-1} (d_u - d_K) \cdot \frac{\partial p_{sc,u}}{\partial \beta_j}$$

for $sc \in SC$ and $1 \leq j \leq r$ while

$$\boldsymbol{E}'(\boldsymbol{\beta}) = -\sum_{s \in S} \boldsymbol{D}_s^{\mathrm{T}} \cdot \boldsymbol{\Sigma}_s^{-1} \cdot \boldsymbol{D}_s.$$

The bias-adjusted estimate of the constant dispersion parameter φ for a given value of the coefficient parameter vector $\boldsymbol{\beta}$ is

$$\varphi(\boldsymbol{\beta}) = \frac{\sum_{s \in S} \boldsymbol{Pres}_s^{\mathrm{T}}(\boldsymbol{\beta}) \cdot \boldsymbol{Pres}_s(\boldsymbol{\beta})}{m(SC) - r}$$

assuming $m(SC) - r > 0$. Compute correlation estimates for the correlation structures of Sect. 2.3 using the formulas of Sect. 2.4.1. Model-based and robust empirical estimates of the covariance matrix for the standard GEE estimate $\boldsymbol{\beta}(SC)$ of the mean coefficient parameter vector $\boldsymbol{\beta}$ can be computed as in Sect. 2.4.2.

12.2.3.2 Partially Modified GEE Modeling

The formulation of Chap. 3 applies with $V(\mu_{sc})$ replaced by $\mathrm{Var}(y_{sc})$. For predictor values $v_{sc,j}$, combine them over $1 \le j \le q$ into the $q \times 1$ vectors $\boldsymbol{v}_{sc}$ for $sc \in SC$, and model the natural log of the non-constant dispersions in terms of these predictor values, that is,

$$\log \varphi_{sc} = \boldsymbol{v}_{sc}^{\mathrm{T}} \cdot \boldsymbol{\gamma}$$

where $\boldsymbol{\gamma}$ is a $q \times 1$ vector of coefficient parameters. Let $\boldsymbol{V}_s$ denote the $m(s) \times q$ predictor matrix with rows $\boldsymbol{v}_{sc}^{\mathrm{T}}$. Define the extended variances as

$$\sigma_{sc}^2 = \varphi_{sc} \cdot V(\mu_{sc})$$

and the standardized residuals as

$$stde_{sc} = e_{sc}/\sigma_{sc}.$$

Combine the extended standard deviations and standardized residuals over $c \in C(s)$ into the $m(s) \times 1$ vectors $\boldsymbol{\sigma}_s$ and $\boldsymbol{stde}_s$ for $s \in S$.

Denote an observation by $O_s = \{\boldsymbol{y}_s, \boldsymbol{X}_s, \boldsymbol{V}_s\}$ and define the likelihood function $L(SC; \boldsymbol{\theta})$ to be the product of terms $L(O_s; \boldsymbol{\theta})$ for $s \in S$ satisfying

$$\ell(O_s;\boldsymbol{\theta}) = \log L(O_s;\boldsymbol{\theta}) = -\boldsymbol{e}_s^{\mathrm{T}} \cdot \boldsymbol{\Sigma}_s^{-1} \cdot \boldsymbol{e}_s/2 - (\log|\boldsymbol{\Sigma}_s|)/2 - (m(s) \cdot \log(2 \cdot \pi))/2$$

where

$$\boldsymbol{\theta} = \begin{pmatrix} \boldsymbol{\beta} \\ \boldsymbol{\gamma} \end{pmatrix}$$

and the $m(s) \times m(s)$ covariance matrix $\boldsymbol{\Sigma}_s$ of $\boldsymbol{y}_s$ satisfies

$$\boldsymbol{\Sigma}_s = \boldsymbol{DIAG}(\boldsymbol{\sigma}_s) \cdot \boldsymbol{R}_s(\boldsymbol{\rho}) \cdot \boldsymbol{DIAG}(\boldsymbol{\sigma}_s)$$

for appropriate choices of the $m(s) \times m(s)$ correlation matrices $\boldsymbol{R}_s(\boldsymbol{\rho})$ for $s \in S$. Estimating equations $\boldsymbol{E}(\boldsymbol{\gamma}) = \boldsymbol{0}$ for the dispersion parameters can be generated by maximizing the likelihood $L(SC; \boldsymbol{\theta})$ in $\boldsymbol{\gamma}$, that is,

$$\boldsymbol{E}(\boldsymbol{\gamma}) = \frac{\partial_0 \ell(SC;\boldsymbol{\theta})}{\partial_0 \boldsymbol{\gamma}}$$

where the operator notation $\frac{\partial_0}{\partial_0 \boldsymbol{\gamma}}$ is used to indicate that this is not the full partial derivative vector for $\ell(SC; \boldsymbol{\theta})$ in $\boldsymbol{\gamma}$ due to not accounting for the effect of $\boldsymbol{\gamma}$ on $\boldsymbol{R}_s(\boldsymbol{\rho})$. $\boldsymbol{E}(\boldsymbol{\gamma})$ is the sum over $s \in S$ of $\boldsymbol{E}_s(\boldsymbol{\gamma})$ with entries

$$E_{s,j}(\gamma)=\boldsymbol{vstde}_{s,j}^{\mathrm{T}}\cdot\boldsymbol{R}_s^{-1}(\rho)\cdot\boldsymbol{stde}_s-\sum_{c\in C(s)}v_{sc,j}/2$$

where $\boldsymbol{vstde}_{s,j}$ is the $m(s)\times 1$ vector with entries

$$vstde_{sc,j}=v_{sc,j}\cdot stde_{sc}/2$$

for $sc\in SC$ and $1\le j\le q$. Now, combine these with the r standard GEE mean estimating equations $\boldsymbol{E}(\boldsymbol{\beta})=\boldsymbol{0}$ to use Newton's method to solve for joint estimates of $\boldsymbol{\beta}$ and $\boldsymbol{\gamma}$. Then, iteratively solve for

$$\boldsymbol{E}(\boldsymbol{\theta})=\begin{pmatrix}E(\beta)\\E(\gamma)\end{pmatrix}=\boldsymbol{0}$$

with $\boldsymbol{E}(\boldsymbol{\theta})$ in the role of the gradient vector and the $(r+q)\times(r+q)$ matrix $\boldsymbol{E}'(\boldsymbol{\theta})$ in the role of the Hessian matrix.

$\boldsymbol{E}'(\boldsymbol{\theta})$ has four component matrices: the $r\times r$ matrix

$$\boldsymbol{E}'(\boldsymbol{\beta})=\frac{\partial_0\boldsymbol{E}(\boldsymbol{\beta})}{\partial_0\boldsymbol{\beta}}$$

for the r mean coefficients as used in standard GEE modeling, the $q\times q$ matrix

$$\boldsymbol{E}'(\boldsymbol{\gamma})=\frac{\partial_0\boldsymbol{E}(\boldsymbol{\gamma})}{\partial_0\boldsymbol{\gamma}}$$

for the q dispersion coefficients, the $r\times q$ matrix

$$\boldsymbol{E}'(\boldsymbol{\beta},\boldsymbol{\gamma})=\frac{\partial_0\boldsymbol{E}(\boldsymbol{\beta})}{\partial_0\boldsymbol{\gamma}},$$

and its transpose $\boldsymbol{E}'(\boldsymbol{\gamma},\boldsymbol{\beta})=\boldsymbol{E}'^{\mathrm{T}}(\boldsymbol{\beta},\boldsymbol{\gamma})$. $\boldsymbol{E}'(\boldsymbol{\gamma})$ is the sum over $s\in S$ of $\boldsymbol{E}'_s(\boldsymbol{\gamma})$ with entries

$$E'_{s,j,j'}(\gamma)=-\boldsymbol{vvstde}_{s,j,j'}^{\mathrm{T}}\cdot\boldsymbol{R}_s^{-1}(\rho)\cdot\boldsymbol{stde}_s-\boldsymbol{vstde}_{s,j}^{\mathrm{T}}\cdot\boldsymbol{R}_s^{-1}(\rho)\cdot\boldsymbol{vstde}_{s,j'}$$

where $\boldsymbol{vvstde}_{s,j,j'}$ is the $m(s)\times 1$ vector with entries

$$vvstde_{sc,j,j'}=v_{sc,j}\cdot v_{sc,j'}\cdot stde_{sc}/4$$

for $sc\in SC$ and $1\le j,j'\le q$. $\boldsymbol{E}'(\boldsymbol{\beta},\boldsymbol{\gamma})$ is the sum over $s\in S$ of $\boldsymbol{E}'_s(\boldsymbol{\beta},\boldsymbol{\gamma})$ with q $r\times 1$ column vectors

$$\boldsymbol{E}'_{s,j}(\boldsymbol{\beta},\boldsymbol{\gamma}) = -\boldsymbol{D}_s^{\mathrm{T}} \cdot \boldsymbol{DIAG}(\boldsymbol{v\sigma inv}_{s,j}) \cdot \boldsymbol{R}_s^{-1}(\boldsymbol{\rho}) \cdot \boldsymbol{stde}_s$$
$$-\boldsymbol{D}_s^{\mathrm{T}} \cdot \boldsymbol{DIAG}(\boldsymbol{1}/\boldsymbol{\sigma}_s) \cdot \boldsymbol{R}_s^{-1}(\boldsymbol{\rho}) \cdot \boldsymbol{vstde}_{s,j}$$

where $\boldsymbol{v\sigma inv}_{s,j}$ is the $m(s) \times 1$ vector with entries

$$v\sigma inv_{sc,j} = \frac{v_{sc,j}}{2 \cdot \sigma_{sc}}$$

for $sc \in SC$ and $1 \leq j \leq q$. Model-based and robust empirical estimates of the covariance matrix for the partially modified GEE estimate $\boldsymbol{\theta}(SC)$ of the mean coefficient parameter vector $\boldsymbol{\theta}$ can be computed as in Sect. 3.4.

Given a value for the vector $\boldsymbol{\theta}$ of all coefficient parameters, an estimate of the correlation parameter vector $\boldsymbol{\rho}$ can be based on the associated standardized residuals $stde_{sc}(\boldsymbol{\theta})$ determined by non-constant dispersions $\varphi_{sc}(\boldsymbol{\gamma})$ computed with the current value for $\boldsymbol{\gamma}$. Calculate the revised correlation estimates for the correlation structures of Sect. 2.3 using the formulas of Sect. 2.4.1 evaluated with the revised standardized residuals $stde_{sc}(\boldsymbol{\theta})$.

12.2.3.3 Fully Modified GEE Modeling

The formulation of Chap. 4 applies with $V(\mu_{sc})$ replaced by $\mathrm{Var}(y_{sc})$ extending the formulation of Sect. 12.2.3.2 using the same likelihood function $L(SC;\boldsymbol{\theta})$ and

$$\boldsymbol{E}(\boldsymbol{\theta}) = \begin{pmatrix} \boldsymbol{E}(\boldsymbol{\beta}) \\ \boldsymbol{E}(\boldsymbol{\gamma}) \end{pmatrix}$$

with $\boldsymbol{E}(\boldsymbol{\gamma})$ computed as in Sect. 12.2.3.2.

$$\boldsymbol{E}(\boldsymbol{\beta}) = \frac{\partial_0 \ell(SC;\boldsymbol{\theta})}{\partial_0 \boldsymbol{\beta}}$$

is the sum over $s \in S$ of $\boldsymbol{E}_s(\boldsymbol{\beta})$ with entries

$$E_{s,j}(\boldsymbol{\beta}) = \boldsymbol{xstde}_{s,j}^{\mathrm{T}} \cdot \boldsymbol{R}_s^{-1}(\boldsymbol{\rho}) \cdot \boldsymbol{stde}_s - \sum_{c \in C(s)} W_{sc,j}/2$$

where $\boldsymbol{xstde}_{s,j}$ is the $m(s) \times 1$ vector with entries

$$xstde_{sc,j} = \frac{\partial \mu_{sc}}{\partial \beta_j} / \sigma_{sc} + stde_{sc} \cdot \frac{W_{sc,j}}{2},$$

$$W_{sc,j} = \frac{\frac{\partial \mathrm{Var}(y_{sc})}{\partial \beta_j}}{\mathrm{Var}(y_{sc})},$$

$$\frac{\partial \mathrm{Var}(y_{sc})}{\partial \beta_j} = \sum_{u=0}^{K-1} \left((d_u - d_K) \cdot (d_u + d_K - 2 \cdot \mu_{sc}) \cdot \frac{\partial p_{sc,u}}{\partial \beta_j} \right),$$

and $\frac{\partial \mu_{sc}}{\partial \beta_j}$ is defined in Sect. 12.2.3.1, for $1 \leq j \leq r$ and $sc \in SC$. As before, use Newton's method to iteratively solve $\boldsymbol{E(\theta)} = \mathbf{0}$. The correlation estimates are the same as those in Sect. 12.2.3.2.

$\boldsymbol{E}'(\boldsymbol{\theta})$ has four component matrices: the $r \times r$ matrix

$$\boldsymbol{E}'(\boldsymbol{\beta}) = \frac{\partial_0 \boldsymbol{E}(\boldsymbol{\beta})}{\partial_0 \boldsymbol{\beta}}$$

for the r mean coefficients, the $q \times q$ matrix

$$\boldsymbol{E}'(\boldsymbol{\gamma}) = \frac{\partial_0 \boldsymbol{E}(\boldsymbol{\gamma})}{\partial_0 \boldsymbol{\gamma}}$$

for the q dispersion coefficients as computed in Sect. 12.2.3.2, the $r \times q$ matrix

$$\boldsymbol{E}'(\boldsymbol{\beta}, \boldsymbol{\gamma}) = \frac{\partial_0 \boldsymbol{E}(\boldsymbol{\beta})}{\partial_0 \boldsymbol{\gamma}},$$

and its transpose $\boldsymbol{E}'(\boldsymbol{\gamma}, \boldsymbol{\beta}) = \boldsymbol{E}'^{\mathrm{T}}(\boldsymbol{\beta}, \boldsymbol{\gamma})$. $\boldsymbol{E}'(\boldsymbol{\beta})$ is the sum over $s \in S$ of $\boldsymbol{E}'_s(\boldsymbol{\beta})$ with entries

$$E'_{s,j,j'}(\boldsymbol{\beta}) = -\boldsymbol{xxstde}^{\mathrm{T}}_{s,j,j'} \cdot \boldsymbol{R}_s^{-1}(\boldsymbol{\rho}) \cdot \boldsymbol{stde}_s - \boldsymbol{xstde}^{\mathrm{T}}_{s,j} \cdot \boldsymbol{R}_s^{-1}(\boldsymbol{\rho}) \cdot \boldsymbol{xstde}_{s,j'} - \sum_{c \in C(s)} W_{sc,j,j'}/2$$

where $\boldsymbol{xxstde}_{s,j,j'}$ is the $m(s) \times 1$ vector with entries

$$xxstde_{sc,j,j'} = -\frac{\frac{\partial^2 \mu_{sc}}{\partial \beta_{j'} \partial \beta_j}}{\sigma_{sc}} + \frac{\partial \mu_{sc}}{\partial \beta_j} \cdot \frac{W_{sc,j'}}{2 \cdot \sigma_{sc}} + xstde_{sc,j'} \cdot \frac{W_{sc,j}}{2} - stde_{sc} \cdot \frac{W_{sc,j,j'}}{2},$$

$$\frac{\partial^2 \mu_{sc}}{\partial \beta_{j'} \partial \beta_j} = \sum_{u=0}^{K-1} (d_u - d_K) \cdot \frac{\partial^2 p_{sc,u}}{\partial \beta_{j'} \partial \beta_j},$$

$$W_{sc,j,j'} = \frac{\partial W_{sc,j}}{\partial \beta_{j'}} = \frac{\frac{\partial^2 \mathrm{Var}(y_{sc})}{\partial \beta_{j'} \partial \beta_j}}{\mathrm{Var}(y_{sc})} - \frac{\frac{\partial \mathrm{Var}(y_{sc})}{\partial \beta_{j'}} \cdot \frac{\partial \mathrm{Var}(y_{sc})}{\partial \beta_j}}{\mathrm{Var}^2(y_{sc})},$$

$$\frac{\partial^2 \mathrm{Var}(y_{sc})}{\partial \beta_{j'} \partial \beta_j} = \sum_{u=0}^{K-1} \left((d_u - d_K) \cdot (d_u + d_K - 2 \cdot \mu_{sc}) \cdot \frac{\partial^2 p_{sc,u}}{\partial \beta_{j'} \partial \beta_j} - 2 \cdot \frac{\partial \mu_{sc}}{\partial \beta_j} \cdot \frac{\partial p_{sc,u}}{\partial \beta_{j'}} \right),$$

for $1 \leq j, j' \leq r$. $\boldsymbol{E}'(\boldsymbol{\beta}, \boldsymbol{\gamma})$ is the sum over $s \in S$ of $\boldsymbol{E}'_s(\boldsymbol{\beta}, \boldsymbol{\gamma})$ with entries

$$E'_{s,j,j'}(\boldsymbol{\beta}, \boldsymbol{\gamma}) = -\boldsymbol{vxstde}^{\mathrm{T}}_{s,j,j'} \cdot \boldsymbol{R}_s^{-1}(\boldsymbol{\rho}) \cdot \boldsymbol{stde}_s - \boldsymbol{xstde}^{\mathrm{T}}_{s,j} \cdot \boldsymbol{R}_s^{-1}(\boldsymbol{\rho}) \cdot \boldsymbol{vstde}_{s,j'}$$

where $\boldsymbol{vxstde}_{s,w,j,j'}$ is the $m(s) \times 1$ vector with entries

$$vxstde_{sc,j,j'} = xstde_{sc,j} \cdot v_{sc,j'}/2$$

and $\boldsymbol{vstde}_{s,j'}$ is defined in Sect. 12.2.3.2 for $sc \in SC$, $1 \leq j \leq r$, and $1 \leq j' \leq q$. Model-based and robust empirical estimates of the covariance matrix for the fully modified GEE estimate $\boldsymbol{\theta}(SC)$ of the mean coefficient parameter vector $\boldsymbol{\theta}$ can be computed as in Sect. 4.1.

12.2.3.4 Extended Linear Mixed Modeling

The formulation of Chap. 5 applies with $V(\mu_{sc})$ replaced by $\mathrm{Var}(y_{sc})$ extending the formulation of Sect. 12.2.3.3. The likelihood function $L(SC; \boldsymbol{\theta})$ is the same as defined in Sect. 12.2.3.2 except that the parameter vector is now

$$\boldsymbol{\theta} = \begin{pmatrix} \boldsymbol{\beta} \\ \boldsymbol{\gamma} \\ \boldsymbol{\rho} \end{pmatrix}$$

with $r + q + p$ entries where p is the number of correlation parameters. The likelihood $L(SC; \boldsymbol{\theta})$ is maximized in the coefficient parameter vector $\boldsymbol{\theta}$. Specifically, use Newton's method to solve the estimating equations

$$\boldsymbol{E}(\boldsymbol{\theta}) = \frac{\partial \ell(SC; \boldsymbol{\theta})}{\partial \boldsymbol{\theta}} = \sum_{s \in S} \boldsymbol{E}_s(\boldsymbol{\theta}) = \sum_{s \in S} \frac{\partial \ell(O_s; \boldsymbol{\theta})}{\partial \boldsymbol{\theta}} = \boldsymbol{0}$$

where the operator notation $\frac{\partial}{\partial \boldsymbol{\theta}}$ is used to indicate that this is a standard partial derivative vector in $\boldsymbol{\theta}$ since $\boldsymbol{\rho}$ is treated as a separate parameter vector. The associated matrix

$$\boldsymbol{E}'(\boldsymbol{\theta}) = \frac{\partial \boldsymbol{E}(\boldsymbol{\theta})}{\partial \boldsymbol{\theta}}.$$

In this case, $\boldsymbol{E}(\boldsymbol{\theta})$ is a true gradient vector and $\boldsymbol{E}'(\boldsymbol{\theta})$ a true Hessian matrix. The four correlation structures of Sect. 2.3 can still be considered. In all cases, there is just one alternative estimate of the correlation vector and not bias-adjusted and bias-unadjusted alternatives as for standard, partially modified, and fully modified GEE. The EC and spatial AR1 cases can be handled without storing associated correlation matrices (Sects. 5.3–5.4), providing efficient computation of associated estimates for data with relatively large numbers m of conditions.

The gradient vector satisfies

$$\boldsymbol{E}(\boldsymbol{\theta}) = \begin{pmatrix} \boldsymbol{E}(\boldsymbol{\beta}) \\ \boldsymbol{E}(\boldsymbol{\gamma}) \\ \boldsymbol{E}(\boldsymbol{\rho}) \end{pmatrix}$$

where $\boldsymbol{E}(\boldsymbol{\gamma})$ is computed as in Sect. 12.2.3.2 for partially modified GEE modeling and $\boldsymbol{E}(\boldsymbol{\beta})$ is computed as in Sect. 12.2.3.3 for fully modified GEE modeling since the correlation matrices do not depend on the dispersion parameters. With the entries of $\boldsymbol{\rho}$ denoted by ρ_j for $1 \le j \le p$,

$$\boldsymbol{E}(\boldsymbol{\rho}) = \frac{\partial \ell(SC;\boldsymbol{\theta})}{\partial \boldsymbol{\rho}}$$

is the sum over $s \in S$ of $\boldsymbol{E}_s(\boldsymbol{\rho})$ with entries

$$E_{s,j}(\boldsymbol{\rho}) = -\,\boldsymbol{stde}_s^{\mathrm{T}} \cdot \frac{\partial \boldsymbol{R}_s^{-1}(\boldsymbol{\rho})}{\partial \rho_j} \cdot \boldsymbol{stde}_s/2 - \frac{\partial \log|\boldsymbol{R}_s(\boldsymbol{\rho})|}{\partial \rho_j}/2$$

where $\boldsymbol{R}_s(\boldsymbol{\rho})$ changes with the correlation structure but does not depend on the mean and dispersion parameters.

$\boldsymbol{E}'(\boldsymbol{\theta})$ has nine component matrices: the $r \times r$ matrix

$$\boldsymbol{E}'(\boldsymbol{\beta}) = \frac{\partial \boldsymbol{E}(\boldsymbol{\beta})}{\partial \boldsymbol{\beta}}$$

for the r mean parameters computed as in Sect. 12.2.3.3 for fully modified GEE modeling, the $q \times q$ matrix

$$\boldsymbol{E}'(\boldsymbol{\gamma}) = \frac{\partial \boldsymbol{E}(\boldsymbol{\gamma})}{\partial \boldsymbol{\gamma}}$$

for the q dispersion parameters computed as in Sect. 12.2.3.2 for partially modified GEE modeling, the $p \times p$ matrix

$$\mathbf{E}'(\boldsymbol{\rho}) = \frac{\partial \mathbf{E}(\boldsymbol{\rho})}{\partial \boldsymbol{\rho}}$$

for the p correlation parameters, the $r \times q$ matrix

$$\mathbf{E}'(\boldsymbol{\beta},\boldsymbol{\gamma}) = \frac{\partial \mathbf{E}(\boldsymbol{\beta})}{\partial \boldsymbol{\gamma}}$$

and its transpose $\mathbf{E}'(\boldsymbol{\gamma},\boldsymbol{\beta}) = \mathbf{E}'^{\mathrm{T}}(\boldsymbol{\beta},\boldsymbol{\gamma})$ computed as in Sect. 12.2.3.3 for fully modified GEE modeling, the $r \times p$ matrix

$$\mathbf{E}'(\boldsymbol{\beta},\boldsymbol{\rho}) = \frac{\partial \mathbf{E}(\boldsymbol{\beta})}{\partial \boldsymbol{\rho}}$$

and its transpose $\mathbf{E}'(\boldsymbol{\rho},\boldsymbol{\beta}) = \mathbf{E}'^{\mathrm{T}}(\boldsymbol{\beta},\boldsymbol{\rho})$, the $q \times p$ matrix

$$\mathbf{E}'(\boldsymbol{\gamma},\boldsymbol{\rho}) = \frac{\partial \mathbf{E}(\boldsymbol{\gamma})}{\partial \boldsymbol{\rho}}$$

and its transpose $\mathbf{E}'(\boldsymbol{\rho},\boldsymbol{\gamma}) = \mathbf{E}'^{\mathrm{T}}(\boldsymbol{\gamma},\boldsymbol{\rho})$. $\mathbf{E}'(\boldsymbol{\rho})$ is the sum over $s \in S$ of $\mathbf{E}'_s(\boldsymbol{\rho})$ with entries satisfying

$$E'_{s,j,j'}(\boldsymbol{\rho}) = -\mathbf{stde}_s^{\mathrm{T}} \cdot \frac{\partial^2 \mathbf{R}_s^{-1}(\boldsymbol{\rho})}{\partial \rho_{j'}\,\partial \rho_j} \cdot \mathbf{stde}_s/2 - \frac{\partial^2 \log|\mathbf{R}_s(\boldsymbol{\rho})|}{\partial \rho_{j'}\,\partial \rho_j}/2.$$

$\mathbf{E}'(\boldsymbol{\beta},\boldsymbol{\rho})$ is the sum over $s \in S$ of $\mathbf{E}'_s(\boldsymbol{\beta},\boldsymbol{\rho})$ with entries

$$E'_{s,j,j'}(\boldsymbol{\beta},\boldsymbol{\rho}) = \mathbf{xstde}_{s,j}^{\mathrm{T}} \cdot \frac{\partial \mathbf{R}_s^{-1}(\boldsymbol{\rho})}{\partial \rho_{j'}} \cdot \mathbf{stde}_s$$

for $1 \le j \le r$ and $1 \le j' \le p$ where $\mathbf{xstde}_{s,w,j}$ is defined in Sect. 12.2.3.3. $\mathbf{E}'(\boldsymbol{\gamma},\boldsymbol{\rho})$ is the sum over $s \in S$ of $\mathbf{E}'_s(\boldsymbol{\gamma},\boldsymbol{\rho})$ with entries

$$E'_{s,j,j'}(\boldsymbol{\gamma},\boldsymbol{\rho}) = \mathbf{vstde}_{s,j}^{\mathrm{T}} \cdot \frac{\partial \mathbf{R}_s^{-1}(\boldsymbol{\rho})}{\partial \rho_{j'}} \cdot \mathbf{stde}_s$$

for $1 \le j \le q$ and $1 \le j' \le p$ where $\mathbf{vstde}_{s,j}$ is defined in Sect. 12.2.3.2. Formulations for first and second partial derivatives of $\log|\mathbf{R}_s(\boldsymbol{\rho})|$ and $\mathbf{R}_s^{-1}(\boldsymbol{\rho})$ with respect to $\boldsymbol{\rho}$ needed to compute $\mathbf{E}(\boldsymbol{\rho})$, $\mathbf{E}'(\boldsymbol{\rho})$, $\mathbf{E}'(\boldsymbol{\beta},\boldsymbol{\rho})$, and $\mathbf{E}'(\boldsymbol{\gamma},\boldsymbol{\rho})$ are provided in Sects. 5.3–5.5 for the EC, spatial AR1, and UN structures. These partial derivatives are dropped for the IND correlation structure. Model-based and robust empirical estimates of the covariance matrix for the ELMM estimate $\boldsymbol{\theta}(SC)$ of the parameter vector $\boldsymbol{\theta}$ can be computed as in Sect. 5.1.

12.2.4 Direct Variance Modeling

This section provides the formulation for direct variance modeling, as first addressed in Sect. 5.7, of correlated univariate discrete outcomes. Section 12.2.4.1 addresses direct variance modeling using multinomial probabilities, Sect. 12.2.4.2 ordinal probabilities, and Sect. 12.2.4.3 censored Poisson probabilities. As in Sect. 5.7, formulations are provided only for the ELMM case.

The variances are $\sigma_{sc}^2 = \varphi_{sc}$ and the standardized residuals $stde_{sc} = e_{sc}/\sigma_{sc}$. The likelihood function $L(SC;\boldsymbol{\theta})$ is the product of terms $L(O_s;\boldsymbol{\theta})$ for $s \in S$ satisfying

$$\ell(O_s;\boldsymbol{\theta}) = \log L(O_s;\boldsymbol{\theta}) = -\boldsymbol{e}_s^{\mathrm{T}} \cdot \boldsymbol{\Sigma}_s^{-1} \cdot \boldsymbol{e}_s/2 - (\log|\boldsymbol{\Sigma}_s|)/2 - (m(s) \cdot \log(2 \cdot \pi))/2$$

where

$$\boldsymbol{\theta} = \begin{pmatrix} \boldsymbol{\beta} \\ \boldsymbol{\gamma} \\ \boldsymbol{\rho} \end{pmatrix}$$

and the $m(s) \times m(s)$ covariance matrix $\boldsymbol{\Sigma}_s$ of $\boldsymbol{y}_s$ satisfies

$$\boldsymbol{\Sigma}_s = \boldsymbol{DIAG}(\boldsymbol{\sigma}_s) \cdot \boldsymbol{R}_s(\boldsymbol{\rho}) \cdot \boldsymbol{DIAG}(\boldsymbol{\sigma}_s)$$

for appropriate choices of the $m(s) \times m(s)$ correlation matrices $\boldsymbol{R}_s(\boldsymbol{\rho})$ for $s \in S$ as addressed in Sect. 2.3. To maximize $L(SC;\boldsymbol{\theta})$, solve

$$\boldsymbol{E}(\boldsymbol{\theta}) = \frac{\partial \ell(SC;\boldsymbol{\theta})}{\partial \boldsymbol{\theta}} = \begin{pmatrix} \boldsymbol{E}(\boldsymbol{\beta}) \\ \boldsymbol{E}(\boldsymbol{\gamma}) \\ \boldsymbol{E}(\boldsymbol{\rho}) \end{pmatrix} = \begin{pmatrix} \dfrac{\partial \ell(S;\boldsymbol{\theta})}{\partial \boldsymbol{\beta}} \\ \dfrac{\partial \ell(S;\boldsymbol{\theta})}{\partial \boldsymbol{\gamma}} \\ \dfrac{\partial \ell(S;\boldsymbol{\theta})}{\partial \boldsymbol{\rho}} \end{pmatrix} = \boldsymbol{0}.$$

12.2.4.1 Multinomial Probabilities

$\boldsymbol{E}(\boldsymbol{\beta})$ is the $(K \cdot r) \times 1$ vector equaling the sum over $s \in S$ of $\boldsymbol{E}_s(\boldsymbol{\beta})$ with entries

$$E_{s,w,j}(\boldsymbol{\beta}) = \boldsymbol{xstde}_{s,w,j}^{\mathrm{T}} \cdot \boldsymbol{R}_s^{-1}(\boldsymbol{\rho}) \cdot \boldsymbol{stde}_s$$

$\boldsymbol{xstde}_{s,w,j}$ is the $m(s) \times 1$ vector with entries

$$xstde_{sc,w,j} = \frac{\partial \mu_{sc}}{\partial \beta_{w,j}} / \sigma_{sc},$$

$$\frac{\partial \mu_{sc}}{\partial \beta_{w,j}} = x_{sc,j} \cdot p_{sc,w} \cdot (d_w - \mu_{sc}),$$

for $1 \leq w \leq K$, $1 \leq j \leq r$, and $sc \in SC$. $\boldsymbol{E}(\boldsymbol{\gamma})$ has the same formulation as in Sect. 12.2.1.2 and $\boldsymbol{E}(\boldsymbol{\rho})$ the same as in Sect. 12.2.1.4. $\boldsymbol{E}'(\boldsymbol{\theta})$ has the same component matrices as defined in Sect. 12.2.1.4. $\boldsymbol{E}'(\boldsymbol{\beta})$ is the sum over $s \in S$ of $\boldsymbol{E}'_s(\boldsymbol{\beta})$ with entries

$$E'_{s,w,j,w',j'}(\boldsymbol{\beta}) = -\boldsymbol{xxstde}^{\mathrm{T}}_{s,wj,w',j'} \cdot \boldsymbol{R}_s^{-1}(\rho) \cdot \boldsymbol{stde}_s - \boldsymbol{xstde}^{\mathrm{T}}_{s,w,j} \cdot \boldsymbol{R}_s^{-1}(\rho) \cdot \boldsymbol{xstde}_{s,w',j'}$$

where $\boldsymbol{xxstde}_{s,w,j,w',j'}$ is the $m(s) \times 1$ vector with entries

$$xxstde_{sc,w,j,w',j'} = -\frac{\partial^2 \mu_{sc}}{\partial \beta_{w',j'} \partial \beta_{w,j}} / \sigma_{sc},$$

$$\frac{\partial^2 \mu_{sc}}{\partial \beta_{w',j'} \partial \beta_{w,j}} = x_{sc,j} \cdot x_{sc,j'} \cdot p_{sc,w} \cdot \left(1 - 2 \cdot p_{sc,w}\right) \cdot (d_w - \mu_{sc}), w' = w,$$

$$\frac{\partial^2 \mu_{sc}}{\partial \beta_{w',j'} \partial \beta_{w,j}} = -x_{sc,j} \cdot x_{sc,j'} \cdot p_{sc,w} \cdot p_{sc,w'} \cdot (d_w + d_{w'} - 2 \cdot \mu_{sc}), w' \neq w,$$

for $1 \leq w, w' \leq K$ and $1 \leq j, j' \leq r$. Component matrices of $\boldsymbol{E}'(\boldsymbol{\theta})$ depending only on $\boldsymbol{\gamma}$ and/or $\boldsymbol{\rho}$ are the same as in Sect. 12.2.1 while those depending on $\boldsymbol{\beta}$ together with $\boldsymbol{\gamma}$ or $\boldsymbol{\rho}$ are computed as in Sect. 12.2.1 but using the above revised formulation for $\boldsymbol{E}(\boldsymbol{\beta})$.

12.2.4.2 Ordinal Probabilities

$\boldsymbol{E}(\boldsymbol{\beta})$ is the $(K + r) \times 1$ vector equaling the sum over $s \in S$ of $\boldsymbol{E}_s(\boldsymbol{\beta})$ with entries

$$E_{s,w}(\boldsymbol{\beta}) = \boldsymbol{xstde}^{\mathrm{T}}_{s,w} \cdot \boldsymbol{R}_s^{-1}(\rho) \cdot \boldsymbol{stde}_s,$$

$$E_{s,K,j}(\boldsymbol{\beta}) = \boldsymbol{xstde}^{\mathrm{T}}_{s,K,j} \cdot \boldsymbol{R}_s^{-1}(\rho) \cdot \boldsymbol{stde}_s$$

$\boldsymbol{xstde}_{s,w}$ and $\boldsymbol{xstde}_{s,K,j}$ are the $m(s) \times 1$ vectors with respective entries

$$xstde_{sc,w} = \frac{\partial \mu_{sc}}{\partial \alpha_w} / \sigma_{sc},$$

$$\frac{\partial \mu_{sc}}{\partial \alpha_w} = p_{sc,\leq w} \cdot \left(1 - p_{sc,\leq w}\right) \cdot \left(d_w - d_{w-1}\right),$$

$$xstde_{sc,K,j} = \frac{\partial \mu_{sc}}{\partial \beta_{K,j}} / \sigma_{sc},$$

$$\frac{\partial \mu_{sc}}{\partial \beta_{K,j}} = x_{sc,j} \cdot \sum_{u=0}^{K-1} \left(p_{sc,\leq u} \cdot \left(1 - p_{sc,\leq u}\right) \cdot \left(d_u - d_{u-1}\right)\right),$$

for $1 \leq w \leq K$, $1 \leq j \leq r$, and $sc \in SC$. $\boldsymbol{E}(\boldsymbol{\gamma})$ has the same formulation as in Sect. 12.2.2.2 and $\boldsymbol{E}(\boldsymbol{\rho})$ the same as in Sect. 12.2.2.4. $\boldsymbol{E}'(\boldsymbol{\theta})$ has the same component matrices as defined in Sect. 12.2.2.4. $\boldsymbol{E}'(\boldsymbol{\beta})$ is the sum over $s \in S$ of $\boldsymbol{E}'_s(\boldsymbol{\beta})$ with entries

$$E'_{s,w,w'}(\boldsymbol{\beta}) = -\boldsymbol{xxstde}^{\mathrm{T}}_{s,w,w'} \cdot \boldsymbol{R}_s^{-1}(\boldsymbol{\rho}) \cdot \boldsymbol{stde}_s - \boldsymbol{xstde}^{\mathrm{T}}_{s,w} \cdot \boldsymbol{R}_s^{-1}(\boldsymbol{\rho}) \cdot \boldsymbol{xstde}_{s,w'},$$

$$E'_{s,w,K,j}(\boldsymbol{\beta}) = -\boldsymbol{xxstde}^{\mathrm{T}}_{s,w,K,j} \cdot \boldsymbol{R}_s^{-1}(\boldsymbol{\rho}) \cdot \boldsymbol{stde}_s - \boldsymbol{xstde}^{\mathrm{T}}_{s,w} \cdot \boldsymbol{R}_s^{-1}(\boldsymbol{\rho}) \cdot \boldsymbol{xstde}_{s,K,j},$$

$$E'_{s,K,j,w'}(\boldsymbol{\beta}) = -\boldsymbol{xxstde}^{\mathrm{T}}_{s,Kj,w'} \cdot \boldsymbol{R}_s^{-1}(\boldsymbol{\rho}) \cdot \boldsymbol{stde}_s - \boldsymbol{xstde}^{\mathrm{T}}_{s,K,j} \cdot \boldsymbol{R}_s^{-1}(\boldsymbol{\rho}) \cdot \boldsymbol{xstde}_{s,w'},$$

$$E'_{s,K,j,j'}(\boldsymbol{\beta}) = -\boldsymbol{xxstde}^{\mathrm{T}}_{s,Kj,j'} \cdot \boldsymbol{R}_s^{-1}(\boldsymbol{\rho}) \cdot \boldsymbol{stde}_s - \boldsymbol{xstde}^{\mathrm{T}}_{s,K,j} \cdot \boldsymbol{R}_s^{-1}(\boldsymbol{\rho}) \cdot \boldsymbol{xstde}_{s,K,j'},$$

where $\boldsymbol{xxstde}_{s,w,w'}$, $\boldsymbol{xxstde}_{s,w,K,j}$, $\boldsymbol{xxstde}_{s,K,j,w'}$, **and** $\boldsymbol{xxstde}_{s,K,j,j'}$ are the $m(s) \times 1$ vectors with respective entries

$$xxstde_{sc,w,w'} = -\frac{\partial^2 \mu_{sc}}{\partial \alpha_{w'} \partial \alpha_w} / \sigma_{sc},$$

$$\frac{\partial^2 \mu_{sc}}{\partial \alpha_{w'} \partial \alpha_w} = p_{sc,\leq w} \cdot \left(1 - p_{sc,\leq w}\right) \cdot \left(1 - 2 \cdot p_{sc,\leq w}\right) \cdot \left(d_w - d_{w+1}\right), w' = w,$$

$$\frac{\partial^2 \mu_{sc}}{\partial \alpha_{w'} \partial \alpha_{w'}} = 0, w' \neq w;$$

$$xxstde_{sc,w,K,j} = -\frac{\partial^2 \mu_{sc}}{\partial \beta_{K,j} \partial \alpha_w} / \sigma_{sc},$$

$$\frac{\partial^2 \mu_{sc}}{\partial \beta_{K,j} \partial \alpha_w} = x_{sc,j} \cdot p_{sc,\leq w} \cdot \left(1 - p_{sc,\leq w}\right) \cdot \left(1 - 2 \cdot p_{sc,\leq w}\right) \cdot \left(d_w - d_{w+1}\right);$$

$$xxstde_{sc,K,j,w'} = -\frac{\partial^2 \mu_{sc}}{\partial \alpha_{w'} \partial \beta_{K,j}} / \sigma_{sc},$$

$$\frac{\partial^2 \mu_{sc}}{\partial \alpha_{w'} \partial \beta_{K,j}} = x_{sc,j} \cdot p_{sc,\le w'} \cdot \left(1 - p_{sc,\le w'}\right) \cdot \left(1 - 2 \cdot p_{sc,\le w'}\right) \cdot \left(d_{w'} - d_{w'+1}\right);$$

$$xxstde_{sc,K,j,j'} = -\frac{\partial^2 \mu_{sc}}{\partial \beta_{K,j'} \partial \beta_{K,j}} / \sigma_{sc},$$

$$\frac{\partial^2 \mu_{sc}}{\partial \beta_{K,j'} \partial \beta_{K,j}} = x_{sc,j} \cdot x_{sc,j'} \cdot \sum_{u=0}^{K-1} \left(p_{sc,\le u} \cdot \left(1 - p_{sc,\le u}\right) \cdot \left(1 - 2 \cdot p_{sc,\le u}\right) \cdot \left(d_u - d_{u+1}\right)\right),$$

for $1 \le w, w' < K$ and $1 \le j, j' \le r$. Component matrices of $\boldsymbol{E}'(\boldsymbol{\theta})$ depending only on $\boldsymbol{\gamma}$ and/or $\boldsymbol{\rho}$ are the same as in Sect. 12.2.2 while those depending on $\boldsymbol{\beta}$ together with $\boldsymbol{\gamma}$ or $\boldsymbol{\rho}$ are computed as in Sect. 12.2.2 but using the above revised formulation for $\boldsymbol{E}(\boldsymbol{\beta})$.

12.2.4.3 Censored Poisson Probabilities

$\boldsymbol{E}(\boldsymbol{\beta})$ is the $r \times 1$ vector equaling the sum over $s \in S$ of $\boldsymbol{E}_s(\boldsymbol{\beta})$ with entries

$$E_{s,j}(\boldsymbol{\beta}) = \boldsymbol{xstde}_{s,j}^{\mathrm{T}} \cdot \boldsymbol{R}_s^{-1}(\rho) \cdot \boldsymbol{stde}_s$$

$\boldsymbol{xstde}_{s,j}$ is the $m(s) \times 1$ vector with entries

$$xstde_{sc,j} = \frac{\partial \mu_{sc}}{\partial \beta_j} / \sigma_{sc},$$

$$\frac{\partial \mu_{sc}}{\partial \beta_j} = \sum_{u=0}^{K-1} \left(d_u - d_K\right) \cdot \frac{\partial p_{sc,u}}{\partial \beta_j},$$

where $\frac{\partial p_{sc,u}}{\partial \beta_j}$ for $0 \le u < K$ are defined in Sect. 12.2.3, for $1 \le j \le r$ and $sc \in SC$. $\boldsymbol{E}(\boldsymbol{\gamma})$ has the same formulation as in Sect. 12.2.3.2 and $\boldsymbol{E}(\boldsymbol{\rho})$ the same as in Sect. 12.2.3.4. $\boldsymbol{E}'(\boldsymbol{\theta})$ has the same component matrices as defined in Sect. 12.2.1.4. $\boldsymbol{E}'(\boldsymbol{\beta})$ is the sum over $s \in S$ of $\boldsymbol{E}'_s(\boldsymbol{\beta})$ with entries

$$E'_{s,j,j'}(\boldsymbol{\beta}) = -\boldsymbol{xxstde}_{s,j,j'}^{\mathrm{T}} \cdot \boldsymbol{R}_s^{-1}(\rho) \cdot \boldsymbol{stde}_s - \boldsymbol{xstde}_{s,j}^{\mathrm{T}} \cdot \boldsymbol{R}_s^{-1}(\rho) \cdot \boldsymbol{xstde}_{s,j'}$$

where $\boldsymbol{xxstde}_{s,j,j'}$ is the $m(s) \times 1$ vector with entries

$$xxstde_{sc,j,j'} = -\frac{\partial^2 \mu_{sc}}{\partial \beta_{j'} \partial \beta_j} / \sigma_{sc},$$

$$\frac{\partial^2 \mu_{sc}}{\partial \beta_{j'} \partial \beta_j} = \sum_{u=0}^{K-1} (d_u - d_K) \cdot \frac{\partial^2 p_{s,u}}{\partial \beta_{j'} \partial \beta_j},$$

where $\frac{\partial^2 p_{s,u}}{\partial \beta_{j'} \partial \beta_j}$ for $0 \le u < K$ are defined in Sect. 12.2.3, for $1 \le j, j' \le r$. Component matrices of $\boldsymbol{E}'(\boldsymbol{\theta})$ depending only on $\boldsymbol{\gamma}$ and/or $\boldsymbol{\rho}$ are the same as in Sect. 12.2.3 while those depending on $\boldsymbol{\beta}$ together with $\boldsymbol{\gamma}$ or $\boldsymbol{\rho}$ are computed as in Sect. 12.2.3 but using the above revised formulation for $\boldsymbol{E}(\boldsymbol{\beta})$.

Chapter 13
Example Multinomial and Ordinal Regression Analyses

Abstract Adaptive analyses are presented of a trichotomous respiratory status data set with an outcome having three possible values over a baseline and four subsequent clinic visits using multinomial regression with the generalized logit link function and ordinal regression with the cumulative logit link function based on either individual or cumulative outcomes. Results are compared for partially modified generalized estimating equations (GEE), fully modified GEE, and extended linear mixed modeling (ELMM). Linearity of the generalized and cumulative logits of the means in visit with constant dispersions is addressed as well as whether unit dispersions are appropriate for these data, a comparison to standard GEE, and the dependence of means and dispersions on visit. Adaptive additive and adaptive moderation models are generated for visit and being on active treatment. A summary of the analysis results is also provided. SAS code for generating these analyses is described along with output generated by that code.

Keywords Extended linear mixed modeling · Generalized estimating equations · Moderation · Multinomial regression · Ordinal regression

Introduction This chapter provides example analyses using a trichotomous respiratory status data set with an outcome having three possible values. The dichotomous respiratory status data of Sect. 2.8.3 analyzed in Chap. 8 have a related outcome. Section 13.1 describes the more general respiratory status data. Section 13.2 provides example analyses of the trichotomous respiratory status data set using multinomial regression, Section 13.3 analyses using ordinal regression based on individual outcomes, and Sect. 13.4 analyses using ordinal regression based on cumulative outcomes. Section 13.5 provides a summary of the analysis results described in prior sections while Sect. 13.6 provides example SAS code for generating such analyses and descriptions of output generated by that code.

Supplementary Information The online version contains supplementary material available at https://doi.org/10.1007/978-3-031-41988-1_13.

G. J. Knafl, *Modeling Correlated Outcomes Using Extensions of Generalized Estimating Equations and Linear Mixed Modeling*,
https://doi.org/10.1007/978-3-031-41988-1_13

The primary purpose of Chap. 13 is to compare adaptive modeling results for partially modified GEE, fully modified GEE, and ELMM applied to polytomous correlated outcomes using multinomial and ordinal regression models (see Chaps. 10–11 respectively for details). Partially modified GEE (see Chap. 3 for details) extends standard GEE (see Chap. 2 for details) by adding extra estimating equations for dispersion parameters to the standard GEE estimating equations for mean parameters. Fully modified GEE (see Chap. 4 for details) extends standard GEE further by providing alternative estimating equations for mean parameters while utilizing the same estimating equations for the dispersions used by partially modified GEE. These new estimating equations are based on minimizing an extended likelihood function, treated as a likelihood function for brevity in what follows. Both partially modified and fully modified GEE use the standard GEE method of estimating correlation parameters using residuals. ELMM (see Chap. 5 for more details) is based on estimating equations for mean, dispersion, and correlation parameters determined by maximizing the likelihood. The estimating equations for the means and dispersions are the same as for fully modified GEE.

13.1 The Polytomous Respiratory Status Data

A data set on respiratory status levels at baseline and at four post-baseline clinic visits, coded as 0–4, for $n = 111$ patients with respiratory disorder are analyzed and are available in Koch et al. (1989). The outcome variable status0_4 for this data set is polytomous with five possible values 0:terrible, 1:poor, 2:fair, 3:good, and 4:excellent. The dichotomous outcome variable statsus0_1 of Sect. 2.8.3 has two possible values corresponding to the values 0:terrible and 1:poor of status0_4 recoded as 0: poor and to the values 2:fair, 3:good, and 4:excellent of status0_4 recoded as 1:good. Analyses reported in this chapter use the trichotomous outcome status0_2 with three possible values corresponding to the values 0:terrible and 1:poor of status0_4 recoded as 0:poor, to the values 2:fair and 3:good of status0_4 recoded to 1:good, and to the value 4:excellent of status0_4 recoded as 2:excellent. This trichotomous outcome is also analyzed by Miller et al. (1993).

There is a total of $m(SC) = 555$ trichotomous outcome measurements with five measurements available for each patient. The measurements are treated as equally spaced due to coding visits as 0–4. The cutoff for a distinct percent decrease in LCV scores (Sect. 2.6.2) for the status0_2 data with $2 \cdot 555 = 1110$ effective measurements is 0.17%, computed using DF $= 1$ degrees of freedom. In the case of multinomial regression, the removal of 1 transform from the model for the means results in $K = 2$ less parameters, and so the cutoff is 0.27%, computed using DF $= 2$ degrees of freedom.

13.2 Multinomial Regression Analyses

13.2.1 Alternative Correlation Structures

Analyses in this section consider multinomial regression modeling. Due to the relatively large number 1110 of effective measurements, fewer alternative models are considered than in example analyses of Chaps. 6–9 to reduce computation times. Also, all LCV scores are computed using $k = 5$ folds.

Table 13.1 contains results for multinomial regression models for probabilities of trichotomous respiratory status in terms of an intercept and untransformed visit assuming constant dispersions. Untransformed visit is used in these models to reduce computation times. Three modeling approaches partially modified GEE, fully modified GEE, and ELMM as well as four correlation structures IND, spatial AR1, EC, and UN are considered. Note that equivalent results would be generated for non-spatial AR1 correlations as for spatial AR1 correlations since outcome measurements are equally spaced in visit. The best LCV score of 0.64721 for partially modified GEE is generated using the spatial AR1 correlation structure. The best LCV score of 0.64952 for fully modified GEE is generated using the spatial AR1 correlation structure. The best LCV score of 0.64778 for ELMM is generated using the spatial AR1 correlation structure. Consequently, all three modeling approaches select the spatial AR1 correlation structure.

Table 13.1 also contains clock times for generated models. Clock times for partially modified GEE range from 0.1 to 2.0 min with a total over all four cases of about 5.2 min, for fully modified GEE from 0.1 to 0.8 min for a total of about

Table 13.1 Multinomial regression models of mean trichotomous respiratory status in terms of an intercept and untransformed visit assuming constant dispersions for alternate modeling approaches and correlation structures

Modeling approach	Correlation	LCV score[a]	clock time (min)
Partially modified GEE	IND	0.58737	0.1
	AR1	0.64721	1.6
	EC	0.64489	1.5
	UN	0.63338	2.0
Fully modified GEE	IND	0.58746	0.1
	AR1	0.64952	0.7
	EC	0.64576	0.4
	UN	0.63266	0.8
ELMM	IND	0.58742	0.1
	AR1	0.64778	2.9
	EC	0.64581	0.7
	UN	0.63675	11.6

AR1 spatial autoregressive order 1; *EC* exchangeable correlations; *ELMM* extended linear mixed modeling; *GEE* generalized estimating equations; *IND* independent; *LCV* likelihood cross-validation; *UN* unstructured

[a]Computed using 5 folds

Table 13.2 Estimated unstructured correlation parameters generated by partially modified generalized estimating equations using multinomial regression[a]

			visit							
			2		3		4		5	
		y	1	2	1	2	1	2	1	2
visit	1	1	0.197	−0.141	0.130	0.005	0.114	−0.007	0.166	−0.086
		2	−0.230	0.356	−0.147	0.216	−0.125	0.201	−0.255	0.342
	2	1			0.359	−0.259	0.298	−0.294	0.234	−0.175
		2			−0.304	0.521	−0.292	0.514	−0.180	0.364
	3	1					0.421	−0.386	0.275	−0.259
		2					−0.349	0.680	−0.240	0.573
	4	1							0.340	−0.246
		2							−0.228	0.567

[a]With means depending on untransformed visit and an intercept assuming constant dispersions

2.0 min, and for ELMM from 0.1 to 11.6 min for a total of about 15.3 min (totals not reported in Table 13.1). Consequently, fully modified GEE requires less time, with partially modified GEE requiring about 2.6 times as much and ELMM requiring about 7.7 times as much. The larger amount of time for ELMM is primarily due to a longer time to estimate the 40 UN correlation parameters. This suggests that the GEE approach for estimating the UN correlation structure is more efficient timewise than the ELMM approach as the number of such parameters increases. Moreover, the approach for estimating the mean parameters used by fully modified GEE, and by ELMM as well, is also more efficient timewise than the standard GEE approach to estimating those parameters as used by partially modified GEE.

Table 13.2 contains estimates of UN correlation parameters $r_{\mathrm{UN},c,c',u,u'}$ for $1 \le c, c' \le 5$ and $1 \le u, u' \le 2$ by the model of Table 13.1 generated using partially modified GEE. Similar estimates of UN correlation parameters are generated using fully modified GEE and ELMM for the associated models of Table 13.1. For each pair of visits $c < c'$, with only one exception, estimates of $r_{\mathrm{UN},c,c',u,u'}$ are positive for $u = u'$ and negative for $u \ne u'$. The one exception occurs for $c = 1$, $c' = 2$, $u = 1$, and $u' = 2$, which has a positive estimate, while $r_{\mathrm{UN},c,c',1,2}$ is negative for other pairs $c < c'$ of visits, but that one positive estimated value equals 0.005 and so is close to being negative. These results support the use of sign-preserving power transforms of spatial AR1 correlation parameter estimates (Sect. 10.3.3).

13.2.2 Adaptive Modeling of Means in Visit with Constant Dispersions

Table 13.3 contains results for adaptive multinomial regression models of trichotomous respiratory status for means in visit assuming constant dispersions using spatial AR1 correlations as justified in Sect. 13.2.1. Models for means generated

Table 13.3 Adaptive multinomial regression models of trichotomous respiratory status for means in visit with constant dispersions[a]

Modeling approach	Transforms of visit for means[b]	LCV score	Clock time (min)
Partially modified GEE	1, $\text{visit}^{0.3}$	0.65015	146.7
Fully modified GEE	1, $\text{visit}^{-0.49}$, $\text{visit}^{0.989}$	0.65279	209.2
ELMM	1, $\text{visit}^{-0.4}$	0.65273	486.7

ELMM extended linear mixed modeling; *GEE* generalized estimating equations; *LCV* likelihood cross-validation

[a]Computed with spatial AR1 correlations and 5 folds

[b]A value of 1 corresponds to an intercept parameter; otherwise, the model has a zero intercept

by partially modified GEE and ELMM are based on one transform of visit with an intercept while the model for the means generated by fully modified GEE is based on two transforms of visit with an intercept.

The model generated by partially modified GEE computed using ELMM has 5-fold LCV score 0.64961 with distinct PD 0.48% (i.e., larger than the cutoff 0.27% for a distinct PD in the LCV score using DF = 2 and so also the cutoff 0.17% using DF = 1). The model generated by fully modified GEE using ELMM has 5-fold LCV score 0.65164 with non-distinct PD 0.17% (and so less than or equal to the cutoff of 0.17% using DF = 1 as well as the cutoff 0.27% using DF = 2). Consequently, partially modified GEE modeling generates an inferior model while fully modified GEE modeling and ELMM generate competitive models. However, the model generated by ELMM is simpler based on one transform of visit with an intercept while the model based on fully modified GEE is based on two transforms of visit with an intercept, and so the ELMM model is the more preferable of these two models as a parsimonious, competitive alternative.

Table 13.3 also contains clock times for generated models. The clock time for partially modified GEE is 146.7 min or about 2.5 h, for fully modified GEE 209.2 min or about 3.5 h, and for ELMM 486.7 min or about 8.1 h. Consequently, partially modified GEE requires less time, with fully modified GEE requiring about 1.4 times as much and ELMM requiring about 3.3 times as much. However, all these times are excessively long, especially considering that adaptive modeling of only the means in terms of a single predictor is the simplest possible adaptive analysis that could be considered. These times indicate that adaptive multinomial regression modeling of correlated polytomous outcomes can be impractical, even in the case of a polytomous outcome with only three possible values. In such cases, only theory-based models can be computed in acceptable amounts of time. Consequently, no further adaptive multinomial regression models are considered.

13.2.3 Assessing Linearity of Generalized Logits of the Means in Visit

The three models of Table 13.1 for the means based on the linear polynomial model in visit using spatial AR1 correlations have LCV scores 0.64721, 0.64952, and 0.64778 with PDs 0.45%, 0.50%, and 0.76% compared to the associated models of Table 13.3, respectively. For partially modified GEE and ELMM, both models are based on one transform of visit plus an intercept and so have the same number of parameters, indicating they are more appropriately assessed using the cutoff of 0.17% based on smallest possible non-zero DF = 1. For fully modified GEE, the adaptive model has one more transform of visit and so has two more parameters, and so is more appropriately assessed using the cutoff of 0.27% based on DF = 2. In all cases, the PDs are distinct. Consequently, the generalized logits for trichotomous respiratory status levels are distinctly nonlinear in visit.

13.2.4 Assessing Constant Versus Unit Dispersions

The models of Table 13.3 for partially modified GEE, fully modified GEE, and ELMM have estimated constant dispersions 1.00, 0.99, and 1.00, respectively. These results indicate that unit dispersions are appropriate for modeling trichotomous respiratory status levels. This is consistent with results for dichotomous respiratory status reported in Chap. 8.

13.2.5 Estimated Probabilities for Trichotomous Respiratory Status Levels

Figure 13.1 provides the plot of estimated probabilities for the three respiratory status levels using the ELMM model of Table 13.3. The probability of a 1:good respiratory level decreases from 0.56 at visit 0 to 0.48 at visit 1 and then increases to 0.52 at visit 4. The probability of a 2:excellent respiratory status level increases from 0.21 at visit 0 to 0.37 at visit 1 and then decreases to 0.30 at visit 4. The probability of a 0:poor respiratory status level decreases from 0.23 at visit 0 to 0.15 at visit 1 and then increases to 0.18 at visit 4. Estimated spatial AR1 correlations for this model rounded to two decimal digits are $r_{\text{AR1},1,1} = 0.34$, $r_{\text{AR1},1,2} = -0.28$, $r_{\text{AR1},2,1} = -0.27$, and $r_{\text{AR1},2,2} = 0.52$ (and so are close to symmetric).

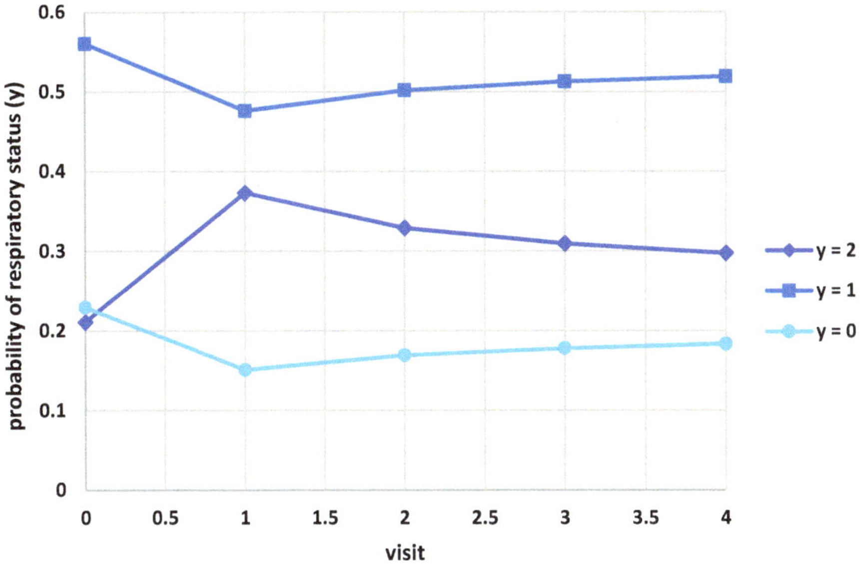

Fig. 13.1 Estimated probabilities for respiratory status levels using multinomial regression

13.3 Ordinal Regression Analyses Using Individual Outcomes

Analyses in this section consider ordinal regression modeling based on individual outcomes. Due to the relatively large number 1110 of effective measurements, fewer alternative models are considered than in example analyses of Chaps. 6–9 to reduce computation times. Also, all LCV scores are computed using $k = 5$ folds.

13.3.1 Alternative Correlation Structures

Table 13.4 contains results for ordinal regression models for mean trichotomous respiratory status using individual outcomes in terms of an intercept and untransformed visit assuming constant dispersions. Untransformed visit is used in these models to reduce computation times. Three modeling approaches partially modified GEE, fully modified GEE, and ELMM as well as four correlation structures IND, spatial AR1, EC, and UN are considered. Note that equivalent results would be generated for non-spatial AR1 correlations as for spatial AR1 correlations since outcome measurements are equally spaced in visit. The best LCV score of 0.63665 for partially modified GEE is generated using the EC correlation structure. The best LCV score of 0.64062 for fully modified GEE is generated using the spatial AR1 correlation structure. The best LCV score of 0.64728 for ELMM is generated using

Table 13.4 Ordinal regression models of mean trichotomous respiratory status using individual outcomes in terms of an intercept and untransformed visit assuming constant dispersions for alternate modeling approaches and correlation structures

Modeling approach	Correlation	LCV score[a]	Clock time (min)
Partially modified GEE	IND	0.58326	0.1
	AR1	0.63607	3.1
	EC	0.63665	4.1
	UN	0.61249	2.0
Fully modified GEE	IND	0.58357	0.1
	AR1	0.64062	0.5
	EC	0.64039	0.2
	UN	0.62876	0.6
ELMM	IND	0.58390	0.1
	AR1	0.64728	1.0
	EC	0.64087	0.5
	UN	0.62833	9.6

AR1 spatial autoregressive order 1; *EC* exchangeable correlations; *ELMM* extended linear mixed modeling; *GEE* generalized estimating equations; *IND* independent; *LCV* likelihood cross-validation; *UN* unstructured

[a]Computed using 5 folds

the spatial AR1 correlation structure. Consequently, partially modified GEE selects the EC correlation structure while fully modified GEE and ELMM select the spatial AR1 correlation structure. The EC model generated with partially modified GEE has ELMM score 0.64087 (Table 13.4) and distinct PD 0.99% compared to the ELMM spatial AR1 model. These results indicate that spatial AR1 correlations are more preferable for ordinal regression modeling using individual outcomes for the trichotomous respiratory status data.

Table 13.4 also contains clock times for generated models. Clock times for partially modified GEE range from 0.1 to 4.1 min with a total over all 4 cases of about 9.3 min, for fully modified GEE from 0.1 to 0.6 min for a total of about 1.4 min, and for ELMM from 0.1 to 9.6 min for a total of about 11.2 min (totals not reported in Table 13.4). Consequently, fully modified GEE requires less time, with partially modified GEE requiring about 6.6 times as much and ELMM requiring about 8.0 times as much. The larger amount of time for ELMM is primarily due to a much longer time to estimate the 40 UN correlation parameters. This suggests that the GEE approach for estimating the UN correlation structure is more efficient timewise than the ELMM approach as the number of such parameters increases. Moreover, the approach for estimating the mean parameters used by fully modified GEE, and by ELMM as well, is also more efficient timewise than the standard GEE approach to estimating those parameters as used by partially modified GEE.

Table 13.5 contains estimates of UN correlation parameters $r_{\mathrm{UN},c,c',u,u'}$ for $1 \le c, c' \le 5$ and $1 \le u, u' \le 2$ by the model of Table 13.4 generated using partially modified GEE. Similar estimates of UN correlation parameters are generated using

Table 13.5 Estimated unstructured correlation parameters generated by partially modified generalized estimating equations using ordinal regression with individual outcomes[a]

			visit							
			2		3		4		5	
		y	1	2	1	2	1	2	1	2
visit	1	1	0.214	−0.003	0.259	0.002	0.243	−0.004	0.227	0.054
		2	−0.112	0.194	−0.159	0.104	−0.115	0.077	−0.068	0.116
	2	1			0.411	−0.099	0.282	−0.026	0.321	−0.054
		2			−0.147	0.328	−0.016	0.265	−0.062	0.201
	3	1					0.526	−0.123	0.521	−0.063
		2					−0.074	0.404	−0.035	0.269
	4	1							0.711	−0.162
		2							−0.144	0.335

[a]With means depending on untransformed visit and an intercept assuming constant dispersions

Table 13.6 Adaptive ordinal regression models of trichotomous respiratory status using individual outcomes for means in visit with constant dispersions[a]

Modeling approach	Transforms of visit for means[b]	LCV score	Clock time (min)
Partially modified GEE	1, $\text{visit}^{-0.5}$	0.64772	173.5
Fully modified GEE	1, $\text{visit}^{-0.397}$	0.65047	33.6
ELMM	1, $\text{visit}^{-0.4}$	0.65302	62.9

ELMM extended linear mixed modeling; *GEE* generalized estimating equations; *LCV* likelihood cross-validation

[a]Computed with spatial AR1 correlations and 5 folds

[b]A power of 0 corresponds to an intercept parameter; otherwise, the model has a zero intercept. A zero intercept for the probabilities means the intercept for $y \leq 0$ is set to zero but not the intercept for $y \leq 1$

fully modified GEE and ELMM for the associated models of Table 13.4. For each pair of visits $c < c'$ with two exceptions, estimates of $r_{\text{UN},c,c',u,u'}$ are positive for $u = u'$ and negative for $u \neq u'$. One exception occurs for $c = 1$, $c' = 2$, $u = 1$, and $u' = 2$, which has a positive estimate, but that estimated value equals 0.002 and so is close to being negative. The other exception occurs for $c = 1$, $c' = 5$, $u = 1$, and $u' = 2$, which has a positive estimate; that estimated value equals 0.054 and so is not that close to being negative, which might be part of the reason that the EC correlation structure is more preferable for these data than the spatial AR1 correlation structure using partially modified GEE. These results support the use of sign-preserving power transforms of spatial AR1 correlation parameter estimates (Sect. 10.3.3), but less strongly than for multinomial regression (Table 13.2).

13.3.2 Adaptive Modeling of Means in Visit with Constant Dispersions

Table 13.6 contains results for adaptive ordinal regression models of trichotomous respiratory status for means in visit with individual outcomes and assuming constant dispersions using spatial AR1 correlations as justified in Sect. 13.3.1. Models for means generated by all three modeling approaches are based on one transform of visit with an intercept. The model generated by partially modified GEE computed using ELMM has 5-fold LCV score 0.65295 with non-distinct PD 0.01%. The model generated by fully modified GEE using ELMM has 5-fold LCV score 0.65300 with non-distinct PD less than 0.01% (not surprising since the powers for visit in these two models differ by 0.003). Consequently, all three modeling approaches generate competitive models.

Table 13.6 also contains clock times for generated models. The clock time for partially modified GEE is 173.5 min or about 2.9 h, for fully modified GEE 31.2 min or about 0.5 h, and for ELMM 55.8 min or about 0.9 h. Consequently, fully modified GEE requires less time, with partially modified GEE requiring about 5.5 times as much and ELMM requiring about 2.0 times as much. Note also that the multinomial regression models of Table 13.3 require 146.7, 209.2, and 486.7 min for partially modified GEE, fully modified GEE, and ELMM, respectively, for a total of 842.6 min compared to a total of 260.5 for the models of Table 13.6 or about 3.2 times as much. Consequently, ordinal regression using individual outcomes is more efficient timewise than multinomial regression.

LCV scores for multinomial regression and ordinal regression using individual outcomes are both based on likelihoods for individual outcomes, and so are comparable. Partially modified GEE, fully modified GEE, and ELMM generated adaptive multinomial regression models for means in visit of Table 13.3 with LCV scores 0.65015, 0.65279, and 0.65273, respectively. Associated ordinal regression models of Table 13.6 for partially modified GEE and fully modified GEE generate distinct PDs of 0.37% and 0.36% (even using the more conservative cutoff 0.27% computed using $DF = 2$), indicating that multinomial regression modeling generates preferable models for these two modeling approaches. On the other hand, the LCV score for the ELMM model of Table 13.3 generates a non-distinct PD 0.04% compared to the associated score of Table 13.6. While the ELMM multinomial regression model is competitive, that model is more complex with 4 parameters (2 intercepts and 2 slopes) for the means compared to 3 parameters (2 intercepts and 1 slope) for the ELMM model of Table 13.6. Consequently, ordinal regression ELMM modeling using individual outcomes is more preferable than multinomial regression ELMM modeling for the trichotomous respiratory status data. For this reason and because ELMM and fully modified GEE generate competitive ordinal regression models, ELMM is preferable over fully modified GEE for ordinal regression modeling using individual outcomes even though ELMM requires more computation time. Only ELMM is considered in any further adaptive analyses using ordinal regression with individual outcomes.

13.3.3 Assessing Linearity of Cumulative Logits of the Means in Visit

The three models of Table 13.4 for the means based on the linear polynomial model in visit using spatial AR1 correlations have LCV scores 0.63607, 0.64062, and 0.64087 with distinct PDs 1.80%, 1.51%, and 1.86% compared to the associated models of Table 13.6, respectively. The partially modified GEE linear polynomial model based on EC correlations has a larger LCV score 0.63665, but the associated PD compared to the partially modified GEE adaptive model of Table 13.6 is distinct at 1.71%. Consequently, the cumulative logits for trichotomous respiratory status levels are distinctly nonlinear in visit.

13.3.4 Assessing Constant Versus Unit Dispersions

The models of Table 13.6 for partially modified GEE, fully modified GEE, and ELMM have estimated constant dispersions 1.01, 1.01, and 1.00, respectively. These results indicate that unit dispersions are appropriate for modeling trichotomous respiratory status levels. This is consistent with results for dichotomous respiratory status reported in Chap. 8. For this reason, subsequent analyses assume unit dispersions.

13.3.5 Adaptive Models for Means in Visit and Active

In this section, ordinal regression with individual outcomes is used to model trichotomous respiratory status with means depending on visit and the indicator active for being on active treatment and assuming unit dispersions as supported by the results of Sect. 13.3.4. Only ELMM is considered as justified by the results of Sect. 13.3.2.

The adaptive additive model for means in visit and active is based on the single transform $\text{visit}^{-0.61}$ with an intercept. Consequently, the indicator active is reasonably considered not to have an additive effect on mean trichotomous respiratory status. The associated ELMM model of Table 13.6 is based on a different transform $\text{visit}^{-0.4}$, which is because the Table 13.6 model assumes constant dispersions as opposed to unit dispersions. The LCV score for the unit dispersion model is 0.65395 so that the associated Table 13.6 model is a competitive alternative with LCV score 0.65302 and non-distinct PD 0.14%. However, the unit dispersion model is simpler while generating a larger LCV score and so is preferable over the constant dispersion model. Clock time for the adaptive additive model is long at 107.0 min or about 1.8 h.

The adaptive moderation model for means in visit, active, and geometric combinations is based on an intercept, the transform $\text{visit}^{-0.61}$, and the geometric combination

$$\left(\text{visit}^{0.5}\cdot\text{active}\right)^{0.99}=\text{visit}^{0.495}\cdot\text{active}.$$

The LCV score is 0.65736 so that the adaptive additive model generates the distinct PD 0.52%. Consequently, the effect of visit on mean trichotomous respiratory status is distinctly moderated by being on active treatment. Clock time for the adaptive moderation model is very long at 620.4 min or about 10.3 h.

13.3.6 Estimated Probabilities for Trichotomous Respiratory Status Levels

Figure 13.2 provides the plot of estimated probabilities for the three respiratory status levels for patients on a placebo. Figure 13.3 provides the plot of estimated probabilities for the three respiratory status levels for patients on active treatment. For patients on a placebo, the probability of a 0:poor respiratory status level decreases from 0.27 at visit 0 to 0.18 at visit 1, and then increases to 0.23 by visit 4. The probability of a 1:good respiratory status level is relatively constant at 0.52 or

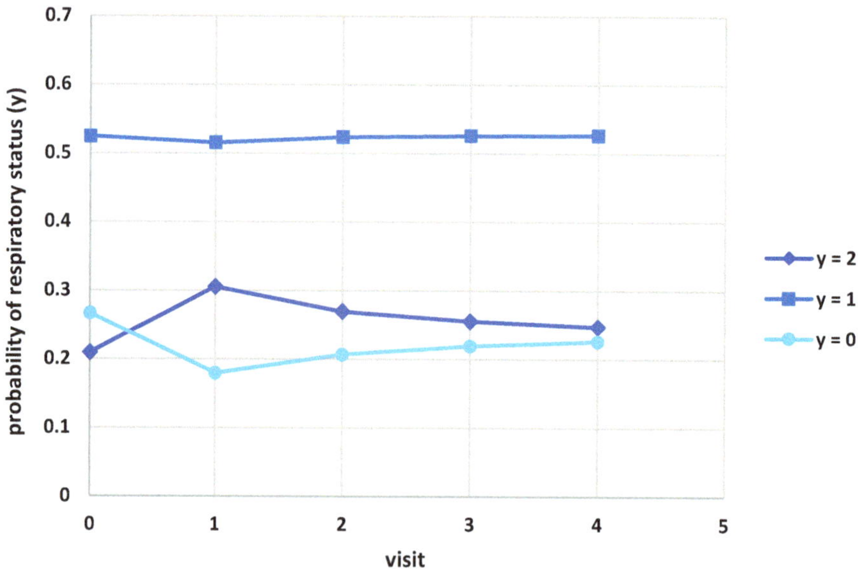

Fig. 13.2 Estimated probabilities for trichotomous respiratory status levels using ordinal regression with individual outcomes for patients on a placebo

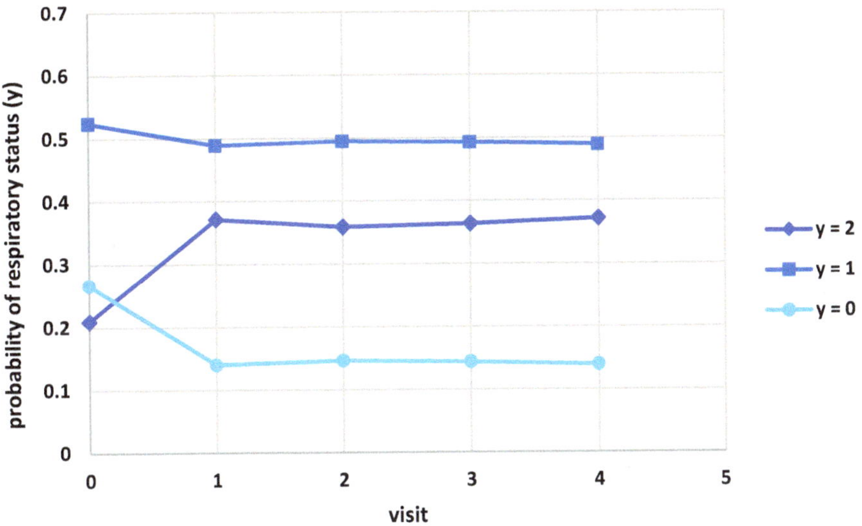

Fig. 13.3 Estimated probabilities for trichotomous respiratory status levels using ordinal regression with individual outcomes for patients on active treatment

0.53 over visits 0–4. The probability of a 2:excellent respiratory status level increases from 0.21 at visit 0 to 0.31 at visit 1, and then decreases to 0.25 by visit 4. On the other hand, for patients on active treatment, probabilities start at visit 0 at the same values for patients on a placebo. The probability of a 0:poor respiratory status level then decreases to between 0.14–0.15 at visits 1–4. The probability of a 1: good respiratory status level then decreases to 0.49 at visits 1–4. The probability of a 2:excellent respiratory status level then increases to between 0.36–0.37 at visits 1–4. Consequently, being on active treatment increases the probability of having excellent respiratory status while decreasing the probabilities of having lower respiratory status with only a small decrease for having good respiratory status. Estimated spatial AR1 correlations for this model rounded to two decimal digits are $r_{\text{AR1},0,0} = 0.51$, $r_{\text{AR1},0.1} = -0.16$, $r_{\text{AR1},1,0} = -0.16$, and $r_{\text{AR1},1,1} = 0.33$ (and so are close to symmetric).

13.4 Ordinal Regression Analyses Using Cumulative Outcomes

Analyses in this section consider ordinal regression modeling based on cumulative outcomes. Due to the relatively large number 1110 of effective measurements, fewer alternative models are considered than in example analyses of Chaps. 6–9 to reduce computation times. Also, all LCV scores are computed using $k = 5$ folds.

13.4.1 Alternative Correlation Structures

Table 13.7 contains results for ordinal regression models for mean trichotomous respiratory status using cumulative outcomes in terms of an intercept and untransformed visit and assuming constant dispersions. Untransformed visit is used in these models to reduce computation times. Three modeling approaches partially modified GEE, fully modified GEE, and ELMM as well as four correlation structures IND, spatial AR1, EC, and UN are considered. Note that equivalent results would be generated for non-spatial AR1 correlations as for spatial AR1 correlations since outcome measurements are equally spaced in visit. The best LCV score of 0.64066 for partially modified GEE is generated using the EC correlation structure. The best LCV score of 0.64263 for fully modified GEE is generated using the EC correlation structure. The best LCV score of 0.64290 for ELMM is generated using the EC correlation structure. Consequently, all three modeling approaches select the EC correlation structure.

Table 13.7 also contains clock times for generated models. Clock times for partially modified GEE range from 0.2 to 4.8 min with a total over all four cases of about 8.2 min, for fully modified GEE from 0.1 to 0.8 min for a total of about 1.9 min, and for ELMM from 0.1 to 11.5 min for a total of about 13.3 min (totals not reported in Table 13.7). Consequently, fully modified GEE requires less time, with partially modified GEE requiring about 4.3 times as much and ELMM requiring about 7.0 times as much. The larger amount of time for ELMM is primarily due to a much longer time to estimate the 40 UN correlation parameters. This suggests that the GEE approach for estimating the UN correlation structure is more efficient

Table 13.7 Ordinal regression models of mean trichotomous respiratory status using cumulative outcomes in terms of an intercept and untransformed visit assuming constant dispersions for alternate modeling approaches and correlation structures

Modeling approach	Correlation	LCV score[a]	Clock time (min)
Partially modified GEE	IND	0.58326	0.2
	AR1	0.63684	0.5
	EC	0.64066	4.8
	UN	0.61249	2.7
Fully modified GEE	IND	0.58389	0.1
	AR1	0.63884	0.7
	EC	0.64263	0.3
	UN	0.62785	0.8
ELMM	IND	0.58390	0.1
	AR1	0.64073	0.9
	EC	0.64290	0.8
	UN	0.62824	11.5

AR1 spatial autoregressive order 1; *EC* exchangeable correlations; *ELMM* extended linear mixed modeling; *GEE* generalized estimating equations; *IND* independent; *LCV* likelihood cross-validation; *UN* unstructured

[a]Computed using 5 folds

Table 13.8 Estimated unstructured correlation parameters generated by partially modified generalized estimating equations using ordinal regression with cumulative outcomes[a]

			visit							
			2		3		4		5	
		y	1	2	1	2	1	2	1	2
visit	1	1	0.214	0.187	0.259	0.221	0.243	0.191	0.227	0.231
		2	0.073	0.309	0.061	0.184	0.097	0.168	0.135	0.296
	2	1			0.411	0.526	0.282	0.200	0.321	0.189
		2			0.202	0.364	0.234	0.482	0.216	0.351
	3	1					0.526	0.292	0.521	0.351
		2					0.364	0.656	0.403	0.333
	4	1							0.711	0.374
		2							0.418	0.563

[a]With means depending on untransformed visit and an intercept assuming constant dispersions

timewise than the ELMM approach as the number of such parameters increases. Moreover, the approach for estimating the mean parameters used by fully modified GEE, and by ELMM as well, is also more efficient timewise than the standard GEE approach used by partially modified GEE.

Table 13.8 contains estimates of UN correlation parameters $r_{\mathrm{UN},c,c',u,u'}$ for $1 \le c, c' \le 5$ and $1 \le u, u' \le 2$ by the model of Table 13.7 generated using partially modified GEE. Similar estimates of UN correlation parameters are generated using fully modified GEE and ELMM for the associated models of Table 13.7. For each pair of visits $c < c'$, with no exceptions, estimates of $r_{\mathrm{UN},c,c',u,u'}$ are all positive for $u = u'$ and for $u \ne u'$. These results suggest that how signs are handled in computing spatial AR1 correlations is not an issue for ordinal regression using cumulative outcomes.

13.4.2 Adaptive Modeling of Means in Visit with Constant Dispersions

Table 13.9 contains results for adaptive ordinal regression models of trichotomous respiratory status for means in visit with cumulative outcomes and assuming constant dispersions using EC correlations as justified in Sect. 13.4.1. Models for means generated by partially modified GEE, fully modified GEE, and ELMM are all based on one transform of visit with an intercept.

The model generated by partially modified GEE computed using ELMM has 5-fold LCV score 0.64888, the same as for the model generated by ELMM. The model generated by fully modified GEE is the same as the model generated by ELMM. Consequently, all three modeling approaches generate competitive models.

Table 13.9 Adaptive ordinal regression models of trichotomous respiratory status using cumulative outcomes for means in visit with constant dispersions[a]

Modeling approach	Transforms of visit for means[b]	LCV score	Clock time (min)
Partially modified GEE	1, $\text{visit}^{-0.29}$	0.64663	165.5
Fully modified GEE	1, $\text{visit}^{-0.2}$	0.64835	20.5
ELMM	1, $\text{visit}^{-0.2}$	0.64888	33.9

ELMM extended linear mixed modeling; *GEE* generalized estimating equations; *LCV* likelihood cross-validation

[a]Computed with spatial EC correlations and 5 folds

[b]A power of 0 corresponds to an intercept parameter; otherwise, the model has a zero intercept. A zero intercept for the probabilities means the intercept for $y \leq 0$ is set to zero but not the intercept for $y \leq 1$

Table 13.9 also contains clock times for generated models. The clock time for partially modified GEE is 165.5 min or about 2.8 h, for fully modified GEE 20.5 min or about 0.3 h, and for ELMM 33.9 min or about 0.6 h. Consequently, fully modified GEE requires less time, with partially modified GEE requiring about 8.1 times as much and ELMM requiring about 1.7 times as much.

13.4.3 Assessing Linearity of Cumulative Logits of the Means in Visit

The three models of Table 13.7 for the means based on the linear polynomial model in visit using EC correlations have LCV scores 0.64066, 0.64263, and 0.64290 with distinct PDs 0.92%, 0.88%, and 0.92% compared to the associated models of Table 13.9, respectively. Consequently, the cumulative logits for trichotomous respiratory status levels are distinctly nonlinear in visit, as is also the case in Sect. 13.3.3.

13.4.4 Assessing Constant Versus Unit Dispersions

The models of Table 13.9 for partially modified GEE, fully modified GEE, and ELMM have estimated constant dispersions 1.00, 1.00, and 1.00, respectively. These results indicate that unit dispersions are appropriate for modeling trichotomous respiratory status levels. This is consistent with results for dichotomous respiratory status reported in Chap. 8.

13.4.5 Adaptive Models for Means in Visit and Active

In this section, ordinal regression with cumulative outcomes is used to model trichotomous respiratory status with means depending on visit and the indicator active for being on active treatment and assuming unit dispersions as supported by the results of Sect. 13.4.4. Only ELMM is considered in order to compare results to those of Sect. 13.3.5.

The adaptive additive model for means in visit and active is based on the transform $\text{visit}^{-0.3}$ and the indicator active with an intercept. The LCV score is 0.65681 so that the associated Table 13.9 model with LCV score 0.64888 generates a distinct PD of 1.21%. Consequently, the indicator active has an additive effect on mean trichotomous respiratory status when modeled using ordinal regression with cumulative outcomes. Clock time for the adaptive additive model is 11.2 min or about 0.2 h. In comparison, the clock time for the additive model using ordinal regression with individual outcomes of Sect. 13.3.5 is much longer at 107.0 min or 1.8 h and so about 9.6 times longer.

The adaptive moderation model for means in visit, active, and geometric combinations is based on an intercept and the geometric combination

$$\left(\text{active}\cdot\text{visit}^3\right)^{-0.06} = \text{active}\cdot\text{visit}^{-0.18}.$$

The LCV score is 0.65987 so that the adaptive additive model generates the distinct PD 0.46%. Consequently, the effect of visit on mean trichotomous respiratory status is distinctly moderated by being on active treatment.

Clock time for the adaptive moderation model is 164.8 min or about 2.4 h. In comparison, the clock time for the moderation model using ordinal regression with individual outcomes of Sect. 13.3.5 is much longer at 620.4 min or about 10.3 h and so about 3.8 times longer.

This moderation model and the associated moderation model generated by ordinal regression with individual outcomes described in Sect. 13.3.5 do not have comparable LCV scores because they are computed using different likelihoods, based, respectively, on cumulative and individual outcomes. They also are based on different correlation structures, EC and spatial AR1, respectively. However, a subjective comparison of means for these models is possible. The model for the means generated by ordinal regression with cumulative outcomes is based on an intercept plus a geometric combination and is more parsimonious than the model for the means generated by ordinal regression with individual outcomes based on an intercept, a transform of visit, and a geometric combination. Also, ordinal regression with cumulative outcomes requires quite a bit less time for the above additive and moderation models generated by ordinal regression with individual outcomes, and so seems preferable.

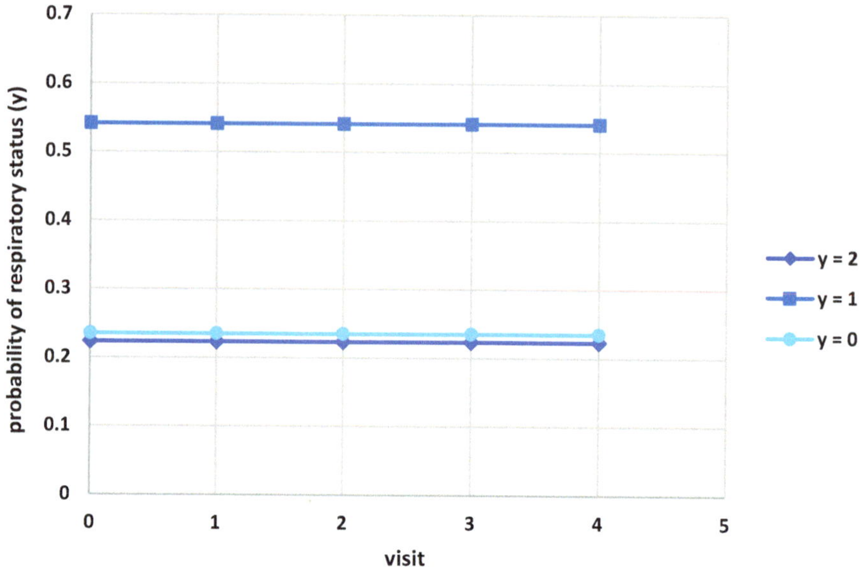

Fig. 13.4 Estimated probabilities for respiratory status levels using ordinal regression with cumulative outcomes for patients on a placebo

13.4.6 Estimated Probabilities for Trichotomous Respiratory Status Levels

Figure 13.4 provides the plot of estimated probabilities for the three respiratory status levels for patients on a placebo. Figure 13.5 provides the plot of estimated probabilities for the three respiratory status levels for patients on active treatment. For patients on a placebo, the probabilities of all three respiratory status levels are constant over visits 0–4 at 0.24 for a 0:poor respiratory status level, 0.54 for a 1:good respiratory status level, and 0.22 for a 2:excellent respiratory status level. On the other hand, for patients on active treatment, probabilities start at visit 0 at the same values for patients on a placebo. The probability of a 0:poor respiratory status level then decreases to 0.09 at visit 1 and increases a little to 0.11 by visit 4. The probability of a 1:good respiratory status level then decreases to 0.44 at visit 1 and increases a little to 0.47 by visit 4. The probability of a 2:excellent respiratory status level, on the other hand, then increases to 0.47 at visit 1 and decreases to 0.41 by visit 4. Consequently, being on active treatment increases the probability of having excellent respiratory status while decreasing the probabilities of having lower respiratory status. Estimated EC correlations for this model rounded to two decimal digits are $r_{\mathrm{AR1},0,0} = 0.37$, $r_{\mathrm{AR1},0.1} = 0.24$, $r_{\mathrm{AR1},1,0} = 0.23$, and $r_{\mathrm{AR1},1,1} = 0.42$ (and so are close to symmetric).

Figures 13.6–13.7 display standardized residuals $stde_{sc,\leq u}$ for respiratory status levels by visit and active for $u = 0$ and $u = 1$, respectively. Standardized residuals for

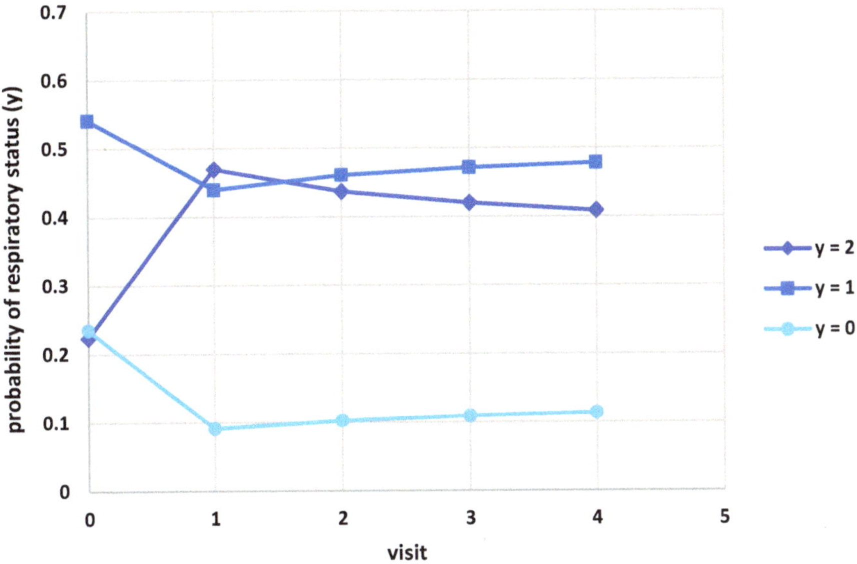

Fig. 13.5 Estimated probabilities for respiratory status levels using ordinal regression with cumulative outcomes for patients on active treatment

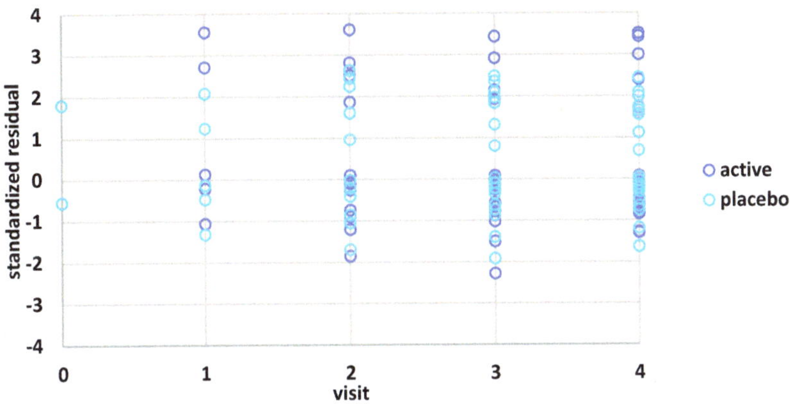

Fig. 13.6 Standardized residuals for 0:poor respiratory status levels using ordinal regression with cumulative outcomes for patients on a placebo and on active treatment

a 0:poor respiratory level (the same as ≤0:poor) of Fig. 13.6 are within ±2 with 8 exceptions. These outlying measurements all occur for patients on active treatment with a respiratory level at one time different from respiratory levels at the other times (actual values not reported). On the other hand, standardized residuals for a ≤ 1:good respiratory level (that is, 0:poor or 1:good) of Fig. 13.7 are all well within ±3 and most within ±2.

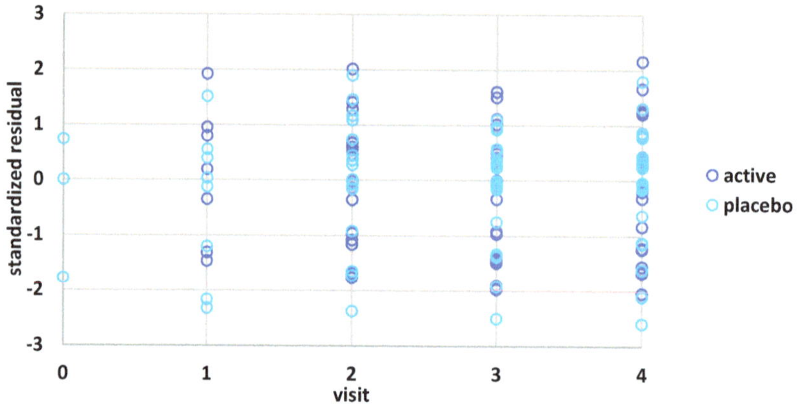

Fig. 13.7 Standardized residuals for ≤1:good respiratory status levels using ordinal regression with cumulative outcomes for patients on a placebo and on active treatment

13.5 Analysis Summary

All LCV scores are computed using $k = 5$ folds.

13.5.1 Multinomial Regression Analyses

A summary of the results of analyses of the trichotomous respiratory status data based on multinomial regression is provided broken down into two categories of results.

1. Models for Means in Untransformed Visit with Constant Dispersions

The preferable model for the trichotomous respiratory status data has spatial AR1 correlations. Fully modified GEE requires less time with partially modified GEE requiring about 2.6 times as much and ELMM requiring about 7.7 times as much.

2. Adaptive Models for Means in Visit Assuming Constant Dispersions

Models selected by fully modified GEE and ELMM are competitive alternatives while the model selected by partially modified GEE is distinctly inferior. However, the ELMM model is simpler than the fully modified GEE model. Estimated probabilities for trichotomous respiratory status are plotted in Fig. 13.1. The generalized logits for trichotomous respiratory status are distinctly nonlinear in visit assuming constant dispersions. Unit dispersions are appropriate for modeling trichotomous respiratory status. Partially modified GEE requires less time with fully modified GEE requiring about 1.4 times as much and ELMM requiring about 3.3 times as much. However, all modeling procedures require excessive amounts of time for what is a relatively simple adaptive analysis, and so no further multinomial regression analyses are conducted.

13.5.2 Ordinal Regression Analyses Based on Individual Outcomes

A summary of the results of analyses of the trichotomous respiratory status data based on ordinal regression using individual outcomes is provided broken down into three categories of results.

1. Models for Means in Untransformed Visit with Constant Dispersions

   The preferable model for the trichotomous respiratory status data has spatial AR1 correlations. Fully modified GEE requires less time with partially modified GEE requiring about 6.6 times as much and ELMM requiring about 8.0 times as much.

2. Adaptive Models for Means in Visit Assuming Constant Dispersions

   Models selected by partially modified GEE, fully modified GEE, and ELMM are all competitive alternatives. The cumulative logits for trichotomous respiratory status are distinctly nonlinear in visit assuming constant dispersions. Unit dispersions are appropriate for modeling trichotomous respiratory status. Fully modified GEE requires less time with partially modified GEE requiring about 5.5 times as much and ELMM requiring about 2.0 times as much.

   Ordinal regression ELMM modeling using individual outcomes is preferable over multinomial regression ELMM modeling for the trichotomous respiratory status data. ELMM is preferable over fully modified GEE for ordinal regression modeling using individual outcomes even though ELMM requires more computation time. Only ELMM is considered in further adaptive analyses using ordinal regression with individual outcomes.

3. Adaptive Models in Visit and Being on Active Treatment Assuming Unit Dispersions

   The indicator active is reasonably considered not to have an additive effect on mean trichotomous respiratory status. The effect of visit on mean trichotomous respiratory status is distinctly moderated by being on active treatment. Clock times for the adaptive additive and moderation models are overly long. Estimated probabilities for trichotomous respiratory status for patients on a placebo are plotted in Fig. 13.2 and for patients on active treatment in Fig. 13.3.

13.5.3 Ordinal Regression Analyses Based on Cumulative Outcomes

A summary of the results of analyses of the trichotomous respiratory status data based on ordinal regression using cumulative outcomes is provided broken down into three categories of results.

1. Models for Means in Untransformed Visit with Constant Dispersions

   The preferable model for the trichotomous respiratory status data has EC correlations. Fully modified GEE requires less time with partially modified GEE requiring about 4.3 times as much and ELMM requiring about 7.0 times as much.

2. Adaptive Models for Means in Visit Assuming Constant Dispersions

   Models selected by partially modified GEE, fully modified GEE, and ELMM are all competitive alternatives. The cumulative logits for trichotomous respiratory status are distinctly nonlinear in visit assuming constant dispersions. Unit dispersions are appropriate for modeling trichotomous respiratory status. Fully modified GEE requires less time with partially modified GEE requiring about 8.1 times as much and ELMM requiring about 1.7 times as much.

3. Adaptive Models in Visit and Being on Active Treatment Assuming Unit Dispersions

   Only ELMM is considered in these adaptive analyses using ordinal regression with cumulative outcomes as is also the case for associated adaptive analyses using ordinal regression with individual outcomes. The indicator active is reasonably considered to have an additive effect on mean trichotomous respiratory status. The effect of visit on mean trichotomous respiratory status is distinctly moderated by being on active treatment. Adaptive additive and moderation models for ordinal regression based on individual outcomes require more time, about 9.6 times longer for additive modeling and about 3.8 times longer for moderation modeling. The moderation model for the means generated by ordinal regression using cumulative outcomes is more parsimonious while requiring less time and so is preferable over ordinal regression modeling using individual outcomes for the trichotomous respiratory status data.

13.5.4 All Models for Trichotomous Respiratory Status

In two cases (Tables 13.6 and 13.9), partially modified GEE, fully modified GEE, and ELMM generate competitive models for means in visit assuming constant dispersions while partially modified GEE is distinctly inferior in one case (Table 13.3). Multinomial regression requires excessive times for all of these three cases while partially modified GEE also requires excessive times for ordinal regression with individual outcomes and with cumulative outcomes. For ordinal regression with individual outcomes and with cumulative outcomes (Tables 13.6 and 13.9), fully modified GEE requires less time than ELMM, 0.9 h compared to 1.5 h, but the fully modified GEE model can be more complex (Table 13.6).

Using ELMM, ordinal regression using individual outcomes generates a more complex moderation model compared to ordinal regression using cumulative outcomes for means in visit. Ordinal regression using individual outcomes also requires much more time to generate all three of the models for the means in visit, the additive model, and the moderation model about 12.1 h compared to 2.9 h or about 4.2 times as much. For these reasons, ordinal regression using cumulative outcomes is more preferable for modeling trichotomous respiratory status.

In general, correlations between different outcome values for multinomial regression, ordinal regression with individual outcomes, and ordinal regression with cumulative outcomes are all distinct from each other. However, for the trichotomous respiratory data, estimated spatial AR1 correlations for multinomial regression and ordinal regression with individual outcomes as well as estimated EC correlations for ordinal regression with cumulative outcomes are close to being symmetric, suggesting consideration of symmetric correlation models for these two structures with fewer parameters. However, this issue has not been addressed.

The approach used by partially modified GEE and fully modified GEE for estimating UN correlation parameters using standardized residuals can be more efficient timewise than the ELMM approach based on maximizing the likelihood, primarily due to the large number of such parameters. On the other hand, the approach used by fully modified GEE, as also used by ELMM, for estimating the mean parameters by maximizing a likelihood function can be more efficient timewise than the approach used by standard GEE and partially modified GEE specifying estimating equations directly without basing them on maximizing a likelihood function.

13.5.5 Selected Model for Trichotomous Respiratory Status in Visit and Being on Active Treatment

Under the most appropriate model for trichotomous respiratory status based on ordinal regression using cumulative outcomes with EC correlations and assuming unit dispersions, estimated probabilities for patients on a placebo are plotted in Fig. 13.4 and for patients on active treatment in Fig. 13.5. Standardized residuals for 0:poor trichotomous respiratory status are plotted in Fig. 13.6 and for ≤1:good trichotomous respiratory status in Fig. 13.7.

13.6 Example SAS Code for Analyzing the Trichotomous Respiratory Status Data

Example SAS code is presented in this section for conducting analyses of trichotomous respiratory status levels as a function of clinic visit and treatment group (either on active treatment or taking a placebo). The code assumes that a data set called longresp has been created in the SAS default library containing the trichotomous respiratory status data (Sect. 13.1) in long format, that is, with one measurement (or row) for each trichotomous respiratory status level at each clinic visit for each patient. This data set contains variables (or columns) called id loaded with unique identifiers for patients; status0_2 loaded with trichotomous respiratory status levels coded as 0:poor, 1;good, or 2:excellent; visit loaded with visit indexes of 0–4; and the indicator active set to 1 for patients on active treatment and to 0 for patients in the control group. Altogether, there are five trichotomous respiratory status levels at different clinic visits for each of 111 different patients, 54 on active treatment and 57 on a placebo, for a total of 555 measurements.

The code also assumes that a %include statement has been executed to load in the current version of the genreg macro for use in conducting adaptive analyses. The genreg macro supports a wide variety of macro parameters, some of which are described here. The interface for this macro contains the complete list of macro parameters along with their default settings. Default settings are used by the macro if a value for the macro parameter has not been specified in the code invoking the macro. Macro parameter settings are case insensitive. The cutoff for a distinct percent decrease in LCV scores (Sect. 2.6.2) for these data with $2 \cdot 555 = 1110$ effective measurements is 0.17%, computed using DF $= 1$ degrees of freedom. In the case of multinomial regression, the removal of 1 transform from the model for the means results in 2 less parameters, and so the cutoff is 0.27%, computed using DF $= 2$ degrees of freedom.

13.6.1 Modeling Means in Visit Assuming Constant Dispersions

The following code uses the genreg macro to generate the adaptive model for trichotomous respiratory status means as a possibly nonlinear function of visit using $k = 5$ folds, exchangeable correlations (EC), extended linear mixed modeling (ELMM), and ordinal regression based on cumulative outcomes as in Sect. 13.4.2 assuming constant dispersions.

```
%genreg(modtype=logis,datain=longresp,yvar=status0_2,matchvar=id,
withinvr=visit,foldcnt=5,corrtype=EC,GEE=n,srchtype=logL,
propodds=y,cumordnl=y,expand=y,expxvars=visit,contract=y);
```

The modtype macro parameter specifies the model type, in this case "modtype=logis" means treat the polytomous outcome variable as categorically distributed. This is the same modtype setting as used in Sect. 8.11 for dichotomous respiratory status. The macro distinguishes between these two cases using the number of observed outcome values. The datain macro parameter indicates that the data to be analyzed is contained in the longresp data set loaded in the SAS default library. The yvar macro parameter specifies the name of the outcome variable, in this case the variable status0_2. The matchvar and withinvr macro parameters specify, respectively, the variable containing unique identifiers for different matched sets, in this case the variable id identifying different patients, and the variable containing within matched set values, in this case the variable visit. The corrtype macro parameter specifies the correlation structure, in this case the EC structure. The other possible corrtype settings are "corrtype=IND", "corrtype=AR1", and "corrtype=UN" for independent, spatial autoregressive order 1, and unstructured correlations, respectively. To request that the clock time for an invocation of the macro be printed in the output, add the setting "rprttime=y" where the value "y" is short for "yes" while the default setting is "rprttime=n" with "n" short for "no".

The modeling approach used by genreg is determined by the combination of the GEE and srchtype macro parameters. In this case, "GEE=n" means use ELMM while "srchtype=logL" means base estimation on maximizing the log-likelihood (as described in Sects. 4.3 and 5.2). These are the default settings for these two macro parameters. Setting "GEE=y" requests GEE modeling. Combining "GEE=y" with "srchtype=GEE" requests partially modified GEE with estimation based on the minimizing the maximum absolute value of the gradient (as described in Sect. 3.7). Combining "GEE=y" with "srchtype=logL" requests fully modified GEE. By default, partially modified and fully modified GEE use bias-unadjusted dispersion estimates. Bias-adjusted dispersion estimates, as used in standard GEE modeling (Sect. 2.4), are requested by adding the setting "biasadj=y".

The macro parameters propodds and cumordnl control the type of regression used in analyzing the outcome variable. The default settings are "propodds=n" and "cumordnl=n" requesting multinomial regression using generalized logits. Changing to "propodds=y" requests ordinal regression using cumulative logits, also called proportional odds modeling. Combining "propodds=y" with the default setting "cumordn=n" requests ordinal regression with individual outcomes while combining it with the setting "cumordn=y" as in the above code requests ordinal regression with cumulative outcomes.

Adaptive modeling is requested using "expand=y" together with "contract=y", meaning first expand the base model and then contract the expanded model. In this case, the base model has constant means and constant dispersions based on only intercept parameters (but this can be changed). The expxvars macro parameter specifies the primary predictor variables for modeling the means to consider in the expansion. In this case, the expansion grows the model for the means by systematically adding in power transforms of the single variable visit while holding the dispersions constant. The maximum number of transforms added by the expansion to the model for the means is controlled by the expxmax parameter with default value "expxmax=5" meaning at most 5 transforms can be added to the means. Changing to the empty setting "expxmax=" removes the restriction on the number of such transforms.

The contraction systematically removes transforms from the expanded model for the means, possibly the constant transform corresponding to the intercept, and adjusts the powers of the remaining transforms to increase the LCV score, which in this case is computed with 5 folds as specified by the setting of the foldcnt macro parameter. It is also computed using matched-set-wise deletion corresponding to the default setting "measdlte=n". Measurement-wise deletion is requested using "measdlte=y". The contraction can optionally be restricted not to remove the intercept for the means in order to generate a non-zero intercept model. An LCV ratio test is used to decide when to stop the contraction. The contraction also stops when there is only one transform remaining in the model for the means. When the contraction leaves the expanded model unchanged, that expanded model has its powers adjusted to increase the LCV score.

The following code directly generates the above adaptive model selected with $k = 5$ folds, EC correlations, and ELMM, including parameter estimates and LCV score.

```
%genreg(modtype=logis,datain=longresp,yvar=status0_2,matchvar=id,
withinvr=visit,foldcnt=5,corrtype=EC,GEE=n,srchtype=logL,
propodds=y,cumordnl=y,xintrcpt=y,xvars=visit,xpowers=−0.2);
```

The xintrcpt macro parameter specifies whether or not the base model for the means includes an intercept, the xvars macro parameter provides the list of primary predictors for the base model for the means, and the xpowers macro parameter the powers for transforming those primary predictors. In this case, the model for the means has a non-zero intercept along with the single transform visit$^{-0.2}$. The default values for these macro parameters are "xintrcpt=y", "xvars=", and "xpowers=" requesting constant means. An empty setting for the xvars macro parameter means includes no transforms for the means, and an empty setting for the xpowers macro parameter means power transform xvars variables if any with the power 1 (and so include them untransformed). The model for the dispersions is based on macro parameters vintrcpt, vvars, and vpowers with analogous meanings and with the same default settings requesting constant dispersions. The xvalid macro parameter is not set in the above code and so has its default setting "xvalid=y" meaning to compute the LCV score for the requested model. In this case, the model has LCV score 0.64888. Adding the setting "xvalid=n" means compute only parameter estimates for the requested model and not the LCV score.

The above code can be changed to generate the standard linear polynomial model for the means based on untransformed visit as follows. Just change the setting for the xpowers macro parameter to "xpowers=1" or remove the setting for the xpowers macro parameter so that it has its default empty value, which means to use the power 1 to transform all variables listed in the setting of the xvars macro parameter. Note that the cumulative logits of the means are linear in visit, but the means are nonlinear due to using the cumulative logit link function. To request the standard quadratic polynomial model for the means, use the settings "xintrcpt=y", "xvars=visit visit", and "xpowers=1 2".

As reported in Sect. 13.4.4, the above model has estimated constant dispersions equal to 1.00, suggesting that unit dispersions are appropriate for the dichotomous respiratory status levels. The following code uses the genreg macro to generate the adaptive model for trichotomous respiratory status means as a possibly nonlinear function of visit using $k = 5$ folds, EC correlations, and ELMM assuming unit dispersions.

```
%genreg(modtype=logis,datain=longresp,yvar=status0_2,matchvar=id,
withinvr=visit,foldcnt=5,corrtype=EC,GEE=n,srchtype=logL,
propodds=y,cumordnl=y,vintrcpt=n,expand=y,expxvars=visit,
contract=y);
```

The base model for the dispersions has a zero intercept, due to the setting "vintrcpt=n", and it remains that way because the model for the dispersions does not change. Since the dispersions are modeled using the natural log link function, all models generated as part of the adaptive process have unit dispersions. The generated unit dispersion model has means based on an intercept and visit$^{-0.3}$ with LCV score 0.64890 (not reported earlier), a little better than the LCV score 0.64888 for the associated constant dispersion model, supporting the use of unit dispersions in subsequent models. The following code directly generates the adaptive unit dispersion model.

```
%genreg(modtype=logis,datain=longresp,yvar=status0_2,matchvar=id,
withinvr=visit,foldcnt=5,corrtype=EC,GEE=n,srchtype=logL,
propodds=y,cumordnl=y,xintrcpt=y,xvars=visit,xpowers=−0.3,
vintrcpt=n);
```

13.6.2 Modeling Means and Dispersions in Visit

The following code uses the genreg macro to generate the adaptive model for trichotomous respiratory level means and dispersions as possibly nonlinear functions of visit using $k = 5$ folds, EC correlations, and ELMM, starting from constant dispersions and allowing for unit dispersions.

```
%genreg(modtype=logis,datain=longresp,yvar=status0_2,matchvar=id,
withinvr=visit,foldcnt=5,corrtype=EC,GEE=n,srchtype=logL,
propodds=y,cumordnl=y,expand=y,expxvars=visit,expvvars=visit,
contract=y,cnvzero=y);
```

As before, adaptive modeling is requested using "expand=y" together with "contract=y" meaning first expand the base model with constant means and constant dispersions and then contract the expanded model. The expxvars and expvvars macro parameters specify the primary predictor variables to consider in the expansion for the means and dispersions, respectively. In this case, the same set of primary predictors is used for the means and for the dispersions, but different sets of primary predictors can be specified. The expansion grows the model for the means and the dispersions in combination by systematically adding in power transforms of the single variable visit one-at-a-time to either the means or to the dispersions, whichever generates the better LCV score. Similar to the expxmax parameter, the expvmax parameter specifies the maximum number of transforms added by the expansion to the model for the dispersions with default value "expvmax=5" meaning at most 5 transforms can be added to the dispersions. Changing to the empty setting "expvmax=" removes the restriction on the number of such transforms.

The contraction systematically removes transforms from the expanded model for the means and dispersions in combination, possibly the constant transforms corresponding to intercepts, and adjusts the powers of the remaining transforms to increase the LCV score. Transforms are removed one-at-a-time from either the means or the dispersions, whichever generates the better LCV score after adjusting all the powers of the remaining transforms for both the means and the dispersions. An LCV ratio test is used to decide when to stop the contraction. By default, the contraction stops removing transforms from the means when there is only one transform remaining in the model for the means and stops removing transforms from the dispersions when there is only one transform remaining in the model for the dispersions. However, in this case, the contraction is allowed to remove all the transforms from the dispersions due to the setting "cnvzero=y". This does not happen otherwise because the default setting is "cnvzero=n". When the contraction leaves the expanded model unchanged, that expanded model has its powers adjusted to increase the LCV score. The above code shows how to conduct adaptive modeling of means and dispersions for polytomous outcomes, but results have not been reported earlier since reported results assumed unit dispersions.

13.6.3 Additive Models in Visit and Being on Active Treatment

The following code uses the genreg macro to generate the adaptive additive model for trichotomous respiratory status means as a possibly nonlinear function of visit and being on active treatment using $k = 5$ folds, EC correlations, and ELMM assuming unit dispersions.

```
%genreg(modtype=logis,datain=longresp,yvar=status0_2,matchvar=id,
withinvr=visit,foldcnt=5,corrtype=EC,GEE=n,srchtype=logL,
propodds=y,cumordnl=y,vintrcpt=n,expand=y,expxvars=visit active,
contract=y);
```

In this case, the expxvars macro parameter specifies the variables visit and active to be the primary predictor variables to consider in the expansion for the means. The expansion grows the model for the means by systematically adding in power transforms of visit or the indicator variable active one-at-a-time. Note that indicator variables like active are not transformed and are included at most once in the model for the means. The contraction then systematically removes transforms from the expanded model for the means, possibly the constant transform corresponding to the intercept, and adjusts the powers of the remaining transforms to increase the LCV score. The model is additive because by default geometric combinations are not considered in the expansion.

The following code directly generates the adaptive additive model for the means assuming unit dispersions.

```
%genreg(modtype=logis,datain=longresp,yvar=status0_2,matchvar=id,
withinvr=visit,foldcnt=5,corrtype=EC,GEE=n,srchtype=logL,
propodds=y,cumordnl=y,xintrcpt=y,xvars=visit active,xpowers=−0.3 1,
vintrcpt=n);
```

As for the unit dispersion model in only visit, the means are based on an intercept and $\text{visit}^{-0.3}$, but now they also depend on the indicator active. The LCV score is 0.65681 so that the model in only visit with LCV score 0.64890 is distinctly inferior generating a distinct PD 1.20% (not reported earlier). Consequently, being on active treatment is reasonably considered to have an additive effect on the means assuming unit dispersions.

13.6.4 Moderation Models in Visit and Being on Active Treatment

The following code uses the genreg macro to generate the adaptive moderation model for trichotomous respiratory status means as a possibly nonlinear function of visit, being on active treatment, and geometric combinations in visit and being on active treatment using $k = 5$ folds, EC correlations, and ELMM assuming unit dispersions.

```
%genreg(modtype=logis,datain=longresp,yvar=status0_2,matchvar=id,
withinvr=visit,foldcnt=5,corrtype=EC,GEE=n,srchtype=logL,
propodds=y,cumordnl=y,vintrcpt=n,expand=y,expxvars=visit active,
geomcmbn=y,contract=y);
```

In this case, the expxvars macro parameter specifies the variables visit and active to be the primary predictor variables to consider in the expansion for the means. The expansion grows the model for the means by systematically adding in power transforms of visit, the indicator variable active, or geometric combinations in visit and active one-at-a-time. Geometric combinations are considered due to adding the setting "geomcmbn=y" to the code for generating the associated additive model in visit and active. The default setting for the geomcmbn macro parameter is "geomcmbn=n" meaning to restrict the expansion to an additive model in the variables specified in the expxvars. The contraction systematically removes transforms from the expanded model for the means, possibly the constant transform corresponding to the intercept, and adjusts the powers of the remaining transforms to increase the LCV score. Note that when a geometric combination of the form $(\text{visit}^p \cdot \text{active})^q$ or $(\text{active} \cdot \text{visit}^p)^q$ is generated by the expansion, the contraction only adjusts the power q and leaves the power p unchanged. When there are more than two primary predictors for the means and/or dispersions, geometric combinations can be generated based on any number of two or more of those primary predictors.

The following code directly generates the adaptive moderation model for the means assuming unit dispersions.

```
%genreg(modtype=logis,datain=longresp,yvar=status0_2,matchvar=id,
withinvr=visit,foldcnt=5,corrtype=EC,GEE=n,srchtype=logL,
propodds=y,cumordnl=y,xintrcpt=y,xgcs=active 1 visit 3,
xgcpowrs=-0.06,vintrcpt=n);
```

In this case, the model for the means is based on an intercept and the geometric combination

$$\left(\text{active} \cdot \text{visit}^3\right)^{-0.06} = \text{active} \cdot \text{visit}^{-0.18}.$$

The LCV score is 0.65987 while the associated additive model has LCV score 0.65681 with distinct PD 0.46%. Consequently, being on active treatment is reasonably considered to moderate the effect of visit on the means assuming unit dispersions.

The macro parameters xgcs and xgcpowrs are used to specify geometric combinations for the means. The setting "xgcs=active 1 visit 3" specifies the untransformed geometric combination $\text{active} \cdot \text{visit}^3$ while the setting "xgcpowrs=−0.06" means to transform $\text{active} \cdot \text{visit}^3$ to the power −0.06. The xgcpowrs setting is needed in this case because its default empty setting "xgcpowrs=" means to leave all the geometric combinations specified by the xgcs macro parameter untransformed. Multiple geometric combinations are specified by separating them by colons (:). For example, use the following code to generate the model with means based on an intercept and the two geometric combinations $(\text{visit}^2 \cdot \text{active})^{0.1}$ and $(\text{visit}^{0.5} \cdot \text{active})^{0.5}$ along with unit dispersions.

```
%genreg(modtype=logis,datain=longresp,yvar=status0_2,matchvar=id,
withinvr=visit,foldcnt=5,corrtype=EC,GEE=n,srchtype=logL,
propodds=y,cumordnl=y,xintrcpt=y,xgcs=visit 2 active 1 : visit 0.5 active 1,
xgcpowrs=0.1 0.5,vintrcpt=n);
```

The macro parameters vgcs and vgcpowrs are used in the same way to specify geometric combinations for the dispersions.

The standard linear moderation model has means based on an intercept, visit, active, and the interaction visit · active. While it would usually have constant dispersions, unit dispersions are more appropriate for trichotomous respiratory status. The standard linear moderation model with unit dispersions can be generated using ELMM with the following code:

```
%genreg(modtype=logis,datain=longresp,yvar=status0_2,matchvar=id,
withinvr=visit,foldcnt=5,corrtype=EC,GEE=n,srchtype=logL,
propodds=y,cumordnl=y,xintrcpt=y,xvars=visit active,
xgcs=visit 1 active 1,vintrcpt=n);
```

The LCV score is 0.64939 with distinct PD 1.59% (not reported earlier) compared to the adaptive moderation model with unit dispersions with LCV score 0.65987, indicating that in this case moderation is distinctly nonlinear.

13.6.5 Example Output

As also considered in Sect. 13.6.4, the following code uses the genreg macro to generate the adaptive moderation model for means of trichotomous respiratory status as a possibly nonlinear function of visit, being in the intervention group, and geometric combinations in visit and being in the intervention group assuming unit dispersions.

```
%genreg(modtype=logis,datain=longresp,yvar=status0_2,matchvar=id,
withinvr=visit,foldcnt=5,corrtype=EC,GEE=n,srchtype=logL,
propodds=y,cumordnl=y,vintrcpt=n,expand=y,expxvars=visit active,
geomcmbn=y,contract=y);
```

The output generated by this code starts with descriptions of settings controlling what kind of model has been generated including the cutoff for a distinct percent decrease in LCV scores followed by a description of the base model. Table 13.10 contains SAS listing output describing the base model.

Table 13.10 Part of the SAS listing output describing the base model for the generation of the adaptive moderation model

```
                 base logit expectation component

      parameter estimates for smaller vs. larger cumulative logits

          predictor     power    status0_2=0     status0_2<=1

          XINTRCPT          1      -1.479776        0.8135739

                   base log dispersion component

                   predictor      power   estimate

                   VZERO              1          0

mth root of extended likelihood using deleted predictions: 0.6411984
```

Table 13.11 Part of the SAS listing output describing the expanded model for the generation of the adaptive moderation model

```
geometric combination logit expectation variables:
         XGC_1    visit**(-0.3)*active
         XGC_2    active*visit**(-6)
         XGC_3    active*visit**(3)
         XGC_4    active*visit

         expanded logit expectation component

parameter estimates for smaller vs. larger cumulative logits

predictor     power   status0_2=0    status0_2<=1      score   order

XINTRCPT          1     -1.16158     1.2660071  0.6411984       0
XGC_1           0.6    -1.181073     -1.181073  0.6598662       1
visit             5    -0.000097     -0.000097  0.6593388       2
XGC_2             2    0.3628847     0.3628847  0.6592624       3
XGC_3             1    0.0160581     0.0160581  0.6589575       4
XGC_4             1    -0.178065     -0.178065  0.6583384       5

         expanded log dispersion component

      VZERO             1            0   0.6411984        0

mth root of extended likelihood using deleted predictions: 0.6583384
```

The means or the probabilities for status0_2 $= 0$ and for status0_2 ≤ 1 (i.e., the logit expectation component) are based only on an intercept term XINTRCPT with estimated values -1.48 and 0.81, respectively, while the dispersions (i.e., the log dispersion component) are based only on a zero-intercept parameter labeled VZERO. The LCV score rounds to 0.64120 (called the "mth root of the extended likelihood using deleted predictions" in the output).

The output then describes the parameters controlling the expansion followed by the expanded model as described in Table 13.11. The output uses the SAS power operator "**". The base model (order 0) has LCV score 0.64120. First, the geometric combination

$$\text{XGC\_1}^{0.6} = \left(\text{visit}^{-0.3} \cdot \text{active}\right)^{0.6} = \text{visit}^{-0.18} \cdot \text{active (order 1)}$$

is added to the means generating LCV score 0.65987. Next, the transform visit^5 (order 2) is added to the model for the means with LCV score 0.65934. Finally, three geometric combinations are added to the means:

$$\text{XGC\_2}^2 = \left(\text{active} \cdot \text{visit}^{-6}\right)^2 = \text{active} \cdot \text{visit}^{-12} \text{ (order 3)},$$

$$\text{XGC\_3}^1 = \text{active} \cdot \text{visit}^3 \text{ (order 4)},$$

and

Table 13.12 Part of the SAS listing output describing the contracted model for the generation of the adaptive moderation model

```
                 contracted logit expectation component

     parameter estimates for smaller vs. larger cumulative logits

                    predictor old power new power

                    XINTRCPT            1         1
                    XGC_3               1     -0.06

        predictor      power   status0_2=0     status0_2<=1

        XINTRCPT           1     -1.179839       1.2458633
        XGC_3          -0.06     -1.12345        -1.12345

           discarded   old power         score    order

                                .    0.6583384        0
           XGC_2                2    0.6596162        1
           XGC_1              0.6    0.6603851        2
           visit                5     0.660476        3
           XGC_4                1    0.6598662        4

                contracted log dispersion component

           predictor old power new power    estimate

           VZERO               1        1           0

                 log dispersion component unchanged

  mth root of extended likelihood using deleted predictions: 0.6598662
```

$$\mathrm{XGC\_4}^1 = \mathrm{active} \cdot \mathrm{visit}\ (\mathrm{order}\ 5),$$

with LCV scores 0.0.65926, 0.65896, and 0.65834, which is the LCV score for the expanded model. Each transform is added to the model without adjusting the powers for previously added transforms. The LCV score is allowed to decrease, and so expanded models usually require contraction. However, in cases where the contraction leaves the expanded model unchanged, a conditional transformation step is executed to adjust the powers of the expanded model to improve its LCV score.

The output then describes the parameters controlling the contraction followed by the contracted model as described in Table 13.12. The expanded model (order 0) has LCV score 0.65834. First, two geometric combinations $\mathrm{XGC\_2}^2$ (order 1) and $\mathrm{XGC\_1}^{0.6}$ (order 2) are removed from the means generating the LCV scores 0.65962 and 0.66039. Then, the transform visit^5 (order 3) is removed from the means with LCV score 0.66048. Finally, the geometric combination $\mathrm{XGC\_4}^1$ (order 4) is removed from the means with LCV score 0.65987, which is the LCV score for the contracted model. With the removal of each transform from the model, the powers for the other transforms are adjusted to improve the LCV score. In this case, the power for XGC _ 3 in the means changes from 1 to −0.06 while the other powers are unchanged. Details on how the powers change at each step of the contraction are not provided in the contraction output, but are available in the SAS log output if that is of interest. Note that the LCV score increased with the removal of the first three transforms and then decreased with the removal of the fourth

Table 13.13 Part of the SAS listing output describing the estimated EC correlation submatrix of the contracted model for the generation of the adaptive moderation model

```
estimated correlation submatrix

              y1        y2

y1 0.3682997 0.2359298
y2 0.2287447 0.4166685

y1, y2, ... are yvar values from smallest to largest
```

transform. In this way, a parsimonious model is generated by the contraction. The contraction stopped because the removal of the next transform would have generated a model with a distinct PD in the LCV score using an LCV ratio test.

The estimated EC correlation submatrix for the contracted model is generated but not included in Table 13.12; it is displayed in Table 13.13. Rounded values for the estimated correlations are 0.37, 0.24, 0.23, and 0.42 as also reported in Sect. 13.4.6. Outcome values are denoted as y1 and y2 representing in this case 0:poor and ≤ 1: good, respectively. The full EC correlation matrix has $5 \cdot 4/2 = 10$ off-diagonal component matrices all equal to this submatrix. The diagonal component matrices are functions of the means and so change with the values of visit and active.

References

Koch, G. G., Carr, C. F., Amara, I. A., Stokes, M. E., & Uryniak, T. J. (1989). Categorical data analysis. In D. A. Berry (Ed.), *Statistical methodology in the pharmaceutical sciences* (pp. 391–475). Marcel Dekker.

Miller, M. E., Davis, C. S., & Landis, J. R. (1993). The analysis of longitudinal polytomous data: Generalized estimating equations and connections with weighted least squares. *Biometrics, 49*, 1033–1044.

Chapter 14
Example Discrete Regression Analyses

Abstract Adaptive analyses are presented of a trichotomous respiratory status data set with an outcome having three possible values over a baseline and four subsequent clinic visits using discrete regression with multinomial, ordinal, or censored Poisson probabilities. Results are compared for partially modified generalized estimating equations (GEE), fully modified GEE, and extended linear mixed modeling (ELMM). Linearity for the probabilities in visit with constant dispersions is addressed as well as whether unit dispersions are appropriate for these data, a comparison to standard GEE, and the dependence of means and dispersions on visit. Adaptive additive and adaptive moderation models are generated for visit and being on active treatment. A comparison to the standard linear moderation model is provided as well as direct variance modeling of trichotomous respiratory status levels. A summary of the analysis results is also provided. SAS code for generating these analyses is described along with output generated by that code.

Keywords Direct variance modeling · Discrete regression · Extended linear mixed modeling · Generalized estimating equations · Moderation · Non-constant dispersions

Introduction Adaptive discrete regression analyses are presented in this chapter of the trichotomous respiratory status data of Sect. 13.1 with $K + 1 = 3$ possible outcome values as also analyzed in Chap. 13 (Koch et al., 1989). The dichotomous respiratory status data of Sect. 2.8.3 analyzed in Chap. 8 have a related outcome. Section 14.1 provides example analyses using multinomial probabilities, Sect. 14.2 analyses using ordinal probabilities, and Sect. 14.3 analyses using censored Poisson probabilities. Section 14.4 provides a summary of the analysis results described in prior sections while Sect. 14.5 provides example SAS code for generating such analyses and descriptions of output generated by that code. The cutoff for a distinct percent decrease in LCV scores (Sect. 2.6.2) for the trichotomous respiratory status

Supplementary Information The online version contains supplementary material available at https://doi.org/10.1007/978-3-031-41988-1_14.

G. J. Knafl, *Modeling Correlated Outcomes Using Extensions of Generalized Estimating Equations and Linear Mixed Modeling*,
https://doi.org/10.1007/978-3-031-41988-1_14

data is 0.35%, computed using DF = 1 degrees of freedom. In the case of multinomial probabilities, the removal of one transform from the model for the means results in $K = 2$ less parameters, and so the cutoff in that case is 0.54%, computed using DF = 2 degrees of freedom.

The primary purpose of Chap. 14 is to compare adaptive modeling results for partially modified GEE, fully modified GEE, and ELMM applied to discrete numeric correlated outcomes using discrete regression models (see Chap. 12 for details). Partially modified GEE (see Chap. 3 for details) extends standard GEE (see Chap. 2 for details) by adding extra estimating equations for dispersion parameters to the standard GEE estimating equations for mean parameters. Fully modified GEE (see Chap. 4 for details) extends standard GEE further by providing alternative estimating equations for mean parameters while utilizing the same estimating equations for the dispersions used by partially modified GEE. These new estimating equations are based on minimizing an extended likelihood function, treated as a likelihood function for brevity in what follows. Both partially modified and fully modified GEE use the standard GEE method of estimating correlation parameters using residuals. ELMM (see Chap. 5 for more details) is based on estimating equations for mean, dispersion, and correlation parameters determined by maximizing the likelihood. The estimating equations for the means and dispersions are the same as for fully modified GEE.

14.1 Multinomial Probabilities

Analyses in this section consider discrete regression modeling based on multinomial probabilities. Section 14.1.1 addresses choosing the correlation structure from among those described in Sect. 2.3 and choosing the number k of folds as described in Sect. 2.6.1. Results are compared for partially modified GEE, fully modified GEE, and ELMM. Section 14.1.2 addresses linearity of the generalized logits of the probabilities in visit with constant dispersions and Sect. 14.1.3 addresses the dependence of probabilities and dispersions on visit. Adaptive additive and adaptive moderation models in visit and being on active treatment assuming constant dispersions are provided in Sect. 14.1.4. Further multinomial probability analyses are not provided due to excessive times for prior analyses.

14.1.1 Choosing the Number of Folds and the Correlation Structure

Analyses reported in this section assume constant dispersions. The effects of the correlation structure on estimation by partially modified GEE, fully modified GEE, and ELMM are assessed as well as the effects of the number k of folds.

Table 14.1 Adaptive discrete regression models of multinomial probabilities for trichotomous respiratory status in power transforms of visit for alternate modeling approaches and correlation structures assuming constant dispersions

Modeling approach	Correlation	Powers of visit[a]	5-fold LCV score	Clock time (min)
Partially modified GEE	IND	0.2	0.35118	71.9
	AR1	−1.01	0.41764	54.3
	EC	0, −2.99, 1.501	0.32069	189.2
	UN	0, 0.41	0.42504	52.4
Fully modified GEE	IND	0.2	0.35123	1.2
	AR1	−0.2	0.41815	11.5
	EC	−0.2	0.41410	6.3
	UN	0.21	0.42337	4.6
ELMM	IND	0.2	0.35123	0.5
	AR1	−0.2	0.41791	1.5
	EC	0.1	0.41449	2.1
	UN	−0.2	0.42434	5.3

AR1 spatial autoregressive order 1; *EC* exchangeable correlations; *ELMM* extended linear mixed modeling; *GEE* generalized estimating equations; *IND* independent; *LCV* likelihood cross-validation; *UN* unstructured

[a]A power of 0 corresponds to an intercept parameter; otherwise, the model has a zero intercept

Table 14.1 contains results for adaptive discrete regression models based on multinomial probabilities for trichotomous respiratory status levels with constant dispersions generated for 12 cases corresponding to each of the three modeling approaches partially modified GEE, fully modified GEE, and ELMM and each of the four correlation structures IND, spatial AR1, EC, and UN with LCV scores based on $k = 5$ folds. Note that equivalent results would be generated for non-spatial AR1 correlations as for spatial AR1 correlations since outcome measurements are equally spaced in visit. The best LCV score of 0.42504 for the four partially modified GEE models is achieved with UN correlations. The best LCV score of 0.42337 for the four fully modified GEE models is achieved with UN correlations. The best LCV score of 0.42434 for the four ELMM models is achieved with UN correlations. Consequently, all three modeling approaches select UN as the most appropriate of the four correlation structures for the trichotomous respiratory status data using $k = 5$ folds.

The 5-fold LCV score for the partially modified GEE model using ELMM is 0.42233 with non-distinct percent decrease (PD) 0.47% (i.e., less than or equal to the cutoff 0.54% for a distinct PD in the LCV score based on DF = 2) compared to the associated ELMM model of Table 14.1. While the partially modified GEE model has a competitive LCV score, it is based on an intercept and a transform of visit and so is more complex than the ELMM model based on a transform of visit without an intercept and with a larger LCV score. Consequently, the ELMM model is preferable. The fully modified GEE model of Table 14.1 is the same as generated by ELMM, and so these two models are competitive alternatives.

Table 14.2 Adaptive discrete regression models of multinomial probabilities for trichotomous respiratory status in power transforms of visit for alternate modeling approaches, correlation structures, and numbers of folds assuming constant dispersions

Modeling approach	Correlation	10 folds			15 folds		
		Powers of visit[a]	LCV score	Clock time (min)	Powers of visit[1]	LCV score	Clock time (min)
Fully modified GEE	IND	−0.3	0.35142	5.0	−0.4	0.35170	6.9
	AR1	−0.3	0.41878	8.0	−0.401	0.42011	13.4
	EC	0.14	0.41445	18.7	−0.28	0.41536	23.5
	UN	0.4	0.42436	9.1	0.18	0.42384	15.4
ELMM	IND	−0.3	0.35142	2.1	−0.4	0.35170	2.9
	AR1	−0.19	0.42022	3.4	−0.2	0.42057	5.6
	EC	0.09	0.41453	5.7	−0.33	0.41529	8.8
	UN	−0.26	0.42553	16.1	−0.3	0.42640	17.0

AR1 spatial autoregressive order 1; *EC* exchangeable correlations; *ELMM* extended linear mixed modeling; *GEE* generalized estimating equations; *IND* independent; *LCV* likelihood cross-validation; *UN* unstructured

[a]A power of 0 corresponds to an intercept parameter; otherwise, the model has a zero intercept

Table 14.1 also contains clock times for generated models. Clock times for partially modified GEE range from 52.4 to 189.2 min with a total over all 4 cases of about 6.1 h, for fully modified GEE from 1.2 to 11.5 min for a total of about 0.4 hours, and for ELMM from 0.5 to 5.3 min for a total of about 0.2 h (totals not reported in Table 14.1). Note that clock times are rounded to 1 decimal digit, but sums are based on unrounded values and so may not be the same as the sum of the rounded values. Consequently, ELMM requires less computation time, with partially modified GEE taking about 30.5 times as much and fully modified GEE about 2.0 times as much. The times for partially modified GEE are excessive, and so partially modified GEE modeling is not considered in subsequent analyses. A comparison of partially modified GEE to standard GEE is also not provided.

Table 14.2 contains results for adaptive discrete regression models based on multinomial probabilities for trichotomous respiratory status levels with constant dispersions generated for 16 cases corresponding to each of the two modeling approaches fully modified GEE and ELMM; each of the four correlation structures IND, spatial AR1, EC, and UN; and each of the two numbers k of folds 10 and 15. Note that equivalent results would be generated for non-spatial AR1 correlations as for spatial AR1 correlations since outcome measurements are equally spaced in visit. The best LCV score of 0.42384 for the eight fully modified GEE models is achieved with UN correlations and $k = 15$ folds, and this is better than the associated LCV scores of Table 14.1 using $k = 5$ folds. The best LCV score of 0.42640 for the eight ELMM models is achieved with UN correlations and $k = 15$ folds, and this is better than the associated LCV scores of Table 14.1 using $k = 5$ folds. Consequently, both modeling approaches select UN as the most appropriate of the four correlation structures for the trichotomous respiratory status data. They also select $k = 15$ as the most appropriate of the three numbers of folds considered in Tables 14.1–14.2.

The 15-fold LCV score for the fully modified GEE model of Table 14.2 using ELMM is 0.42508 so that the associated ELMM model of Table 14.1 generates a non-distinct PD of 0.31%. Consequently, both modeling approaches generate competitive constant dispersion models.

Table 14.2 also contains clock times for generated models. Clock times for fully modified GEE range from 13.4 to 23.5 min for a total of about 1.7 h and for ELMM from 2.9 to 17.0 min for a total of about 1.0 h (totals not reported in Table 14.2). Note that clock times are rounded to 1 decimal digit, but sums are based on unrounded values and so may not be the same as the sum of the rounded values. Consequently, ELMM requires less computation time, with fully modified GEE about 1.7 times as much.

It is possible that a larger number of folds than $k = 15$ is more appropriate to use. This is assessed using ELMM. The associated model with $k = 20$ and UN correlations has smaller LCV score 0.42609, indicating that $k = 15$ is an appropriate choice for selecting discrete regression models based on multinomial probabilities for the trichotomous respiratory status data. For this reason, subsequent analyses use $k = 15$ folds and UN correlations.

Using ELMM because it generates a competitive model in less time, the adaptive model has means based on visit$^{-0.3}$ without an intercept and estimated constant dispersion 0.5. Figure 14.1 provides the plot of estimated mean trichotomous respiratory status over visits 0–4. Mean trichotomous respiratory status increases from 1 at visit 0 to 1.2 at visit 1 and then remains relatively constant after that up to visit 4. Figure 14.2 provides the plot of estimated probabilities for the ELMM model over visits 0–4. The estimated baseline probabilities at visit 0 equal the same value 0.33 for outcome values 0–2. Post-baseline estimated probabilities for 0:poor increase gradually to 0.42 by visit 4, for 1:good respiratory status decrease to 0 at visits 1–4, and for 2:excellent respiratory status increase to 0.61 at visit 2 and then decrease gradually to 0.58 by visit 4. Table 14.3 provides estimates of UN correlation parameters. These range from 0.30 between visits 0 and 3 to 0.69 between visits 3 and 4.

14.1.2 Assessing Linearity of the Generalized Logits for the Probabilities in Visit

Using ELMM with constant dispersions, $k = 15$ folds, and UN correlations identified as an appropriate alternative in Sect. 14.1.1, the linear polynomial model in visit has LCV = 0.42193 with distinct PD 1.05% compared to the adaptive model in visit with LCV score 0.42640. Consequently, the generalized logits for the probabilities of trichotomous respiratory status are distinctly nonlinear in visit when the dispersions are treated as constant.

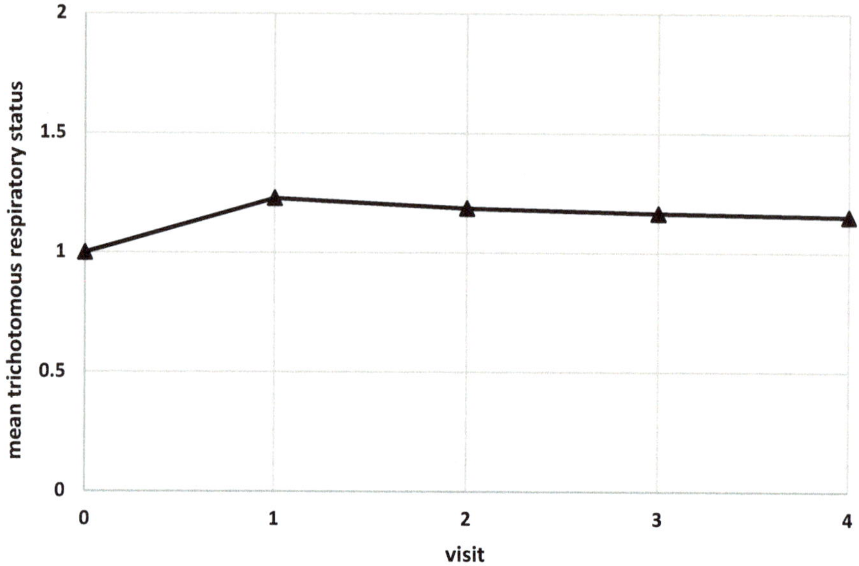

Fig. 14.1 Estimated mean trichotomous respiratory status over visits 0–4 under the discrete regression model based on multinomial probabilities as a function of visit with constant dispersions using ELMM

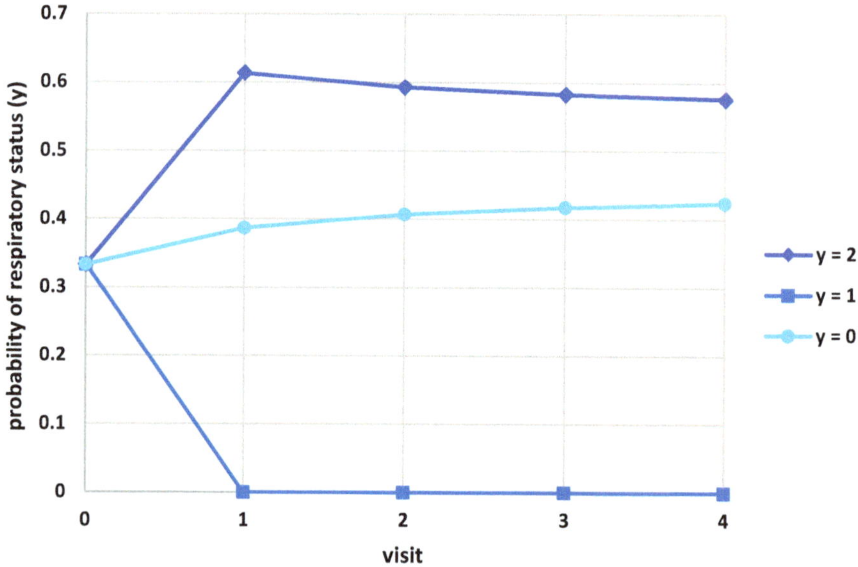

Fig. 14.2 Estimated probabilities for trichotomous respiratory status over visits 0–4 under the discrete regression model based on multinomial probabilities as a function of visit with constant dispersions using ELMM

Table 14.3 Estimated unstructured correlations for trichotomous respiratory status using the adaptive discrete regression model based on multinomial probabilities as a function of visit[a]

visit	1	2	3	4
0	0.43	0.34	0.30	0.37
1		0.59	0.52	0.44
2			0.68	0.65
3				0.69

[a]Using extended linear mixed modeling with 15 folds

Table 14.4 Adaptive discrete regression models of trichotomous respiratory status for multinomial probabilities and dispersions as a function of visit[a]

Modeling approach	Transforms of visit for probabilities[2]	Transforms of visit for dispersions[b]	LCV score	Clock time (min)
Fully modified GEE	$\text{visit}^{-0.32}$	1	0.42540	46.5
ELMM	$\text{visit}^{-0.28}$	1	0.42640	50.1

ELMM extended linear mixed modeling; *GEE* generalized estimating equations; *LCV* likelihood cross-validation
[a]Computed with unstructured correlations and 15 folds
[b]A value of 1 corresponds to an intercept parameter; otherwise, the model has a zero intercept

14.1.3 Modeling Probabilities and Dispersions in Visit

Adaptive analyses of trichotomous respiratory status are presented in this section using $k = 15$ folds and the UN correlation structure as determined in Sect. 14.1.1. Adaptive models for probabilities and non-constant dispersions in visit are generated to assess the usual assumption of constant dispersions. Table 14.4 provides results for adaptive models for probabilities and dispersions in visit. The two modeling approaches fully modified GEE and ELMM are considered.

The models generated by fully modified GEE and ELMM have means based on one transform of visit without an intercept and with constant dispersions. The ELMM model has LCV score 0.42640. The fully modified GEE model computed using ELMM has LCV score 0.42540 with non-distinct PD of 0.23%. Consequently, both modeling approaches generate competitive adaptive models for means and dispersions in visit. Moreover, both models have constant dispersions and so dispersions are reasonably considered not to change with visit.

Table 14.4 also contains clock times for generated models. The clock time is 46.5 min or about 0.8 h for fully modified GEE and 50.1 min or about 0.9 h for ELMM. Consequently, fully modified GEE requires less computation time, with ELMM about 1.1 times as much.

14.1.4 Adaptive Models in Visit and Active Treatment Assuming Constant Dispersions

Table 14.5 contains results for adaptive additive models and adaptive moderation models for mean trichotomous respiratory status in terms of visit and the indicator active for being on active treatment assuming constant dispersions based on fully modified GEE and ELMM. The additive ELMM model is the same as the associated model of Table 14.2. The fully modified GEE model is not the same as the associated Table 14.2 model, but has one transform of visit plus an intercept while the associated Table 14.2 model has one transform of visit without an intercept. The expanded model from which the Table 14.2 model is generated also has a single transform with an intercept and LCV score 0.42596 with non-distinct PD 0.09% and so is a competitive alternative. In any case, these results indicate that an additive effect to being on active treatment is not supported using discrete regression modeling based on multinomial probabilities and assuming constant dispersions.

Table 14.5 contains results for adaptive moderation models for mean trichotomous respiratory status in terms of visit and the indicator active for being on active treatment assuming constant dispersions based on fully modified GEE and ELMM. The fully modified GEE moderation model has LCV score 0.42981 while the associated additive model has LCV score 0.42636 with distinct PD 0.80%, indicating that moderation is supported using discrete regression modeling based on multinomial probabilities and assuming constant dispersions. On the other hand, the ELMM moderation model has LCV score 0.42758 while the ELMM additive model has LCV score 0.42640 with non-distinct PD 0.28%, indicating that, even though a geometric combination is included in the model, moderation is not supported using discrete regression modeling based on multinomial probabilities and assuming constant dispersions. The fully modified GEE model has LCV score 0.42957 computed using ELMM so that the ELMM moderation generates a non-distinct PD 0.46%, indicating that the two moderation models are competitive

Table 14.5 Adaptive discrete regression models for multinomial probabilities of trichotomous respiratory status in visit and the indicator for being on active treatment assuming constant dispersions[a]

	Additive models			Moderation models[b]		
Modeling approach	Transforms for probabilities[3]	LCV score	Clock time (min)	Transforms for probabilities[c]	LCV score	Clock time (min)
Fully modified GEE	1, $\text{visit}^{0.0799}$	0.42636	28.9	$(\text{active}\cdot\text{visit}^{-1})^{-0.001}$, $(\text{active}\cdot\text{visit}^{3})^{0.8}$	0.42981	861.9
ELMM	$\text{visit}^{-0.3}$	0.42640	32.5	$(\text{visit}^{-1}\cdot\text{active})^{0.0001}$	0.42759	348.5

ELMM extended linear mixed modeling; *GEE* generalized estimating equations; *LCV* likelihood cross-validation.

[a]Computed with unstructured correlations and 15 folds

[b]Partially modified GEE not considered due to requiring excessive time in prior analyses

[c]All models have zero intercepts. The variable active is the indicator for being on active treatment

alternatives. Since the ELMM model is simpler, it is preferable, supporting the conclusion that moderation is not supported.

Table 14.5 also contains clock times for adaptive additive and moderation models for the means generated assuming constant dispersions. For additive models, the clock times are 28.9 min or about 0.5 h for fully modified GEE and 32.5 min or also about 0.5 h for ELMM. Consequently, fully modified GEE requires less computation time, with ELMM about 1.1 times as much. The fully modified GEE moderation model requires 861.9 min or about 14.4 h while ELMM moderation modeling requires 348.5 min or about 5.8 h. Consequently, ELMM requires less time, with fully modified GEE requiring about 2.5 times as much. Since both moderation models require excessive amounts of time, no further adaptive discrete regression analyses based on multinomial probabilities are conducted.

The preferable adaptive additive ELMM model of Table 14.4 is the same as the associated model of Table 14.2. Moreover, the adaptive ELMM model of Table 14.3 has the same LCV score, indicating that the preferable model based on multinomial probabilities is described in Sect. 14.1.1 using Figs. 14.1-14.2 and Table 14.3.

14.2 Ordinal Probabilities

Analyses in this section consider discrete regression modeling based on ordinal probabilities. Section 14.2.1 addresses choosing the correlation structure from among those described in Sect. 2.3 and choosing the number *k* of folds as described in Sect. 2.6.1. Results are compared for partially modified GEE, fully modified GEE, and ELMM. Section 14.2.2 addresses linearity of the cumulative logits of the probabilities in visit with constant dispersions, Sect. 14.2.3 provides a comparison to standard GEE, and Sect. 14.2.4 the dependence of probabilities and dispersions on visit. Adaptive additive and adaptive moderation models for means assuming constant dispersions are generated for visit and being on active treatment in Sect. 14.2.5. A comparison to standard linear additive and moderation models is provided in Sect. 14.2.6. Adaptive additive and adaptive moderation models for means and dispersions are generated for visit and being on active treatment in Sect. 14.2.7. Section 14.2.8 addresses direct variance modeling of the trichotomous respiratory status data and Sect. 14.2.9 covers unit dispersion modeling.

14.2.1 Choosing the Number of Folds and the Correlation Structure

Analyses reported in this section assume constant dispersions. The effects of the number *k* of folds and of the correlation structure on estimation by partially modified GEE, fully modified GEE, and ELMM are assessed. Table 14.6 contains results for adaptive discrete regression models of ordinal probabilities for trichotomous respiratory status levels with constant dispersions generated for 36 cases corresponding to each of the three modeling approaches partially modified GEE, fully modified GEE, and ELMM; each of the four correlation structures IND, spatial AR1, EC, and UN; and each of the three numbers k of folds 5, 10, and 15. Note that equivalent results would be generated for non-spatial AR1 correlations as for spatial AR1 correlations since outcome measurements are equally spaced in visit.

The best LCV score of 0.42467 for the 12 partially modified GEE models is achieved at $k = 5$ under UN correlations. The best LCV score of 0.42736 for the 12 fully modified GEE models is achieved at $k = 10$ under UN correlations. The best LCV score of 0.42450 for the 12 ELMM models is achieved at $k = 10$ under UN correlations. Consequently, all three modeling approaches select UN as the most appropriate of the four correlation structures for the trichotomous respiratory status data. Partially modified GEE selects 5 folds while fully modified GEE and ELMM select 10 folds. Subsequent analyses use the conservative choice of 10 folds.

The partially modified GEE model selected using 5 folds has 10-fold LCV score 0.42447 computed using ELMM with non-distinct percent decrease (PD) 0.01% compared to the selected ELMM model. The fully modified GEE model selected using 10 folds has 10-fold LCV score 0.42469 computed using ELMM while the selected ELMM has LCV score 0.42450 and non-distinct PD 0.04% compared to the fully modified GEE model. Consequently, all three modeling procedures generate competitive models. Note that LCV scores for associated multinomial probability models are computed using $k = 15$ fold and so are not comparable to LCV scores for associated ordinal probability models computed with $k = 10$ folds

Table 14.6 also contains clock times for generated models. Clock times for partially modified GEE range from 21.7 to 268.4 min with a total over all 12 cases of about 18.8 h, for fully modified GEE from 1.5 to 24.0 min for a total of about 1.7 h, and for ELMM from 0.2 to 10.5 min for a total of about 0.6 h (totals not reported in Table 14.6). Note that clock times are rounded to 1 decimal digit, but sums are based on unrounded values and so may not be the same as the sum of the rounded values. Consequently, ELMM requires less computation time, with partially modified GEE taking about 31.3 times as much and fully modified GEE about 2.8 times as much. The times for partially modified GEE are excessive, and so partially modified GEE is not considered in subsequent analyses.

Using ELMM because it generates a competitive model in less time, the adaptive model has means based on visit$^{0.4}$ with an intercept and estimated constant dispersion 2.9. Figure 14.3 provides the plot of estimated mean trichotomous respiratory status over visits 0–4. Mean trichotomous respiratory status gradually increases from 1.0 at visit 0 to 1.2 by visit 4. Figure 14.4 provides the plot of estimated probabilities for the ELMM model over visits 0–4. Estimated probabilities for a 0:poor respiratory status decrease from 0.07 at visit 0 to 0.02 by visit 4, for a 1:good respiratory status decrease from 0.87 at visit 0 to 0.77 at visit 4, and for a 2:excellent respiratory status increase from 0.06 at visit 0 to 0.21 at visit 4. Table 14.7 provides estimates of UN correlation parameters. These range from 0.30 between visits 0 and 3 to 0.69 between visits 2 and 3 and also between visits 3 and 4.

Table 14.6 Adaptive discrete regression models of ordinal probabilities for trichotomous respiratory status in power transforms of visit for alternate modeling approaches, correlation structures, and numbers of folds assuming constant dispersions

Modeling approach	Correlation	5 folds			10 folds			15 folds		
		Powers of visit[1]	LCV score	Clock time (min)	Powers of visit[1]	LCV score	Clock time (min)	Powers of visit[a]	LCV score	Clock time (min)
Partially modified GEE	IND	0, 0.08	0.35257	82.1	0, 0.19	0.35151	103.6	0, 0.29	0.35093	74.0
	AR1	−0.1	0.41985	65.1	0, −0.49	0.19850	75.1	0, −0.5	0.41991	106.1
	EC	0	0.31074	21.7	0	0.31119	46.7	0	0.31113	59.6
	UN	0, 0.3	0.42467	54.0	0, 0.402	0.42466	268.4	0, 0.4	0.42448	172.2
Fully modified GEE	IND	0, 0.3	0.35137	1.5	0, 0.21	0.35131	3.1	0, 0.21	0.35214	5.7
	AR1	−0.1	0.41966	10.7	−0.1	0.42027	11.1	0, −0.201	0.42034	8.3
	EC	−0.16	0.41590	5.0	0, −0.27	0.41523	3.9	0, −0.3	0.41573	6.2
	UN	0, 0.097	0.42615	6.7	0, 0.09	0.42736	24.0	0, 0.41	0.42513	15.5
ELMM	IND	0, 0.3	0.35137	0.2	0, 0.1	0.35205	0.5	0, 0.29	0.35102	0.7
	AR1	−0.4	0.41987	1.9	0.01	0.42018	4.1	0, −0.6	0.41974	2.3
	EC	0, −0.36	0.41556	0.6	0, −0.29	0.41521	0.9	0, −0.3	0.41574	1.6
	UN	−0.7	0.42372	6.5	0, 0.4	0.42450	6.0	0, −0.39	0.42426	10.5

AR1 spatial autoregressive order 1; *EC* exchangeable correlations; *ELMM* extended linear mixed modeling; *GEE* generalized estimating equations; *IND* independent; *LCV* likelihood cross-validation; *UN* unstructured.

[a]A power of 0 corresponds to an intercept parameter; otherwise, the model has a zero intercept. A zero intercept for the probabilities means the intercept for $y \leq 0$ is set to zero but not the intercept for $y \leq 1$

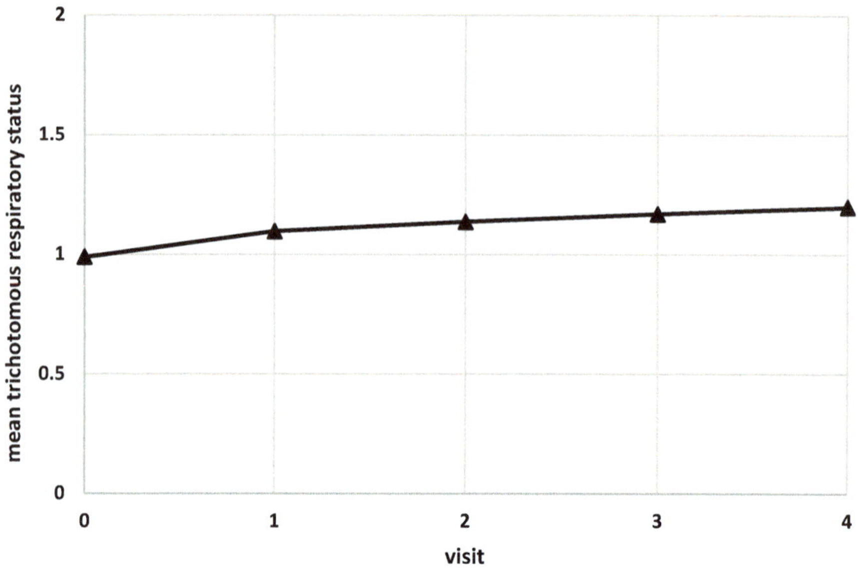

Fig. 14.3 Estimated mean trichotomous respiratory status over visits 0–4 under the discrete regression model for ordinal probabilities in visit with constant dispersions using ELMM

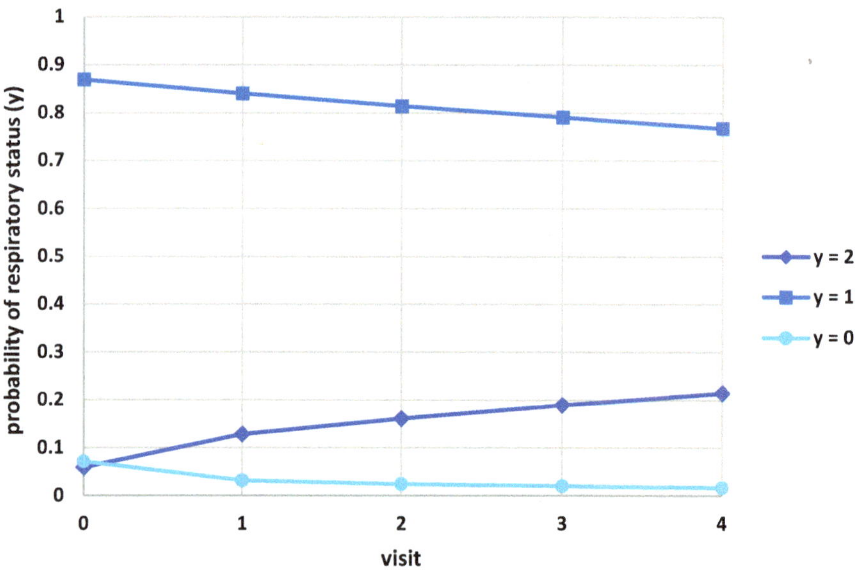

Fig. 14.4 Estimated probabilities for trichotomous respiratory status over visits 0–4 under the discrete regression model for ordinal probabilities in visit with constant dispersions using ELMM

Table 14.7 Estimated unstructured correlations for trichotomous respiratory status using the discrete regression model for ordinal probabilities in visit[a]

visit	1	2	3	4
0	0.42	0.33	0.30	0.38
1		0.56	0.50	0.42
2			0.68	0.65
3				0.69

[a]Using extended linear mixed modeling with 10 folds

14.2.2 Assessing Linearity of the Cumulative Logits of the Probabilities in Visit

Using ELMM with constant dispersions, $k = 10$ folds, and UN correlations as identified as an appropriate choice in Sect. 14.2.1, the linear polynomial model in visit has LCV = 0.42297 with distinct PD of 0.36% compared to the adaptive model in visit with LCV score 0.42450. Consequently, the cumulative logits for the probabilities of mean trichotomous respiratory status are distinctly nonlinear in visit when dispersions are treated as constant.

14.2.3 Comparison to Standard GEE Modeling

When dispersions are treated as constant, the only difference between partially modified GEE and standard GEE is how the constant dispersion parameter is estimated. Partially modified GEE uses a bias-unadjusted estimate (Sect. 3.5) while standard GEE uses a bias-adjusted estimate (Sect. 2.4). Standard GEE is thus a possible alternative to partially modified GEE for modeling means with constant dispersions. For the trichotomous respiratory status data, the adaptively generated standard GEE model for the ordinal probabilities assuming unit dispersions (to reduce the computations; see Sect. 3.5) has constant probabilities based on only an intercept and LCV score 0.39978 with distinct PD 5.86% compared to the associated partially modified GEE model with LCV score 0.42466, indicating that in this case partially modified GEE modeling distinctly outperforms standard GEE modeling. In contrast, standard GEE modeling requires 0.5 min of clock time compared to 268.4 min or about 536.9 times more for partially modified GEE modeling. On the other hand, the model for the probabilities generated by standard GEE modeling computed using ELMM and constant dispersions has LCV score 0.42065 with distinct PD 0.91% compared to the LCV score of 0.42450 for the associated ELMM model (Table 14.6). However, ELMM requires about 15.4 times more time than standard GEE modeling.

Table 14.8 Adaptive discrete regression models of trichotomous respiratory status for ordinal probabilities and dispersions in visit[a]

Modeling approach	Transforms of visit for probabilities[b]	Transforms of visit for dispersions[b]	LCV score	Clock time (min)
Fully modified GEE	1, $visit^{0.088}$	1	0.42742	63.6
ELMM	1, $visit^{-0.4}$	1, $visit^{1.1}$	0.42553	20.4

ELMM extended linear mixed modeling; *GEE* generalized estimating equations; *LCV* likelihood cross-validation

[a]Computed with unstructured correlations and 10 folds

[b]A value of 1 corresponds to an intercept parameter; otherwise, the model has a zero intercept. A zero intercept for the probabilities means the intercept for $y \leq 0$ is set to zero but not the intercept for $y \leq 1$

14.2.4 Modeling Probabilities and Dispersions in Visit

Adaptive analyses of trichotomous respiratory status levels are presented in this section using $k = 10$ folds and the UN correlation structure as determined in Sect. 14.2.1. Adaptive models for probabilities and non-constant dispersions in visit are generated to assess the common assumption of constant dispersions. Table 14.8 provides results for adaptive models for probabilities and dispersions in visit. Only the two modeling approaches fully modified GEE and ELMM are considered in subsequent analyses due to excessive times for partially modified GEE in the analyses of Sect. 14.2.1.

The fully modified GEE model has LCV score 0.42742 while the associated constant dispersion model selected using 10 folds of Table 14.5 has LCV score 0.42736 with non-distinct PD 0.01%. The ELMM model has LCV score 0.42553 while the associated constant dispersion model of Table 14.6 has LCV score 0.42450 with non-distinct PD 0.24%. Consequently, fully modified GEE modeling and ELMM both suggest that dispersions are reasonably considered as constant in visit.

The fully modified GEE model computed using ELMM has LCV score 0.42471 with non-distinct PD 0.19%. Consequently, both modeling approaches generate competitive adaptive models for means and dispersions in visit.

Table 14.8 also contains clock times for generated models. The clock time is 63.6 min or about 1.1 h for fully modified GEE and 20.4 min or about 0.3 h for ELMM. Consequently, ELMM requires less computation time, with fully modified GEE taking about 3.1 times as much.

14.2.5 Adaptive Models in Visit and Active Treatment Assuming Constant Dispersions

Table 14.9 contains results for discrete regression adaptive additive models and adaptive moderation models of ordinal probabilities for trichotomous respiratory

Table 14.9 Adaptive discrete regression models of ordinal probabilities for trichotomous respiratory status in visit and the indicator for being on active treatment assuming constant dispersions[a]

	Additive models			Moderation models		
Modeling approach	Transforms for probabilities[b]	LCV score	Clock time (min)	Transforms for probabilities[b]	LCV score	Clock time (min)
Fully modified GEE	1, $\text{visit}^{0.09}$	0.42736	25.2	1, $\text{visit}^{0.09}$	0.42736	105.0
ELMM	$\text{visit}^{-0.2}$	0.42434	8.4	$(\text{active}\cdot\text{visit}^{-0.21})^{0.99}$	0.42691	102.1

ELMM extended linear mixed modeling; *GEE* generalized estimating equations; *LCV* likelihood cross-validation

[a]Computed with unstructured correlations and 10 folds

[b]A value of 1 corresponds to an intercept parameter; otherwise, the model has a zero intercept. A zero intercept for the probabilities means the intercept for $y \le 0$ is set to zero but not the intercept for $y \le 1$

status in terms of visit and the indicator active for being on active treatment assuming constant dispersions based on fully modified GEE and ELMM. The fully modified GEE and ELMM additive models do not contain the indicator active. Consequently, an additive effect to being on active treatment is not supported using discrete regression modeling of ordinal probabilities assuming constant dispersions. The fully modified GEE moderation model is the same as the associated additive model of Table 14.9, and so moderation is not supported by fully modified GEE assuming constant dispersions. On the other hand, the ELMM moderation model of Table 14.8 has LCV score 0.42691 while the ELMM additive model of Table 14.9 has LCV score 0.42434 with distinct PD 0.60%. Consequently, moderation is supported by discrete regression modeling of ordinal probabilities using ELMM assuming constant dispersions.

The adaptive moderation model generated using fully modified GEE of Table 14.9 computed using ELMM has LCV score 0.42469 with distinct PD 0.52% compared to the ELMM moderation model of Table 14.9. Consequently, ELMM outperforms fully modified GEE in generating moderation models assuming constant dispersions. For this reason, subsequent analyses use only ELMM.

Table 14.9 also contains clock times for adaptive additive and moderation models for the ordinal probabilities generated assuming constant dispersions. For additive models, the clock times are 25.2 min for fully modified GEE and 8.4 min for ELMM. Consequently, ELMM additive modeling requires less computation time, with fully modified GEE additive modeling requiring about 3.0 times as much. For moderation models, fully modified GEE requires 105.0 min while ELMM requires 102.1 min. Consequently, ELMM moderation modeling requires slightly less computation time.

14.2.6 Comparison to Linear Additive and Moderation Models with Constant Dispersions

The standard linear additive model has cumulative logits of the probabilities based on an intercept together with main effects to the linear polynomial model in visit and active along with constant dispersions. This model computed using ELMM has LCV score 0.42233. The standard linear moderation model has the cumulative logits of the probabilities based on an intercept, main effects to untransformed visit and active, and the interaction of visit and active along with constant dispersions. This moderation model computed using ELMM has smaller LCV score 0.42159, indicating that standard linear moderation is not supported. On the other hand, as indicated in Sect. 14.2.5, moderation is supported allowing for nonlinearity and assuming constant dispersions. Consequently, adaptive ELMM modeling is required in this case to identify moderation.

14.2.7 Adaptive Models in Visit and Active Treatment for Probabilities and Dispersions

Only ELMM is considered for generating adaptive models for ordinal probabilities and dispersions of trichotomous respiratory status in terms of visit and the indicator active for being on active treatment. Results for partially modified GEE are not reported due to requiring long times while results for fully modified GEE are not reported because it generates a distinctly inferior moderation model with constant dispersions.

The ELMM additive model has probabilities based on $\text{visit}^{-0.2}$ with an intercept, dispersions based on $\text{visit}^{1.2}$ without an intercept, and LCV score 0.42635, and so does not depend on the indicator active. The associated model of Table 14.8 has LCV score 0.42553 with non-distinct PD 0.19%. Consequently, an additive effect to being on active treatment is not supported using discrete regression modeling of ordinal probabilities and dispersions.

The ELMM adaptive moderation model for ordinal probabilities and dispersions of trichotomous respiratory status in terms of visit and the indicator active for being on active treatment has LCV score 0.43067 while the associated additive model has LCV score 0.42635 with distinct PD 1.00%. Consequently, moderation of the effect to being on active treatment is supported by discrete regression modeling of ordinal probabilities and dispersions using ELMM.

The ELMM moderation model assuming constant dispersions of Table 14.9 has LCV score 0.42691 with distinct PD 0.87% compared to the associated non-constant dispersion model with LCV score 0.43067. Consequently, nonlinearity of dispersions is supported by discrete regression moderation modeling of ordinal probabilities and dispersions using ELMM. However, the non-constant moderation model has dispersions depending only on a transform of visit, indicating that the

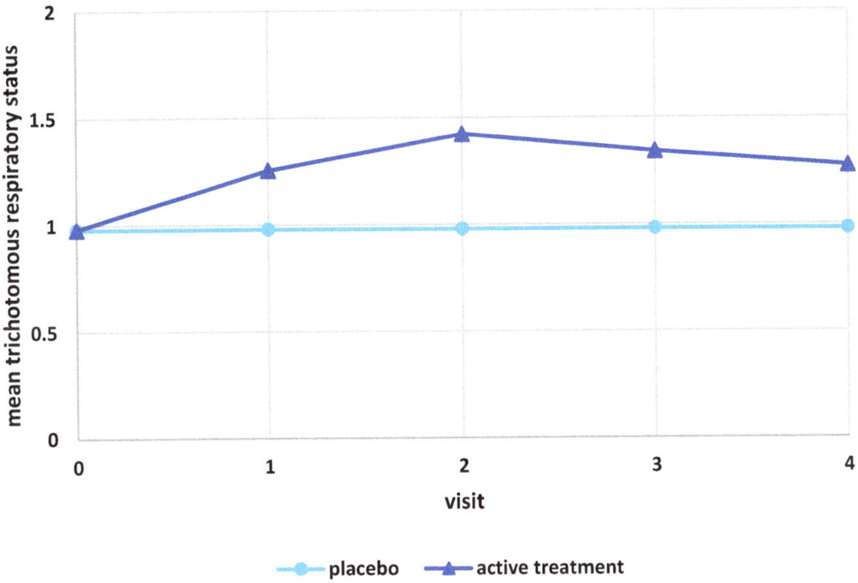

Fig. 14.5 Estimated means for trichotomous respiratory status under the discrete regression model of ordinal probabilities and dispersions in terms of visits and the indicator for being on active treatment using ELMM

dispersions do not depend on the indicator of being on active treatment either as an additive effect or interacting with the effect of visit.

The ELMM discrete regression moderation model of ordinal probabilities and dispersions for trichotomous respiratory status has probabilities based on the two geometric combinations

$$\left(\text{active} \cdot \text{visit}^{-0.21}\right)^{9.99} = \text{active} \cdot \text{visit}^{-2.0979}$$

and

$$\text{active} \cdot \text{visit}^{-1}$$

with an intercept as well as dispersions based on $\text{visit}^{1.68}$ without an intercept. Estimated means for this model are plotted in Fig. 14.5. For patients on a placebo, estimated mean trichotomous respiratory status is constant at 1.0 over visits 0–4. For patients on active treatment, estimated mean trichotomous respiratory status is 1.0 visit 0, the same as for patients on a placebo, and then increases to 1.4 at visit 2 and decreases to 1.3 at visit 4. Figure 14.6 contains the plot of estimated dispersions for trichotomous respiratory status. Estimated dispersions increase nonlinearly from 1.0 at visit 0 to a rounded value of 1.4 by visit 4 and are the same for patients on a placebo and patients on active treatment.

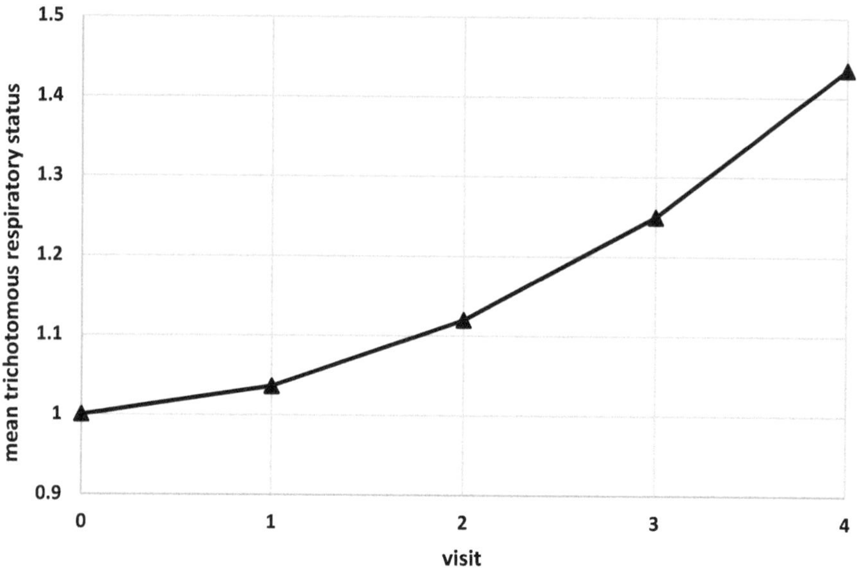

Fig. 14.6 Estimated dispersions for trichotomous respiratory status over visits 0–4 under the discrete regression model of ordinal probabilities and dispersions using ELMM

Figures 14.7-14.8 provide plots of probabilities for trichotomous respiratory status levels 0–2 (that is, 0:poor, 1:good, and 2:excellent) using the ELMM discrete regression model of Table 14.10 for patients on a placebo and patients on active treatment, respectively. For patients on a placebo, probabilities for respiratory status levels 0–2 are constant at 0.20, 0.62, and 0.18, respectively. For patients on active treatment, probabilities for respiratory status levels 0–2 are the same at baseline as for patients on a placebo. The probability of a 0 level decreases to 0.06 by visit 2 and then increases to 0.09 at visit 4. The probability of a 1 level decreases to 0.46 by visit 2 and then increases to 0.55 at visit 4. The probability of a 2 level increases to 0.48 by visit 2 and then decreases to 0.36 at visit 4. Consequently, being on active treatment increases the probability of having 2:excellent respiratory status while decreasing the probabilities of having both 0:poor and 1:good respiratory status from visit 0 to visit 2 while decreasing somewhat less from visit 2 to visit 4.

Figure 14.9 displays standardized residuals by visit and type of treatment. These are all within ±3 except for two measurements, one for a patient on a placebo with standardized residual −3.01 and one for a patient on active treatment with standardized residual −3.37. Table 14.10 contains estimated unstructured correlations for the trichotomous respiratory status outcome. These range from 0.30 for outcomes at visits 0 and 3 to 0.68 for outcomes at visits 3 and 4.

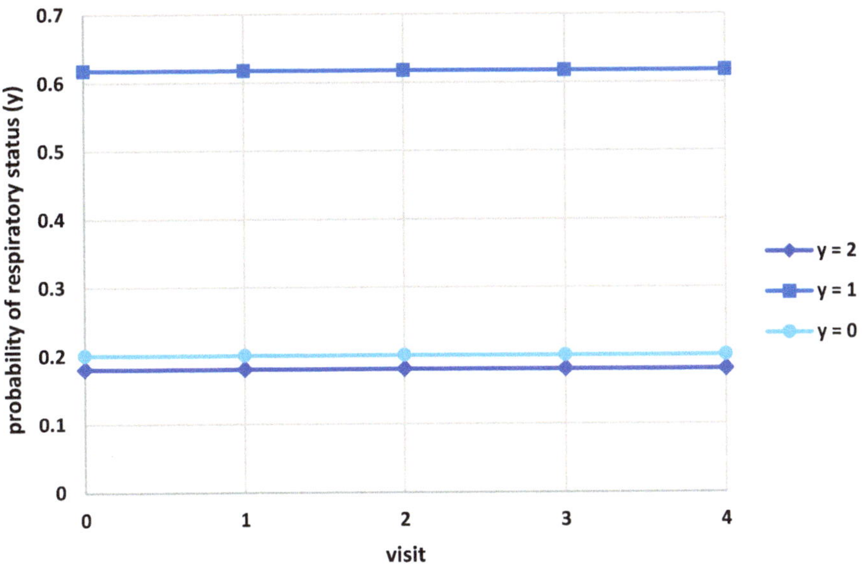

Fig. 14.7 Estimated ordinal probabilities for trichotomous respiratory status over visits 0–4 under the discrete regression moderation model in visit for patients on a placebo using ELMM

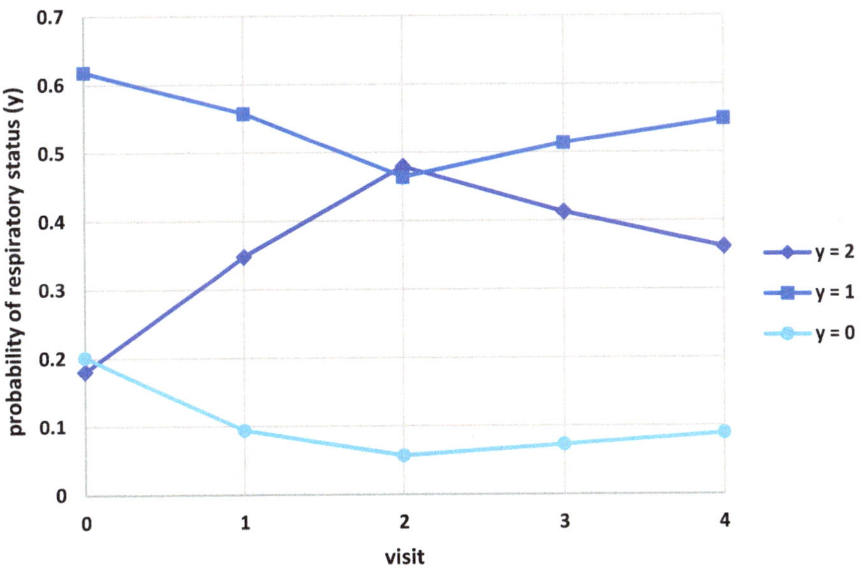

Fig. 14.8 Estimated ordinal probabilities for trichotomous respiratory status over visits 0–4 under the discrete regression moderation model in visit for patients on active treatment using ELMM

Table 14.10 Estimated unstructured correlations for trichotomous respiratory status using the adaptive discrete regression model of ordinal probabilities and dispersions in visit, the indicator active, and geometric combinations[a]

visit	1	2	3	4
0	0.41	0.35	0.30	0.37
1		0.53	0.47	0.42
2			0.64	0.64
3				0.68

[a]Using extended linear mixed modeling with 10 folds

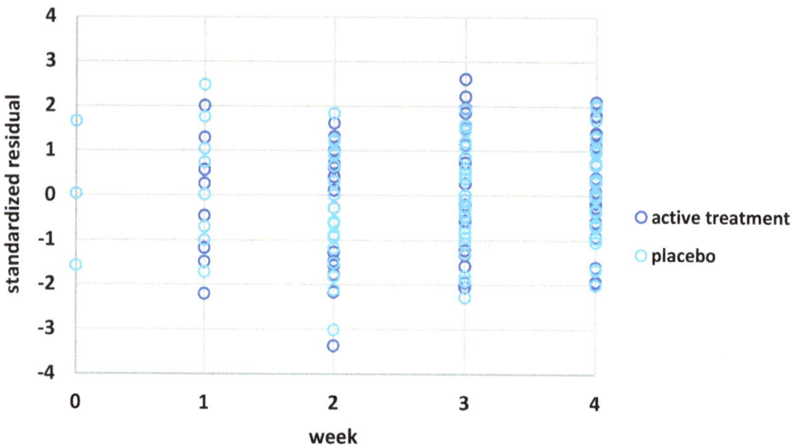

Fig. 14.9 Standardized residuals for trichotomous respiratory status under the discrete regression model for ordinal probabilities in visit for patients on active treatment using ELMM

14.2.8 Direct Variance Discrete Regression Modeling of Trichotomous Respiratory Status

Direct variance modeling treats the variance function as $V(\mu) = 1$ so that variances are the same as dispersions. Using ELMM, the adaptive discrete regression model for ordinal probabilities and dispersions of trichotomous respiratory status in visit using direct variance modeling has probabilities based on visit$^{-1.022}$ with an intercept along with dispersions, and so also variances, based on an intercept and visit^3. The LCV score is 0.41865 with distinct PD 1.62% compared to the associated extended variance model of Table 14.8 with LCV score 0.42553. The direct variance model requires 44.6 min of clock time or about 2.2 times as much as the 20.4 min required for the associated extended variance model of Table 14.8. The adaptive additive and moderation models for the probabilities and dispersions in visit and the indicator active using direct variance modeling are the same model as generated by direct variance modeling in only visit. Consequently, in this case, direct variance modeling is an ineffective alternative to extended variance modeling accounting for the dependence of variances on probabilities along with dispersions.

14.2.9 Unit Dispersion Modeling

So far, discrete regression models for ordinal probabilities have included dispersions either as constant or changing with visit and/or the indicator active for being on active treatment. A comparison of these prior models to corresponding models generated assuming unit dispersions is provided in this section. Only models generated using ELMM are considered.

The adaptive model for ordinal probabilities in visit assuming unit dispersions has means based on $\text{visit}^{-0.2}$ and an intercept with LCV score 0.42442 and non-distinct PD 0.26% compared to the associated model also allowing for dispersions depending on visit of Table 14.9 with LCV score 0.42553. The unit dispersion model requires 5.9 min compared to 20.4 min or about 3.5 times more for the non-constant dispersion model.

The adaptive additive model for ordinal probabilities in visit and the indicator active assuming unit dispersions is the same model as generated for visit alone with LCV score 0.42442 and distinct PD 0.46% compared to the associated additive model allowing for non-unit dispersions with LCV score 0.42635. The unit dispersion model requires 7.9 min compared to 45.3 min (not reported earlier) or about 5.7 times more for the non-constant dispersion model.

The adaptive moderation model for ordinal probabilities in visit, the indicator active, and geometric combinations assuming unit dispersions has ordinal probabilities based on the two geometric combinations:

$$\left(\text{active}\cdot\text{visit}^{-0.1}\right)^{8} = \text{active}\cdot\text{visit}^{-0.8},$$

$$\left(\text{active}\cdot\text{visit}^{=6}\right)^{0.5} = \text{active}\cdot\text{visit}^{-3},$$

and an intercept with LCV score 0.42865 and distinct PD 0.47% compared to the associated moderation model also allowing for dispersions depending on visit, the indicator active, and geometric combinations with LCV score 0.43067. The unit dispersion model requires 84.9 min or about 1.4 h compared to 266.3 min or about 4.4 h (not reported earlier) or about 3.1 times more for the non-constant dispersion model. The additive model assuming unit dispersions generates an LCV score with distinct PD 0.99%, supporting the conclusion that the effect of visit on the probabilities is moderated by the indicator for being on active treatment, as is also the case allowing for constant dispersions in Sect. 14.2.5 and allowing for non-constant dispersions in Sect. 14.2.7.

Unit dispersion modeling generates a competitive alternative model in one of the three cases considered and generates a distinctly inferior model in the other two cases. Consequently, unit dispersion modeling is not a reasonable alternative for the ordinal probabilities case even though it requires less time.

14.3 Censored Poisson Probabilities

Analyses in this section consider discrete regression modeling based on censored Poisson probabilities. Section 14.3.1 addresses choosing the correlation structure from among those described in Sect. 2.3 and choosing the number k of folds as described in Sect. 2.6.1. Results are compared for partially modified GEE, fully modified GEE, and ELMM. Section 14.3.2 addresses linearity of the $\log\lambda_{sc}$ terms (see Sect. 12.2.3) in visit with constant dispersions, Sect. 14.3.3 provides a comparison to standard GEE, and Sect. 14.3.4 the dependence of probabilities and dispersions on visit. Adaptive additive and moderation models for means assuming constant dispersions are generated for visit and being on active treatment in Sect. 14.3.5. A comparison to standard linear additive and moderation models is provided in Sect. 14.3.6. Adaptive additive and adaptive moderation models for means and dispersions are generated for visit and being on active treatment in Sect. 14.3.7. Section 14.3.8 addresses direct variance modeling of the trichotomous respiratory status data and Sect. 14.3.9 covers unit dispersion modeling.

14.3.1 Choosing the Number of Folds and the Correlation Structure

Analyses reported in this section assume constant dispersions. The effects of the number k of folds and of the correlation structure on estimation by partially modified GEE, fully modified GEE, and ELMM are assessed. Table 14.11 contains results for adaptive discrete regression models of censored Poisson probabilities for trichotomous respiratory status levels with constant dispersions generated for 36 cases corresponding to each of the three modeling approaches partially modified GEE, fully modified GEE, and ELMM; each of the four correlation structures IND, spatial AR1, EC, and UN; and each of the three numbers k of folds 5, 10, and 15. Note that equivalent results would be generated for non-spatial AR1 correlations as for spatial AR1 correlations since outcome measurements are equally spaced in visit.

The best LCV score of 0.42143 for the 12 partially modified GEE models is achieved at $k = 15$ under spatial AR1 correlations. The best LCV score of 0.42263 for the 12 fully modified GEE models is achieved at $k = 15$ under UN correlations. The best LCV score of 0.42536 for the 12 ELMM models is achieved at $k = 15$ under UN correlations. Consequently, partially modified GEE selects spatial AR1 as the most appropriate of the four correlation structures for the trichotomous respiratory status data while fully modified GEE and ELMM select UN. The spatial AR1

Table 14.11 Adaptive discrete regression models of censored Poisson probabilities for trichotomous respiratory status in power transforms of visit for alternate modeling approaches, correlation structures, and numbers of folds assuming constant dispersions

Modeling approach	Correlation	5 folds			10 folds			15 folds		
		Powers of visit[a]	LCV score	Clock time (min)	Powers of visit[a]	LCV score	Clock time (min)	Powers of visit[a]	LCV score	Clock time (min)
Partially modified GEE	IND	−0.2	0.35109	4.7	−0.2	0.35066	9.8	−0.2	0.35046	13.7
	AR1	−0.1	0.42075	10.3	−0.1	0.42115	18.6	−0.1	0.42143	27.6
	EC	−0.1	0.41642	10.1	−0.2	0.41585	18.2	−0.2	0.41648	27.6
	UN	−0.15	0.41855	9.9	−0.13	0.41960	18.3	−0.2	0.41956	26.5
Fully modified GEE	IND	−0.2	0.35115	1.6	−0.2	0.35068	3.5	−0.2	0.35048	4.7
	AR1	−0.1	0.42069	2.7	−0.1	0.42115	5.3	−0.1	0.42139	8.0
	EC	−0.1	0.41649	2.9	−0.1	0.41594	5.3	−0.2	0.41648	8.1
	UN	−0.2	0.42226	5.7	−0.2	0.42243	11.1	−0.2	0.42263	16.3
ELMM	IND	−0.2	0.35115	0.1	−0.2	0.35068	0.3	−0.2	0.35048	0.4
	AR1	−0.1	0.42074	0.6	−0.1	0.42113	1.1	−0.1	0.42139	1.6
	EC	−0.1	0.41649	0.4	−0.1	0.41594	0.8	−0.2	0.41648	1.1
	UN	−0.2	0.42487	2.7	−0.1	0.42513	5.0	−0.2	0.42536	8.3

AR1 spatial autoregressive order 1; *EC* exchangeable correlations; *ELMM* extended linear mixed modeling; *GEE* generalized estimating equations; *IND* independent; *LCV* likelihood cross-validation; *UN* unstructured

[a]A power of 0 corresponds to an intercept parameter; otherwise, the model has a zero intercept

Table 14.12 Estimated unstructured correlations for trichotomous respiratory status using the discrete regression model for censored Poisson probabilities in visit[a]

visit	1	2	3	4
0	0.46	0.34	0.30	0.37
1		0.56	0.49	0.42
2			0.66	0.62
3				0.67

[a]Using extended linear mixed modeling with 15 folds

model selected by partially modified GEE model using 15 folds is the same model as selected by ELMM using spatial AR1 correlations and so has smaller 15-fold LCV score computed using ELMM compared to the selected ELMM model with UN correlations. Consequently, UN correlations are used in subsequent censored Poisson analyses. Also, all three modeling approaches select 15 folds.

The model selected by fully modified GEE using 15 folds is the same model as selected by ELMM using 15 folds. Consequently, fully modified GEE and ELMM generate competitive models.

Table 14.11 also contains clock times for generated models. Clock times for partially modified GEE range from 4.7 to 27.6 min with a total over all 12 cases of 195.3 min or about 3.3 h, for fully modified GEE from 1.6 to 16.3 min for a total of 75.4 min or about 1.2 h, and for ELMM from 0.1 to 8.3 min for a total of 22.4 min or about 0.4 h (totals not reported in Table 14.12). Clock times are rounded to 1 decimal digit, but sums are based on unrounded values and so may not be the same as the sum of the rounded values. Consequently, ELMM requires less computation time, with partially modified GEE taking about 8.7 times as much and fully modified GEE about 3.4 times as much.

The 20-fold ELMM model using UN correlations has LCV score 0.42511. Since this is smaller than the associated 15-fold LCV score of Table 14.11, $k = 15$ folds are used in subsequent analyses.

Using ELMM since it generates a competitive model in less time, the adaptive model has probabilities based on $\text{visit}^{-0.2}$ without an intercept and estimated constant dispersion 0.7. Figure 14.10 provides the plot of estimated mean trichotomous respiratory status over visits 0–4. Mean trichotomous respiratory status changes from 0.9 at visit 0 to 1.1 by visit 4. Figure 14.11 provides the plot of estimated probabilities for the ELMM model over visits 0–4. Estimated probabilities for a 0: poor respiratory status decrease from 0.37 at visit 0 to 0.27 by visit 4, for a 1:good respiratory status change only a little from 0.37 at visit 0 to 0.36 at visit 4, and for a 2: excellent respiratory status increase from 0.26 at visit 0 to 0.41 at visit 1 and then decrease a little to 0.37 at visit 4. Table 14.12 provides estimates of UN correlation parameters. These range from 0.30 between visits 0 and 3 to 0.67 between visits 3 and 4.

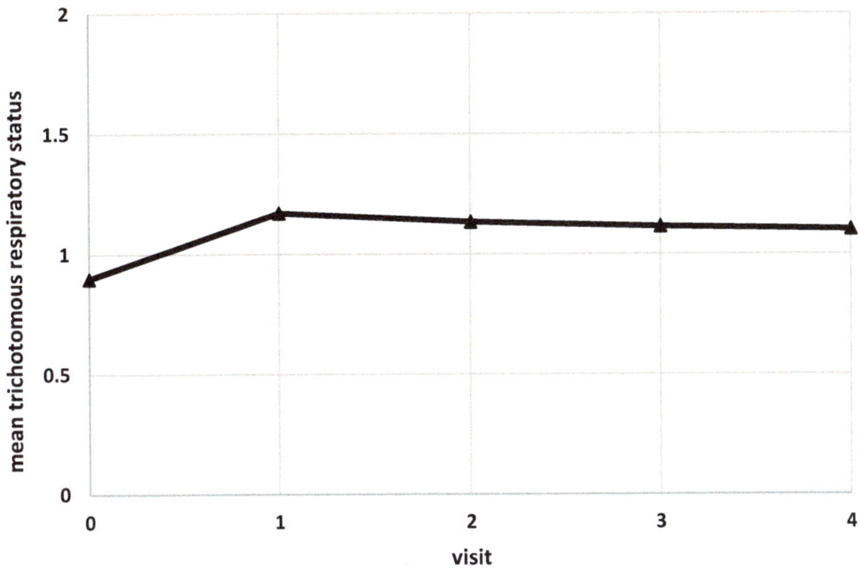

Fig. 14.10 Estimated mean trichotomous respiratory status over visits 0–4 under the discrete regression model for censored Poisson probabilities in visit with constant dispersions using ELMM

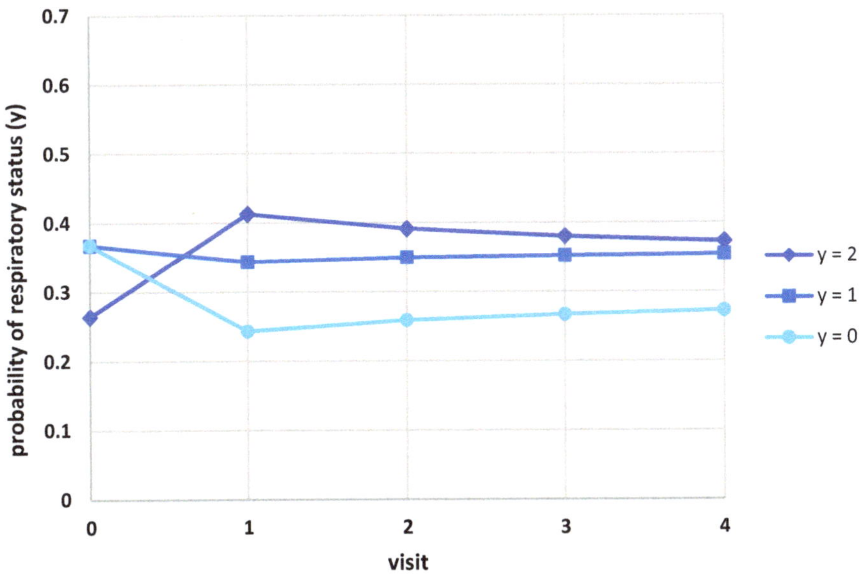

Fig. 14.11 Estimated probabilities for trichotomous respiratory status over visits 0–4 under the discrete regression model for censored Poisson probabilities in visit with constant dispersions using ELMM

14.3.2 Assessing Linearity in Visit

Using ELMM with constant dispersions, $k = 15$ folds, and UN correlations as identified as an appropriate choice in Sect. 14.3.1, the linear polynomial model in visit has LCV = 0.42095 with distinct percent decrease (PD) 1.04% (that is, greater than the cutoff 0.35% for a distinct PD using DF = 1) compared to the adaptive model in visit with LCV score 0.42536. Consequently, the $\log\lambda_{sc}$ terms for the probabilities of trichotomous respiratory status are distinctly nonlinear in visit when dispersions are treated as constant.

14.3.3 Comparison to Standard GEE Modeling

When dispersions are treated as constant, the only difference between partially modified GEE and standard GEE is how the constant dispersion parameter is estimated. Partially modified GEE uses a bias-unadjusted estimate (Sect. 3.5) while standard GEE uses a bias-adjusted estimate (Sect. 2.4). Standard GEE is thus a possible alternative to partially modified GEE for modeling means with constant dispersions. For the trichotomous respiratory status data, the adaptively generated standard GEE model for the censored Poisson probabilities assuming unit dispersions (to reduce the computations; see Sect. 3.5) has probabilities based on $\text{visit}^{0.7}$ without an intercept and with LCV score 0.40632 and distinct PD 3.16% compared to the associated partially modified GEE model with LCV score 0.41956, indicating that in this case partially modified GEE modeling outperforms standard GEE modeling. Standard GEE modeling requires 13.0 min of clock time compared to 26.5 min or about 2.0 times more for partially modified GEE modeling. Furthermore, the model for the probabilities generated by standard GEE modeling computed using ELMM and constant dispersions has LCV score 0.42064 with distinct PD 1.11% compared to the LCV score of 0.42536 for the associated ELMM model (Table 14.12). Also, it requires about 1.6 times more time than the 8.3 min for the ELMM model.

14.3.4 Modeling Probabilities and Dispersions in Visit

Adaptive analyses of trichotomous respiratory status levels are presented in this section using $k = 15$ folds and the UN correlation structure as determined in Sect. 14.3.1. Adaptive models for probabilities and non-constant dispersions in visit are generated to assess the common assumption of constant dispersions. Table 14.13 provides results for adaptive models for probabilities and dispersions in visit. Three modeling approaches partially modified GEE, fully modified GEE, and ELMM are considered.

Table 14.13 Adaptive discrete regression models of trichotomous respiratory status for censored Poisson probabilities and dispersions in visit[a]

Modeling approach	Transforms of visit for probabilities[b]	Transforms of visit for dispersions[b]	LCV score	Clock time (min)
Partially modified GEE	$visit^{-0.2}$	1, $visit^{0.9}$	0.42653	119.6
Fully modified GEE	$visit^{-0.11}$	1, visit	0.42685	36.3
ELMM	$visit^{-0.2}$	1, visit	0.42696	25.0

ELMM extended linear mixed modeling; *GEE* generalized estimating equations; *LCV* likelihood cross-validation
[a]Computed with unstructured correlations and 15 folds
[b]A value of 1 corresponds to an intercept parameter; otherwise, the model has a zero intercept

The partially modified GEE model has LCV score 0.42653 while the associated constant dispersion model of Table 14.11 with UN correlations has LCV score 0.41956 with distinct PD 1.63%. The fully modified GEE model has LCV score 0.42685 while the associated constant dispersion model of Table 14.11 has LCV score 0.42263 with distinct PD 0.99%. The ELMM model has LCV score 0.42696 while the associated constant dispersion model of Table 14.11 has LCV score 0.42536 with distinct PD 0.37%. Consequently, all three modeling approaches indicate that dispersions are distinctly non-constant in visit.

The partially modified GEE model computed using ELMM has LCV score 0.42694 with non-distinct PD less than 0.01% compared to the LCV score 0.42696 for the ELMM model. The fully modified GEE model computed using ELMM has LCV score 0.42685 with non-distinct PD 0.03% compared to the ELMM model. Consequently, all three modeling approaches generate competitive adaptive models for means and dispersions in visit.

Table 14.13 also contains clock times for generated models. The clock time is 119.6 min or about 2.0 h for partially modified GEE, 36.3 min or about 0.6 h for fully modified GEE, and 25.0 min or about 0.4 h for ELMM. Consequently, ELMM requires less computation time, with partially modified GEE taking about 4.8 times as much and fully modified GEE taking about 1.5 times as much.

14.3.5 Adaptive Models in Visit and Active Treatment Assuming Constant Dispersions

Table 14.14 contains results for discrete regression adaptive additive models and adaptive moderation models of censored Poisson probabilities for trichotomous respiratory status in terms of visit and the indicator active for being on active treatment assuming constant dispersions based on partially modified GEE, fully modified GEE, and ELMM. All three additive models contain the indicator active. The LCV scores for the partially modified GEE, fully modified GEE, and ELMM

Table 14.14 Adaptive discrete regression models of censored Poisson probabilities for trichotomous respiratory status in visit and the indicator for being on active treatment assuming constant dispersions[a]

	Additive models			Moderation models		
Modeling approach	Transforms for probabilities[b]	LCV score	Clock time (min)	Transforms for probabilities[b]	LCV score	Clock time (min)
Partially modified GEE	$\text{visit}^{-0.3}$, active	0.42219	36.5	$(\text{visit}^{-0.5}\cdot\text{active})^{0.2}$	0.42255	301.2
Fully modified GEE	$\text{visit}^{-0.3}$, active	0.42480	18.5	$(\text{visit}^{-3}\cdot\text{active})^{0.06}$	0.42508	271.6
ELMM	$\text{visit}^{-0.2}$, active	0.42702	10.7	$(\text{active}\cdot\text{visit}^{-7})^{0.23}$, visit^{-7}, $(\text{visit}\cdot\text{active})^{-1.1}$	0.43049	130.3

ELMM extended linear mixed modeling; *GEE* generalized estimating equations; *LCV* likelihood cross-validation
[a]Computed with unstructured correlations and 15 folds
[b]A value of 1 corresponds to an intercept parameter; otherwise, the model has a zero intercept. Active is the indicator for being on active treatment

models, respectively, are 0.42219, 0.42480, and 0.42702 while the associated constant dispersion models in only visit of Table 14.11 are 0.41956, 0.42263, and 0.42536 with distinct PDs 0.62%, 0.51%, and 0.39%. Consequently, an additive effect to being on active treatment is supported using discrete regression modeling of censored Poisson probabilities assuming constant dispersions. Partially and fully modified GEE generate the same model with LCV score 0.42704 computed using ELMM while the ELMM model has LCV score 0.42702 with non-distinct PD less than 0.01%. Consequently, all three modeling approaches generate competitive additive models with constant dispersions.

The partially modified GEE and fully modified GEE moderation models of Table 14.14 have LCV scores 0.42255 and 0.42522, respectively, while the associated additive models have LCV scores 0.42219 and 0.42480 with non-distinct PDs 0.09% and 0.10%. On the other hand, the ELMM moderation model of Table 14.14 has LCV score 0.43049 while the ELMM additive model has LCV score 0.42702 with distinct PD 0.81%. Consequently, moderation is supported using discrete regression modeling of censored Poisson probabilities using ELMM but not by partially and fully modified GEE, assuming constant dispersions.

The adaptive moderation models generated using partially and fully modified GEE of Table 14.14 computed using ELMM have LCV scores 0.42733 and 0.42709, respectively, with distinct PDs 0.73% and 0.79% compared to the ELMM moderation model of Table 14.14 with LCV score 0.43049. Consequently, partially modified GEE and fully modified GEE generate distinctly inferior moderation models compared to ELMM assuming constant dispersions.

Table 14.14 also contains clock times for adaptive additive and moderation models for the censored Poisson probabilities generated assuming constant dispersions. For additive models, the clock times are 36.5 min for fully modified GEE, 18.5 min for fully modified GEE, and 10.7 min for ELMM. Consequently, ELMM additive modeling requires less computation time, with partially modified GEE additive modeling requiring about 3.4 times as much and fully modified GEE about 1.7 times as much. For moderation models, partially modified GEE requires 301.2 min or about 5.0 h, fully modified GEE requires 271.6 min or about 4.5 h, and ELMM requires 130.3 min or about 2.2 h. Consequently, ELMM moderation modeling requires less time, with partially modified GEE moderation modeling requiring about 2.3 times as much and fully modified GEE moderation modeling about 2.1 times as much. These are relatively long times, and so only ELMM is considered in subsequent analyses.

14.3.6 Comparison to Linear Additive and Moderation Models with Constant Dispersions

The standard linear additive model has $\log\lambda_{sc}$ terms for the probabilities based on an intercept together with main effects to untransformed visit and active along with constant dispersions. This model computed using ELMM has LCV score 0.42119. The standard linear moderation model has $\log\lambda_{sc}$ terms for the probabilities based on an intercept, main effects to untransformed visit and active, and the interaction of visit and active along with constant dispersions. This moderation model computed using ELMM has smaller LCV score 0.42099, indicating that standard linear moderation is not supported. On the other hand, as indicated in Sect. 14.3.5, moderation is supported using ELMM allowing for nonlinearity and assuming constant dispersions. Consequently, adaptive modeling is required in this case to identify moderation.

14.3.7 Adaptive Models in Visit and Active Treatment for Probabilities and Dispersions

Only ELMM is considered for generating adaptive models for censored Poisson probabilities and non-constant dispersions of trichotomous respiratory status in terms of visit and the indicator active for being on active treatment. Results for partially and fully modified GEE are not reported to reduce the amount of computation time. The ELMM additive model has probabilities based on visit$^{-0.2}$ and the indicator active without an intercept, constant dispersions, LCV score 0.42702 and requires 47.9 min or about 0.8 h of clock time. This is the same additive model as in Table 14.14. Consequently, an additive effect to being on active treatment is supported using discrete regression modeling for censored Poisson probabilities but dispersions are reasonably treated as not depending on either visit or active.

The ELMM adaptive moderation model for censored Poisson probabilities and non-constant dispersions of trichotomous respiratory status in terms of visit and the indicator active for being on active treatment has LCV score 0.43238 and requires 462.0 min or about 7.7 h of clock time. The associated additive model has LCV score 0.42702 with distinct PD 1.24%. Consequently, moderation of the effect to being on active treatment is supported by discrete regression modeling of censored Poisson probabilities and dispersions using ELMM.

The ELMM moderation model assuming constant dispersions of Table 14.14 has LCV score 0.43049 with distinct PD 0.44% compared to the associated moderation model of allowing for non-constant dispersions with LCV score 0.43238. Consequently, nonlinearity of dispersions is supported by discrete regression moderation modeling of censored Poisson probabilities and dispersions using ELMM. However, the non-constant moderation model has dispersions depending only on a transform of visit, indicating that the dispersions do not depend on the indicator of being on active treatment either as an additive effect or interacting with the effect of visit.

The ELMM discrete regression model of censored Poisson probabilities and dispersions for trichotomous respiratory status has probabilities based on the transform visit^{-7} and the geometric combinations

$$\left(\text{visit}^{-3} \cdot \text{active}\right)^{0.5} = \text{visit}^{-1.5} \cdot \text{active}$$

and

$$(\text{active} \cdot \text{visit})^{-1} = \text{active} \cdot \text{visit}^{-1}$$

without an intercept as well as dispersions based on $\text{visit}^{1.5}$ with an intercept. Estimated means for this model are plotted in Fig. 14.12. For patients on a placebo, estimated mean trichotomous respiratory status is 0.9 visit 0, increases to 1.1 at visit 1 and then decreases to 0.9 at visit 2 and remains at 0.9 for visits 3–4. For patients on active treatment, estimated mean trichotomous respiratory status is 0.9 visit 0, the same as for patients on a placebo, and then increases to 1.0 at visit 1, then to 1.4 at visit 2 and the decreases to 1.3 by visit 4. Figure 14.13 contains the plot of estimated dispersions for trichotomous respiratory status. Estimated dispersions increase nonlinearly from 0.6 at visit 0 gradually to 2.3 by visit 3 and then quickly to 13.9 by visit 4 and are the same for patients on a placebo and patients on active treatment.

Figures 14.14–14.15 provide plots of probabilities for trichotomous respiratory status levels 0–2 (that is, 0:poor, 1:good, and 2:excellent) using the ELMM discrete regression moderation model for patients on a placebo and patients on active treatment, respectively. For patients on a placebo, probabilities for 0:poor respiratory status are constant at 0.37 over visits 0 and 2–4 with lower probability 0.28 at visit 1, for 1:good respiratory status are close to constant at 0.36–0.37 over visits 0–4, and for 2:excellent respiratory status are 0.26 at visit 0, increase to 0.36 at visit 1, then

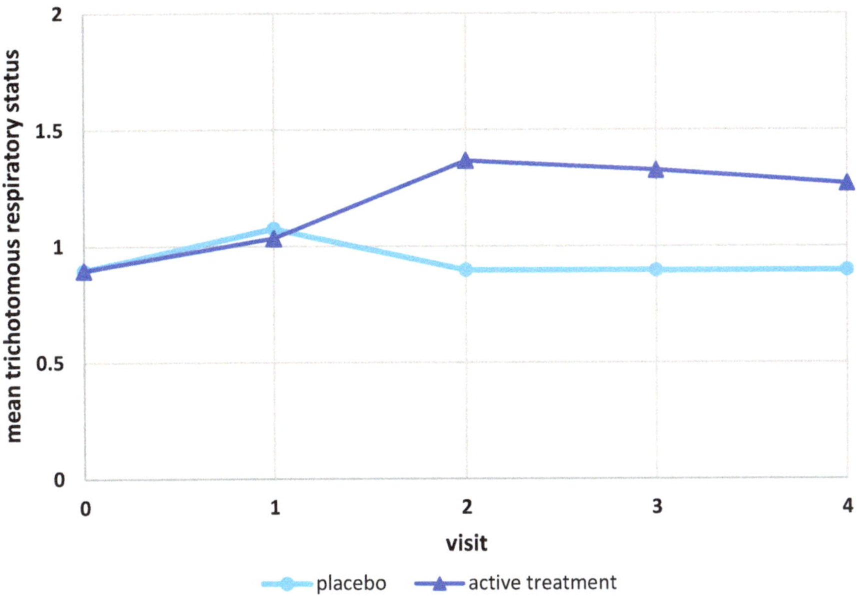

Fig. 14.12 Estimated means for trichotomous respiratory status under the discrete regression model of censored Poisson probabilities and dispersions in terms of visits and the indicator for being on active treatment using ELMM

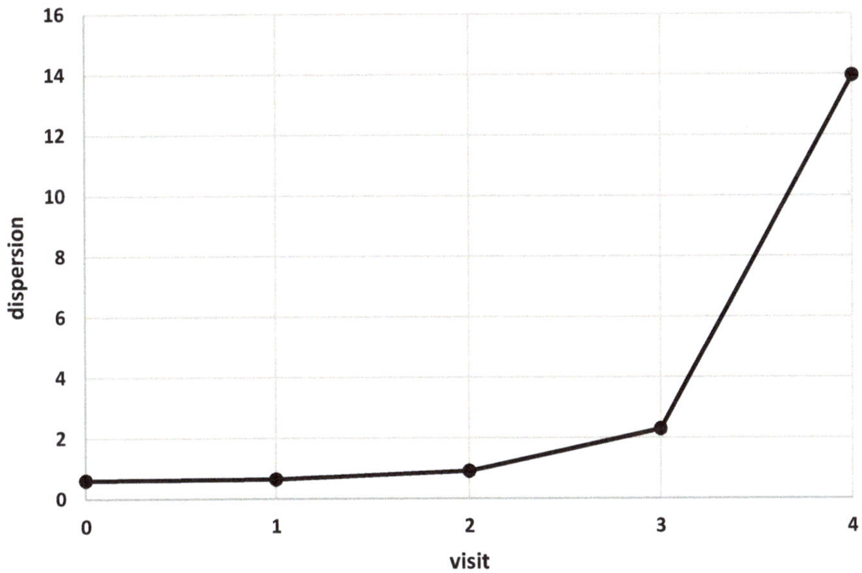

Fig. 14.13 Estimated dispersions for trichotomous respiratory status over visits 0–4 under the discrete regression moderation model of censored Poisson probabilities and dispersions using ELMM

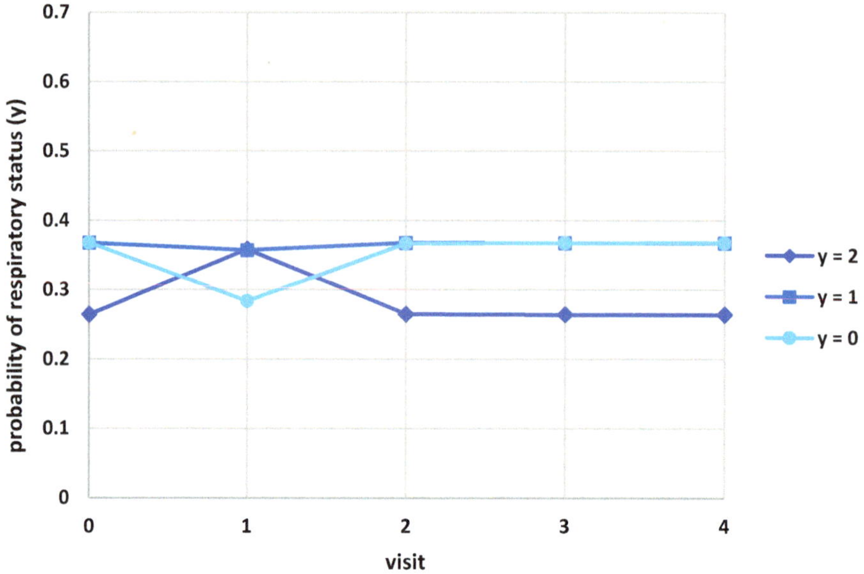

Fig. 14.14 Estimated censored Poisson probabilities for trichotomous respiratory status over visits 0–4 under the discrete regression moderation model in visit for patients on a placebo using ELMM

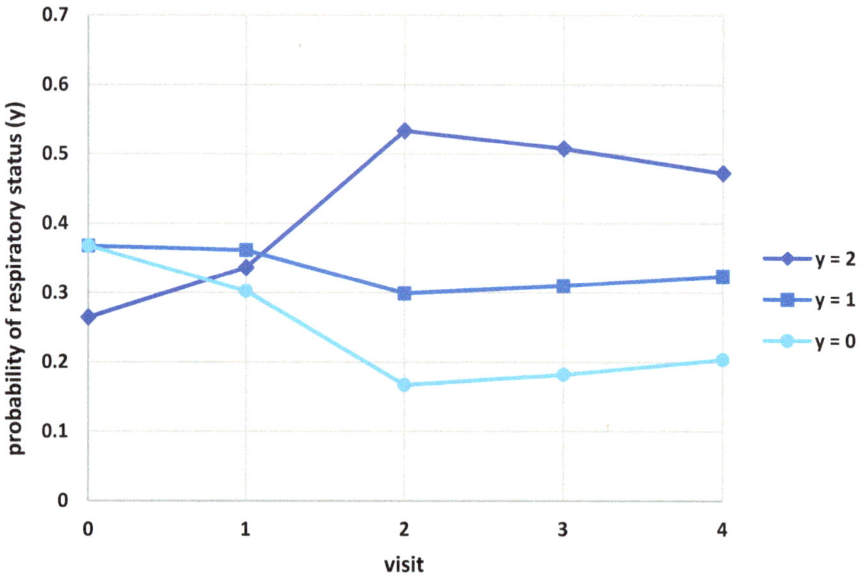

Fig. 14.15 Estimated censored Poisson probabilities for trichotomous respiratory status over visits 0–4 under the discrete regression moderation model in visit for patients on active treatment using ELMM

Table 14.15 Estimated unstructured correlations for trichotomous respiratory status using the discrete regression moderation model for censored Poisson probabilities in visit[a]

visit	1	2	3	4
0	0.43	0.35	0.31	0.38
1		0.56	0.49	0.43
2			0.64	0.64
3				0.69

[a]Using extended linear mixed modeling with 15 folds

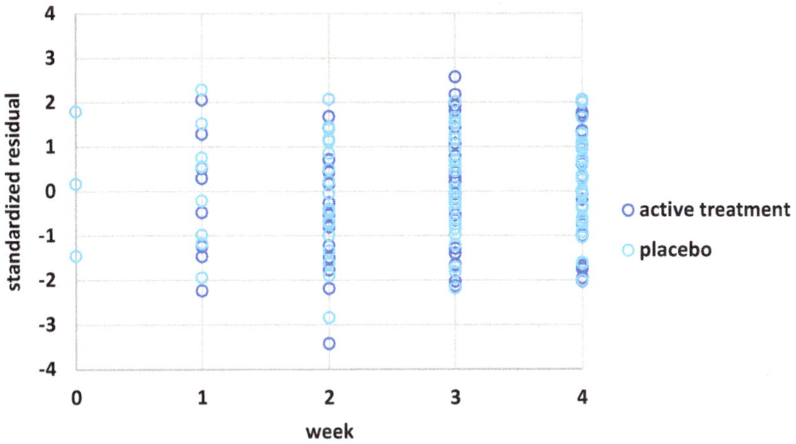

Fig. 14.16 Standardized residuals for trichotomous respiratory status under the discrete regression model for censored Poisson probabilities in visit for patients on active treatment using ELMM

decrease to 0.26 at visit 2 and remain there to visit 4. For patients on active treatment, probabilities for 0:poor respiratory status decrease from 0.37 at visit 0 to 0.17 at visit 2 and then increase to 0.20 at visit 4, for 1:good respiratory status decrease from 0.37 at visit 0 to 0.30 at visit 2 and then increase to 0.32 at visit 4, and for 2:excellent respiratory status increase from 0.26 at visit 0 to 0.53 at visit 2 and then decrease to 0.47 at visit 4. Table 14.15 contains estimated unstructured correlations for the trichotomous respiratory status outcome. These range from 0.31 for outcomes at visits 0 and 3 to 0.69 for outcomes at visits 3 and 4.

Figure 14.16 displays standardized residuals by visit and type of treatment. These are all within ±3 except for one measurement with standardized residual −3.42. This occurs for the patient with ID 21 at visit 2 who was on active treatment and had respiratory status levels 1, 2, 0, 2, 1 at visits 0–3, respectively. This measurement is also identified as outlying in Sect. 14.2.7.

14.3.8 Direct Variance Discrete Regression Modeling of Trichotomous Respiratory Status

Direct variance modeling treats the variance function as $V(\mu) = 1$ so that the extended variances are the same as the dispersions. Using ELMM, the adaptive discrete regression model for the censored Poisson probabilities and dispersions of trichotomous respiratory status in visit using direct variance modeling has probabilities based on $\text{visit}^{-0.3}$ without an intercept along with dispersions, and so also variances, based on $\text{visit}^{4.1002}$ without an intercept. The LCV score is 0.39799 with distinct PD 6.79% compared to the associated extended variance model of Table 14.14 with LCV score 0.42696. The direct variance model requires 67.8 min of clock time or about 2.7 times as much as the 25.0 min required for the associated extended variance model of Table 14.13.

The adaptive additive model for the probabilities and dispersions in visit and the indicator active using direct variance modeling is almost the same model and has probabilities based on $\text{visit}^{-0.32}$ without an intercept along with dispersions, and so also variances, based on $\text{visit}^{1.189}$ without an intercept. It has a little smaller LCV score 0.39762 and so with distinct PD 6.68% compared to the additive extended variance model of Sect. 14.3.7. The direct variance additive model requires 107.7 min or about 1.9 h of clock time or about 2.2 times as much as the 47.9 min or about 0.8 h required for the associated extended variance additive model.

The adaptive moderation model using direct variance modeling has probabilities based on the transform $\text{visit}^{-0.4}$ and the geometric combinations

$$\left(\text{visit}^{-0.3} \cdot \text{active}\right)^{1.3} = \text{visit}^{-0.39} \cdot \text{active}$$

and

$$\left(\text{active} \cdot \text{visit}^{2}\right)^{-1.2899} = \text{active} \cdot \text{visit}^{-2.5798}$$

with an intercept as well as dispersions based on $\text{visit}^{4.4991}$ without an intercept. The LCV score is 0.40133 while the direct variance additive model has LCV score 0.39762 with distinct PD 0.92% so that moderation is supported by direct variance modeling. On the other hand, the direct variance model generates a distinct PD 7.18% in the LCV score compared to the associated extended variance moderation model of Sect. 14.3.7 allowing variances to also depend on the probabilities with LCV score 0.43238. The direct variance moderation model requires 936.8 min or about 15.6 h of clock time, an excessive amount of time, or about 2.0 times as much as the 462.0 min or about 7.7 h required for the associated extended variance moderation model of Sect. 14.3.7.

Consequently, in this case, direct variance modeling is an ineffective alternative to extended variance modeling accounting for the dependence of variances on probabilities along with dispersions. It also requires much more time.

14.3.9 Unit Dispersion Modeling

So far, discrete regression models for censored Poisson probabilities have included dispersions either as constant or changing with visit and/or the indicator active for being on active treatment. A comparison of these prior models to corresponding models generated assuming unit dispersions is provided in the section. Only models generated using ELMM are considered.

The adaptive model for censored Poisson probabilities in visit assuming unit dispersions has means based on $\text{visit}^{-0.2}$ without an intercept and LCV score 0.42142 and distinct PD 1.30% compared to the associated model also allowing for non-constant dispersions of Table 14.14 with LCV score 0.42696. The unit dispersion model requires 6.5 min compared to 25.0 min or about 3.8 times more for the non-constant dispersion model.

The adaptive additive model for censored Poisson probabilities in visit and the indicator active assuming unit dispersions is the same model as generated for visit alone with LCV score 0.42142 and distinct PD 1.31% compared to the associated additive model also allowing for non-constant dispersions with LCV score 0.42702. The unit dispersion model requires 8.5 min compared to 47.9 min or about 5.6 times more for the non-constant dispersion model.

The adaptive moderation model for censored Poisson probabilities in visit, the indicator active, and geometric combinations assuming unit dispersions has censored Poisson probabilities based on the transform visit^{-8} and the two geometric combinations

$$\left(\text{visit}^{-0.2}\cdot\text{active}\right)^{7.5}=\text{visit}^{-1.5}\cdot\text{active}$$

and

$$\left(\text{active}\cdot\text{visit}^{-2}\right)^{0.6}=\text{active}\cdot\text{visit}^{-1.2}$$

without an intercept. The LCV score is 0.42593 with distinct PD 1.49% compared to the associated moderation model also allowing for non-constant dispersions with LCV score 0.43238. The unit dispersion model requires 95.7 min or about 1.6 h compared to 462.0 min or about 7.7 h and so about 4.8 times more for the non-constant dispersion model. The additive model assuming unit dispersions generates an LCV score with distinct PD 1.06%, supporting the conclusion that the effect of visit on the probabilities is moderated by the indicator for being on active treatment, as is also the case allowing for constant dispersions in Sect. 14.3.5 and allowing for non-constant dispersions in Sect. 14.3.7.

Consequently, unit dispersion modeling requires less computation time in all three cases considered here for an overall time of 110.7 min or about 1.8 h compared to 534.9 min or about 8.9 h, so about 4.8 times more for non-constant dispersion modeling. However, unit dispersion modeling generates distinctly inferior models in all three cases.

14.3.10 Comparison to Ordinal Probability Modeling

LCV scores for censored Poisson probability models are based on $k = 15$ folds and so are not comparable to LCV scores for ordinal probability models based on $k = 10$ folds. Ordinal and censored Poisson probability models can be compared by computing the 10-fold LCV score for the censored Poisson model and the 15-fold score for the ordinal model. The most preferable ordinal and censored Poisson models are the adaptive moderation models for both probabilities and dispersions of Sects. 14.2.7 and 14.3.7, respectively. The censored Poisson moderation model has 10-fold LCV score 0.43210 while the ordinal moderation model has 10-fold LCV score 0.43067 with non-distinct PD 0.33%, indicating that censored Poisson modeling generates a model that is a competitive alternative to the ordinal model as a 10-fold model, but more preferable since its 10-fold LCV score is larger. On the other hand, the ordinal model has 15-fold LCV score 0.42839 with distinct PD 0.92% compared to the censored Poisson model, indicating that the ordinal model is distinctly inferior as a 15-fold model.

The adaptive moderation model for censored Poisson probabilities has 5 parameters, 3 slopes for the probabilities, and 1 slope plus an intercept for the dispersions. The associated adaptive moderation model for ordinal probabilities also has 5 parameters, 2 intercepts, and 2 slopes for the probabilities and 1 slope for the dispersions.

The censored Poisson probability moderation model requires 462.0 min or about 7.7 h. The associated ordinal probability moderation model requires 266.3 min or about 4.4 h, and so the censored Poisson probability moderation model requires about 1.8 times more.

Consequently, the model selected using censored Poisson probabilities is preferable to the model selected using ordinal probabilities. Censored Poisson probability modeling generates a better 10-fold LCV score and a distinctly better 15-fold LCV score, with the same number of parameters, but requires more time.

14.4 Analysis Summary

14.4.1 Multinomial Probability Analyses

A summary of the results of analyses of the trichotomous respiratory status data based on discrete regression using multinomial probabilities is provided broken down into three categories of results.

1. Adaptive Models for Probabilities in Visit Assuming Constant Dispersions

The preferable model for the trichotomous respiratory status data has UN correlations with LCV scores based on $k = 15$ folds

For $k = 5$ folds, models selected by partially modified GEE, fully modified GEE, and ELMM are all competitive alternatives. However, the fully modified GEE and

ELMM models are simpler than the partially modified GEE model. For $k = 5$ folds, ELMM requires less time with partially modified GEE requiring about 30.5 times as much and fully modified GEE requiring about 2.0 times as much. Partially modified GEE modeling is not considered further due to excessive times.

For $k = 15$ folds, models selected by fully modified GEE and ELMM are competitive alternatives. Estimated mean trichotomous respiratory status is plotted in Fig. 14.1 and estimated probabilities for trichotomous respiratory status in Fig. 14.2. The generalized logits for probabilities of trichotomous respiratory status are distinctly nonlinear in visit assuming constant dispersions. ELMM requires less time with fully modified GEE requiring about 1.7 times more.

2. Models for Probabilities and Dispersions in Visit

Models selected by fully modified GEE and ELMM are competitive alternatives. Dispersions are reasonably considered to be constant in visit. Fully modified GEE requires less time with ELMM requiring about 1.1 times more.

3. Models for Probabilities in Visit and Being on Active Treatment with Constant Dispersions.

The indicator active is reasonably considered not to have an additive effect on probabilities for trichotomous respiratory status. The effect of visit on mean trichotomous respiratory status is reasonably considered not to be moderated by being on active treatment. For additive modeling, fully modified GEE requires less time with ELMM requiring about 1.1 times more. For moderation modeling, ELMM requires less time, but times are excessive for both modeling procedures, and so multinomial probabilities are not modeled any further.

14.4.2 Ordinal Probability Analyses

A summary of the results of analyses of the trichotomous respiratory status data based on discrete regression using ordinal probabilities is provided broken down into six categories of results.

1. Adaptive Models for Probabilities in Visit Assuming Constant Dispersions

The preferable model for the trichotomous respiratory status data has UN correlations with LCV scores based on $k = 10$ folds. Models selected by partially modified GEE, fully modified GEE, and ELMM are all competitive alternatives. Estimated mean trichotomous respiratory status is plotted in Fig. 14.3 and associated probabilities in Fig. 14.4. The cumulative logits for trichotomous respiratory status are distinctly nonlinear in visit assuming constant dispersions. The model generated by standard GEE is distinctly outperformed by the model generated by partially modified GEE and by the ELMM model. ELMM requires less time with partially modified GEE requiring about 31.3 times as much and fully modified GEE about 2.8

times as much. Partially modified GEE modeling is not considered further due to excessive times.

2. Models for Probabilities and Dispersions in Visit

Models selected by fully modified GEE and ELMM are competitive alternatives. Moreover, fully modified GEE and ELMM both suggest dispersions are constant in visit. ELMM requires less time with fully modified GEE requiring about 3.1 times as much.

3. Adaptive Models in Visit and Being on Active Treatment Assuming Constant Dispersions

The indicator active is reasonably considered not to have an additive effect on the ordinal probabilities for trichotomous respiratory status. For additive modeling, ELMM requires less time with fully modified GEE requiring about 3.0 times as much.

The moderation model selected by fully modified GEE is distinctly inferior to the ELMM moderation model. Moreover, fully modified GEE suggests that the effect of visit on mean trichotomous respiratory status is not moderated by being on active treatment while ELMM suggests that it is moderated. Using ELMM, standard linear moderation is not supported. ELMM requires less time but fully modified GEE requires almost the same amount of time. Fully modified GEE modeling is not considered further due to generating a distinctly inferior moderation model, and so only ELMM is considered in subsequent analyses.

4. Adaptive Models for Probabilities and Dispersions in Visit and Being on Active Treatment

The indicator active is reasonably considered not to have an additive effect on the probabilities of trichotomous respiratory status. The effect of visit on probabilities of trichotomous respiratory status is reasonably considered to be moderated by being on active treatment. Dispersions are reasonably considered to be non-constant in visit and not to depend on being on active treatment. Estimated mean trichotomous respiratory status for patients on a placebo and on active treatment is plotted in Fig. 14.5 and estimated dispersions in Fig. 14.6. Estimated probabilities for trichotomous respiratory status for patients on a placebo are plotted in Fig. 14.7 and for patients on active treatment in Fig. 14.8. Standardized residuals are plotted in Fig. 14.9. There are two outliers with one mild.

5. Direct Variance Modeling of Trichotomous Respiratory Status

The same direct variance model is generated accounting only for the effect to visit, allowing also for an additive effect to being in the intervention group, and allowing for moderation of the effect of visit by being in the intervention group. Direct variance modeling is an ineffective alternative to extended variance modeling accounting for the dependence of variances on probabilities as well as dispersions.

6. Unit Dispersion Modeling of Trichotomous Respiratory Status

Compared to modeling allowing for non-constant dispersions, unit dispersion modeling generates a competitive model in visit but distinctly inferior additive and moderation models.

14.4.3 Censored Poisson Probability Analyses

A summary of the results of analyses of the trichotomous respiratory status data based on discrete regression using censored Poisson probabilities is provided broken down into six categories of results.

1. Adaptive Models for Probabilities in Visit Assuming Constant Dispersions

The preferable model for the trichotomous respiratory status data has UN correlations with LCV scores based on $k = 15$ folds. Models selected by fully modified GEE and ELMM are based on the same UN correlation structure and are competitive alternatives while the model selected by partially modified GEE is based on a different correlation structure. Estimated mean trichotomous respiratory status is plotted in Fig. 14.10 and associated probabilities in Fig. 14.11. The $\log\lambda_{sc}$ terms for the probabilities of trichotomous respiratory status are distinctly nonlinear in visit when dispersions are treated as constant. The model generated by standard GEE is outperformed by the model generated by partially modified GEE and by the ELMM model. ELMM requires less time with partially modified GEE requiring about 8.7 times as much and fully modified GEE about 3.4 times as much.

2. Models for Probabilities and Dispersions in Visit

Models selected by partially modified GEE, fully modified GEE, and ELMM are competitive alternatives. All three modeling procedures indicate that dispersions are distinctly non-constant in visit. ELMM requires less time with partially modified GEE requiring about 4.8 times as much and fully modified GEE requiring about 1.5 times as much.

3. Adaptive Models in Visit and Being on Active Treatment Assuming Constant Dispersions

Additive models selected by partially modified GEE, fully modified GEE, and ELMM are competitive alternatives. The indicator active is reasonably considered to have an additive effect on the censored Poisson probabilities for trichotomous respiratory status. For additive modeling, ELMM requires less time with partially modified GEE requiring about 3.4 times as much and fully modified GEE about 1.7 times as much.

The moderation model selected by ELMM is distinctly superior to the moderation models selected by partially modified GEE and fully modified GEE. Moreover, ELMM suggests that the effect of visit on mean trichotomous respiratory status is moderated by being on active treatment while partially modified GEE and fully modified GEE suggest that it is not moderated. Using ELMM, standard linear moderation is not supported. ELMM requires less time with partially modified GEE requiring about 2.3 times as much and fully modified GEE about 2.1 times as much. Partially modified GEE and fully modified GEE modeling are not considered further to reduce the computation time, and so only ELMM is considered in subsequent analyses.

4. Adaptive Models for Probabilities and Dispersions in Visit and Being on Active Treatment

The indicator active is reasonably considered to have an additive effect on the probabilities of trichotomous respiratory status. However, dispersions are reasonably considered to be constant in additive effects to visit and being on active treatment.

The effect of visit on probabilities of trichotomous respiratory status is reasonably considered to be moderated by being on active treatment. Dispersions are reasonably considered to be non-constant in visit but not to depend on being on active treatment.

5. Direct Variance Modeling of Trichotomous Respiratory Status

Using direct variance modeling, an additive effect to being in the intervention group is not supported, but moderation is supported. Direct variance modeling is an ineffective alternative to extended variance modeling accounting for the dependence of variances on probabilities as well as dispersions. It also requires more time.

6. Unit Dispersion Modeling of Trichotomous Respiratory Status

Moderation is supported by unit dispersion modeling. Unit dispersion modeling requires less time with modeling allowing for non-constant dispersions requiring about 4.8 times as much over all three cases of the model based only on visit, the additive model, and the moderation model. However, unit dispersion modeling generates distinctly inferior models in these three cases.

14.4.4 All Models for Trichotomous Respiratory Status

Partially modified GEE, fully modified GEE, and ELMM generate competitive models in all cases when all three are compared with one exception. ELMM generates an adaptive moderation model for censored Poisson probabilities assuming constant dispersions that is distinctly superior to the associated partially and fully modified GEE models. Also, ELMM generates an adaptive model for means and dispersions in visit that is distinctly superior to the associated fully modified GEE model when only those two modeling approaches are compared.

Fewer multinomial probability models are generated for each of the three modeling approaches due to excessive times. Also, fewer ordinal probability models are generated for partially modified GEE due to excessive times. Over all cases for ordinal probabilities (Tables 14.6, 14.8, and 14.9) and for censored Poisson probabilities (Tables 14.12, 14.13, and , 14.14) combined, ELMM requires less time, 5.7 h compared to 11.2 h for fully modified GEE. or about 1.9 times more. Over all cases for censored Poisson probabilities (Tables 14.12, 14.13, and 14.14), ELMM requires less time, 3.0 h compared to 10.9 h or about 5.5 times more for partially modified GEE and 6.2 h or about 2.1 times more for fully modified GEE.

Using ELMM, the model selected using censored Poisson probabilities is distinctly preferable to the model selected using ordinal probabilities. The censored Poisson probability model generates a distinctly better 15-fold LCV score, with the same number of parameters although it requires more time, 7.7 h compared to 4.4 h or 1.8 times more. Multinomial probabilities are not a reasonable alternative due to excessive times.

14.4.5 Selected Model for Trichotomous Respiratory Status in Visit and Being on Active Treatment

Under the most appropriate model for trichotomous respiratory status based on censored Poisson probabilities with UN correlations, estimated means are plotted in Fig. 14.12 and estimated dispersions in Fig. 14.13. Estimated probabilities for patients on a placebo are plotted in Fig. 14.14 and for patients on active treatment in Fig. 14.15. Estimated correlations are provided in Table 14.15. Standardized residuals are plotted in Fig. 14.16.

14.5 Example SAS Code for Analyzing the Trichotomous Respiratory Status Data

Example SAS code is presented in this section for conducting discrete regression analyses of trichotomous respiratory status as a function of clinic visit and treatment group (either on active treatment or taking a placebo). The code assumes that a data set called longresp has been created in the SAS default library containing the trichotomous respiratory status data (Sect. 13.1) in long format, that is, with one measurement (or row) for each trichotomous respiratory status level at each clinic visit for each patient. This data set contains variables (or columns) called id loaded with unique identifiers for patients; status0_2 loaded with trichotomous respiratory status levels coded as 0:poor, 1:good, or 2:excellent; visit loaded with visit indexes of 0–4; and the indicator active set to 1 for patients on active treatment and to 0 for patients in the control group. Altogether, there are five trichotomous respiratory status levels at different clinic visits for each of 111 different patients, 54 on active treatment and 57 on a placebo, for a total of 555 measurements.

The code also assumes that a %include statement has been executed to load in the current version of the genreg macro for use in conducting adaptive analyses. The genreg macro supports a wide variety of macro parameters, some of which are described here. The interface for this macro contains the complete list of macro parameters along with their default settings. Default settings are used by the macro if a value for the macro parameter has not been specified in the code invoking the macro. Macro parameter settings are case insensitive. The cutoff for a distinct percent decrease in LCV scores (Sect. 2.6.2) for these data with 555 measurements is 0.35%, computed using DF = 1 degrees of freedom. In the case of multinomial probabilities, the removal of 1 transform from the model for the probabilities results in 2 less parameters, and so the cutoff is 0.54%, computed using DF = 2 degrees of freedom.

14.5.1 Modeling Probabilities in Visit Assuming Constant Dispersions

The following code uses the genreg macro to generate the adaptive model for trichotomous respiratory status probabilities as a possibly nonlinear function of visit using $k = 15$ folds, unstructured (UN) correlations, extended linear mixed modeling (ELMM), and censored Poisson probabilities as in Sect. 14.3.1 assuming constant dispersions.

```
%genreg(modtype=dscrt,datain=longresp,yvar=status0_2,matchvar=id,
withinvr=visit,foldcnt=15,corrtype=UN,GEE=n,srchtype=logL,
propodds=n,usepoiss=y,expand=y,expxvars=visit,contract=y);
```

The modtype macro parameter specifies the model type, in this case "modtype=dscrt" means treat the polytomous outcome variable as discrete. The datain macro parameter indicates that the data to be analyzed is contained in the longresp data set loaded in the SAS default library. The yvar macro parameter specifies the name of the outcome variable, in this case the variable status0_2. The matchvar and withinvr macro parameters specify, respectively, the variable containing unique identifiers for different matched sets, in this case the variable id identifying different patients, and the variable containing within matched set values, in this case the variable visit. The corrtype macro parameter specifies the correlation structure, in this case the UN structure. The other possible corrtype settings are "corrtype=IND", "corrtype=EC", and "corrtype=AR1" for independent, exchangeable, and spatial autoregressive order 1, respectively. To request that the clock time for an invocation of the macro be printed in the output, add the setting "rprttime=y" where the value "y" is short for "yes" while the default setting is "rprttime=n" with "n" short for "no".

The modeling approach used by genreg is determined by the combination of the GEE and srchtype macro parameters. In this case, "GEE=n" means use ELMM while "srchtype=logL" means base estimation on maximizing the log-likelihood (as described in Sects. 4.3 and 5.2). These are the default settings for these two macro parameters. Setting "GEE=y" requests GEE modeling. Combining "GEE=y" with "srchtype=GEE" requests partially modified GEE with estimation based on the minimizing the maximum absolute value of the gradient (as described in Sect. 3.7). Combining "GEE=y" with "srchtype=logL" requests fully modified GEE. By default, partially modified and fully modified GEE use bias-unadjusted dispersion estimates. Bias-adjusted dispersion estimates, as used in standard GEE modeling (Sect. 2.4), are requested by adding the setting "biasadj=y".

The macro parameters propodds and usepoiss control the type of probabilities for the discrete outcome variable. The default settings are "propodds=n" and "usepoiss=n" requesting multinomial probabilities based on generalized logits. Changing to "propodds=y" requests ordinal probabilities based on cumulative logits, also called proportional odds modeling. Combining "propodds=n" with "usepoiss=y" requests censored Poisson probabilities.

Adaptive modeling is requested using "expand=y" together with "contract=y", meaning first expand the base model and then contract the expanded model. In this case, the base model has constant probabilities and constant dispersions based on only intercept parameters (but this can be changed). The expxvars macro parameter specifies the primary predictor variables for modeling the probabilities to consider in the expansion. In this case, the expansion grows the model for the probabilities by systematically adding in power transforms of the single variable visit while holding the dispersions constant. The maximum number of transforms added by the expansion to the model for the means is controlled by the expxmax parameter with default value "expxmax=5" meaning at most 5 transforms can be added to the means. Changing to the empty setting "expxmax=" removes the restriction on the number of such transforms.

The contraction systematically removes transforms from the expanded model for the probabilities, possibly the constant transform corresponding to the intercept, and adjusts the powers of the remaining transforms to increase the LCV score, which in this case is computed with 15 folds as specified by the setting of the foldcnt macro parameter. It is also computed using matched-set-wise deletion corresponding to the default setting "measdlte=n". Measurement-wise deletion is requested using "measdlte=y". The contraction can optionally be restricted not to remove the intercept for the probabilities in order to generate a non-zero intercept model. An LCV ratio test is used to decide when to stop the contraction. The contraction also stops when there is only one transform remaining in the model for the probabilities. When the contraction leaves the expanded model unchanged, that expanded model has its powers adjusted to increase the LCV score.

The following code directly generates the above adaptive model selected with $k = 15$ folds, UN correlations, and ELMM, including parameter estimates and LCV score.

```
%genreg(modtype=dscrt,datain=longresp,yvar=status0_2,matchvar=id,
withinvr=visit,foldcnt=15,corrtype=UN,GEE=n,srchtype=logL,
propodds=n,usepoiss=y,xintrcpt=n,xvars=visit,xpowers=−0.2);
```

The xintrcpt macro parameter specifies whether or not the base model for the probabilities includes an intercept, the xvars macro parameter provides the list of primary predictors for the base model for the probabilities, and the xpowers macro parameter the powers for transforming those primary predictors. In this case, the model for the probabilities has a zero intercept along with the single transform $\text{visit}^{-0.2}$. The default values for these macro parameters are "xintrcpt=y", "xvars=", and "xpowers=" requesting constant probabilities. An empty setting for the xvars macro parameter means includes no transforms for the probabilities, and an empty setting for the xpowers macro parameter means power transform xvars variables if any with the power 1 (and so include them untransformed). The model for the dispersions is based on macro parameters vintrcpt, vvars, and vpowers with analogous meanings and with the same default settings requesting constant dispersions. The xvalid macro parameter is not set in the above code and so has its default setting "xvalid=y" meaning to compute the LCV score for the requested model. In this case, the model has LCV score 0.42536. Adding the setting "xvalid=n" means compute only parameter estimates for the requested model and not the LCV score.

The above code can be changed to generate the standard linear polynomial model for the probabilities based on untransformed visit as follows. Change the setting for the xintercpt macro parameter to "xintrcpt=y" and the setting for the xpowers macro parameter to "xpowers=1"; alternately, remove the settings for the xintrcpt and xpowers macro parameters so that they have their default values, which mean to include an intercept and to use the power 1 to transform all variables listed in the setting of the xvars macro parameter. Note that $\log\lambda_{sc}$ terms of the probabilities are linear in visit, but the probabilities are nonlinear due to the log transform. To request the standard quadratic polynomial model for the probabilities, use the settings "xintrcpt=y", "xvars=visit visit", and "xpowers=1 2".

14.5.2 Modeling Probabilities and Dispersions in Visit

The following code uses the genreg macro to generate the adaptive model for trichotomous respiratory level probabilities and non-constant dispersions as possibly nonlinear functions of visit using $k = 15$ folds, UN correlations, and ELMM, starting from constant dispersions.

```
%genreg(modtype=dscrt,datain=longresp,yvar=status0_2,matchvar=id,
withinvr=visit,foldcnt=15,corrtype=UN,GEE=n,srchtype=logL,
propodds=n,usepoiss=y,expand=y,expxvars=visit,expvvars=visit,
contract=y);
```

As before, adaptive modeling is requested using "expand=y" together with "contract=y" meaning first expand the base model with constant probabilities and constant dispersions and then contract the expanded model. The expxvars and expvvars macro parameters specify the primary predictor variables to consider in the expansion for the probabilities and dispersions, respectively. In this case, the same set of primary predictors is used for the probabilities and for the dispersions, but different sets of primary predictors can be specified. The expansion grows the model for the probabilities and the dispersions in combination by systematically adding in power transforms of the single variable visit one-at-a-time to either the probabilities or the dispersions, whichever generates the better LCV score. Similar to the expxmax parameter, the expvmax parameter specifies the maximum number of transforms added by the expansion to the model for the dispersions with default value "expvmax=5" meaning at most 5 transforms can be added to the dispersions. Changing to the empty setting "expvmax=" removes the restriction on the number of such transforms.

The contraction systematically removes transforms from the expanded model for the probabilities and dispersions in combination, possibly the constant transforms corresponding to intercepts, and adjusts the powers of the remaining transforms to increase the LCV score. Transforms are removed one-at-a-time from either the probabilities or the dispersions, whichever generates the better LCV score after adjusting all the powers of the remaining transforms for both the probabilities and the dispersions. An LCV ratio test is used to decide when to stop the contraction. The contraction stops removing transforms from the probabilities when there is only one transform remaining in the model for the probabilities. Also, by default, the contraction stops removing transforms from the dispersions when there is only one transform remaining in the model for the dispersions. Unit dispersion models can be considered in the contraction by changing the setting of the cnvzero parameter from its default setting of "cnvzero=n" to "cnvzero=y". When the contraction leaves the expanded model unchanged, that expanded model has its powers adjusted to increase the LCV score.

14.5.3 Additive Models in Visit and Being on Active Treatment

The following code uses the genreg macro to generate the adaptive additive model for trichotomous respiratory status probabilities as a possibly nonlinear function of visit and being on active treatment using $k = 15$ folds, UN correlations, and ELMM assuming constant dispersions.

```
%genreg(modtype=dscrt,datain=longresp,yvar=status0_2,matchvar=id,
withinvr=visit,foldcnt=15,corrtype=UN,GEE=n,srchtype=logL,
propodds=n,usepoiss=y,expand=y,expxvars=visit active,contract=y);
```

In this case, the expxvars macro parameter specifies the variables visit and active to be the primary predictor variables to consider in the expansion for the probabilities. The expansion grows the model for the probabilities by systematically adding in power transforms of visit or the indicator variable active one-at-a-time. Note that indicator variables like active are not transformed and are included at most once in the model for the probabilities. The contraction then systematically removes transforms from the expanded model for the probabilities, possibly the constant transform corresponding to the intercept, and adjusts the powers of the remaining transforms to increase the LCV score. The model is additive because by default geometric combinations are not considered in the expansion.

The following code directly generates the adaptive additive model for the probabilities assuming constant dispersions.

```
%genreg(modtype=dscrt,datain=longresp,yvar=status0_2,matchvar=id,
withinvr=visit,foldcnt=15,corrtype=UN,GEE=n,srchtype=logL,
propodds=n,usepoiss=y,xintrcpt=n,xvars=visit active,xpowers=−0.2 1,
vintrcpt=y);
```

The probabilities are based on a zero intercept, visit$^{-0.2}$, and the indicator active. The LCV score is 0.42702 so that the model in only visit with LCV score 0.42536 is distinctly inferior generating a distinct PD 0.39%. Consequently, being on active treatment is reasonably considered to have an additive effect on the probabilities assuming constant dispersions. Additive models for both probabilities and dispersions can be generated by adding the setting "expvvars=visit active".

14.5.4 Moderation Models in Visit and Being on Active Treatment

The following code uses the genreg macro to generate the adaptive moderation model for trichotomous respiratory status probabilities as a possibly nonlinear function of visit, being on active treatment, and geometric combinations in visit and being on active treatment using $k = 15$ folds, UN correlations, and ELMM assuming constant dispersions.

```
%genreg(modtype=dscrt,datain=longresp,yvar=status0_2,matchvar=id,
withinvr=visit,foldcnt=15,corrtype=UN,GEE=n,srchtype=logL,propodds=n,
usepoiss=y,expand=y,expxvars=visit active,geomcmbn=y,
contract=y);
```

In this case, the expxvars macro parameter specifies the variables visit and active to be the primary predictor variables to consider in the expansion for the probabilities. The expansion grows the model for the probabilities by systematically adding in power transforms of visit, the indicator variable active, or geometric combinations in visit and active one-at-a-time. Geometric combinations are considered due to adding the setting "geomcmbn=y" to the code for generating the associated additive model in visit and active. The default setting for the geomcmbn macro parameter is "geomcmbn=n" meaning to restrict the expansion to an additive model in the variables specified in expxvars. The contraction systematically removes transforms from the expanded model for the probabilities, possibly the constant transform corresponding to the intercept, and adjusts the powers of the remaining transforms to increase the LCV score. Note that when a geometric combination of the form

$(\text{visit}^p \cdot \text{active})^q$ or $(\text{active} \cdot \text{visit}^p)^q$ is generated by the expansion, the contraction only adjusts the power q and leaves the power p unchanged. When there are more than two primary predictors for the probabilities and/or dispersions, geometric combinations can be generated based on any number of two or more of those primary predictors.

The following code directly generates the adaptive moderation model for the probabilities with constant dispersions.

```
%genreg(modtype=dscrt,datain=longresp,yvar=status0_2,matchvar=id,
withinvr=visit,foldcnt=15,corrtype=UN,GEE=n,srchtype=logL,
propodds=n,usepoiss=y,xintrcpt=n,xvars=visit,xpowers=−7,
xgcs=active 1 visit −7: active 1 visit 1,xgcpowrs=0.23 −1.1,
vintrcpt=y);
```

In this case, the model for the probabilities is based on a zero intercept, visit^{-7}, and the two geometric combinations

$$\left(\text{active} \cdot \text{visit}^{-7}\right)^{0.23} = \text{active} \cdot \text{visit}^{-1.61}.$$

and

$$(\text{active} \cdot \text{visit})^{-1.1} = \text{active} \cdot \text{visit}^{-1.1}.$$

The LCV score is 0.43049 while the associated additive model has LCV score 0.42702 with distinct PD 0.81%. Consequently, being on active treatment is reasonably considered to moderate the effect of visit on the censored Poisson probabilities assuming constant dispersions. Moderation models for both probabilities and dispersions can be generated by adding the setting "expvvars=visit active".

The macro parameters xgcs and xgcpowrs are used to specify geometric combinations for the probabilities. The setting "xgcs=visit −0.2 active 1" specifies the untransformed geometric combination $\text{visit}^{-0.2} \cdot \text{active}$ while the setting "xgcpowrs=5.5" means to transform $\text{visit}^{-0.2} \cdot \text{active}$ to the power 5.5. The xgcpowrs setting is needed in this case because its default empty setting "xgcpowrs=" means to leave all the geometric combinations specified by the xgcs macro parameter untransformed. Multiple geometric combinations are specified by separating them by colons (:) as in the above code. The macro parameters vgcs and vgcpowrs are used in the same way to specify geometric combinations for the dispersions.

The standard linear moderation model has probabilities based on an intercept, visit, active, and the interaction visit · active with constant dispersions. The standard linear moderation model can be generated using ELMM with the following code.

```
%genreg(modtype=dscrt,datain=longresp,yvar=status0_2,matchvar=id,
withinvr=visit,foldcnt=15,corrtype=UN,GEE=n,srchtype=logL,
propodds=n,usepoiss=y,xintrcpt=y,xvars=visit active,
xgcs=visit 1 active 1,vintrcpt=y);
```

The LCV score is 0.42099. The associated standard linear additive model is generated by removing the setting "xgcs=visit 1 active 1" from the above code. It has larger LCV score 0.42220, indicating that in this case standard linear moderation is not supported.

14.5.5 Direct Variance Modeling

The dirctvar macro parameter controls whether or not variances are directly modeled. The default setting "dirctvar=n" means use extended variances based on both the dispersions and the variances. Adding the setting "dirctvar=y" treats the variances as 1 so that the extended variances are the same as the dispersions. The following code uses the genreg macro to generate the adaptive direct variance, ELMM model for trichotomous respiratory status probabilities and dispersions as possibly nonlinear functions of visit.

```
%genreg(modtype=logis,datain=longresp,yvar=status0_2,matchvar=id,
withinvr=visit,foldcnt=15,corrtype=UN,GEE=n,srchtype=logL,expand=y,
expxvars=visit,expvvars=visit,contract=y,dirctvar=y);
```

The following code directly generates the above direct variance model.

```
%genreg(modtype=logis,datain=longresp,yvar=status0_2,matchvar=id,
withinvr=visit,foldcnt=15,corrtype=UN,GEE=n,srchtype=logL,
xintrcpt=n,xvars=visit,xpowers=−0.3,vintrcpt=y,vvars=visit,
vpowers=4.1002,dirctvar=y);
```

This model has means based on a zero intercept and the transform $\text{visit}^{-0.3}$ along with dispersions, and so also variances, based on a zero intercept and $\text{visit}^{4.1002}$. It has LCV score 0.39799 with distinct PD 6.79% compared to the associated model accounting for the variance with LCV score 0.42696. Consequently, direct variance modeling in visit generates a distinctly inferior model. The same conclusions hold for direct variance modeling allowing for additive effects to visit and int as well as moderation effects.

14.5.6 Unit Variance Modeling

The following code uses the genreg macro to generate the adaptive model for trichotomous respiratory status probabilities as a possibly nonlinear function of visit using $k = 15$ folds, UN correlations, and ELMM assuming unit dispersions.

```
%genreg(modtype=dscrt,datain=longresp,yvar=status0_2,matchvar=id,
withinvr=visit,foldcnt=15,corrtype=UN,GEE=n,srchtype=logL,
propodds=n,usepoiss=y,vintrcpt=n,expand=y,expxvars=visit,
contract=y);
```

The base model for the dispersions has a zero intercept, due to the setting "vintrcpt=n", and it remains that way because the model for the dispersions does not change. Since the dispersions are modeled using the natural log link function, all models generated as part of the adaptive process have unit dispersions. The generated unit dispersion model has probabilities based on a zero intercept and visit$^{-0.2}$ with LCV score 0.42142 and with distinct PD 1.30% compared to the associated non-constant variance model with LCV score 0.42696. Consequently, unit dispersion modeling in visit generates a distinctly inferior model. The same conclusions hold for unit dispersion modeling allowing for additive effects to visit and int as well as for moderation effects.

14.5.7 Example Output

The following code uses the genreg macro to generate the adaptive moderation model for trichotomous respiratory status probabilities and non-constant dispersions as possibly nonlinear functions of visit, being in the intervention group, and geometric combinations in visit and being in the intervention group starting with constant dispersions.

```
%genreg(modtype=dscrt,datain=longresp,yvar=status0_2,matchvar=id,
withinvr=visit,foldcnt=15,corrtype=UN,GEE=n,srchtype=logL,
propodds=n,usepoiss=y,expand=y,expxvars=visit active,
expvvars=visit active,geomcmbn=y,contract=y);
```

The output generated by this code starts with descriptions of settings controlling what kind of model has been generated including the cutoff for a distinct percent decrease in LCV scores followed by a description of the base model. Table 14.17 contains SAS listing output describing the base model. The probabilities for status0_2 having values 0, 1, and 2 (i.e., the probability component) are based only on an intercept parameter XINTRCPT with estimated value 0.25 while the dispersions (i.e., the log dispersion component) are also based only on an intercept parameter VINTRCPT with estimated value −0.32. The LCV score rounds to 0.42047 (called the "mth root of the extended likelihood using deleted predictions" in the output).

Table 14.17 Part of the SAS listing output describing the base model for the generation of the adaptive moderation model

```
          base probability component

predictor      power     estimate

XINTRCPT           1    0.2525992

          base log dispersion component

predictor      power     estimate

VINTRCPT           1    -0.317327

mth root of extended likelihood using deleted predictions: 0.4204739
```

Table 14.18. Part of the SAS listing output describing the expanded model for the generation of the adaptive moderation model

```
geometric combination expectation variables:
        XGC_1     visit**(-0.2)*active
        XGC_2     active*visit**(-7)
        XGC_3     visit**(-3)*active
        XGC_4     active*visit

geometric combination log dispersion variables:
        VGC_1     active*visit**(2)

          expanded probability component

predictor      power    estimate      score    order

XINTRCPT           1    0.0712337 0.4204739        0
XGC_1            0.5    0.9605426 0.4269854        1
XGC_2              2    0.4044274 0.4291902        3
visit             -4    0.2141834 0.4308172        4
XGC_3              1    -1.098737 0.4309555        5
XGC_4              1    -0.110481 0.4300919        7

          expanded log dispersion component

predictor      power    estimate        score    order

VINTRCPT           1    -0.518513    0.4204739        0
visit            1.5    0.0366099    0.4288488        2
VGC_1            0.8    0.0204969     0.430927        6
active             1    0.0429142    0.4282986        8

mth root of extended likelihood using deleted predictions: 0.4282986
```

The output then describes the parameters controlling the expansion followed by the expanded model as described in Table 14.18. The output uses the SAS power operator "**". The base model (order 0) has LCV score 0.42047. First, the geometric combination

$$\text{XGC\_1}^{0.5} = \left(\text{visit}^{-0.2} \cdot \text{active}\right)^{0.5} = \text{visit}^{-0.1} \cdot \text{active (order 1)}$$

is added to the probabilities generating LCV score 0.42699. Next, the transform $\text{visit}^{1.5}$ (order 2) is added to the model for the dispersions with LCV score 0.42885. Next, three terms are added to the probabilities: visit^{-4} (order 3),

$$\text{XGC\_2}^{2} = \left(\text{active} \cdot \text{visit}^{-7}\right)^{2} = \text{active} \cdot \text{visit}^{-14} \text{ (order 4)},$$

and

$$\text{XGC\_3}^{1} = \text{visit}^{-3} \cdot \text{active (order 5)}$$

with LCV scores 0.0.42919, 0.43082, and 0.43096, respectively. Then, the geometric combination

$$\text{VGC\_2}^{0.8} = \left(\text{active} \cdot \text{visit}^{2}\right)^{0.8} = \text{active} \cdot \text{visit}^{1.6} \text{ (order 6)},$$

Table 14.19 Part of the SAS listing output describing the contracted model for the generation of the adaptive moderation model

```
                 contracted probability component

           predictor old power   new power    estimate

           visit             -4          -7   0.230659
           XGC_3              1         0.5   -3.35567
           XGC_4              1          -1  3.5350274

            discarded   old power        score   order

                                .    0.4282986       0
            XGC_1             0.5    0.4312075       2
            XINTRCPT            1    0.4317962       3
            XGC_2               2    0.4321217       4

               contracted log dispersion component

            predictor old power new power   estimate

            VINTRCPT          1         1  -0.494715
            visit           1.5       1.5  0.0489084

            discarded   old power        score   order

                                .    0.4282986       0
            active              1    0.4301941       1
            VGC_1             0.8    0.4323768       5

mth root of extended likelihood using deleted predictions: 0.4323768
```

is added to model for the dispersions with LCV score 0.43093, followed by the geometric combination

$$\mathrm{XGC\_4}^{1} = \mathrm{active} \cdot \mathrm{visit}\ (\mathrm{order}\ 7)$$

added to the model for the probabilities with LCV score 0.43009. Finally, the indicator active is added to the model for the dispersions with LCV score 0.42830, which is the LCV score for the expanded model. Each transform is added to the model without adjusting the powers for previously added transforms. The LCV score is allowed to decrease, and so expanded models usually require contraction. However, in cases where the contraction leaves the expanded model unchanged, a conditional transformation step is executed to adjust the powers of the expanded model to improve its LCV score.

The output then describes the parameters controlling the contraction followed by the contracted model as described in Table 14.19. The expanded model (order 0) has LCV score 0.42830. First, the indicator active (order1) is removed from the model for the dispersions with LCV score 0.43019 followed by the three terms removed from the model for the probabilities: $\mathrm{XGC\_3}^{1}$ (order 2), XINTRCPT (order 3), and $\mathrm{XGC\_2}^{2}$ (order 4) with LCV scores 0.43121, 0.43180, and 0.43212. Finally, the geometric combination $\mathrm{VGC\_1}^{0.8}$ (order 5) is removed from the model for the dispersions with LCV score 0.43238, which is the LCV score for the contracted model. With the removal of each transform from the model, the powers for the other transforms are adjusted to improve the LCV score. In this case, the powers for visit, XGC_3, and XGC_4 for the probabilities change from −4 to −7, 1 to 0.5, and 1 to

Table 14.20. Part of the SAS listing output describing the estimated EC correlation matrix of the contracted model for the generation of the adaptive moderation model

```
                     estimated correlation matrix:

                   w1         w2         w3         w4         w5

        w1          1  0.4270191 0.3504739  0.309013  0.3768234
        w2  0.4270191          1 0.5553533 0.4869796  0.4265936
        w3  0.3504739  0.5553533         1 0.6428793  0.6395684
        w4   0.309013  0.4869796 0.6428793         1  0.6860829
        w5  0.3768234  0.4265936 0.6395684 0.6860829          1

      w1, w2, ... are withinvr values from smallest to largest
```

−1, respectively, while the other powers are unchanged. Details on how the powers change at each step of the contraction are not provided in the contraction output, but are available in the SAS log output if that is of interest. Note that the LCV score increased with the removal of the four transforms, but can decrease in general. In this way, a parsimonious model is generated by the contraction. The contraction stopped because the removal of the next transform would have generated a model with a distinct PD in the LCV score using an LCV ratio test.

The estimated UN correlation matrix for the contracted model is generated but not included in Table 14.19; it is displayed in Table 14.20. Within values are denoted as w1, w2, w3, w4, and w5 representing in this case visit 0, 1, 2, 3, and 4, respectively.

Reference

Koch, G. G., Carr, C. F., Amara, I. A., Stokes, M. E., & Uryniak, T. J. (1989). Categorical data analysis. In D. A. Berry (Ed.), *Statistical methodology in the pharmaceutical sciences* (pp. 391–475). Marcel Dekker.

Part III
Adaptive Analysis Strategies

Part III describes and demonstrates a systematic approach for conducting adaptive analyses. Chapter 15 describes concise analyses for the data sets previously analyzed more extensively in Chaps. 6–9 and 13–14, specifies systematic strategies for conducting concise adaptive analyses of correlated outcomes justified by the prior analyses reported in the chapter, provides an evaluation of the effectiveness of ELMM for analyzing theory-based models, and addresses future work needed for analyzing correlated outcomes. All the data sets analyzed so far have repeatedly measured outcomes with continuous measurement condition values and no missing outcome measurements. Chapter 16 demonstrates the use of these analysis strategies. It uses data not previously analyzed and of different kinds including correlated outcomes with categorical measurement condition values corresponding to different scales from the same survey instrument (Sect. 16.2) as well as correlated dyadic data with some missing outcome measurements (Sects. 16.3–16.5).

Chapter 15
Alternative Analyses

Abstract Analyses are reported to identify appropriate strategies for modeling correlated outcomes in terms of available predictors, addressing which methods to use and which order to apply them. Analyses are conducted using extended linear mixed modeling (ELMM) of a continuous outcome treated as normally distributed, a count/rate outcome treated as Poisson distributed, a dichotomous outcome treated as Bernoulli distributed, a positive continuous outcome treated as exponentially distributed, and a trichotomous outcome treated as either multinomially, ordinally, or discretely distributed. Whether non-constant or unit dispersions are appropriate is addressed as well as adaptive additive modeling, adaptive moderation modeling, and a comparison of results for extended variance modeling and direct variance modeling. A detailed specification of possible analysis strategies is provided as well as an assessment of ELMM for analyzing theory-based models and future work needed.

Keywords Bootstrapping · Direct variance modeling · Discrete regression · Extended linear mixed modeling · Moderation · Multinomial regression · Ordinal regression

Introduction Analyses are reported in this chapter of the data sets of Sects. 2.8 and 13.1 in order to identify appropriate strategies for efficient modeling of the associated correlated outcomes in terms of available predictors, addressing which methods to use and in which order to apply them. Section 15.1 provides analyses of the dental measurement data of Sect. 2.8.1, Sect. 15.2 of the epilepsy seizure rate data of Sect. 2.8.2, Sect. 15.3 of the dichotomous respiratory status data of Sect. 2.8.3, Sect. 15.4 of the blood lead level data of Sect. 2.8.4, and Sects. 15.5–15.6 of the trichotomous respiratory status data of Sect. 13.1. Section 15.7 provides an overview of results for the analyses of Sects. 15.1–15.6 while Sect. 15.8 describes general analysis strategies for adaptive modeling of correlated outcomes based on prior analyses. Section 15.9 provides an assessment of ELMM for analyzing theory-based models

---

Supplementary Information The online version contains supplementary material available at https://doi.org/10.1007/978-3-031-41988-1_15.

G. J. Knafl, *Modeling Correlated Outcomes Using Extensions of Generalized Estimating Equations and Linear Mixed Modeling*,
https://doi.org/10.1007/978-3-031-41988-1_15

for correlated outcomes while Sect. 15.10 addresses future work needed on analyzing correlated outcomes.

ELMM is demonstrated in Chaps. 6–9 and 14 to be preferable over partially modified generalized estimating equations (GEE) and fully modified GEE for analyzing correlated univariate outcomes since it generates at least a competitive model and, in some cases, a distinctly better model while requiring less time and sometimes much less time. Similar results hold for the multinomial/ordinal regression analyses of correlated multivariate outcomes in Chap. 13, except that ELMM can require more time for UN correlations since they can be based on large numbers of parameters. For these reasons, only ELMM is used in analyses reported in this chapter.

15.1 Analyzing the Dental Measurement Data

There are 108 dental measurements (Potthoff & Roy, 1964). The cutoff for a distinct percent decrease (PD) in the LCV score using DF = 1 is 1.76%. All LCV scores are computed using matched-set-wise deletion since there are no missing dental measurements. Analyses are conducted using linear regression.

15.1.1 Alternative Correlation Structures

As reported in Sect. 6.1, the exchangeable correlation (EC) structure generates the best LCV scores using ELMM for 5, 10, and 15 folds compared to independent (IND), spatial autoregressive order 1 (AR1), and unstructured (UN) correlation structures. However, that decision is based on adaptive models for the means in child age with constant variances. An approach that considers a more general model while requiring a limited amount of computation time is desirable for handling general data sets with possibly different distributions and possibly large numbers of measurements. One possible choice for such a model is the one with different means and different variances for different measurement conditions, in this case, different child ages.

Table 15.1 provides LCV scores for this model computed using 5, 10, and 15 folds for each of the IND, spatial AR1, EC, and UN correlation structures. For all three numbers of folds, EC generates the best LCV score over the four correlation structures. Consequently, only EC correlations are used in subsequent analyses. The 12 models of Table 15.1 require 0.1 min of clock time.

Table 15.1 LCV scores using alternative correlation structures and numbers of folds for the dental measurements[a]

Correlation structure	LCV score[b]		
	5 folds	10 folds	15 folds
IND	0.08965	0.09112	0.08849
AR1	0.09686	0.09753	0.09617
EC	0.11146	0.11163	0.11003
UN	0.06174	0.07357	0.07241

AR1 spatial autoregressive order 1; *EC* exchangeable correlations; *IND* independent; *LCV* likelihood cross-validation; *UN* unstructured
[a]Using models based on assuming different means and different variances for different child ages and computed using linear mixed modeling
[b]Computed using matched-set-wise deletion

Table 15.2 Comparison of LCV scores for adaptively generated models based on child age of dental measurement means and variances[a]

Model in child age			LCV score[b]		
Index	Means	Variances	5 folds	10 folds	15 folds
1	Different	Different	0.11146	0.11163	0.11003
2	Adaptive	Adaptive	0.11881	0.12044	0.11906
PD for model 1 versus model 2			6.19%	7.31%	7.58%

LCV likelihood cross-validation; *PD* percent decrease in the LCV score
[a]Computed using linear mixed modeling and exchangeable correlations
[b]Computed using matched-set-wise deletion

15.1.2 Models Based on Child Age

Table 15.2 contains LCV scores of the same three numbers of folds as in Table 15.1 for two alternative models for dental measurements in terms of child age including the model with different means and different variances and the model with adaptive means and adaptive non-constant variances. It also contains percent decreases (PDs) for comparing these models. For all three numbers of folds, the PD for the model with different means and different variances is distinct (that is, greater than the cutoff 1.76% based on DF = 1) compared to the model with adaptive means and adaptive variances, indicating that adaptive modeling of means and variances provides a distinct improvement.

For each of the two models of Table 15.2, the largest LCV score is achieved with 10 folds (as is also the case for the adaptive models for the means with constant variances with EC correlations of Table 6.1). These results indicate that 10 folds is a reasonable choice for adaptive analyses of the dental measurement data.

Table 15.3 provides power transforms for the adaptive models of Table 15.2 generated using the same three numbers of folds. Models have 1–2 mean parameters and 1 variance parameter. The same model is generated using 10 and 15 folds. Using 10 folds because it maximizes associated LCV scores, models with adaptive means and adaptive variances generated with 5 and 15 folds have 10-fold LCV scores

Table 15.3 Power transforms and clock times for adaptively generated models based on child age of dental measurement means and variances[a]

	Number of folds		
	5	10	15
Means[b]	0, 2	0.32	0.32
Variances[b]	0.1	0.2	0.2
Clock time (min)	0.4	0.6	0.8

[a]Computed using linear mixed modeling, exchangeable correlations, and matched-set-wise deletion with the contraction allowing for unit variances

[b]A power of 0 corresponds to an intercept; otherwise, the model has a zero intercept

0.11880 and 0.12044, respectively, with non-distinct PDs 1.36% and 0.00% compared to the associated model generated with 10 folds and 10-fold LCV score 0.12044. Consequently, the choice of the number of folds has little impact on the generated model. Table 15.3 also contains clock times in minutes for the adaptive models of Table 15.2 generated using the same three numbers of folds. As would be expected, clock times increase with the number of folds with all three models requiring a total of only 1.8 min.

The contraction used in generating the adaptive models of Table 15.3 allowed for the possibility of unit variances, but generated variances for those models are each based on a transform of child age, indicating that unit variances need not be considered further. Models based on the normal distribution are always based on direct variance modeling, and so that is not an issue to consider for the dental measurement data.

15.1.3 Models Based on Child Age and Child Gender

The results of Sect. 15.1.2 indicate that the dental measurement data are appropriately analyzed using EC correlations with LCV scores computed using 10 folds, and so these choices are used in subsequent analyses. This section provides a comparison of adaptive additive and adaptive moderation models for means and variances in child age and child gender.

Table 15.4 provides a comparison of the adaptive additive model and the adaptive moderation model for dental measurement means and variances. The additive model has 10-fold LCV score 0.12798 with distinct PD 4.83% compared to the moderation model with 10-fold LCV score 0.13447. Consequently, a distinct moderation effect is identified. This is also the case for the associated analysis reported in Sect. 6.6, but that moderation model is only close to the model of Table 15.4 because it was generated using 5 folds. The adaptive additive model requires 1.4 min of clock time while the adaptive moderation model requires 7.2 min.

The LMM model of Table 15.4 has estimated correlation 0.71 and estimated standard deviation for girls 1.7 mm which increases to 2.4 mm for boys. Figure 15.1 displays mean dental measurements over child age and child gender. Mean dental

Table 15.4 Adaptively generated models based on child age and child gender of dental measurement means and variances[a]

10-fold LCV score	Mean transforms[b]	Variance transforms[b]
0.12798	$age^{0.27}$	male, $age^{0.6}$
0.13447	$age^{0.23}$ $(male \cdot age^{10})^{0.18}$	1, male

[a]Computed using linear mixed modeling, exchangeable correlations, and matched-set-wise deletion
[b]The transform 1 represents an intercept; otherwise, the intercept is zero. The transform male represents the indicator for the child being male

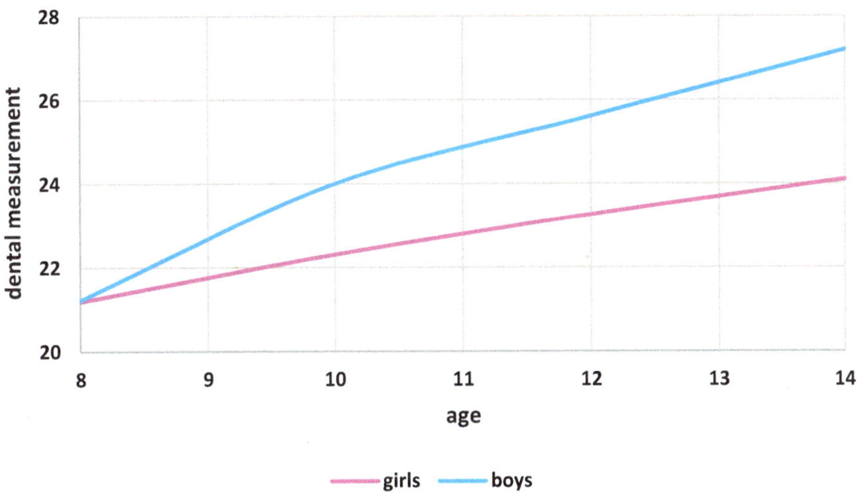

Fig. 15.1 Estimated means for dental measurements for girls and for boys as they age from 8 to 14 years old

measurements increase as children age from a common value of 21.2 mm at age 8 for boys and girls, but to a higher level by age 14 for boys of 27.2 mm than the level for girls at age 14 of 24.1 mm.

15.1.4 Clock Times for Analyses

Clock times for the analyses of Sect. 15.1 include 0.1 min for the models of Table 15.1, 1.8 min for the models of Tables 15.2–15.3, and 8.6 min for the models of Table 15.4. Consequently, analyses of the dental measurement data require 10.5 min altogether.

15.2 Analyzing the Epilepsy Seizure Rate Data

There are 295 epilepsy seizure rates (Thall & Vail, 1990). The cutoff for a distinct percent decrease (PD) in the LCV score using DF = 1 is 0.65%. All LCV scores are computed using matched-set-wise deletion since there are no missing epilepsy seizure rates. Models reported in this section are based on extended variances determined by dispersions combined with means unless explicitly specified to be based on direct variance modeling determined entirely by dispersions. Analyses are conducted using Poisson regression.

15.2.1 Alternative Correlation Structures

As reported in Sect. 7.1, the exchangeable correlation (EC) structure generates the best LCV scores using ELMM for 5, 10, and 15 folds compared to independent (IND), spatial autoregressive order 1 (AR1), and unstructured (UN) correlation structures. However, that decision is based on adaptive models for the means in visit with constant dispersions. An approach that considers a more general model while requiring a limited amount of computation time is desirable for handling general data sets with possibly different distributions and possibly large numbers of measurements. One possible choice for such a model is the one with different means and different dispersions for different measurement conditions, in this case, different visits.

Table 15.5 provides LCV scores for this model computed using 5, 10, and 15 folds for each of the IND, spatial AR1, EC, and UN correlation structures. For all three numbers of folds, EC generates the best LCV score over the four correlation structures. Consequently, only EC correlations are used in subsequent analyses. The 12 models of Table 15.5 require 0.5 min of clock time.

Table 15.5 LCV scores using alternative correlation structures and numbers of folds for the epilepsy seizure rates[a]

Correlation structure	LCV score[b]		
	5 folds	10 folds	15 folds
IND	0.012964	0.012628	0.012290
AR1	0.018173	0.018015	0.017845
EC	0.021549	0.020458	0.020339
UN	0.018259	0.018793	0.018517

AR1 spatial autoregressive order 1; *EC* exchangeable correlations; *IND* independent; *LCV* likelihood cross-validation; *UN* unstructured

[a]Using extended variance models based on assuming different means and different dispersions for different visits and computed using extended linear mixed modeling

[b]Computed using matched-set-wise deletion

15.2.2 Models Based on Visit

Table 15.6 contains LCV scores of the same three numbers of folds as in Table 15.5 for two alternative models for the epilepsy seizure rates in terms of visit including the model with different means and different dispersions and the model with adaptive means and adaptive non-constant dispersions. It also contains percent decreases (PDs) for comparing these models. For all three numbers of folds, the PD for the model with different means and different dispersions is distinct (that is, greater than the cutoff 0.65% based on DF = 1) compared to the model with adaptive means and adaptive dispersions, indicating that adaptive modeling of means and dispersions provides a distinct improvement.

For each of the two models of Table 15.6, the largest LCV score is achieved with 5 folds (as is also the case for the adaptive ELMM models for the means with constant dispersions with EC correlations of Table 7.1). These results indicate that 5 folds is a reasonable choice for adaptive analyses of the epilepsy seizure rate data.

Table 15.7 provides power transforms for the adaptive models of Table 15.6 generated using the same three numbers of folds. Models have 1–2 mean parameters and 2–3 dispersion parameters with a total of 4 mean and dispersion parameters for all three cases. Using 5 folds because it maximizes associated LCV scores, models with adaptive means and adaptive dispersions generated with 10 and 15 folds have 5-fold LCV scores 0.024378 and 0.024410, respectively, with non-distinct PDs 0.24% and 0.11% compared to the associated model generated with 5 folds and

Table 15.6 Comparison of LCV scores for adaptively generated extended variance models based on visit of epilepsy seizure rate means and dispersions[a]

Model in visit			LCV score[b]		
Index	Means	Dispersions	5 folds	10 folds	15 folds
1	Different	Different	0.021549	0.020458	0.020339
2	Adaptive	Adaptive	0.024437	0.023697	0.023562
PD for model 1 versus model 2			11.82%	13.67%	13.68%

LCV likelihood cross-validation; *PD* percent decrease in the LCV score
[a]Computed using extended linear mixed modeling and exchangeable correlations
[b]Computed using matched-set-wise deletion

Table 15.7 Power transforms and clock times for adaptively generated extended variance models based on visit of epilepsy seizure rate means and dispersions[a]

	Number of folds		
	5	10	15
Means[b]	0, 19	0	0
Dispersions[b]	0, −0.01	0, 0.1, 13	0, 0.09, 8
Clock time (min)	3.6	3.6	8.0

[a]Computed using extended linear mixed modeling, exchangeable correlations, and matched-set-wise deletion with the contraction allowing for unit dispersions
[b]A power of 0 corresponds to an intercept; otherwise, the model has a zero intercept

Table 15.8 LCV scores, power transforms, and clock times for adaptively generated direct variance models based on visit of epilepsy seizure rate means and dispersions[a]

	Number of folds		
	5	10	15
LCV score[b]	0.024414	0.023697	0.023562
Means[c]	0	0	0
Dispersions[c]	0, 0.06, 9	0, 0.1, 13	0, 0.09, 12
Clock time (min)	2.2	4.1	7.4

[a]Computed using extended linear mixed modeling and exchangeable correlations with contraction allowing for unit dispersions
[b]Computed using matched-set-wise deletion
[c]A power of 0 corresponds to an intercept; otherwise, the model has a zero intercept

5-fold LCV score 0.024437. Consequently, the choice of the number of folds has little impact on the generated model. The 10-fold and 15-fold models indicate that means for epilepsy seizure rates can be considered constant when combined with more complex dispersions than the 5-fold model. Table 15.7 also contains clock times in minutes for the adaptive models of Table 15.6 generated using the same three numbers of folds. Models for the three numbers of folds require a total of 15.2 min of clock time.

The contraction used in generating the adaptive models of Table 15.7 allowed for the possibility of unit dispersions, but generated dispersions for those models are based on 1–2 transforms of visit together with an intercept, indicating that consideration of unit dispersions is not needed. In any case, the fact that each model has dispersions based on 2–3 transforms means that dispersions could not have been based on a single parameter and so then unit dispersions could not have been chosen.

Models considered in the section so far have been based on extended variances depending on means and dispersions. Direct variance modeling is considered next using EC correlations as selected above.

Table 15.8 contains LCV scores of the same three numbers of folds as in Tables 15.6–15.7 for three alternative direct variance models for epilepsy seizure rates in terms of visit with adaptive means and adaptive dispersions. Over all three numbers of folds, LCV scores are maximized at 5 folds, supporting the use of 5 folds as before.

Table 15.8 also provides power transforms for its direct variance models using the same three numbers of folds. All three models have constant means with dispersions based on two transforms of visit together with an intercept. The model selected using 10 folds has 5-fold LCV score 0.024378 with non-distinct PD 0.15% while the model selected using 15 folds has 5-fold LCV score 0.024391 with non-distinct PD 0.09%, indicating that the three direct variance models are competitive alternatives. Also, the direct variance model of Tables 15.8 based on 5 folds has LCV score 0.024437 so that the extended variance model of Tables 15.6–15.7 with 5-fold LCV score 0.024414 generates a non-distinct PD 0.09%. Consequently, the direct variance model is a competitive alternative. Moreover, direct variance modeling generates more consistent models with all three of the models of Table 15.8 having constant means and similar dispersions based on an intercept and two transforms of visit compared to extended variance modeling with only two of the three models of Table 15.7 consistent in that way. Consequently, only direct variance modeling is used in subsequent analyses. As for extended variance modeling, the contraction used in generating the adaptive direct variance models of Table 15.8 allowed for the possibility of unit dispersions, but non-unit dispersions are generated in all three cases, so unit dispersions are not considered in subsequent analyses.

Table 15.8 also contains clock times in minutes for the direct variance models of Table 15.8. Clock times increase with the number of folds for a total of 13.7 min. In contrast, the associated models of Tables 15.6–15.7 require a total of 15.2 min or about 1.6 times as much as for direct variance modeling. Consequently, in this case direct variance modeling requires less computation time, further supporting its use over extended variance modeling.

15.2.3 Models Based on Visit and Treatment Group

The results of Sect. 15.2.2 indicate that the epilepsy seizure rate data are appropriately analyzed using direct variance modeling based on EC correlations with LCV scores computed with 5 folds. This section provides a comparison of adaptive models for means and dispersions in visit and the indicator int for being in the intervention group using direct variance modeling.

Table 15.9 provides a comparison of the adaptive additive model and the adaptive moderation models for epilepsy seizure rate means and dispersions using direct variance modeling. The additive and moderation models are the same and have 5-fold LCV score 0.024414. The common model does not depend on the indicator int for being in the intervention group and has constant means with dispersions based on two transforms of visit together with an intercept. The same results are generated in Sect. 7.8. The two models of Table 15.9 require a total of 7.8 min of clock time.

The direct variance model of Table 15.9 has constant mean seizure rates per week with value 3.6 at all visits and estimated exchangeable correlation 0.80. Figure 15.2 provides the plot for estimated standard deviations for seizure rates. Estimated

Table 15.9 Adaptively generated direct variance models based on visit and treatment group of epilepsy seizure rate means and dispersions[a]

Model type	5-fold LCV score	Mean transforms[b]	Dispersion transforms[b]	Clock time (min)
Additive	0.024414	1	1, $\text{visit}^{0.06}$, visit^{9}	2.3
Moderation	0.024414	1	1, $\text{visit}^{0.06}$, visit^{9}	5.5

[a]Computed using extended linear mixed modeling, exchangeable correlations, and matched-set-wise deletion

[b]The transform 1 represents an intercept; otherwise, the intercept is zero. The transform int represents the indicator for being in the intervention

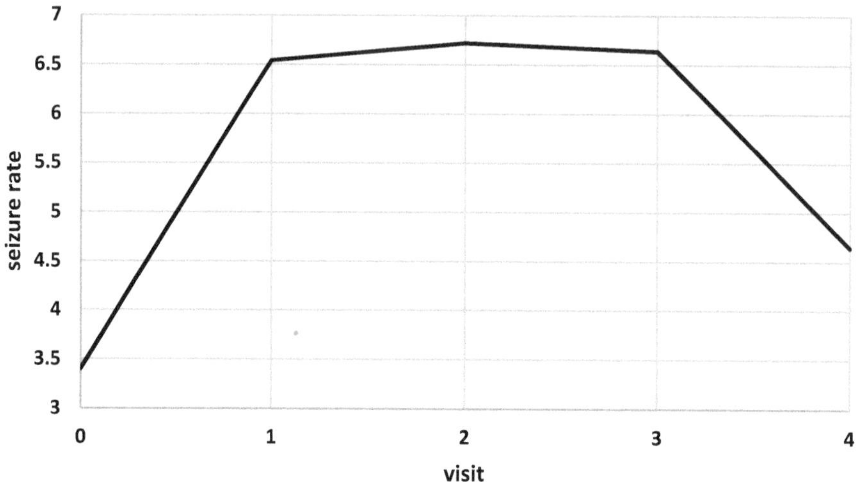

Fig. 15.2 Estimated standard deviations for seizure rates per week over visits based only on dispersions

standard deviations start at 3.4 at visit 0, increase to 6.5 at visit 1, change a little from visit 1 to visit 3, then decrease to 4.6 by visit 4.

15.2.4 Clock Times for Analyses

Clock times for the analyses of Sect. 15.2 include 0.5 min for the models of Table 15.5, 15.2 minutes for the models of Tables 15.6–15.7, 13.7 min for the models of Table 15.8, and 7.8 min for the models of Table 15.9. Consequently, analyses of the epilepsy seizure rate data require 37.2 min altogether.

15.3 Analyzing the Dichotomous Respiratory Status Data

There are 555 dichotomous respiratory status levels (Koch et al., 1989; Stokes et al., 2012). The cutoff for a distinct percent decrease (PD) in the LCV score using DF = 1 is 0.35%. All LCV scores are computed using matched-set-wise deletion since there are no missing dichotomous respiratory status levels. Models reported in this section are based on extended variances determined by dispersions combined with means unless explicitly specified to be based on direct variance modeling determined entirely by dispersions. Analyses are conducted using logistic regression.

15.3.1 Alternative Correlation Structures

As reported in Sect. 7.1, the exchangeable correlation (EC) structure generates the best LCV scores using ELMM for 5, 10, and 15 folds compared to independent (IND), spatial autoregressive order 1 (AR1), and unstructured (UN) correlation structures. However, that decision is based on adaptive models for the means in visit with constant dispersions. An approach that considers a more general model while requiring a limited amount of computation time is desirable for handling general data sets with possibly different distributions and possibly large numbers of measurements. One possible choice for such a model is the one with different means and different dispersions for different measurement conditions, in this case, different visits.

Table 15.10 provides LCV scores for this model computed using 5, 10, and 15 folds for each of the IND, spatial AR1, EC, and UN correlation structures. For all three numbers of folds, EC generates the best LCV score over the four correlation structures. Consequently, only EC correlations are used in subsequent analyses. The 12 models of Table 15.5 require 0.5 min of clock time.

15.3.2 Models Based on Visit

Table 15.11 contains LCV scores of the same three numbers of folds as in Table 15.10 for two alternative models for dichotomous respiratory status levels in terms of visit including the model with different means and different dispersions and the model with adaptive means and adaptive non-constant dispersions. It also contains percent decreases (PDs) for comparing these models. For 10 and 15 folds, the PDs of 0.26% and 0.33%, respectively, for the model with different means and different dispersions are non-distinct (that is, less than or equal to the cutoff 0.35% based on DF = 1) compared to the model with adaptive means and adaptive dispersions. On the other hand, for 5 folds, the PD of 0.38% for the model with

Table 15.10 LCV scores using alternative correlation structures and numbers of folds for the dichotomous respiratory status levels[a]

Correlation structure	LCV score[b]		
	5 folds	10 folds	15 folds
IND	0.48382	0.48440	0.48345
AR1	0.55502	0.55448	0.55328
EC	0.56170	0.56377	0.56283
UN	0.55608	0.55581	0.55619

AR1 spatial autoregressive order 1; *EC* exchangeable correlations; *IND* independent; *LCV* likelihood cross-validation; *UN* unstructured

[a]Using extended variance models based on assuming different means and different dispersions for different visits and computed using extended linear mixed modeling

[b]Computed using matched-set-wise deletion

Table 15.11 Comparison of LCV scores for adaptively generated extended variance models based on visit of dichotomous respiratory status means and dispersions[a]

Model in visit			LCV score[b]		
Index	Means	Dispersions	5 folds	10 folds	15 folds
1	Different	Different	0.56170	0.56377	0.56283
2	Adaptive	Adaptive	0.56385	0.56523	0.56472
PD for model 1 versus model 2			0.38%	0.26%	0.33%

LCV likelihood cross-validation; *PD* percent decrease in the LCV score
[a]Computed using extended linear mixed modeling and exchangeable correlations
[b]Computed using matched-set-wise deletion

Table 15.12 Power transforms and clock times for adaptively generated extended variance models based on visit of dichotomous respiratory status means and dispersions[a]

	Number of folds		
	5	10	15
Means[b]	−0.1	−0.2	−0.3
Dispersions[c]	--	--	--
Clock time (min)	1.1	3.0	2.8

[a]Computed using extended linear mixed modeling, exchangeable correlations, and matched-set-wise deletion with the contraction allowing for unit dispersions
[b]A power of 0 corresponds to an intercept; otherwise, the model has a zero intercept
[c]All models have unit dispersions

different means and different dispersions is distinct. Consequently, adaptive modeling of means and dispersions provides a distinct improvement for 5 folds, but not for 10 and 15 folds.

For each of the two models of Table 15.11, the largest LCV score is achieved with 10 folds (as is also the case for the adaptive ELMM models for the means with constant dispersions with EC correlations of Table 8.1). These results indicate that 10 folds is a reasonable choice for adaptive analyses of the dichotomous respiratory status data.

Table 15.12 provides power transforms for the adaptive models of Table 15.12 generated using the same three numbers of folds. All models have a single mean parameter along with unit dispersions. Using 10 folds because it maximizes associated LCV scores, the model with adaptive means and adaptive dispersions generated with 5 folds has 10-fold LCV score 0.56513 with non-distinct PDs 0.02% compared to the associated model generated with 10 folds and with 10-fold LCV score 0.56532. This latter model generates a non-distinct PD 0.01% compared to the associated model generated with 15 folds and with 10-fold LCV score 0.56526. Consequently, the choice of the number of folds has little impact on the generated model. Table 15.13 also contains clock times in minutes for the adaptive models of Table 15.12 generated using the same three numbers of folds. Models for the three numbers of folds require a total of 6.9 min of clock time.

The contraction used in generating the adaptive models of Tables 15.12–15.13 allowed for the possibility of unit dispersions, and all those models have unit

Table 15.13 Adaptively generated extended variance models based on visit and treatment group of dichotomous respiratory status means assuming unit dispersions[a]

Model type	10-fold LCV score	Mean transforms[b]	Clock time (min)
Additive	0.56523	$\text{visit}^{-0.22}$	0.6
Moderation	0.57350	$(\text{active} \cdot \text{visit}^{-3})^{0.05}$	5.5

[a]Computed using extended linear mixed modeling, exchangeable correlations, and matched-set-wise deletion
[b]The transform 1 represents an intercept; otherwise, the intercept is zero. The transform active represents the indicator for being on active treatment

dispersions. Consequently, the dichotomous respiratory status levels are reasonably treated as having unit dispersions. As this provides a parsimonious description of the variances, it seems reasonable to skip consideration of direct variance modeling of these data. Consequently, only unit dispersion models are considered in subsequent analyses.

15.3.3 Models Based on Visit and Treatment Group

The results of Sect. 15.3.2 indicate that the dichotomous respiratory status data are appropriately analyzed using EC correlations and unit dispersions with LCV scores computed using 10 folds. This section provides a comparison of adaptive models for means in visit and the indicator active for being on active treatment assuming unit dispersions based on 10-fold LCV scores.

Table 15.13 provides a comparison of adaptively generated models for dichotomous respiratory status means assuming unit dispersions using 10-fold LCV scores. The adaptive additive model does not depend on the indicator active, suggesting that being on active treatment does not have an additive effect on dichotomous respiratory status means. On the other hand, the adaptive moderation model is based on a single geometric combination without an intercept. The LCV score for the moderation model is 0.57350 while the additive model has LCV score 0.56523 with distinct PD 1.44%, indicating that being on active treatment distinctly moderates the effect of visit on the dichotomous respiratory status means. The geometric combination is

$$\left(\text{active} \cdot \text{visit}^{-3}\right)^{0.05} = \text{active} \cdot \text{visit}^{-0.15}.$$

The estimated exchangeable correlation 0.47. The same unit dispersion moderation model is generated in Sect. 8.7. The two models of Table 15.13 require a total of 6.1 min of clock time.

Figure 15.3 displays estimated probabilities for good respiratory status over visits for patients on active and placebo treatment. There is no effect to visit for patients on placebo treatment with estimated probabilities of good respiratory status constant at

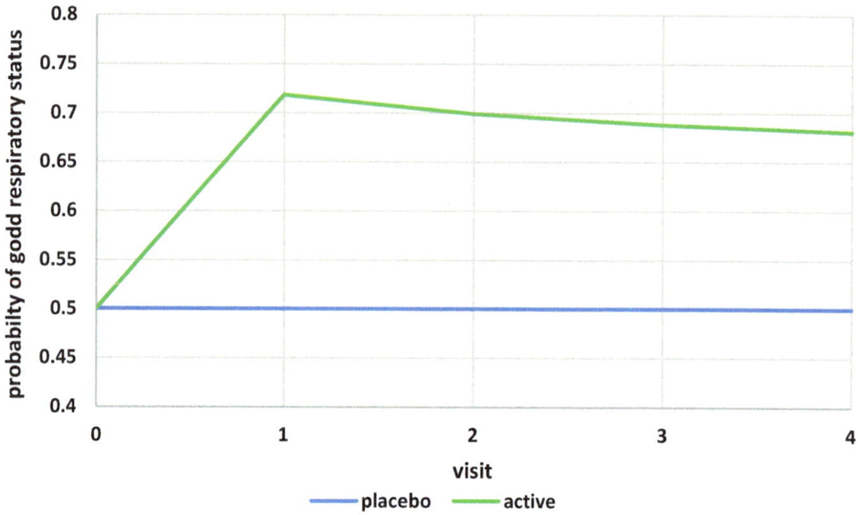

Fig. 15.3 Estimated probability of good respiratory status over visits for patients on active versus placebo treatment

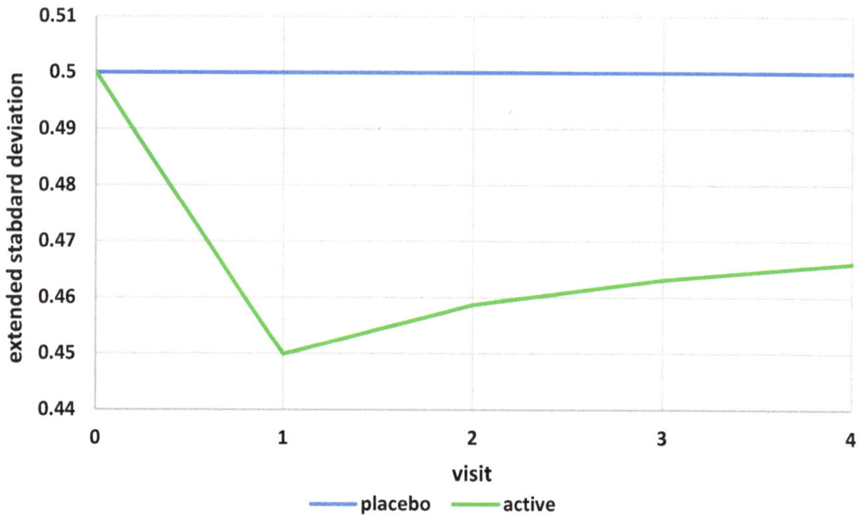

Fig. 15.4 Estimated extended standard deviations for good respiratory status over visits for patients on active versus placebo treatment

0.5 over all visits. On the other hand, the estimated probabilities of good respiratory status increase from 0.50 at baseline to about 0.72 at visit 1 and then decrease slowly over time to 0.68 at visit 4. Figure 15.4 displays estimated extended standard deviations for good respiratory status over visits for patients on active and placebo treatment. There is no effect to visit for patients on placebo treatment with estimated extended standard deviations of good respiratory status constant at 0.5 over all visits. On the other hand, the estimated extended standard deviations of good respiratory status decrease from 0.50 at baseline to about 0.45 at visit 1 and then increase slowly over time to about 0.47 at visit 4.

15.3.4 Clock Times for Analyses

Clock times for the analyses of Sect. 15.3 include 0.5 min for the models of Table 15.10, 6.9 min for the models of Tables 15.11–15.12, and 6.1 min for the models of Table 15.13. Consequently, analyses of the dichotomous respiratory status data require 13.5 min altogether.

15.4 Analyzing the Blood Lead Level Data

There are 400 blood lead levels (Treatment of Lead-exposed Children (TLC) Trial Group, 2000). The cutoff for a distinct percent decrease (PD) in the LCV score using DF $= 1$ is 0.48%. All LCV scores are computed using matched-set-wise deletion since there are no missing blood lead levels. Models reported in this section are based on extended variances determined by dispersions combined with means unless explicitly specified to be based on direct variance modeling determined entirely by dispersions. Analyses are conducted using exponential regression.

15.4.1 Alternative Correlation Structures

As reported in Sect. 9.1, the unstructured (UN) correlation structure generates the best LCV scores using ELMM for 5, 10, and 15 folds compared to independent (IND), spatial autoregressive order 1 (AR1), and exchangeable (EC) correlation structures. However, that decision is based on adaptive models for the means in week with constant dispersions. An approach that considers a more general model while requiring a limited amount of computation time is desirable for handling general data sets with possibly different distributions and possibly large numbers of measurements. One possible choice for such a model is the one with different means and different dispersions for different measurement conditions, in this case, different weeks.

Table 15.14 provides LCV scores for this model computed using 5, 10, and 15 folds for each of the IND, spatial AR1, EC, and UN correlation structures. For all three numbers of folds, UN generates the best LCV score over the four correlation structures. Consequently, only UN correlations are used in subsequent analyses. The 12 models of Table 15.14 require 0.4 min of clock time. For all three numbers of

Table 15.14 LCV scores using alternative correlation structures and numbers of folds for the blood lead levels[a]

Correlation structure	LCV score[b]		
	5 folds	10 folds	15 folds
IND	0.032302	0.032753	0.032629
AR1	0.034989	0.035458	0.035171
EC	0.037946	0.038503	0.038039
UN	0.038606	0.039397	0.038917

AR1 spatial autoregressive order 1; *EC* exchangeable correlations; *IND* independent; *LCV* likelihood cross-validation; *UN* unstructured
[a]Using extended variance models based on assuming different means and different dispersions for different weeks and computed using extended linear mixed modeling
[b]Computed using matched-set-wise deletion

folds, the second-best LCV score is generated using EC correlations, which are based on a single correlation parameter while UN correlations are more complex based on $4{\cdot}3/2 = 6$ parameters and so with 5 more parameters. The cutoff for a distinct PD computed using DF $=$ 5 is 1.37%. The PDs for EC correlations compared to UN correlations for 5, 10, and 15 folds are 1.71%, 2.27%, and 2.26%, respectively, indicating that UN correlations provide a sufficient improvement in LCV scores to justify being based on 5 more parameters.

15.4.2 Models Based on Week

Table 15.15 contains LCV scores of the same three numbers of folds as in Table 15.14 for two alternative models for blood lead levels in terms of week including the model with different means and different dispersions and the model with adaptive means and adaptive dispersions. It also contains percent decreases (PDs) for comparing these models. For 5, 10, and 15 folds, the PDs of 3.78%, 3.11%, and 4.08%, respectively, compared to the model with different means and different non-constant dispersions are distinct (that is, greater than the cutoff 0.48% based on

Table 15.15 Comparison of LCV scores for adaptively generated extended variance models based on week of blood lead level means and dispersions[a]

Model in week			LCV score[b]		
Index	Means	Dispersions	5 folds	10 folds	15 folds
1	Different	Different	0.038606	0.039397	0.038917
2	Adaptive	Adaptive	0.040123	0.040662	0.040572
PD for model 1 versus model 2			3.78%	3.11%	4.08%

LCV likelihood cross-validation; *PD* percent decrease in the LCV score
[a]Computed using extended linear mixed modeling and unstructured correlations
[b]Computed using matched-set-wise deletion

Table 15.16 Power transforms and clock times for adaptively generated extended variance models based on week of blood level means and dispersions[a]

	Number of folds		
	5	10	15
Means[b]	0, −0.19	0, −0.17	0, −0.1981
Dispersions[b]	0, −0.1	0, −0.1	0, −0.13
Clock time (min)	9.7	30.3	35.0

[a]Computed using extended linear mixed modeling, unstructured correlations, and matched-set-wise deletion allowing for unit dispersions

[b]A power of 0 corresponds to an intercept; otherwise, the model has a zero intercept

DF = 1). Consequently, adaptive modeling of means and dispersions provides a distinct improvement for all three numbers of folds.

Table 15.16 provides power transforms for the adaptive models of Table 15.15 generated using the same three numbers of folds. All models have two mean parameters and two dispersion parameters. The largest LCV score for the adaptive models is generated using 10 folds. The 5-fold and 15-fold models have 10-fold LCV scores 0.040663 and 0.040640 with non-distinct PDs 0.01% and 0.05%, respectively. Table 15.16 also contains clock times in minutes for its adaptive models. Clock times for the three numbers of folds require a total of 75.0 min or about 1.3 h.

The contraction used in generating the adaptive models of Tables 15.15–15.16 allowed for the possibility of unit dispersions, but generated dispersions for those models are based on a single transform of visit together with an intercept, indicating that unit dispersions need not be considered further. In any case, the fact that each model has dispersions based on two transforms means that dispersions could not have been based on a single parameter and so unit dispersions could not have been chosen.

Models considered in the section so far have been based on extended variances depending on means and dispersions. Direct variance modeling is considered next using UN correlations as selected above.

Table 15.17 contains LCV scores for alternate numbers of folds for direct variance models for blood lead levels in terms of week with adaptive means and adaptive dispersions. Values are generated for 5, 10, 15, 20, and 25 folds in order to establish that the first local maximum occurs at 20 folds in contrast to the choice of 10 folds for extended variance modeling. Only the first three folds can be compared to extended variance results of Tables 15.15–15.16. Extended variance modeling generates a 10-fold LCV score 0.040662 while direct variance modeling generates a 10-fold LCV score 0.040630 with non-distinct PD 0.08%, indicating that these are competitive alternatives. On the other hand, extended variance modeling generates 5-fold and 15-fold LCV scores 0.040123 and 0.040572 with distinct PD 0.90% and 0.80%, indicating that direct variance modeling generates superior models for these two cases.

Table 15.17 also provides power transforms for its direct variance models using the five alternate numbers of folds. The 10-fold model computed using 20 folds has

Table 15.17 LCV scores, power transforms, and clock times for adaptively generated direct variance models based on week of blood lead level means and dispersions[a]

	Number of folds				
	5	10	15	20	25
LCV score[b]	0.040486	0.040630	0.040900	0.041060	0.040843
Means[c]	0, −5.17, −1.8	0, −0.17	0, −5.18, −1.9	0, −6.18, −1.8	0, −4.18, −1.8
Dispersions[c]	0, −0.07	0, −0.08	0, −0.07	0, −0.08	0, −0.07
Clock time (min)	23.4	39.2	58.2	77.9	88.7

[a]Computed using extended linear mixed modeling and unstructured correlations
[b]Computed using matched-set-wise deletion
[c]A power of 0 corresponds to an intercept; otherwise, the model has a zero intercept

LCV score 0.040686 with distinct PD 0.52% while the 5-fold, 15-fold, and 25-fold models have 20-fold LCV scores 0.040901, 0.041059, and 0.041055 with non-distinct PDs 0.39%, less than 0.01%, and 0.01%, respectively. Consequently, direct variance modeling generates consistent models in most cases and also for large enough numbers of folds, that is, for 15 or more folds.

All five direct variance models have dispersions based on one transform of week with close power values −0.07 or − 0.08 together with an intercept. The 10-fold model for the means is based on only one transform of week plus an intercept while the other four models include one more transform of week. All three extended variance models also have dispersions based on one transform of week with close powers −0.1 or − 0.13 together with an intercept, and so are similar to dispersions for the direct variance models, but generate more complex variances based on both means and dispersions. All three extended variance models also have means based on one transform of week together with an intercept. In contrast, the four direct variance models generating distinctly better LCV scores than the associated extended variance models are based on one more transform of week. In this case, using direct modeling of the variances identifies more complex but also more effective models for the means while generating simpler models for the variances.

Table 15.17 also contains clock times in minutes for the five direct variance models. Clock times increase with the number of folds for a total of 287.4 min or about 4.8 h. The first three of these models require a total of 120.8 min or about 1.6 times as much as the 75.0 min required for the associated extended variance models of Tables 15.15–15.16.

Direct variance modeling generates distinctly better models than extended variance modeling for 5 and 15 folds and a competitive model for 10 folds. Consequently, direct variance modeling is preferable to extended variance modeling for the blood lead level data even though it requires more computation time. For this reason, only direct variance modeling is used in subsequent analyses. While the first local maximum in the LCV score is generated for 20 folds, a consistent model is generated using 15 folds, suggesting that 15 folds could be used in place of 20 folds to reduce computation times. In order to assess this, both 15-fold and 20-fold models are considered in the next stage of the analysis.

As for extended variance modeling, the contraction used in generating the adaptive direct variance models of Table 15.17 allowed for the possibility of unit dispersions, but non-unit dispersions are generated in all three cases, so unit dispersions are not considered in subsequent analyses.

15.4.3 *Additive Models Based on Week and Being on Succimer*

The results of Sect. 15.4.2 indicate that the blood lead level data are appropriately analyzed using UN correlations and direct variance modeling with LCV scores computed using either 15 or 20 folds. This section provides a comparison of adaptive

Table 15.18 Adaptively generated additive direct variance models based on week and being on succimer of blood lead level means and dispersions[a]

Number of folds	LCV score	Mean transforms	Dispersion transforms	Clock time (min)
15	0.044645	1, $\mathrm{week}^{0.04}$	1, succimer, $\mathrm{week}^{-0.1}$	52.2
20	0.044456	1, $\mathrm{week}^{0.03}$	1, succimer, $\mathrm{week}^{-0.1}$	70.1

[a]Computed using extended linear mixed modeling, unstructured correlations, and matched-set-wise deletion. The transform 1 represents an intercept; otherwise, the intercept is zero. The variable succimer represents the indicator for being on the chelating agent succimer

models for means and dispersions in week and the indicator succimer for being on the chelating agent succimer, which are used to further assess the choice of the number of folds.

Table 15.18 provides a comparison of the adaptive additive models for blood lead level means and dispersions using 15-fold and 20-fold LCV scores. For 15 and 20 folds, the additive models have LCV scores 0.044645 and 0.044456, respectively, while the associated models based on only week of Table 15.17 have LCV scores 0.040900 and 0.041060 with distinct PDs of 8.39% and 7.64%. Consequently, both choices for the number of folds support the conclusion that there is an additive effect to being on succimer. Moreover, both models indicate that this additive effect only applies to the dispersions and not to the means.

Dispersion models are the same for the two cases and mean models are very close based on a single transform of week with power values differing only by 0.01. These results suggest that it can be reasonable to base the choice of the number of folds on consistency rather than on having the best LCV score in order to reduce computation times. For these reasons, only 15 folds are used in subsequent analyses of the blood lead level data. In this case, this decision is further supported by a larger LCV score for the smaller number of folds.

Table 15.17 also contains clock times in minutes for its adaptive models. The two models require a total of 122.3 min or about 2.0 h of clock time.

15.4.4 Moderation Model Based on Week and Being on Succimer

The results of Sect. 15.4.3 indicate that the blood lead level data are appropriately analyzed using UN correlations, direct variance modeling, and 15-fold LCV scores. This section provides an assessment of the adaptive moderation model for means and dispersions in week and the indicator succimer for being on the chelating agent succimer.

The generated adaptive moderation model has LCV score 0.049573. As reported in Sect. 15.4.3, the associated additive model has 15-fold LCV score 0.044645 with distinct PD of 9.94% compared to the moderation model. Consequently, succimer

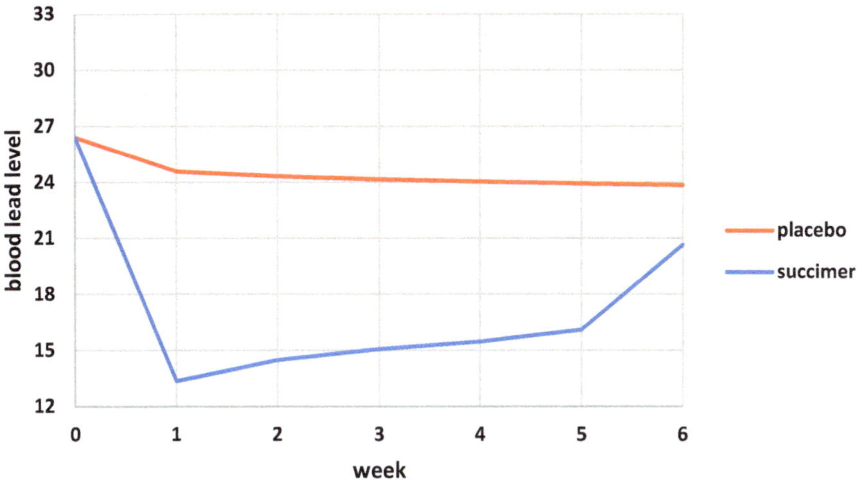

Fig. 15.5 Estimated mean blood level levels in μg/dL over 0–6 weeks under the ELMM model in week, the indicator succimer, and geometric combinations

distinctly moderates the effect of week on blood lead level means and dispersions. This moderation model has means based on an intercept, week$^{0.2}$, and the two geometric combinations

$$\left(\text{succimer} \cdot \text{week}^{-0.29}\right)^{0.8} = \text{succimer} \cdot \text{week}^{-0.232}$$

and

$$\left(\text{succimer} \cdot \text{week}^{12}\right)^{1..1} = \text{succimer} \cdot \text{week}^{13.2}.$$

It has dispersions based on an intercept, the indicator succimer, and the geometric combination

$$\left(\text{week}^{-0.09} \cdot \text{succimer}\right)^{-2.1} = \text{week}^{0.189} \cdot \text{succimer}.$$

Its computation requires 194.4 min or about 3.2 h of clock time.

Figure 15.5 provides the plot of estimated means for blood lead levels over weeks 0–6 based on the above adaptive moderation model. For children on a placebo, mean blood lead levels decrease from 26.4 μg/dL at week 0 to 24.6 μg/dL at week 1 and then continue to decrease gradually to 23.8 μg/dL at week 6. For children on succimer, mean blood lead levels decrease from 26.4 μg/dL at week 0 to lower levels of 13.4 μg/dL at week 1 and then increasing to 20.6 μg/dL at week 6. Figure 15.6 provides the plot of estimated dispersions for blood lead levels over weeks 0–6. For children on a placebo, the estimated dispersions are constant at 22.1 μg/dL

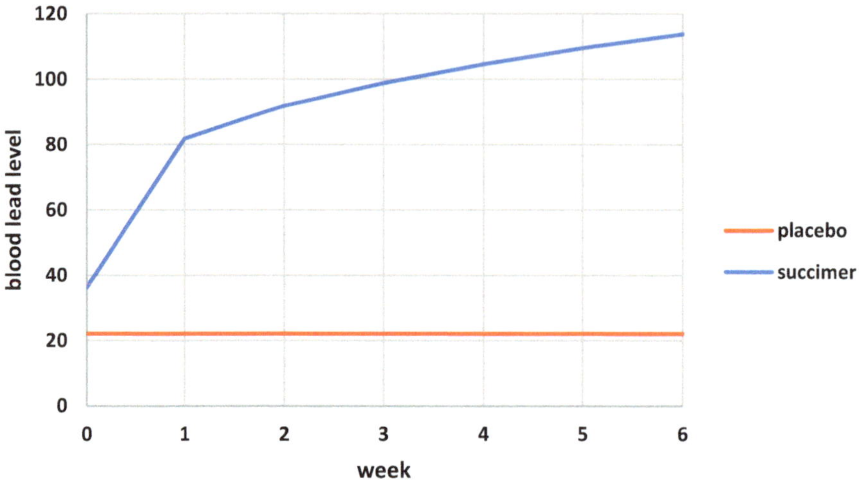

Fig. 15.6 Estimated dispersions for blood lead levels in μg/dL over 0–6 weeks under the ELMM model in week, the indicator succimer, and geometric combinations

at weeks 0–6. On the other hand, for children on succimer, the estimated dispersions increase from 36.2 μg/dL at week 0 to 81.9 μg/dL at week 1, and then continue to increase to 113.8 μg/dL at week 6. Consequently, although post-baseline mean blood lead levels are lower over time for children on succimer, there is much more variability in the post-baseline blood lead levels than for children on a placebo. Estimated UN correlations are not provided, but they are relatively large ranging from 0.66 to 0.82.

The moderation model selected in Chap. 9 for the blood lead level data is based on extended variance modeling and 10-fold LCV scores. Its 15-fold LCV score is 0.049361 with non-distinct PD 0.43% compared to the LCV score of 0.049573 for the moderation model selected in this section. Consequently, they are competitive alternatives. However, a comparison of Figs. 15.5–15.6 to the corresponding Figs. 9.4–9.5 indicates that both models generate similar estimated means in all cases except for week 6 for children on succimer, in which case the estimated mean is much larger at 31.2 μg/dL in Fig. 9.4 compared to 20.6 μg/dL in Fig. 15.6. This difference is compensated for by much larger dispersions for both groups in Fig. 15.6 compared to Fig. 9.5.

15.4.5 Clock Times for Analyses

Clock times for the analyses of Sect. 15.4 include 0.4 min for the models of Table 15.14, 75.0 min for the models of Tables 15.15–15.16, 287.4 min for the direct variance models of Table 15.17, 122.3 min for the additive model of

Table 15.18, and 194.4 min for the moderation models of Sect. 15.4.4. Consequently, analyses of the blood lead level data require 679.5 min or about 11.3 h altogether.

15.5 Analyzing the Trichotomous Respiratory Status Data Using Multinomial/Ordinal Regression

There are 555 trichotomous respiratory status measurements each with three possible outcome values for a total of 1110 effective measurements (Koch et al., 1989; Miller et al., 1993). The cutoff for a distinct percent decrease (PD) in the LCV score is 0.17% using DF = 1 and 0.27% using DF = 2 as needed for multinomial regression. All LCV scores are computed using matched-set-wise deletion since there are no missing dental measurements. To reduce computation times given the large number of effective measurements, LCV scores are only computed using $k = 5$ folds. However, this means that much different results might possibly be generated using larger numbers of folds.

15.5.1 Alternative Correlation Structures

Considering the independent (IND), spatial autoregressive order 1 (AR1), exchangeable (EC), and unstructured (UN) correlation structures, the spatial AR1 correlation structure generates the best LCV score for multinomial regression as reported in Sect. 13.2.1 and for ordinal regression using individual outcomes as reported in Sect. 13.3.1 while the EC correlation structure generates the best LCV score for ordinal regression using cumulative outcomes as reported in Sect. 13.4.1. However, those decisions are based on linear polynomial models for the means in visit with constant dispersions. An approach that considers a more general model while requiring a limited amount of computation time is desirable for handling general data sets with possibly different distributions and possibly large numbers of measurements. One possible choice for such a model is the one with different means for different measurement conditions, in this case, different visits, while assuming constant dispersions. The model for the means is generated using an intercept plus indicators for each of the 4 non-zero visits.

Table 15.19 provides 5-fold LCV scores for this model computed using each of the IND, spatial AR1, EC, and UN correlation structures and each of the modeling methods multinomial regression, ordinal regression using individual outcomes, and ordinal regression using cumulative outcomes. For the four correlation structures, spatial AR1 generates the best LCV score 0.64587 for multinomial regression and 0.65079 for ordinal regression using individual outcomes. These LCV scores are comparable because they are based on the same likelihood function for the individual outcomes. Consequently, ordinal regression using individual outcomes is

Table 15.19 LCV scores using alternative correlation structures and probability types for the trichotomous respiratory status levels[a]

Correlation structure	5-fold LCV score[b]		
	Multinomial regression	Ordinal regression with individual outcomes	Ordinal regression with cumulative outcomes
IND	0.58685	0.58622	0.58622
AR1	0.64587	0.65079	0.64546
EC	0.64501	0.64212	0.64772
UN	0.63752	0.63268	0.63192

AR1 spatial autoregressive order 1; *EC* exchangeable correlations; *IND* independent; *LCV* likelihood cross-validation; *UN* unstructured

[a]Using extended variance models assuming different means for different visits and assuming constant dispersions and computed using extended linear mixed modeling

[b]Computed using matched-set-wise deletion

preferable to multinomial regression since it generates the larger LCV score. It is also simpler with 2 intercept and 4 slope parameters for the means compared to 2 intercept and 8 slope parameters for multinomial regression. On the other hand, EC generates the best LCV score 0.64772 for ordinal regression using cumulative outcomes. This LCV score is not comparable to LCV scores for multinomial regression and ordinal regression using individual outcomes since it is based on a different likelihood, the one for cumulative rather than individual outcomes. Consequently, ordinal regression using individual outcomes with spatial AR1 correlations along with ordinal regression using cumulative outcomes with EC correlations are used in subsequent analyses. The four models of Table 15.19 for multinomial regression require 29.0 min compared to 12.2 min for ordinal regression using individual outcomes and 15.5 min for ordinal regression using cumulative outcomes, and so ordinal regression using individual outcomes requires the least amount of time for these analyses. The total clock time is 51.7 min or about 0.9 h.

15.5.2 Models Based on Visit

The adaptive ordinal regression model using individual outcomes for means and dispersions starting with constant dispersions and allowing for unit dispersions is based on $\text{visit}^{-0.49}$ with an intercept along with dispersions based on $\text{visit}^{0.6}$ without an intercept and LCV score 0.65539 while requiring 396.8 min or about 6.6 h. The associated adaptive model for the means with constant dispersions of Sect. 13.3.2 has LCV score 0.65302 with distinct PD 0.36%, indicating that dispersions are distinctly non-constant in visit. On the other hand, the adaptive ordinal regression model using cumulative outcomes for means and dispersions starting with constant dispersions and allowing for unit dispersions means is based on $\text{visit}^{-0.2}$ with an intercept along with unit dispersions and LCV score 0.64891 while requiring

94.0 min or about 1.6 h. This LCV score is a little larger than the LCV score 0.64888 for the constant dispersion model as reported in Sect. 13.4.2, indicating that in this case unit dispersions are reasonably assumed to hold.

Adaptive ordinal regression models based on individual and cumulative outcomes are based on different likelihoods and so their LCV scores are not comparable. In this case, they are also based on different correlation structures with different conclusions about the dispersions. However, the models they generate for the means are similar based on an intercept and a transform of visit. Moreover, clock time for the individual outcomes model is about 4.2 times more than for cumulative outcomes. For these reasons, only ordinal regression using cumulative outcomes is considered in subsequent analyses in order to reduce computation times. As justified above for that case, only unit dispersions are considered as well.

15.5.3 Models Based on Visit and Being on Active Treatment

Models reported in this section are based on ordinal regression using cumulative outcomes and unit dispersions. The adaptive additive model in visit and active has means based on the transform $\text{visit}^{-0.3}$ and the indicator active with an intercept, LCV score 0.65681, and clock time 11.2 min or about 0.2 h. The adaptive moderation model in visit, active, and geometric combinations has means based on an intercept and the geometric combination

$$\left(\text{active} \cdot \text{visit}^3\right)^{-0.06} = \text{active} \cdot \text{visit}^{-0.18}.$$

The LCV score is 0.65987 so that the adaptive additive model generates the distinct PD 0.46%. Consequently, the effect of visit on mean trichotomous respiratory status is distinctly moderated by being on active treatment. Estimated EC correlations for this model rounded to two decimal digits are $r_{\text{AR1},0,0} = 0.37$, $r_{\text{AR1},0.1} = 0.24$, $r_{\text{AR1},1,0} = 0.23$, and $r_{\text{AR1},1,1} = 0.42$ (and so are close to symmetric). Clock time for the adaptive moderation model is 164.8 min or about 2.4 h. These are the same models generated in Sect. 13.4.5.

Figures 15.7–15.8 provide the plots of estimated probabilities for the three respiratory status levels for patients on a placebo and on active treatment, respectively. For patients on a placebo, the probabilities of all three respiratory status levels are constant over visits 0–4 at 0.24 for a 0:poor respiratory status level, 0.54 for a 1: good respiratory status level, and 0.22 for a 2:excellent respiratory status level. On the other hand, for patients on active treatment, probabilities start at visit 0 at the same values for patients on a placebo. The probability of a 0:poor respiratory status level then decreases to 0.09 at visit 1 and increases a little to 0.11 by visit 4. The probability of a 1:good respiratory status level then decreases to 0.44 at visit 1 and increases a little to 0.47 by visit 4. The probability of a 2:excellent respiratory status level then increases to 0.47 at visit 1 and decreases to 0.41 by visit 4. Consequently,

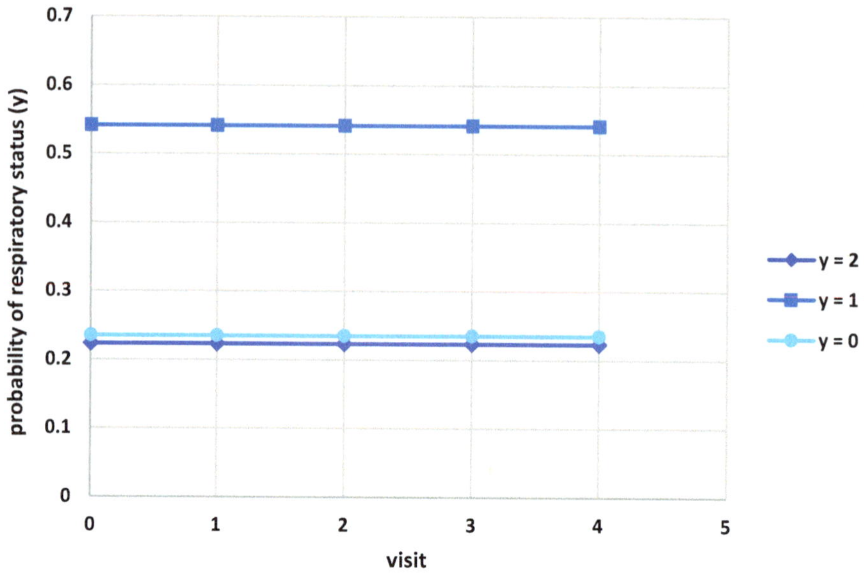

Fig. 15.7 Estimated probabilities for respiratory status levels using ordinal regression with cumulative outcomes for patients on a placebo

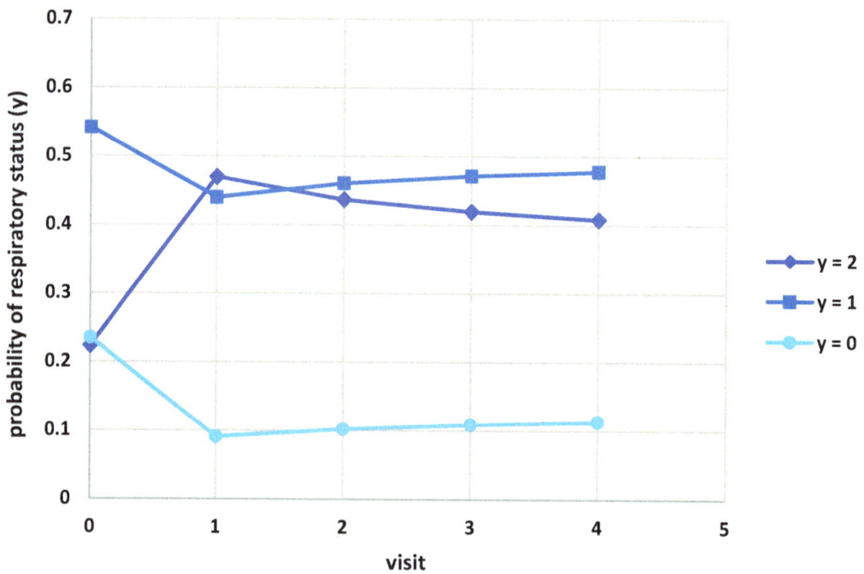

Fig. 15.8 Estimated probabilities for respiratory status levels using ordinal regression with cumulative outcomes for patients on active treatment

being on active treatment increases the probability of having excellent respiratory status while decreasing the probabilities of having lower respiratory status levels.

15.5.4 Clock Times for Analyses

Clock times for the analyses of Sect. 15.5 include 51.7 min for the models of Table 15.19, 490.8 min for the two adaptive models of Sect. 15.5.2, and 176.0 min for the two models of Sect. 15.5.3. Consequently, multinomial and ordinal regression analyses of the trichotomous respiratory status data require altogether 718.5 min or about 12.0 h of clock time.

15.6 Analyzing the Trichotomous Respiratory Status Data Using Discrete Regression

There are 555 trichotomous respiratory status levels (Koch et al., 1989; Miller et al., 1993). The cutoff for a distinct percent decrease (PD) in the LCV score using DF = 1 is 0.35% while it is 0.54% for DF = 2 as needed for multinomial probability models. All LCV scores are computed using matched-set-wise deletion since there are no missing trichotomous respiratory status levels. Models reported in this section are based on extended variances determined by dispersions combined with probabilities unless explicitly specified to be based on direct variance modeling determined entirely by dispersions. Analyses are conducted using discrete regression.

15.6.1 Alternative Correlation Structures

As reported in Sects. 14.1.1, 14.2.1, and 14.3.1 for multinomial probabilities, ordinal probabilities, and censored Poisson probabilities, the unstructured (UN) correlation structure generates the best LCV scores using ELMM for 5, 10, and 15 folds compared to independent (IND), spatial autoregressive order 1 (AR1), and exchangeable (EC) correlation structures. However, that decision is based on adaptive models for the probabilities in visit with constant dispersions. An approach that considers a more general model while requiring a limited amount of computation time is desirable for handling general data sets with possibly different distributions and possibly large numbers of measurements. One possible choice for such a model is the one with different probabilities and different dispersions for different measurement conditions, in this case, different visits.

Table 15.20 provides LCV scores for this model computed using 5, 10, and 15 folds for each of the IND, spatial AR1, EC, and UN correlation structures and

Table 15.20 LCV scores using alternative probability types, correlation structures, and numbers of folds for the trichotomous respiratory status levels[a]

Probability type	Correlation structure	LCV score[b]		
		5 folds	10 folds	15 folds
Multinomial	IND	0.35053	0.35028	0.35036
	AR1	0.41559	0.41641	0.41700
	EC	0.41325	0.41281	0.41370
	UN	0.42268	0.42306	0.42348
Ordinal	IND	0.35051	0.35028	0.35036
	AR1	0.41559	0.41641	0.41700
	EC	0.41325	0.41281	0.41370
	UN	0.42264	0.42306	0.42348
Censored Poisson	IND	0.35053	0.35028	0.35036
	AR1	0.41559	0.41641	0.41700
	EC	0.41325	0.41281	0.41370
	UN	0.42268	0.42306	0.42348

AR1 spatial autoregressive order 1; *EC* exchangeable correlations; *IND* independent; *LCV* likelihood cross-validation; *UN* unstructured

[a]Using extended variance models based on different probabilities and different dispersions for different visits and computed using extended linear mixed modeling

[b]Computed using matched-set-wise deletion

each of the multinomial, ordinal, and censored Poisson probability types. For multinomial and censored Poisson probabilities, LCV scores are all the same as each other for each of the 12 cases of three numbers of folds and four correlation structure while LCV scores for ordinal probabilities agree with LCV scores for the other two types of probabilities in all but two cases, but only differ in the fifth decimal digit for those two cases. For all three numbers of folds, UN generates the best LCV score over the four correlation structures. There are $5 \cdot 4/2 = 10$ UN correlation parameters. Spatial AR1 generates the next largest LCV score but using 9 less correlation parameters. However, using ordinal probability models, the LCV scores for the spatial AR1 models generate PDs 1.67%, 1.57%, and 1.53% for 5, 10, and 15 folds, respectively, which are greater than the cutoff of 1.51% for DF = 9. Corresponding PDs for the other two probability types are 1.68%, 1.57%, and 1.53%. Consequently, only UN correlations are used in subsequent analyses. The models of Table 15.5 require 1.0 min for multinomial probabilities, 0.7 min for ordinal probabilities, and 0.6 min for ordinal probabilities for a total of 2.3 min.

15.6.2 Models Based on Visit

Table 15.21 contains LCV scores of the same three numbers of folds and three probability types as in Table 15.20 for models of trichotomous respiratory status levels in terms of visit with adaptive probabilities, adaptive non-constant

Table 15.21 LCV scores, power transforms, and clock times for adaptively generated extended variance models based on visit of trichotomous respiratory status means and dispersions[a]

Probability type		Number of folds		
		5	10	15
	LCV score	0.42605	0.42553	0.42640
Multinomial	Means[b]	−0.2	−0.26	−0.28
	Dispersions[b]	0, −1	0	0
	Clock time (min)	20.2	25.7	51.1
	LCV score	0.42620	0.42492	0.42604
Ordinal	Means[b]	−0.11	0, 0.4	0, −0.39
	Dispersions[b]	0, 1.2	0, 1.1	0, 0.9
	Clock time (min)	39.0	20.9	30.4
	LCV score	0.42672	0.42691	0.42696
Censored Poisson	Means[b]	−0.2	−0.1	−0.2
	Dispersions[b]	0, 1.3	0, 1.1	0, 1
	Clock time (min)	9.1	15.1	24.8

[a]Computed using extended linear mixed modeling, unstructured correlations, and matched-set-wise deletion with contraction allowing for unit dispersions
[b]A power of 0 corresponds to an intercept; otherwise, the model has a zero intercept

dispersions, and UN correlations. For all three numbers of folds, censored Poisson probabilities generate the best LCV scores, supporting their use instead of the other two probability types. For each of the three models of Table 15.11, the largest LCV score is achieved with 15 folds. Table 15.21 also provides power transforms of visit for probabilities and dispersions. Similar multinomial probability models are generated for 10 and 15 folds as is also the case for ordinal probability models while similar censored Poisson probability models are generated for 5, 10, and 15 folds.

Table 15.21 also provides clock times. The multinomial probability models require a total of 97.0 min or about 1.6 h, ordinal probability models require a total of 90.3 min or about 1.5 h, and censored Poisson probability models require a total of 49.0 min or about 0.8 h, and so altogether 236.3 min or about 3.9 h. Censored Poisson probabilities require less total time with multinomial probability models requiring about 2.0 as much time and ordinal probability models about 1.8 as much time. Consequently, censored Poisson probabilities generate better LCV scores, relatively consistent models for different numbers of folds, and require less time, and so only censored Poisson probabilities are used in subsequent analyses.

Models considered in the section so far have been based on extended variances depending on probabilities and dispersions. Direct variance modeling is considered next using UN correlations as selected above.

Table 15.22 contains LCV scores of the same three numbers of folds as in Table 15.21 for three alternative direct variance models for trichotomous respiratory status in terms of visit with adaptive censored Poisson probabilities and adaptive dispersions. Table 15.22 also provides power transforms for its direct variance models. All three models have probabilities and dispersions each based on one transform of visit without an intercept. LCV scores for 5, 10, and 15 folds are

Table 15.22 LCV scores, power transforms, and clock times for adaptively generated direct variance models based on visit of trichotomous respiratory status probabilities and dispersions[a]

	Number of folds		
	5	10	15
LCV score[b]	0.39578	0.39616	0.39799
Means[c]	−0.24	0	−0.3
Dispersions[c]	6.4	3.501	4.1002
Clock time (min)	22.6	35.6	66.5

[a]Computed using extended linear mixed modeling, unstructured correlations, and censored Poisson probabilities with contraction allowing for unit dispersions

[b]Computed using matched-set-wise deletion

[c]A power of 0 corresponds to an intercept; otherwise, the model has a zero intercept

0.39578, 0.39616, and 0.39799 with distinct PDs 7.25%, 7.20%, and 6.79%, respectively, compared to associated extended variance models of Table 15.21. Consequently, extended variance modeling distinctly outperforms direct variance modeling in this case, and so only extended variance models are considered in subsequent analyses.

Table 15.22 also contains clock times in minutes for the direct variance models of Table 15.8. Clock times increase with the number of folds for a total of 124.7 min or about 2.1 h. In contrast, the associated models of Table 15.21 require a total of 49.0 min so that direct variance modeling requires about 2.5 times as much. Consequently, in this case extended variance modeling requires less computation time, further supporting its use over direct variance modeling.

The largest LCV score for the extended variance models based on censored Poisson probabilities of Table 15.21 is 0.42696 for 15 folds. The associated model generated using 20 folds has smaller 20-fold LCV score 0.42695 so that the 15-fold LCV score is the first local maximum. The 20-fold model has probabilities based on $\text{visit}^{-0.1}$ without an intercept and dispersions based on untransformed visit with an intercept, and so is similar to the 15-fold model. The 20-fold model requires 30.9 min. Subsequent models are based on LCV score computed with 15 folds.

15.6.3 Models Based on Visit and Treatment Group

The results of Sect. 15.6.2 indicate that the trichotomous respiratory status data are appropriately analyzed using UN correlations, censored Poisson probabilities, and extended variance models with LCV scores computed using 15 folds. This section provides a comparison of adaptive models for probabilities in visit and the indicator active for being on active treatment based on these modeling choices.

Table 15.23 provides a comparison of adaptively generated models for trichotomous respiratory status probabilities and dispersions. The adaptive additive model has probabilities based on the transform $\text{visit}^{-0.2}$ and the indicator active, supporting

Table 15.23 Adaptively generated extended variance models based on visit and treatment group of trichotomous respiratory status probabilities and dispersions[a]

Model type	15-fold LCV score	Probability transforms[b]	Dispersion transforms[b]	Clock time (min)
Additive	0.42702	$\text{visit}^{-0.2}$, active	1	50.5
Moderation	0.43238	visit^{-7}, $(\text{visit}^{-3} \cdot \text{active})^{0.5}$, $(\text{active} \cdot \text{visit})^{-1}$	1, $\text{visit}^{1.5}$	461.0

[a]Computed using extended linear mixed modeling, unstructured correlations, censored Poisson probabilities, and matched-set-wise deletion
[b]A value of 1 represents an intercept; otherwise, the intercept is zero. Active represents the indicator for being on active treatment

an additive effect on the probabilities to being on active treatment, along with constant dispersions. On the other hand, the adaptive moderation model has probabilities based on the two geometric combinations

$$\left(\text{visit}^{-3} \cdot \text{active}\right)^{0.5} = \text{visit}^{-1.5} \cdot \text{active}$$

and

$$(\text{active} \cdot \text{visit})^{-1} = \text{active} \cdot \text{visit}^{-1}$$

as well as the transform visit^{-7} without an intercept while the dispersions are based on the transform $\text{visit}^{1.5}$ with an intercept. The LCV score for the moderation model is 0.43238 while the additive model has LCV score 0.42702 with distinct PD 1.24%, indicating that being on active treatment distinctly moderates the effect of visit on the trichotomous respiratory status probabilities. The same moderation model is generated in Sect. 14.3.7. The two models of Table 15.22 require a total of 511.5 min of clock time or about 8.5 h.

Estimated means for the moderation model are plotted in Fig. 15.9. For patients on a placebo, estimated mean trichotomous respiratory status is 0.9 at visit 0, increases to 1.1 at visit 1 and then decreases to 0.9 at visit 2 and remains at 0.9 for visits 3–4. For patients on active treatment, estimated mean trichotomous respiratory status is 0.9 at visit 0, the same as for patients on a placebo, and then increases to 1.0 at visit 1, then to 1.4 at visit 2 and then decreases to 1.3 by visit 4. Figure 15.10 contains the plot of estimated dispersions for trichotomous respiratory status. Estimated dispersions increase nonlinearly from 0.6 at visit 0 gradually to 2.3 by visit 3 and then quickly to 13.9 by visit 4 and are the same for patients on a placebo and patients on active treatment.

Figures 15.11–15.12 provide plots of probabilities for trichotomous respiratory status levels 0–2 (that is, 0:poor, 1:good, and 2:excellent) using the moderation model for patients on a placebo and patients on active treatment, respectively. For patients on a placebo, probabilities for 0:poor respiratory status are constant at 0.37 over visits 0 and 2–4 with lower probability 0.28 at visit 1, for 1:good respiratory status are close to constant at 0.36–0.37 over visits 0–4, and for 2:excellent

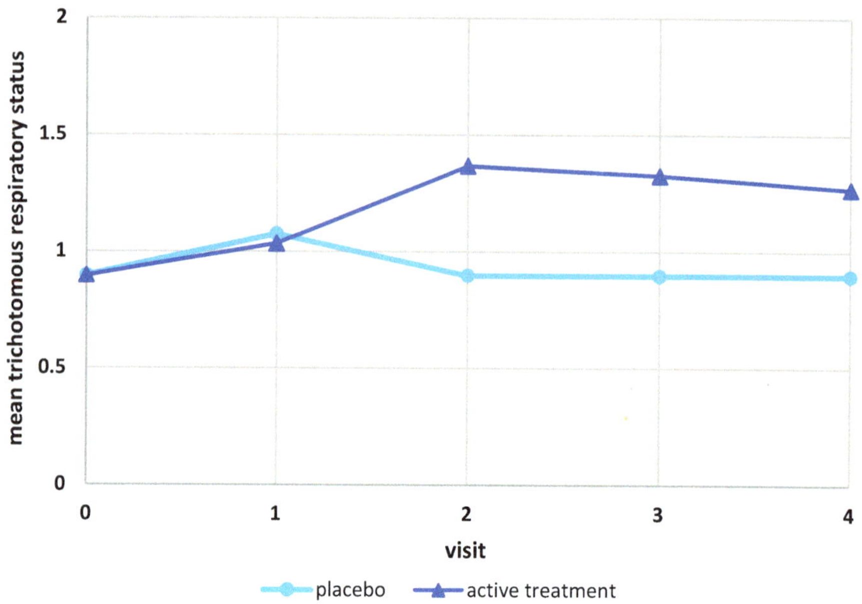

Fig. 15.9 Estimated means for trichotomous respiratory status under the discrete regression model of censored Poisson probabilities and dispersions in terms of visits and the indicator for being on active treatment using ELMM

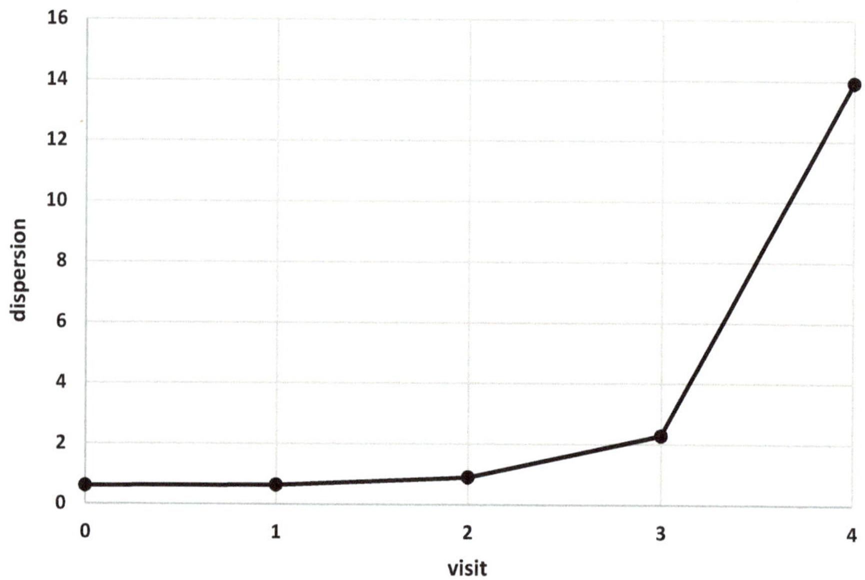

Fig. 15.10 Estimated dispersions for trichotomous respiratory status over visits 0–4 under the discrete regression moderation model of censored Poisson probabilities and dispersions using ELMM

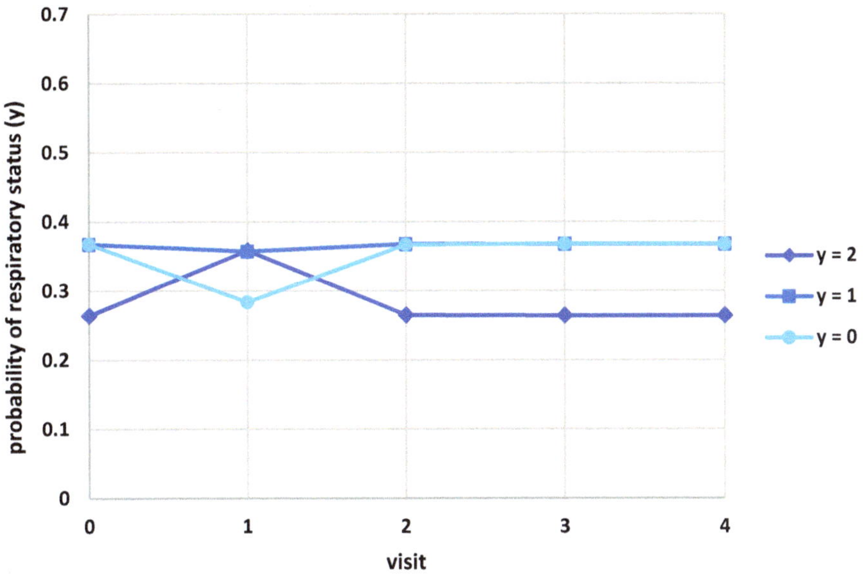

Fig. 15.11 Estimated censored Poisson probabilities for trichotomous respiratory status over visits 0–4 under the discrete regression moderation model in visit for patients on a placebo using ELMM

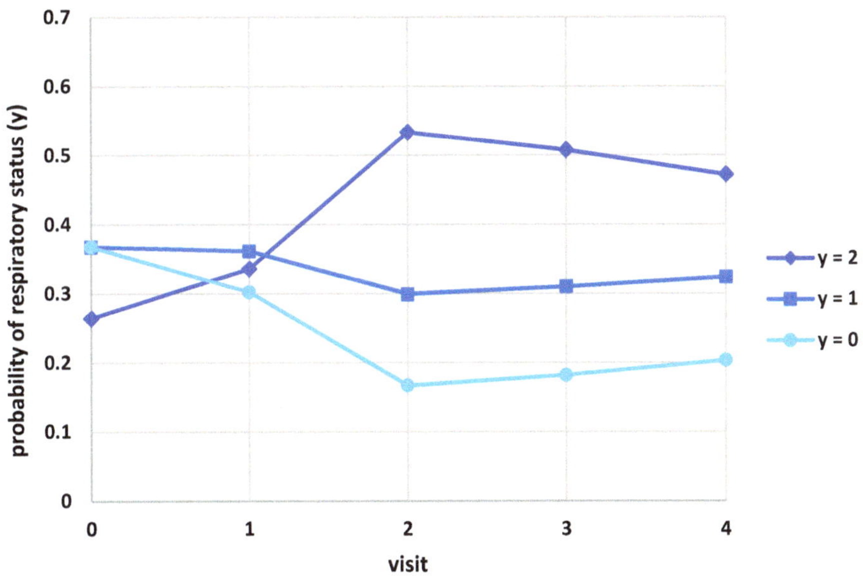

Fig. 15.12 Estimated censored Poisson probabilities for trichotomous respiratory status over visits 0–4 under the discrete regression moderation model in visit for patients on active treatment using ELMM

respiratory status are 0.26 at visit 0, increase to 0.36 at visit 1, then decrease to 0.26 at visit 2 and remain there to visit 4. For patients on active treatment, probabilities for 0:poor respiratory status decrease from 0.37 at visit 0 to 0.17 at visit 2 and then increase to 0.20 at visit 4, for 1:good respiratory status decrease from 0.37 at visit 0 to 0.30 at visit 2 and then increase to 0.32 at visit 4, and for 2:excellent respiratory status increase from 0.26 at visit 0 to 0.53 at visit 2 and then decrease to 0.47 at visit 4.

15.6.4 Clock Times for Analyses

Clock times for the analyses of Sect. 15.6 include 2.3 min for the models of Table 15.20, 236.3 min for the models of Table 15.21, 30.9 min for the associated 20-fold model of Sect. 15.6.2, 124.7 min for the direct variance models of Table 15.12, and 511.5 min for the models of Table 15.23. Consequently, analyses of the trichotomous respiratory status data using discrete regression require 905.7 min or about 15.1 h altogether.

15.6.5 Comparison of Discrete Regression to Multinomial/Ordinal Regression

Multinomial regression and ordinal regression analyses of Sect. 15.5 and discrete regression analyses of Sect. 15.6 use the same trichotomous respiratory status outcome. However, LCV scores for these two types of analyses are based on different likelihoods and so are not comparable. Estimated probabilities for the moderation model generated by ordinal regression using cumulative outcomes are displayed in Figs. 15.7–15.8 while estimated censored Poisson probabilities generated by discrete regression are displayed in Figs. 15.11–15.12. While both analyses identify a moderation effect, that effect is quite different for the two cases although both models identify that being on active treatment tends to increase the post-baseline chance of having 2:excellent respiratory status level compared to the chance of having the other two respiratory status levels.

The multinomial/ordinal regression analyses require 12.0 h compared to 15.1 h for the discrete regression analyses. However, only 5-fold LCV scores are considered in the multinomial/ordinal regression analyses while the discrete regression analyses consider LCV scores based on 5, 10, 15, and 20 folds. A consideration of alternative numbers of folds for multinomial/ordinal regression analyses could require substantially more clock time, especially if a number of folds larger than 5 is identified as more appropriate to use in such analyses.

LCV scores for ordinal regression using cumulative outcomes are not comparable to LCV scores for multinomial regression and ordinal regression using individual outcomes so that the choice between these three alternatives cannot be based on objective considerations. In contrast, discrete regression has the advantage that LCV scores for multinomial, ordinal, and censored Poisson probabilities are comparable allowing for an objective choice between these three alternatives.

Standardized residuals for the moderation models generated by ordinal regression using cumulative outcomes and by censored Poisson probabilities are not displayed here (but see Figs. 13.6–13.7 and 14.16). The ordinal regression model using cumulative outcomes generates eight outlying observations with value outside of ± 3 compared to only one outlying observation for censored Poisson model, indicating that the censored Poisson model provides a better fit to the trichotomous respiratory status data.

In summary, multinomial/ordinal regression requires less time than discrete regression, but a full assessment of the impact of the number of folds is not addressed in multinomial/ordinal regression analyses, which could require longer times than for discrete regression. Results for the three multinomial/ordinal regression alternatives cannot be compared objectively using LCV scores while the three discrete regression alternatives can be. Also, discrete regression provides in this case for a better fit to the data than multinomial/ordinal regression. Consequently, discrete regression seems the preferable choice for analyzing the trichotomous respiratory status data.

15.7 Overview of Analysis Results

Child age has an effect on the 108 dental measurements that is moderated by child gender using models based on linear regression, 10-fold LCV scores, and EC correlations while requiring 10.5 min (see Fig. 15.1). Visit has an effect on the 295 epilepsy seizure rates, but being in the intervention group does not have an additive or a moderation effect using models based on Poisson regression, 5-fold LCV scores, direct variance modeling, and EC correlations while requiring 37.2 min (see Fig. 15.2). Visit has an effect on the 555 dichotomous respiratory status levels that is moderated by being on active treatment using models based on logistic regression, 10-fold LCV scores, unit dispersions, and EC correlations while requiring 13.5 min (see Figs. 15.3–15.4). Week has an effect on the 400 blood lead levels that is moderated by being on the chelating agent succimer using models based on exponential regression, 15-fold LCV scores, direct variance modeling, and UN correlations while requiring 11.3 h (see Figs. 15.5–15.6). Visit has an effect on the 555 trichotomous respiratory status levels recoded as 1110 dichotomous measurements that is moderated by being on active treatment using models based on ordinal regression with cumulative outcomes, 5-fold LCV scores, unit dispersions, and spatial AR1 correlations while requiring 12.0 h (see Figs. 15.7–15.8). Visit has an effect on the 555 trichotomous respiratory status levels that is moderated by being on active treatment using models based on discrete regression, censored Poisson probabilities, 15-fold LCV scores, extended variance modeling, and UN correlations while requiring 15.1 h (see Figs. 15.9–15.12).

Computation time increases with the number of (effective) measurements, the number of folds used to compute LCV scores, and when UN correlations are more appropriate to use than the other correlation structures. Analyses of the trichotomous respiratory status levels require more time using discrete regression than using multinomial/ordinal regression, but the discrete regression analyses provide a much more complete assessment of those data and a better fit. Consequently, discrete regression seems preferable to use instead of multinomial/ordinal regression. Multinomial regression can require excessive times (as reported in Chap. 13), and so it seems reasonable not to consider that method in general for analyzing correlated multivariate outcomes, using only ordinal regression instead.

The spatial AR1, EC, and UN correlation structures are each selected in one or more of the reported analyses, indicating the need in general to consider all of these alternatives. Although IND correlations are not selected in the reported analyses, the extra computation time to compute such models can be negligible. Consideration of unit dispersions is important to consider, but may only be needed when outcomes are dichotomous as for logistic, multinomial, and ordinal regression. Consideration of direct variance modeling can also be important to consider.

15.8 Strategies for Analyzing Correlated Outcomes

Strategies are provided in this section as a series of steps for conducting adaptive analyses of correlated outcomes based on the results of analyses reported in Sects. 15.1–15.6. These adaptive analysis strategies generate effective adaptive models, but might need adjustment in some cases due to extraordinary circumstances.

1. The modeling approach

Use ELMM to conduct adaptive analyses of correlated outcomes rather than partially or fully modified GEE. One exception is that fully modified GEE can be used instead of ELMM in analyzing correlated polytomous outcomes recoded as multivariate dichotomous outcomes using UN correlations in order to substantially reduce computation times. Maximum likelihood estimation of the large number of UN correlation parameters can require longer computation times than the GEE approach for estimating those correlation parameters. Generalized linear mixed modeling is another alternative for modeling correlated outcomes, but this is currently only appropriate to use with theory-based models since adaptive generalized linear mixed modeling methods still need development.

Use extended variance modeling to start with and change to direct variance modeling when appropriate as addressed in Strategy Step 7.

2. Computing LCV scores

Use measurement-wise deletion for data with some matched sets having missing measurements (i.e., less than the maximum number m of measurements), for data having only 1 matched set, and for data having a small number n of matched sets (not clear what constitutes a small number of matched sets). Otherwise, use matched-set-wise deletion.

3. Choosing the correlation structure

Consider the IND, spatial AR1, EC, and UN correlation structures for most analyses. IND correlations can be dropped to reduce computation time and only considered when EC or AR1 correlations are chosen with a small estimate of the correlation parameter (not clear what constitutes a small estimate), but can be considered in any case without much effect on computation times. Spatial AR1 can only be considered when measurements within matched sets are ordered, for example, when the conditions correspond to times or dosages. When matched sets correspond to classes of individuals, or of other types of entities, of varying sizes, for example, patients of the same provider, nurses working on the same hospital unit, or children in the same classroom, only the IND and EC correlation structures should usually be considered. In such cases, the constant correlation is commonly called the intra-class correlation. The UN correlation structure in this case seems only reasonable to consider when the maximum number m of within measurements for matched sets is small (not clear what constitutes a small maximum number of measurements), but that number is likely not to be small in most cases. When the measurement conditions are ordered and the number of conditions is large (not clear what constitutes large enough), the same correlation for each distance apart as assumed with EC correlations is unlikely to hold and AR1 correlations are more likely to be preferable. UN correlations are also impractical for large enough numbers m of measurement conditions since the number of correlation parameters equals $m \cdot (m - 1)/2$. For example, when $m = 5$, there are 10 correlation parameters which seems reasonable. However, an increase of 1 unit to $m = 6$ results in a 50% increase in the number of correlation parameters to 15, which may be unacceptably large.

Selection of a correlation structure to use in subsequent analyses can be based on LCV scores for models based on different means/probabilities and different variances/dispersions for different measurement conditions and computed using alternative correlation structures and 5, 10, and 15 folds. See also Strategy Step 5.

When UN correlations generate the largest overall k-fold LCV score, compare that LCV score to the better of the two k-fold LCV scores for spatial AR1 and EC correlations (or only EC when spatial AR1 is not under consideration) using an LCV ratio test. When the numbers of the non-correlation parameters are the same, base the cutoff on $\text{DF} = m \cdot (m - 1)/2 - 1$ degrees of freedom. Adjust this DF appropriately when the numbers of non-correlation parameters differ. When the percent decrease (PD) is greater than this cutoff, the extra number of correlation parameters provides a distinct improvement, and so it is reasonable to use UN correlations in subsequent analyses. Otherwise, the correlation structure generating the second largest LCV score provides a competitive alternative and can be used instead of UN correlations to reduce computation times. This reduction in computation times can be substantial. In the unusual case with the IND correlation structure generating a better LCV score than both the spatial AR1 and EC correlation structures, the above assessment of the UN structure can be conducted using 1 more degree of freedom.

A general approach for selecting the correlation structure would be to choose the least complex correlation structure with a competitive LCV score. Treat the IND, EC, AR1, and UN correlation structures as increasingly complex with associated numbers of correlation parameters of 0, 1, 1, and $m \cdot (m - 1)/2$, respectively. If UN generates the largest LCV score, compare it to the IND, EC, and AR1 correlation structures in that order using DF set to $m \cdot (m - 1)/2$, $m \cdot (m - 1)/2 - 1$, and $m \cdot (m - 1)/2 - 1$, respectively. Use the simplest of these three correlation structures generating a competitive LCV score, if any, in subsequent analyses. Otherwise, use the UN correlation structure. Next if AR1 generates the largest LCV score, compare it to the IND and EC correlation structures in that order using DF set to 1 and 1, respectively. Use the simplest of these two correlation structures generating a competitive LCV score, if any, in subsequent analyses. Otherwise, use the AR1 correlation structure. Next, if EC generates the largest LCV score, compare it to the IND correlation structure using DF set to 1. Use IND in subsequent analyses if it generates a competitive LCV score. Otherwise, use the EC correlation structure. Finally, if IND generates the largest LCV score, use it in subsequent analyses.

For polytomous outcomes, the assessment of the correlation structure needs also to consider multiple modeling methods. When recoded as multiple dichotomous outcomes, consider results for multinomial regression, ordinal regression using individual outcomes, and ordinal regression using cumulative outcomes. When analyzed as discrete outcomes, consider results for multinomial, ordinal, and censored Poisson probabilities. When multinomial regression generates a better LCV score than ordinal regression using individual outcomes, an LCV ratio test can be used to assess whether the better LCV score for multinomial regression provides a distinct improvement; if not, ordinal regression using individual outcomes is preferable. However, LCV scores for ordinal regression using cumulative outcomes are based on a different likelihood and so are not appropriately compared to LCV scores for multinomial regression and ordinal regression using individual outcomes. A subjective comparison is required (see Sects. 13.4.5 and 15.5.1). For discrete regression, an LCV ratio test can be used to assess whether a probability type with fewer probability parameters and a smaller LCV score is a preferable alternative to one with more probability parameters and a larger LCV score. LCV scores for discrete regression models based on multinomial, ordinal, and censored Poisson probabilities are appropriately compared.

4. Choosing the number of folds for computing LCV scores

Use LCV scores for models based on adaptive means/probabilities and adaptive variances/dispersions for different measurement conditions, possibly adjusted as in Strategy Step 5, and with LCV scores computed using 5, 10, and 15 folds to select the number of folds to use in subsequent analyses. If 5 or 10 folds generates the best of the three LCV scores, use that number of folds in subsequent analyses. If 15 folds generates the largest LCV score, compute LCV scores for larger multiples of 5 folds until the first local maximum is identified and use that number of folds in subsequent analyses. Results for associated models with different means/probabilities and different variances/dispersions are available from the assessment of the correlation structure and so can be used for further assessment of the impact of the number of folds. Increased support for the choice of the number of folds based on the adaptive model is provided when the same maximum over 5, 10, and 15 folds also occurs for the model with different means/probabilities and different variances/dispersions. However, in cases where the maximum occurs at different numbers of folds for the two models, the results for the adaptive model are more appropriate to use in setting the number of folds.

It is also important that models generated using different folds generate consistent models in the sense that models generated with numbers of folds other than the number *k* generating the best LCV score are competitive alternatives to the model generated using *k* folds. Assess this using *k*-fold LCV scores for the models generated by the other numbers of folds. In cases where models are not consistent, continue assessing the impact of the number of folds using adaptive additive models based on adding another available predictor (an example is provided in the analyses of Sect. 15.4). In cases where models are consistent, a value for the number of folds smaller than the number *k* can be used instead of *k* to reduce computation times. This is especially important for cases where the UN correlation structure has been chosen.

When UN correlations are selected in Strategy Step 3, the next best correlation structure (EC or AR1) might still provide a reasonable alternative requiring less computation time. This can be assessed by comparing the adaptive models for the means/probabilities and variances/dispersions using these two correlation structures generated using the number of folds selected using the UN correlation structure. If these two models are very similar except for the correlation parameters, the simple correlation structure using that number of folds could provide an acceptable, more efficient alternative to UN correlations.

For polytomous outcomes, the assessment of the number of folds needs also to consider multiple modeling methods. When recoded as multiple dichotomous outcomes, consider results for multinomial regression, ordinal regression using individual outcomes, and ordinal regression using cumulative outcomes. The analyses used to determine the correlation structure can be used for these purposes to reduce the computation times. When analyzed as discrete outcomes, consider results for multinomial, ordinal, and censored Poisson probabilities. Use the results of these analyses to choose between these modeling methods to use in subsequent analyses. Objective comparison of results for different probability types is possible for discrete regression modeling, but not for all multinomial/ordinal regression modeling approaches (see Strategy Step 3), and so only discrete regression modeling could be considered to reduce computation times.

Analyses assessing the choice of the number of folds also need to address the need for unit variances/dispersions and/or for direct variance modeling as described in Strategy Steps 6–7.

5. Adjusting for missingness

For data sets with some missing outcome measurements (such as reported in Sects. 16.2–16.4), one or more measures of missingness (e.g., some measurements missing or not; the number of missing measurements) can be included in analyses for selecting the correlation structure and the number of folds.

6. Assessing the need for unit variances/dispersions

For adaptive analyses of means/probabilities and variances/dispersions used to assess the number of folds (Strategy Step 4), use contractions that allow for the possibility of unit variances/unit dispersions. Should unit variances/dispersions be generated, it can be reasonable to only consider unit variance/dispersion models in subsequent analyses.

In reported analyses, unit dispersions are identified as appropriate for logistic regression modeling of the dichotomous respiratory status levels and for multinomial modeling and ordinal regression modeling using cumulative outcomes of the trichotomous respiratory status levels recoded as multiple dichotomous outcomes. These results, as well as the fact that extended variances for dichotomous outcomes combined with unit dispersions are necessarily equal to the associated variance function of the means, suggest that this may hold generally for these kinds of analyses. This is further supported by the results of Sect. 16.4. However, non-constant dispersions are identified using ordinal regression based on individual outcomes indicating that unit dispersions may not always be appropriate in these cases.

When unit variances/dispersions are identified as above as a reasonable choice for any type of outcome, a more extensive assessment of the appropriateness of unit variances/dispersions may be conducted for completeness. For example, unit variances/dispersions may be a reasonable alternative to non-constant variances/dispersions for different measurement conditions but not for non-constant variances/dispersions based on a larger set of predictors.

7. Choosing between extended and direct variance modeling

Direct variance modeling is always used for linear regression analyses, and so only needs to be considered for other types of regression analyses. When unit dispersions are identified as appropriate for some other type of outcome as part of assessing the number of folds, direct variance modeling can be reasonably dropped from consideration or conducted for completeness. In other cases, a choice is needed between extended and direct variance modeling because a direct variance model can sometimes be preferable to the associated extended variance model (see Sects. 15.2.2 and 15.4.4 for examples).

When Strategy Step 4 using extended variance modeling generates a clear-cut choice for the number of folds (as in Sect. 15.2.2), compare those results to associated results generated with direct variance modeling using alternative numbers of folds. If the direct variance model with the best LCV score generates a distinctly better LCV score than the associated extended variance model, use direct variance modeling in subsequent analyses. Computation time can be reduced by generating a direct variance model using only the number of folds selected using extended variances. Direct variance modeling can also be used instead of extended variance modeling if it generates a competitive model along with more consistent models across different numbers of k and/or in less time (see Sect. 15.2.2 for an example). Otherwise, use extended variance modeling in subsequent analyses.

In cases when Strategy Step 4 using extended variance modeling does not generate a clear-cut choice for the number of folds (as in Sect. 15.4.2), use extended variance additive models to identify the appropriate number of folds (as in Sect. 15.4.3). Then compare moderation models based on extended and direct variance modeling to choose between these two alternatives (as in Sect. 15.4.4).

8. Alternatives for reducing computation times for large data sets

When the number m of measurements or, for multinomial/ordinal regression modeling, the number of effective measurements $m \cdot K$ is large (not clear what constitutes a large number), computation times can be reduced by adjusting the analysis strategy as follows.

The use of 5 folds for all analyses can reduce computation times. However, this means that much different results might possibly be generated using larger number of folds.

Consideration of only constant and unit variances/dispersions can also reduce computation times. This can generate effective models for means/probabilities, but models based on non-constant variances/dispersions might possibly generate distinctly better models.

Consideration of only extended variance modeling can also reduce computations.

When additive modeling requires large computation times, moderation models are likely to require excessive times, and so can be dropped from consideration as impractical to generate. However, moderation models often provide unique information about relationships not identifiable using only additive models.

For polytomous outcomes recoded as multiple dichotomous outcomes, computation times can be reduced by considering only ordinal regression using cumulative outcomes. For polytomous outcomes with truly numeric outcome values, discrete regression is likely to provide for a more complete analysis and so computation times can be reduced by not also considered multinomial or ordinal regression methods. Computation times for discrete regression analyses can be reduced by considering only censored Poisson probabilities.

Computation times can be substantively reduced by using adjusted AIC/BIC scores (Sect. 2.6.3) in place of LCV scores. For very large numbers of measurements (not clear what constitutes very large), adjusted AIC scores approximate LCV scores, and so in those cases models generated using adjusted AIC scores are likely to be comparable to models generated with LCV scores while requiring much less computation time. Also, in those cases, more complex models can be feasibly generated than with LCV scores.

9. Further adaptive analyses

The data analyzed in this chapter have only two predictors. Correlated outcomes with more than two available predictors require further adaptive analyses to assess the impact of these extra predictors. First, use analyses based on the measurement condition (e.g., age, visit, or week) and a measure of missing measurements when appropriate (as for analyses of Sects. 16.2–16.4) to select choices for the correlation structure, the number of folds, unit versus adaptive variances/dispersions, extended versus direct variance modeling, and the modeling method in the case of polytomous outcomes. Second, conduct additive and moderation analyses also accounting for an appropriate choice for one of the other predictors of importance (e.g., gender and treatment group as for analyses reported in this chapter). Third conduct additive and moderation analyses accounting for the other predictors. However, the most general adaptive analyses might not always be possible due to requiring very long computation times. Geometric combinations can be restricted to use only two or three of the available predictors to reduce computations.

Categorical predictors may need to be addressed in adaptive analyses. The analyses of this chapter only involve categorical predictors with two levels (i.e., gender; treatment versus control). Categorical predictors with more than two levels can be addressed by recoding them as indicators for subsets of values. Examples are provided in Chap. 16.

Analyses based on more than two predictors may not be feasible due to large computation times. Computation times can be reduced by only considering additive models in all available predictors and not any moderation models. Alternately, a series of additive and moderation models can be generated for varying subsets of small numbers of predictors. How many predictors can be considered in these latter analyses would depend on issues such as the sample size, the correlation structure, and the number of folds.

15.9 Evaluation of ELMM for Theory-Based Models of Correlated Outcomes

Theory-based models typically address relationships represented by means for outcomes in terms of specific predictors. When such outcomes are correlated, a correlation structure needs to be selected in order to generate estimates for the theory-based mean parameters and tests for whether they are zero. Strategy Step 3 above is needed in this case, not just for adaptive modeling situations. The model recommended for use in this step is a specific fixed model that is also a reasonable choice for identifying a correlation structure for theory-based modeling of a correlated outcome. For this reason, an assessment of the performance of ELMM modeling for theory-based modeling cases is appropriately begun using this model. The correlated dichotomous respiratory status outcome analyzed in Chap. 8 and Sect. 15.3 has been selected to conduct this evaluation in what follows.

Table 15.24 Comparison of estimates and 95% confidence intervals for mean dichotomous respiratory status as a function of visit[a]

Type	Correlation	visit			
		1	2	3	4
Slope estimate		0.54	0.36	0.54	0.29
Model-based 95% CI	IND	0.01–1.07	−0.17 - 0.89	0.01–1.07	−0.24 - 0.82
	AR1	0.17–0.91	−0.09 - 0.81	0.15–1.03	−0.22 - 0.80
	EC	0.15–0.93	−0.03 - 0.75	0.15–0.93	−0.10 - 0.68
	UN	0.15–0.93	−0.07 - 0.79	0.13–0.95	−0.12 - 0.70
Robust empirical 95% CI		0.17–0.91	−0.07 - 0.79	0.15–0.93	−0.12 - 0.70
Bootstrap median[b]		0.54	0.36	0.54	0.29
Bootstrap 95% CI[b]		0.20–0.90	−0.07 - 0.79	0.16–0.96	−0.11 - 0.69

AR1 spatial autoregressive order 1; *CI* confidence interval; *EC* exchangeable correlations; *IND* independent; *UN* unstructured

[a]Using models based on assuming different means and different variances for different visits and computed using extended linear mixed modeling

[b]Using 500 bootstrapped resamples

The Strategy Step 3 model for the mean respiratory status over visits 0–4 is the one based on an intercept parameter and four indicators for the outcome being measured at visits 1–4. The intercept represents the mean for the outcome at the baseline visit 0 while the slopes for the four indicator variables represent how much of a difference there is between the means at the post-baseline visits and the baseline mean. This is also the case for the model for the dispersions. The number of folds used to compute LCV score for models for this outcome has no effect on mean and dispersion parameter estimates, but can be used to select an appropriate correlation structure. Tests for zero mean slope parameters are generated as part of ELMM (as described in Sect. 5.1) for any correlated outcome, including model-based and robust empirical tests. Another more general approach for conducting such tests is based on bootstrapped confidence intervals (Efron, 1982).

Table 15.24 contains results for estimates of the four mean slope parameters of the Strategy Step 3 model for dichotomous respiratory status as a function of visit along with model-based, robust empirical, and bootstrapped 95% confidence intervals for those parameters under alternative correlation structures. The slope estimates are the same for the four correlation structures. The 95% model-based confidence intervals change with the correlation structure but the robust empirical and the bootstrapped confidence intervals are the same for all correlation structures. The bootstrapped medians and the ELMM mean parameter estimates rounded to two decimal digits are all equal to each other. The 95% confidence intervals all produce the same conclusions that the means for visits 1 and 3 are significantly different from the baseline mean while the means are visits 2 and 4 are not. The 95% confidence intervals for the IND correlation structure are much less precise than the other model-based and robust empirical 95% confidence intervals and the bootstrapped 95% confidence intervals, which are all reasonably close to each other.

Table 15.25 Choice of a correlation structure using LCV scores based on alternate numbers of folds[a]

Number of folds	Chosen from data	Percent chosen from resamples[b]			
		IND	EC	AR1	UN
5	EC	0.0%	88.6%	4.2%	7.2%
10	EC	0.0%	87.8%	3.0%	9.2%
15	EC	0.0%	89.0%	2.8%	8.2%
20	EC	0.0%	88.8%	2.0%	9.2%
overall[c]	EC	0.0%	86.8%	3.6%	9.6%

AR1 spatial autoregressive order 1; *EC* exchangeable correlations; *IND* independent; *LCV* likelihood cross-validation; *UN* unstructured

[a]Using models based on assuming different means and different variances for different visits and computed using extended linear mixed modeling. Correlation structure chosen so that it is the least complex alternative generating a competitive LCV score computed using the associated number of folds

[b]Using 500 bootstrapped resamples

[c]The choice based on the best LCV score over the four numbers 5, 10, 15, and 20 folds

Table 15.25 provides an assessment of how consistent the choice of the correlation structure is over bootstrapped resamples using LCV scores based on alternate numbers of folds. The EC correlation structure is chosen for all four choices (5, 10, 15, and 20) of the numbers of folds using the dichotomous respiratory status data. This same correlation structure is also selected for about 88% to 89% of the bootstrapped resamples using these four numbers of folds. It is also selected for about 87% of the time over all of the four numbers of folds.

The above results for the Strategy Step 1 model indicate that estimates and confidence intervals generated by ELMM provide highly consistent results to those for bootstrapped resamples. The choice of the correlation structure using this model is also highly consistent with that choice based on bootstrapped resamples.

The dichotomous respiratory status data have been collected as part of a randomized clinical trial testing the efficacy of an intervention involving active treatment versus a placebo, and so the most natural theory-based model in need of testing involves assessing whether active treatment has a positive interaction effect on the probability of good respiratory status over visits. This is addressed by the linear moderation model with effects to visit, the indicator active, and the interaction between the two, more specifically, using an intercept, indicators visit1–visit4 for being measured at the post-baseline visits 1–4, the indicator active, and the four interactions equal to products of the indicators visit1–visit4 with the indicator active. A positive impact to active treatment is indicated by one or more positive slopes for the four interactions. In what follows, EC correlations are assumed as justified by the results of Table 15.25 as well as unit dispersions as justified in Sect. 15.3.2.

Table 15.26 contains results for estimates of the four interaction slope parameters of the linear moderation model for dichotomous respiratory status along with model-based, robust empirical, and bootstrapped 95% confidence intervals for those parameters under alternative correlation structures. The bootstrapped medians and

Table 15.26 Comparison of estimates and 95% confidence intervals for mean dichotomous respiratory status as a function of post-baseline visits for participants on active treatment[a]

Type	Interaction of active and visit			
	1	2	3	4
Slope estimate	0.87	1.38	1.20	0.75
Model-based 95% CI	0.11–1.63	0.62–2.14	0.44–1.96	−0.01–1.51
Robust 95% CI	0.16–1.58	0.52–2.24	0.42–1.98	−0.07–1.57
Bootstrap median[b]	0.89	1.45	1.20	0.78
Bootstrap 95% CI[b]	0.20–1.67	0.48–2.30	0.36–2.09	−0.03–1.62

CI confidence interval
[a]Using models based on an intercept, indicators visit1-visit4 for being measured at post-baseline visits, the indicator active for being on active versus placebo treatment, and the four interactions between active and visit1-visit4 assuming exchangeable correlations and unit variances and computed using extended linear mixed modeling
[b]Using 500 bootstrapped resamples

the ELMM mean parameter estimates rounded to two decimal digits are close to each other. The 95% confidence intervals all produce the same conclusions that the interactions for visits 1 to visit 3 with active treatment are significantly non-zero while the interaction for visit 4 is not. These results indicate that estimates and confidence intervals generated by ELMM provide highly consistent results to those for bootstrapped resamples with all approaches supporting a positive effect to active treatment for three post-baseline visits, but that then is diminished by visit 4.

15.10 Future Work

ELMM has been developed for modeling of categorical correlated outcomes and has been demonstrated to be preferable to standard, partially modified, and fully modified GEE. However, future research on other alternative methods is still needed. Covariance structures for ELMM have been based on only a limited number of directly specified correlation structures. Random effects and random coefficients models provide for more extensive sets of possible covariance structures. They are already used in linear mixed modeling. Random effects/coefficients can be incorporated into extended likelihoods for categorical correlated outcomes in the same way as they are incorporated into the multivariate normal density for linear mixed modeling. However, in order to conduct adaptive modeling allowing for such covariance structures requires generating and testing code to compute random effects/coefficients models in the contexts covered in this book and to incorporate searches through alternative models of that kind in combination with the kinds of models addressed in reported analyses.

Future research is also needed to conduct adaptive generalized linear mixed modeling and compare results to those for ELMM. This also requires generating and testing code to compute generalized linear mixed models and incorporating searches through those models in combination with the kinds of models addressed in reported analyses.

References

Efron, B. (1982). *The jackknife, the bootstrap, and other resampling plans, CBMS 38, SIAM-NSF*. Society for Industrial and Applied Mathematics.

Koch, G. G., Carr, C. F., Amara, I. A., Stokes, M. E., & Uryniak, T. J. (1989). Categorical data analysis. In D. A. Berry (Ed.), *Statistical methodology in the pharmaceutical sciences* (pp. 391–475). Marcel Dekker.

Miller, M. E., Davis, C. S., & Landis, J. R. (1993). The analysis of longitudinal polytomous data: Generalized estimating equations and connections with weighted least squares. *Biometrics, 49*, 1033–1044.

Potthoff, R. F., & Roy, S. N. (1964). A generalized multivariate analysis of variance model useful especially for growth curve problems. *Biometrika, 51*, 313–326.

Stokes, M. E., Davis, C. S., & Koch, G. G. (2012). *Categorical data analysis using the SAS system* (3rd ed.). SAS Institute.

Thall, P. F., & Vail, S. C. (1990). Some covariance models for longitudinal count data with overdispersion. *Biometrics, 46*, 657–671.

Treatment of Lead-exposed Children (TLC) Trial Group. (2000). Safety and efficacy of succimer in toddlers with blood lead levels of 20-44 μg/dL. *Pediatric Research, 48*, 593–599.

Chapter 16
Additional Example Analyses

Abstract Adaptive analyses are conducted in this chapter of data sets not considered in prior analyses using analysis strategies determined from those prior analyses. Analyses are conducted of cross-sectionally measured correlated outcomes provided by single mothers on three scales measuring family management of a child's chronic condition (e.g., diabetes, Crohn's disease, cystic fibrosis). Analyses are also provided of cross-sectionally measured correlated dyadic outcomes with some missing outcome values as provided by partnered parents of a child having a chronic condition using measures assessing the child's conduct-disordered behaviors. These dyadic analyses are based on three related outcomes including a continuous outcome treated as normally distributed, a count outcome treated as Poisson distributed, and a dichotomous outcome treated as Bernoulli distributed. Extended linear mixed modeling (ELMM) is used to conduct all analyses. Whether non-constant or unit dispersions are appropriate is addressed as well as adaptive additive and adaptive moderation modeling. A comparison of results for extended variance modeling and direct variance modeling is also provided when appropriate.

Keywords Childhood chronic conditions · Direct variance modeling · Extended linear mixed modeling · Moderation · Non-constant dispersions

Introduction Adaptive analysis strategies are formulated in Sect. 15.8 based on analyses of the data sets of Sects. 2.8 and 13.1. These strategies are demonstrated in this chapter using data not considered in those prior analyses. Section 16.1 provides analyses of cross-sectionally measured correlated outcomes based on multiple related scales measuring a common concept. Measurement conditions correspond to scale type, an analysis of variance factor. Prior analyses have not addressed this case. There are no missing outcome values. Sections 16.2–16.4 provide analyses of cross-sectionally measured correlated dyadic outcomes with some missing outcome values. Prior analyses all use data with no missing outcome values. Section 16.2

Supplementary Information The online version contains supplementary material available at https://doi.org/10.1007/978-3-031-41988-1_16.

G. J. Knafl, *Modeling Correlated Outcomes Using Extensions of Generalized Estimating Equations and Linear Mixed Modeling*, https://doi.org/10.1007/978-3-031-41988-1_16

analyzes a continuous outcome treated as normally distributed, Sect. 16.3 analyzes a count outcome treated as Poisson distributed, and Sect. 16.4 analyzes a dichotomous outcome treated as Bernoulli distributed. All analyses are conducted using ELMM.

16.1 Analyses of Data for Single Mothers on Managing a Child's Chronic Condition

Analyses are provided in this section of data provided by single mothers on three scales measuring family management of a child's chronic condition (e.g., diabetes, Crohn's disease, cystic fibrosis). Section 16.1.1 describes the data used in these analyses. Section 16.1.2 addresses the choice of a correlation structure for these data. Sections 16.1.3–16.1.4 provide analyses assessing, respectively, the impact of different scales and the impact of both the scales and a measure of general family functioning. Section 16.1.5 provides a summary of clock times required for the analyses of the section.

16.1.1 The Single Mothers Data

Data are available for 65 single mothers on dimensions of family management of a child's chronic condition. The Family Management Measure (FaMM) consists of six scales related to the family's management of a child's chronic condition (Knafl et al. 2011). Three of these scales address problematic aspects of family management especially pertinent to single mothers including family life difficulty, condition management effort, and view of condition impact; referred to as difficulty, effort, and impact for short. Larger scores indicate higher levels of difficulty, effort, and impact for family management of the child's chronic condition. These scales are usually computed as sums of items rated with values 1–5. Different numbers of items are summed to compute each scale so that larger values can be a consequence of scales being based on more items. For this reason, reported results are based on normalized values of the three scales computed using the average of the scale's item values so that the range for all scale values is 1–5. In this way, larger values for different scales indicate more problematic effects on family management of a child's chronic condition.

The measurement conditions for outcomes in each matched set correspond to a single mother and have indexes 1, 2, and 3 corresponding to the values for that mother of the normalized difficulty, effort, and impact scales, respectively. There is a total of 195 outcome measurements, three for each of the 65 single mothers, and so with no missing outcome measurements. For this reason, reported LCV scores are computed using matched-set-wise deletion. The cutoff for a distinct percent decrease (PD) in the LCV score using DF = 1 is 0.98%.

Indicator variables are available in the data set for measurements corresponding to the three FaMM scales; these variables have the same names difficulty, effort, and impact as the scales. Indicator variables are also available for being a measurement for one of two of the scales including the indicator diffeff for being either the difficulty or the effort scale, the indicator diffimp for being either the difficulty or the impact scale, and the indicator effimp for being either the effort or the impact scale. A predictor variable named famfunct is also available for a measure of general family functioning, not specifically addressing family management, using the McMaster Family Assessment Device (Epstein et al. 1983) based on the average of 12 items rated 1–4 with larger values indicating worse levels of family functioning.

All models are based on linear regression treating continuous outcomes as normally distributed with identity link function. For such models, extended variance modeling is the same as direct variance modeling.

16.1.2 Alternate Correlation Structures

The model with different means and different variances for the single mothers data is based on the two indicators difficulty and effort together with an intercept. For the means, the intercept represents the mean for the impact scale while the slopes for the indicators difficulty and effort represent how much of a difference there is for the means for these two scales compared to the impact scale. The intercept and slopes for the variances have the same interpretation for the log of the variances. Table 16.1 provides LCV scores for this model computed using 5, 10, and 15 folds for each of the IND, EC, and UN correlation structures. The spatial AR1 correlation structure is not relevant since the measurement conditions have nominal values corresponding to different scales and are not truly ordered. For all three numbers of folds, EC generates the best LCV score over the three correlation structures. Consequently, only EC correlations are used in subsequent analyses. The nine models of Table 16.1 require 0.2 min of clock time.

Table 16.1 LCV scores using alternative correlation structures and numbers of folds for the single mothers data[a]

Correlation structure	LCV score[b]		
	5 folds	10 folds	15 folds
IND	0.27265	0.27444	0.27459
EC	0.32002	0.32140	0.32158
UN	0.31785	0.31842	0.31795

EC exchangeable correlations; *IND* independent; *LCV* likelihood cross-validation; *UN* unstructured

[a]Using models based on assuming different means and different variances for different scales and computed using linear mixed modeling

[b]Computed using matched-set-wise deletion

16.1.3 Models Based on Scale

Table 16.2 contains LCV scores for 5, 10, and 15 folds for the model for the three FaMM scale measurements with adaptive means and adaptive non-constant variances. The base model has constant means and variances, is expanded based on the six indicator variables difficulty, effort, impact, diffeff, diffimp, and effimp, and then contracted allowing for unit dispersions. In this way, the adaptive modeling process takes into account the possibility of different means and variances for each of the three scales and for the possibility of the same means and variances for the three possible pairs of scales. The largest LCV score is achieved with 10 folds. The same model is generated for the means for all three numbers of folds while different models are generated for the variances of each of those three numbers of folds. The model generated with 15 folds has 10-fold LCV score 0.32162 with non-distinct PD 0.0.07% (i.e., less than or equal to the cutoff 0.98% using DF = 1). On the other hand, the model generated with 5 folds has 10-fold LCV score 0.31689 with distinct PD 1.54%. These results indicate that 10 folds is a reasonable choice for adaptive analyses of the single mothers data since it generates the best LCV score and a model consistent with the model generated using 15 folds and distinctly outperforms the model generated using 5 folds. The three models of Table 16.2 require 1.2 min of clock time.

For the model generated by 10 folds of Table 16.2, estimated mean difficulty is 2.5, estimated mean impact 2.8, and estimated mean effort 3.7. The estimated standard deviation for impact is 0.8 and the common estimated standard deviation for difficulty and effort is 1.0. The estimated exchangeable correlation is 0.62.

16.1.4 Models Based on Scale and Family Functioning

The results of Sects. 16.1.2–16.1.3 indicate that the single mothers data are appropriately analyzed using EC correlations with LCV scores computed using 10 folds,

Table 16.2 Predictor variables and clock times for adaptively generated models based on scales for means and variances of the single mothers data[a]

	Number of folds		
	5	10	15
LCV score	0.31701	0.32187	0.32185
Means[b]	1, effort, difficulty	1, effort, difficulty	1, effort, difficulty
Variances[b]	--[c]	impact	1, effort
Clock time (min)	0.2	0.4	0.6

[a]Computed using linear mixed modeling, exchangeable correlations, and matched-set-wise deletion with the contraction allowing for unit variances

[b]A value of 1 corresponds to an intercept; otherwise, the model has a zero intercept. The variables difficulty, effort, and impact are the indicators for being the associated scale

[c]Has unit variances

Table 16.3 Adaptively generated models based on scales and family functioning for means and variances of the single mothers data[a]

Model type	10-fold LCV score	Mean transforms[b]	Variance transforms[b]	Clock time (min)
Additive	0.33112	effort, difficulty, $\text{famfunct}^{0.33}$	effort, $\text{famfunct}^{0.3}$	5.3
Moderation	0.33490	$(\text{famfunct}^{-3}\cdot\text{diffimp})^{0.23}$, $(\text{famfunct}^{-1.5}\cdot\text{diffeff})^{0.9}$	1, effort	98.2

[a]Computed using linear mixed modeling, exchangeable correlations, and matched-set-wise deletion
[b]The transform 1 represents an intercept; otherwise, the intercept is zero. The variables difficulty and effort are the indicators for being the associated scale while diffimp is the indicator for being either the difficulty or the impact scales and diffeff is the indicator for being either the difficulty or the effort scales; famfunct represents the family functioning predictor

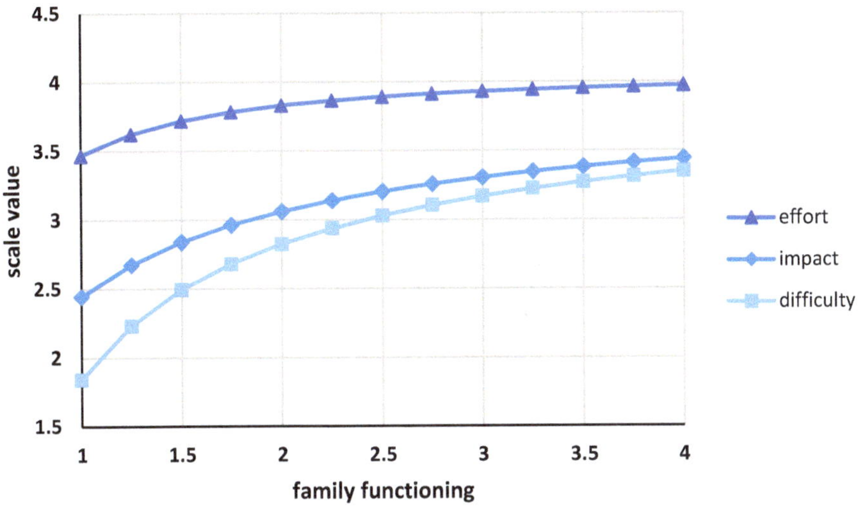

Fig. 16.1 Estimated mean scale values as a function of family functioning by scale type

and so these choices are used in subsequent analyses. This section provides a comparison of the adaptive additive model and the adaptive moderation model for means and variances in scale and family functioning.

Table 16.3 provides a comparison of adaptively generated additive and moderation models for means and variances of the single mothers data. The additive model has 10-fold LCV score 0.33112 with distinct PD 1.13% compared to the moderation model with 10-fold LCV score 0.33490. Consequently, a distinct moderation effect is identified. The adaptive additive model requires 5.3 min of clock time while the adaptive moderation model requires 98.2 min for a total of 103.5 min or about 1.7 h, almost all of which is required to compute the moderation model.

The moderation model of Table 16.3 has estimated exchangeable correlation 0.55. Figure 16.1 provides plots of estimated mean scale values as a function of family functioning for the three different scales based on the moderation model.

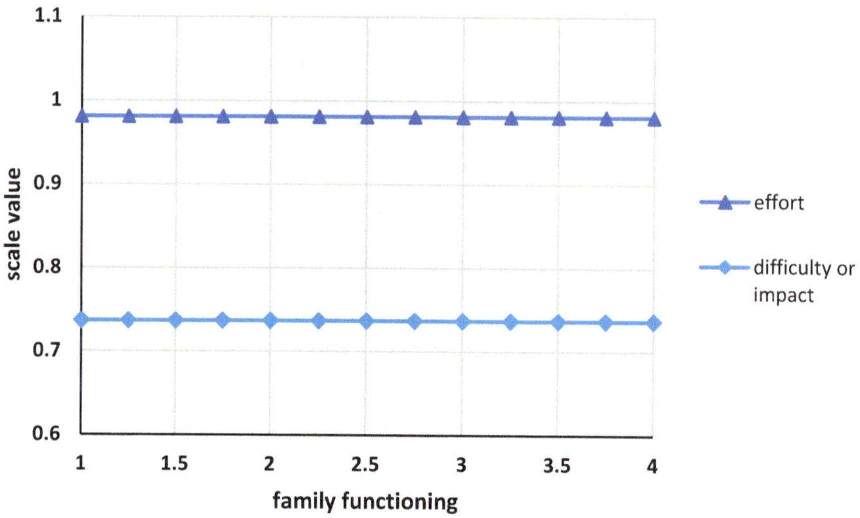

Fig. 16.2 Estimated standard deviations of scale values as a function of family functioning by scale type

Mean scale values increase (worsen) nonlinearly with increased (worse) family functioning with the lowest level for the difficulty scale, an intermediate level for the impact scale, and the highest level for the effort scale. These results indicate that effort is the most problematic of the three aspects of family management for single mothers of their child with a chronic condition followed by impact and then difficulty. Figure 16.2 provides plots of the estimated standard deviations for scale values as a function of family functioning for the three different scales based on the moderation model. Effort scale values have constant variability in family functioning larger than the common constant variability for the difficulty and impact scales. Figure 16.3 provides the plot of standardized residuals of the moderation model for the three scales. All standardized residuals are well within ±3, and so there are no outlying measurements.

16.1.5 Clock Times for Analyses

Clock times for the analyses of Sect. 16.1 include 0.2 min for the models of Table 16.1, 1.2 min for the models of Table 16.2, and 103.5 min for the models of Table 16.3. Consequently, analyses of the single mothers data require 104.9 min or about 1.7 h altogether.

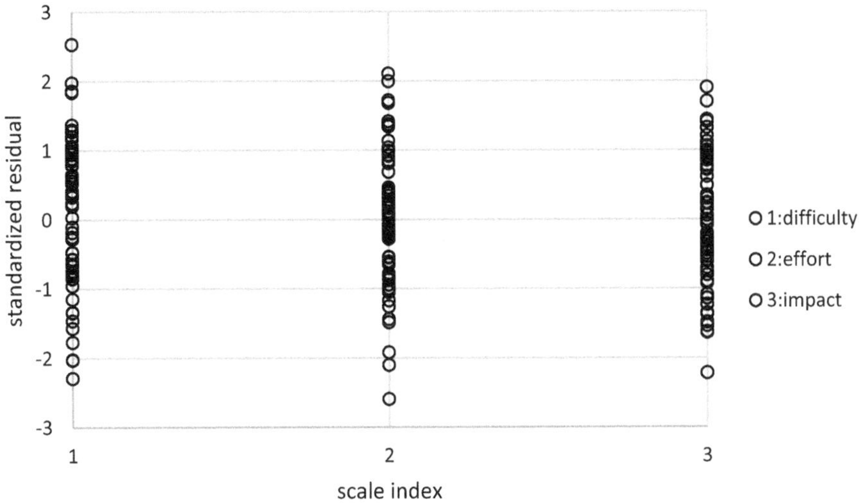

Fig. 16.3 Standardized residuals for the moderation model in scale and family functioning

16.2 Analyses of the Intensity of Conduct-Disordered Behaviors

Analyses are provided in this section of data provided by partnered parents of a child having a chronic condition (e.g., diabetes, Crohn's disease, cystic fibrosis) on a measure of the intensity of the child's conduct-disordered behaviors. Section 16.2.1 describes the data used in these analyses (and also used in the analyses of Sects. 16.3–16.4). These are dyadic data with a maximum of two outcome measurements per matched set requiring only a single correlation parameter, and so all models use exchangeable correlations (EC). Section 16.2.2 addresses the choice of the number of folds for computing LCV scores. Section 16.2.3 provides analyses assessing the impact of types based on parent, family, and how the family manages the child's condition. Section 16.2.4 expands these analyses to also account for the impact of a measure of general family functioning. Section 16.2.5 provides a summary of clock times required for the analyses of the section.

All models of the intensity of conduct-disordered behaviors are based on linear regression treating continuous outcomes as normally distributed with identity link function. For such models, extended variance modeling is the same as direct variance modeling.

16.2.1 The Partnered Parents Data

Data are available for 471 partnered parents. Three different outcome measurements are available based on the Eyberg Child Behavior Inventory (Eyberg and Pincus 1999). Section. 16.2 provides analyses of the intensity of conduct-disordered behaviors for that child based on the sum of 36 items rated 1–7. Larger values indicate more frequent occurrence of conduct-disordered behaviors. Section 16.3 provides analyses of the number of these 36 items the parent considers problematic. Section 16.4 provides analyses of the occurrence of a high level of intensity of conduct-disordered behaviors, that is, larger than the cutoff of 127 provided by Eyberg and Ross (1978). In all three cases, outcome measurements are available for mothers from 328 families and from fathers for 143 of those families, and so only for mothers for 185 of the families.

The matched sets correspond to families and the measurement conditions to parents of those families. Matched sets contain one outcome measurement for just the mother or two outcome measurements for the mother and the father. Indicator variables named father and momonly are available in the data set for an outcome measurement provided by a father and provided by a mother for which the outcome measurement for the father is missing, respectively. There is a total of 471 outcome measurements with 185 families having a missing outcome measurement, and so LCV scores are computed using measurement-wise deletion. The cutoff for a distinct percent decrease (PD) in the LCV score using $\mathrm{DF} = 1$ is 0.40%.

The Family Management Measure (FaMM) consists of six scales related to the family's management of a child's chronic condition (Knafl et al. 2011), three of which are considered in the analyses of Sect. 16.1. The partnered parent families are categorized on the basis of values for these six scales into four family management types (Knafl et al. 2013) on a scale of better to poorer family management including family focused (120 parents from 83 families), somewhat family focused (166 parents from 115 families), somewhat condition focused (156 parents from 109 families), and condition focused (29 parents from 21 families). Indicator variables called Ffocus, SFfocus, SCfocus, and Cfocus are available for families being in each of these four family management types, respectively. An indicator variable named F_SFfocus is also available for families being either family focused or somewhat family focused as well as an indicator variable named SC_Cfocus for families being somewhat condition focused or condition focused. A predictor variable named famfunct is also available for a measure of general family functioning (Epstein, Baldwin, & Bishop, 1983), not specifically addressing family management, with larger values indicating worse levels of family functioning as also used in the analyses of Sect. 16.1.

16.2.2 Alternate Numbers of Folds

The model with adaptive means and adaptive non-constant variances for the intensity of conduct-disordered behaviors is determined using the two indicators father and momonly. This accounts for possible effects to both the measurement condition and for missingness. Table 16.4 provides LCV scores for this model computed using 5, 10, and 15 folds and the EC correlation structure. The largest LCV score is achieved for 5 folds. For all three numbers of folds, the same model is generated based on constant means and constant variances. Consequently, 5 folds generate the best LCV score as well as a model consistent with the ones generated with 10 and 15 folds, and so subsequent models are computed using 5-fold LCV scores. The three models of Table 16.4 require 2.0 min of clock time.

The expanded model for all three numbers of folds has means and variances based on the two indicators father and momonly together with an intercept. For the means of this expanded model, the intercept represents the mean intensity of conduct-disordered behaviors for mothers with participating fathers while the slopes for the indicators father and momonly represent how much of a difference there is in the means for fathers and for mothers without participating fathers, respectively, compared to mothers with participating fathers. The intercept and slopes for the variances have the same interpretation for the log of the variances.

For the adaptive model of Table 16.4, estimated mean intensity of the child's conduct-disordered behaviors is 86.8 for all parents. This is a relatively low value as compared to the cutoff of 127 for a high level of intensity of conduct-disordered behaviors provided by Eyberg and Ross (1978). The estimated standard deviation is 28.5 for all parents. The estimated correlation is 0.64.

Table 16.4 Predictors and clock times for adaptively generated models based on parent type and family type for means and variances of the intensity of conduct-disordered behaviors for the partnered parents data[a]

	Number of folds		
	5	10	15
LCV score	0.0091155	0.0091089	0.0091000
Means[b]	0	0	0
Variances[b]	0	0	0
Clock time (min)	0.3	0.7	1.0

[a]Computed using linear mixed modeling, exchangeable correlations, and measurement-wise deletion with the contraction allowing for unit variances. Parent type is represented by the indicator for being a father while family type is represented by the indicator for a family with only the mother participating

[b]A power of 0 corresponds to an intercept

16.2.3 Models Based on Parent, Family, and Family Management Types

The results of Sect. 16.2.2 indicate that the intensity of conduct-disordered behaviors is appropriately analyzed using EC correlations with LCV scores computed using 5 folds, and so these choices are used in subsequent analyses. This section provides a comparison of the adaptive additive model and the adaptive moderation model for means and variances in parent, family, and family management types. Parent type is represented by the indicator father, family type by the indicator momonly, and family management type by the six indicator variables Ffocus, SFfocus, SCfocus, Cfocus, F_SFfocus, and SC_Cfocus. Geometric combinations based on these indicator variables are standard interactions based on products of two or more of the indicator variables, and so are also indicator variables.

Table 16.5 provides a comparison of adaptively generated additive and moderation models based on parent, family, and family management types for means and variances of the intensity of conduct-disordered behaviors. The additive model has 5-fold LCV score 0.0.0094728. In comparison, the model of Table 16.4 based on only parent and family types has 5-fold LCV score 0.0091157 with distinct PD 3.77% (i.e., greater than the cutoff of 0.40%). Consequently, family management type provides for a distinct improvement. The LCV score for the additive model of Table 16.5 has distinct PD 0.41% compared to the moderation model with 5-fold LCV score 0.0.0095117. Consequently, a distinct moderation effect is identified. The adaptive additive model requires 1.5 min of clock time while the adaptive moderation model requires 10.2 min for a total of 11.7 min.

For the moderation model of Table 16.5, estimated mean intensity of the child's conduct-disordered behaviors is 96.9 for parents in conditioned or somewhat condition focused families, which decreases (improves) to 78.9 for parents in family focused families and for mothers in somewhat family focused families and increases (worsens) from there to 85.6 for fathers in somewhat family focused families. The estimated standard deviation is 26.3 for parents in family focused, somewhat family

Table 16.5 Adaptively generated models based on parent, family, and family management types for means and variances of the intensity of conduct-disordered behaviors for the partnered parents data[a]

Model type	5-fold LCV score	Mean transforms[b]	Variance transforms[b]	Clock time (min)
Additive	0.0094728	1, F_SFfocus	1, Cfocus	1.5
Moderation	0.0095117	1, F_SFfocus, father·SFfocus	1, Cfocus	10.2

[a]Computed using linear mixed modeling, exchangeable correlations, and measurement-wise deletion

[b]The transform 1 represents an intercept; otherwise, the intercept is zero. Father is the indicator for the parent being a father. F_SFfocus, SFfocus, and Cfocus are indicators for the family being family focused or somewhat family focused, being somewhat family focused, and being condition focused, respectively

focused, and somewhat condition focused families, which increases to 37.4 for parents in condition focused families. The estimated correlation is 0.61.

16.2.4 Models Based on Parent, Family, and Family Management Types and on Family Functioning

This section provides a comparison of the adaptive additive model and the adaptive moderation model for means and variances in parent, family, and family management types together with family functioning. Parent, family, and family management type are represented by the same indicator variables as in Sect. 16.2.3.

Table 16.6 provides a comparison of adaptively generated additive and moderation models based on parent, family, and family management types together with family functioning for means and variances of the intensity of conduct-disordered behaviors. The additive model has 5-fold LCV score 0.0096569 while the moderation model has 5-fold LCV score 0.0098480. In comparison, the associated models of Table 16.5 based on only parent, family, and family management types have 5-fold LCV scores 0.0094728 and 0.0095117 with distinct PDs 1.91% and 3.41%. Consequently, family functioning provides for a distinct improvement in both cases. The LCV score for the additive model of Table 16.6 has distinct PD 1.94% compared to the LCV score for moderation model of Table 16.6. Consequently, a distinct moderation effect is identified. The adaptive additive model requires 26.0 min of clock time while the adaptive moderation model requires 99.3 min for a total of 125.3 min or about 2.1 h.

The moderation model of Table 16.3 has estimated exchangeable correlation 0.62. Figure 16.4 provides plots of estimated mean intensity of the child's conduct-disordered behaviors as a function of family functioning for parent type and family management type combinations based on the moderation model. Mean intensity of the child's conduct-disordered behaviors increases (worsens) nonlinearly with increased (worse) family functioning. The lowest level is achieved for family focused parents and somewhat family focused mothers (225 or 49.9% of the parents), the next higher level for somewhat family focused fathers (51 or 10.8% of the parents), then somewhat condition focused parents and condition focused mothers (177 or 37.6% of the parents), followed by the highest level for condition focused fathers (8 or 1.7% of the parents). Values are plotted for the maximum range of 1–4 for family functioning except for condition focused fathers. Values in that case are plotted for the range 1–2.5 with 2.5 the maximum observed value for that case because of a large increase in the estimated mean at 2.5. This is a consequence of a highly influential outcome measurement value of 186 for one condition focused father at a family functioning value of 2.2. This is the largest observed outcome value in the data set; the next largest value is 169. The mother for this family also provided a family functioning value of 2.2 but a much lower outcome measurement value of 106.

Table 16.6 Adaptively generated models based on parent, family, and family management types and on family functioning for means and variances of the intensity of conduct-disordered behaviors for the partnered parents data[a]

Model type	5-fold LCV score	Mean transforms[b]	Variance transforms[b]	Clock time (min)
Additive	0.0096569	F_SFfocus, $\text{famfunct}^{0.21}$	$\text{famfunct}^{0.09}$	26.0
Moderation	0.0098480	$(\text{F\_SFfocus} \cdot \text{famfunct}^{-1.1})^{-0.19}$, $\text{Cfocus} \cdot \text{father} \cdot \text{famfunct}^{16}$ $(\text{SC\_Cfocus} \cdot \text{famfunct}^{3})^{0.07}$, $\text{father} \cdot \text{SFfocus}$	1, $\left(\text{momonly} \cdot \text{SC\_Cfocus} \cdot \text{famfunct}^{2}\right)^{0.9}$	99.3

[a]Computed using linear mixed modeling, exchangeable correlations, and measurement-wise deletion

[b]The transform 1 represents an intercept; otherwise, the intercept is zero. The variable father is the indicator for the parent being a father. The variable momonly is the indicator for a family with only the mother participating. F_SFfocus, SC_Cfocus, and Cfocus are indicators for the family being family focused or somewhat family focused, being somewhat conditioned focused or condition focused, and being condition focused, respectively. The variable famfunct represents general family functioning

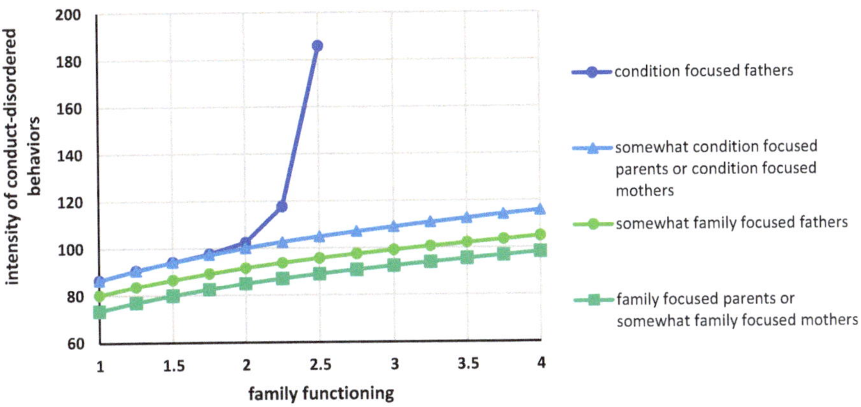

Fig. 16.4 Estimated mean intensity of conduct-disordered behaviors in terms of family functioning by combinations of parent type and family management type

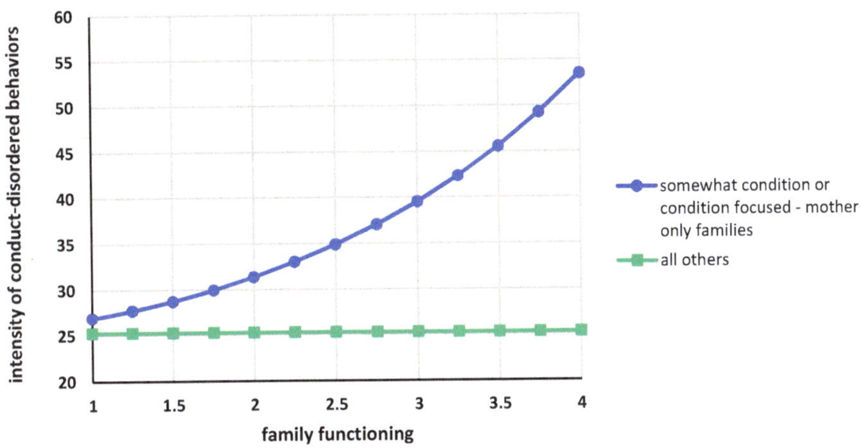

Fig. 16.5 Estimated standard deviation of intensity of conduct-disordered behaviors in terms of family functioning by combinations of family type and family management type

Figure 16.5 provides plots of the estimated standard deviation of intensity of conduct-disordered behaviors as a function of family functioning for family type and family management type combinations based on the moderation model. The estimated standard deviation increases nonlinearly from 26.9 to 53.5 for mothers in somewhat condition and condition focused families without participating fathers (75 or 15.9% of the parents) while it is constant at a lower level of 25.3 for the other parents (396 or 84.1% of the parents).

Figure 16.6 provides the plot of standardized residuals of the moderation model. All standardized residuals are within ±3 except for one measurement with standardized residual 3.11. The exceptional measurement is for a somewhat condition

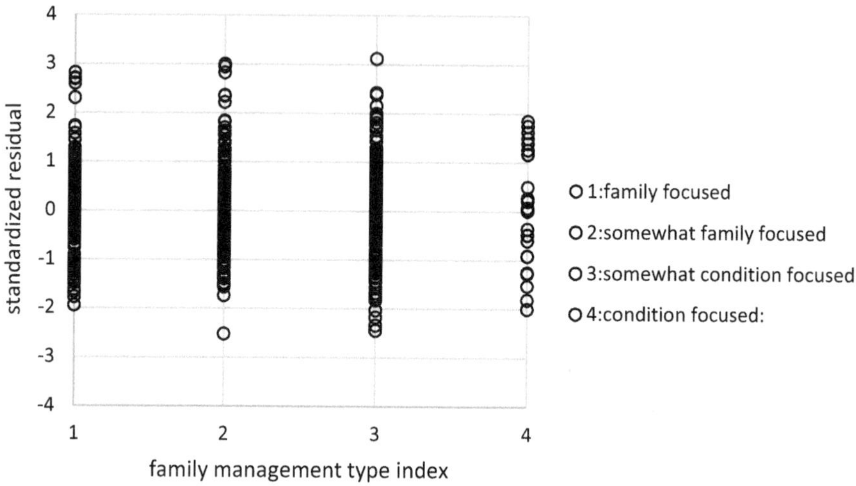

Fig. 16.6 Standardized residuals for the moderation model in parent, family, and family management type together with family functioning

focused mother with relatively high value 141 for the intensity of conduct-disordered behaviors together with family functioning value 1.8. In contrast, the outcome measurement for the associated father is only 61 with family functioning value 1.3.

16.2.5 Clock Times for Analyses

Clock times for the analyses of Sect. 16.2 include 2.0 min for the models of Table 16.4, 11.7 min for the models of Table 16.5, and 125.3 min for the models of Table 16.6. Consequently, analyses of the intensity of conduct-disordered behaviors for the partnered parents data require 139.0 min or about 2.3 h altogether.

16.3 Analyses of the Number of Problematic Conduct-Disordered Behaviors

Analyses reported in this section use the partnered parents data of Sect. 16.2.1 with outcome measurements given by the number of a child's problematic conduct-disordered behaviors. The maximum possible range for the outcome measurements is 0–36 while the observed range is 0–33. As in Sect. 16.2, outcome measurements are available for mothers from 328 families and from fathers for 143 of those families, and so only for mothers for 185 of the families. There is a total of 471 outcome measurements with 185 families having a missing outcome measurement, and so LCV scores are computed using measurement-wise deletion. The cutoff for a distinct percent decrease (PD) in the LCV score using DF = 1 is 0.40%. The available predictors are the same as described in Sect. 16.2.1 including indicator variables based on parent, family, and family management types and the measure famfunct of general family functioning.

All models are based on Poisson regression treating count outcomes as Poisson distributed with natural log link function. Models can be converted to address the proportion of problematic conduct-disordered behaviors, but are not since this would be based on an offset variable with constant value log36 and so would not provide any extra value. Models reported in this section are based on extended variances determined by dispersions combined with means unless explicitly specified to be based on direct variance modeling determined entirely by dispersions. Dyadic data like the partnered parents data with a maximum of two outcome measurements per matched set require only a single correlation parameter so that all models use exchangeable correlations (EC).

Section 16.3.1 addresses the choice of the number of folds for computing LCV scores. Section 16.3.2 provides analyses assessing the impact of types based on parent, family, and how the family manages the child's condition. Section 16.3.3 expands these analyses to also account for the impact of a measure of general family functioning. Section 16.3.4 provides a summary of clock times required for the analyses of the section.

16.3.1 *Alternate Numbers of Folds*

The model with adaptive means and adaptive dispersions for the number of problematic conduct-disordered behaviors is determined by the two indicators father and momonly. This accounts for possible effects to both the measurement condition and whether or not a measurement is missing. Table 16.7 provides LCV scores for this

Table 16.7 Predictors and clock times for adaptively generated models based on parent type and family type for means and dispersions of the number of problematic conduct-disordered behaviors for the partnered parents data[a]

	Number of folds		
	5	10	15
LCV score	0.037589	0.037451	0.037575
Means[b]	0	0	0
Dispersions[b]	0	0	0
Clock time (min)	0.2	0.4	0.7

[a]Computed using extended linear mixed modeling, exchangeable correlations, and measurement-wise deletion with the contraction allowing for unit dispersions. Parent type is represented by the indicator for being a father while family type is represented by the indicator for a family with only the mother participating

[b]A power of 0 corresponds to an intercept

model computed using 5, 10, and 15 folds and the EC correlation structure. The largest LCV score is achieved for 5 folds. For all three numbers of folds, the same model is generated based on constant means and constant dispersions. Consequently, 5 folds generate the best LCV score as well as a model consistent with the models generated with 10 and 15 folds, and so subsequent models are computed using 5-fold LCV scores. The three models of Table 16.7 require 1.3 min of clock time.

For the adaptive model of Table 16.7, estimated mean number of the child's problematic conduct-disordered behaviors is 6.9 for all parents. This is a relatively low value as compared to the cutoff of 11 for a high level of number of problematic conduct-disordered behaviors given by Eyberg and Ross (1978). The estimated dispersion is 6.5 for all parents. The estimated correlation is 0.51.

16.3.2 Models Based on Parent, Family, and Family Management Types

The results of Sect. 16.3.1 indicate that the number of problematic conduct-disordered behaviors is appropriately analyzed using EC correlations with LCV scores computed using 5 folds, and so these choices are used in subsequent analyses. This section provides a comparison of the adaptive additive model and the adaptive moderation model for means and dispersions in parent, family, and family management types. Parent type is represented by the indicator father, family type by the indicator momonly, and family management type by the six indicator variables Ffocus, SFfocus, SCfocus, Cfocus, F_SFfocus, and SC_Cfocus.

Table 16.8 provides a comparison of adaptively generated additive and moderation models based on parent, family, and family management types for means and non-constant dispersions of the number of problematic conduct-disordered behaviors. The additive model has 5-fold LCV score 0.039332. In comparison, the model

Table 16.8 Adaptively generated models based on parent, family, and family management types for means and dispersions of the number of problematic conduct-disordered behaviors for the partnered parents data[a]

Model type	5-fold LCV score	Mean transforms[b]	Dispersion transforms[b]	Clock time (min)
Additive	0.039332	1, F_SFfocus	1	2.0
Moderation	0.039623	1, F_SFfocus	1, SCfocus, momonly · F _ SFfocus	9.1

[a]Computed using extended linear mixed modeling, exchangeable correlations, and measurement-wise deletion

[b]The transform 1 represents an intercept; otherwise, the intercept is zero. The variable momonly is the indicator for a family with only the mother participating. F_SFfocus and SCfocus are indicators for the family being family focused or somewhat family focused and being somewhat condition focused, respectively

Table 16.9 Adaptively generated direct variance models based on parent, family, and family management types for means and dispersions of the number of problematic conduct-disordered behaviors for the partnered parents data[a]

Model type	5-fold LCV score	Mean transforms[b]	Dispersion transforms[b]	Clock time (minutes)
Additive	0.039305	1, F_SFfocus	1, Ffocus	1.7
Moderation	0.039698	1, F_SFfocus	1, momonly · F _ SFfocus, Ffocus	15.0

[a]Computed using extended linear mixed modeling, exchangeable correlations, and measurement-wise deletion

[b]The transform 1 represents an intercept; otherwise, the intercept is zero. The variable momonly is the indicator for a family with only the mother participating. F_SFfocus and Ffocus are indicators for the family being family focused or somewhat family focused and being family focused, respectively

of Table 16.7 based on only parent and family types has 5-fold LCV score 0.037589 with distinct PD 4.43% (i.e., greater than the cutoff of 0.40%). Consequently, family management type provides for a distinct improvement. The LCV score for the additive model of Table 16.8 has distinct PD 0.73% compared to the moderation model with 5-fold LCV score 0.039623. Consequently, a distinct moderation effect is identified, but only for the dispersions. The adaptive additive model requires 2.0 min of clock time while the adaptive moderation model requires 9.1 min for a total of 11.1 min.

For the moderation model of Table 16.8, the estimated mean number of the child's problematic conduct-disordered behaviors is 9.3 for parents in somewhat condition focused or conditioned focused families (185 or 39.3% of the parents), which decreases (improves) to 5.2 for parents in family focused or somewhat family focused families (286 or 60.7% of the parents). The estimated dispersion is 7.5 for parents in family or somewhat family focused families with participating fathers and in condition focused families (205 or 43.5% of the parents), which decreases to 5.4 for parents in somewhat condition focused families (156 or 33.1% of the parents), and then to 4.7 for mothers in family focused or somewhat family focused families without participating fathers (110 or 23.4% of the parents). The estimated correlation is 0.51.

So far models have been based on extended variance modeling. Table 16.9 provides results for direct variance modeling analogous to the results of Table 16.8. Models for the means in the two tables are the same while models for the dispersions differ somewhat. The direct variance additive model has LCV score 0.039305 with non-distinct PD 0.07% compared to the LCV score of 0.039332 for the extended variance additive model. The extended variance moderation model has LCV score 0.039623 with non-distinct PD 0.19% compared to the LCV score of 0.039698 for the direct variance adaptive moderation model. Consequently, direct variance and extended variance modeling generate competitive models. The two direct variance models require 16.7 min of clock time or about 1.5 times as much as the 11.1 min for the extended variance models. Only extended variance modeling is considered in subsequent analyses since it generates competitive models in less time.

16.3.3 Models Based on Parent, Family, and Family Management Types and on Family Functioning

This section provides a comparison of adaptive additive and moderation models for means and dispersions in parent, family, and family management types together with family functioning. Parent, family, and family management type are represented by the same indicator variables as in Sect. 16.3.2.

Table 16.10 provides a comparison of adaptively generated additive and moderation models based on parent, family, and family management types together with family functioning for means and dispersions of the number of problematic conduct-disordered behaviors. The adaptive additive model has 5-fold LCV score 0.039960 while the adaptive moderation model has 5-fold LCV score 0.041083. In comparison, the associated models of Table 16.8 based on only parent, family, and family management types have 5-fold LCV scores 0.039332 and 0.039623 with distinct PDs 1.57% and 3.55%. Consequently, family functioning provides for a distinct improvement in both cases. The LCV score for the additive model of Table 16.10 has distinct PD 2.73% compared to the LCV score for moderation model of Table 16.10. Consequently, a distinct moderation effect is identified. The adaptive additive model requires 13.4 min of clock time while the adaptive moderation model requires 116.1 min for a total of 129.5 min or about 2.2 h.

Table 16.10 Adaptively generated models based on parent, family, and family management types and on family functioning for means and dispersions of the number of problematic conduct-disordered behaviors for the partnered parents data[a]

Model type	5-fold LCV score	Mean transforms[b]	Dispersion transforms[b]	Clock time (min)
Additive	0.039960	F_SFfocus, $\text{famfunct}^{0.24}$	$\text{famfunct}^{-0.06}$	13.4
Moderation	0.041083	$\text{SC\_Cfocus}\cdot\text{famfunct}^{1.2}$, $(\text{SCfocus}\cdot\text{famfunct}^{-3}\cdot\text{father})^{3.7}$, $(\text{famfunct}^{-6}\cdot\text{F\_SFfocus}\cdot\text{momonly})^{0.3}$, $\text{famfunct}^{0.15}$	1, $\text{SCfocus}\cdot\text{famfunct}^{7}$	116.1

[a]Computed using extended linear mixed modeling, exchangeable correlations, and measurement-wise deletion

[b]The transform 1 represents an intercept; otherwise, the intercept is zero. The variable father is the indicator for the parent being a father. The variable momonly is the indicator for a family with only the mother participating. F_SFfocus, SC_Cfocus, and SCfocus are indicators for the family being family focused or somewhat family focused, and being somewhat conditioned focused or condition focused. The variable famfunct represents general family functioning

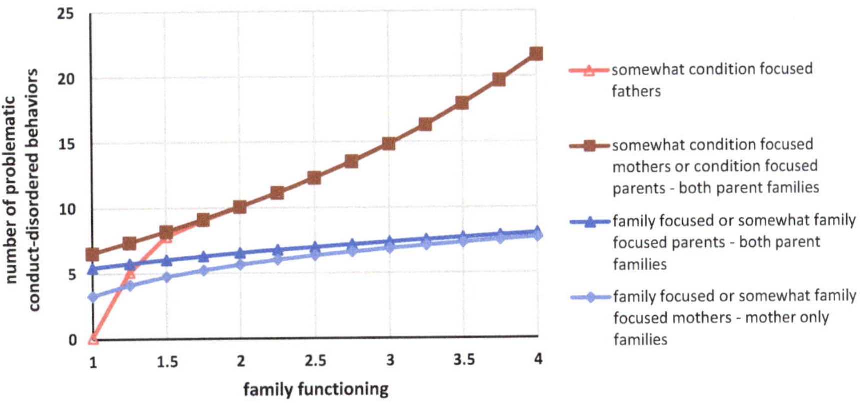

Fig. 16.7 Estimated mean number of problematic conduct-disordered behaviors in terms of family functioning by combinations of parent type and family management type

The moderation model of Table 16.10 has estimated exchangeable correlation 0.51. Figure 16.7 provides the plot of estimated mean number of problematic conduct-disordered behaviors as a function of family functioning for parent type and family management type combinations based on the moderation model. For parents in somewhat conditioned focused and condition focused families, mean number of the child's problematic conduct-disordered behaviors increases (worsen) nonlinearly with increased (worse) family functioning along two different patterns starting at different levels but increasing to a common value about 21.6 at high values for family functioning (including 13 or 2.8% parents in conditioned focused families with only mothers participating, 47 or 10.0% fathers in somewhat conditioned families, and 125 or 26.5% parents in the remaining somewhat condition and condition focused families). On the other hand, for parents in family focused and somewhat family focused families, mean number of the child's problematic conduct-disordered behaviors has lower levels increasing somewhat from 3.3 to 7.7 for mothers without participating fathers and from 5.4 to 8.0 for mothers and fathers when both are participating (including 110 or 23.4% mothers in families with only mothers participating and 176 or 37.4% parents in families with both parents participating).

Figure 16.8 provides the plot of estimated dispersions for the number of problematic conduct-disordered behaviors as a function of family functioning for family type and family management type combinations based on the moderation model. The estimated dispersions start at 6.0 for the lowest value of 1.0 for family functioning and then decrease nonlinearly to essentially zero by a family functioning value of 3.5 for mothers in somewhat condition focused families (156 or 33.1% of the parents). For all other parents (315 or 66.9% of the parents), the estimated dispersions are constant at 6.0, the initial level for mothers in somewhat condition focused families.

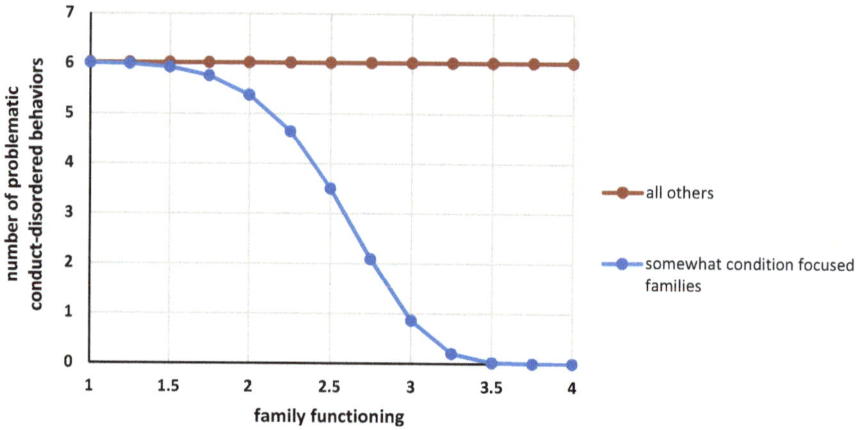

Fig. 16.8 Estimated dispersions for the number of problematic conduct-disordered behaviors in terms of family functioning by combinations of family type and family management type

Figure 16.9 provides the plot of standardized residuals of the moderation model. Standardized residuals are within ±3 except for three measurements including a standardized residual 3.07 based on an outcome value of 24 for a father in a family focused family, a standardized residual 3.68 based on an outcome value of 29 for a mother in a somewhat family focused family, and a standardized residual 3.49 based on an outcome value of 32 for a mother in a somewhat family focused family. These are three of the largest four values for the number of problematic conduct-disordered behaviors. The largest observed value is 33.

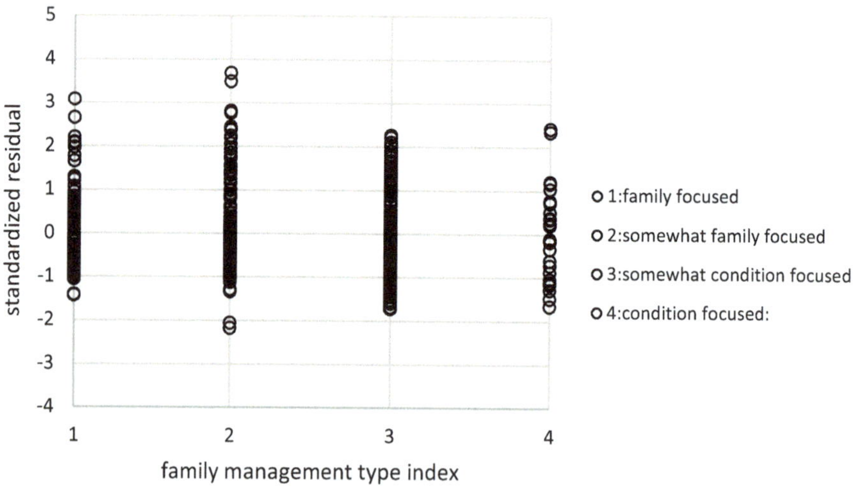

Fig. 16.9 Standardized residuals for the moderation model in parent, family, and family management type together with family functioning

16.3.4 Clock Times for Analyses

Clock times for the analyses of Sect. 16.3 include 1.3 min for the models of Table 16.7, 11.1 min for the models of Table 16.8, 16.7 min for the models of Table 16.9, and 129.5 min for the models of Table 16.10. Consequently, analyses of the number of problematic conduct-disordered behaviors for the partnered parent data require 158.6 min or about 2.6 h altogether.

16.4 Analyses of a High Level of Intensity of Conduct-Disordered Behaviors

Analyses reported in this section use the partnered parents data of Sect. 16.2.1 with outcome measurements representing a high level (i.e., greater than or equal to 127) of the intensity of a child's conduct-disordered behaviors. As in Sect. 16.2, outcome measurements are available for mothers from 328 families and from fathers for 143 of those families, and so only for mothers for 185 of the families. There is a total of 471 outcome measurements with 185 families having a missing outcome measurement, and so LCV scores are computed using measurement-wise deletion. The cutoff for a distinct percent decrease (PD) in the LCV score using DF = 1 is 0.40%. The available predictors are the same as described in Sect. 16.2.1 including indicator variables based on parent, family, and family management types and the measure famfunct of general family functioning.

All models are based on logistic regression treating dichotomous outcomes as Bernoulli distributed with logit link function. Models reported in this section are based on extended variances determined by dispersions combined with means unless explicitly specified to be based on direct variance modeling determined entirely by dispersions. Dyadic data like the partnered parents data with a maximum of two outcome measurements per matched set require only a single correlation parameter so that all models use exchangeable correlations (EC).

Section 16.4.1 addresses the choice of the number of folds for computing LCV scores. Section 16.4.2 provides analyses assessing the impact of types based on parent, family, and how the family manages the child's condition. Section 16.4.3 expands these analyses to also account for the impact of a measure of general family functioning. Section 16.4.4 provides a summary of clock times required for the analyses of the section.

16.4.1 Alternate Numbers of Folds

The model with adaptive means and adaptive dispersions for a high level of intensity of conduct-disordered behaviors is based on the two indicators father and momonly.

Table 16.11 Predictors and clock times for adaptively generated models based on parent type and family type for means and dispersions of a high level of intensity of conduct-disordered behaviors for the partnered parents data[a]

	Number of folds		
	5	10	15
LCV score	0.84992	0.83957	0.84192
Means[b]	0	0	0
Dispersions[c]	--	--	--
Clock time (min)	0.3	0.6	0.8

[a]Computed using extended linear mixed modeling, exchangeable correlations, and measurement-wise deletion with the contraction allowing for unit dispersions. Parent type is represented by the indicator for being a father while family type is represented by the indicator for a family with only the mother participating
[b]A power of 0 corresponds to an intercept
[c]All models have unit dispersions

This accounts for possible effects to both the measurement condition and for missingness. Table 16.11 provides LCV scores for this model computed using 5, 10, and 15 folds and the EC correlation structure. The largest LCV score is achieved for 5 folds. For all three numbers of folds, the same model is generated based on constant means and unit dispersions. Consequently, 5 folds generate the best LCV score as well as a model consistent with the ones generated with 10 and 15 folds, and so subsequent models are computed using 5-fold LCV scores. Based on the models of Table 16.11, subsequent models are also computed assuming unit dispersions, and so direct variance modeling is not considered in subsequent analyses. The three models of Table 16.11 require 1.7 min of clock time.

For the adaptive model of Table 16.11, the estimated probability of a high level of intensity of the child's conduct-disordered behaviors is 0.09 for all parents. The estimated dispersion is 1 for all parents. The estimated correlation is 0.45.

16.4.2 Models Based on Parent, Family, and Family Management Types

The results of Sect. 16.4.1 indicate that a high level of intensity of conduct-disordered behaviors is reasonably analyzed using EC correlations with unit dispersions and LCV scores computed using 5 folds, and so these choices are used in subsequent analyses. This section provides a comparison of the adaptive additive model and the adaptive moderation model for means in parent, family, and family management types. Parent type is represented by the indicator father, family type by the indicator momonly, and family management type by the six indicator variables Ffocus, SFfocus, SCfocus, Cfocus, F_SFfocus, and SC_Cfocus.

Table 16.12 provides a comparison of adaptively generated additive and moderation models based on parent, family, and family management types for means of the

Table 16.12 Adaptively generated unit dispersion models based on parent, family, and family management types for means of the number of problematic conduct-disordered behaviors for the partnered parents data[a]

Model type	5-fold LCV score	Mean transforms[b]	Clock time (min)
Additive	0.88578	F_SFfocus, SCfocus	0.2
Moderation	0.91322	1, momonly · F _ SFfocus, Cfocus	2.0

[a]Computed using extended linear mixed modeling, exchangeable correlations, and measurement-wise deletion
[b]The transform 1 represents an intercept; otherwise, the intercept is zero. The variable momonly is the indicator for a family with only the mother participating. F_SFfocus and Cfocus are indicators for the family being family focused or somewhat family focused and being condition focused, respectively

high level of intensity of conduct-disordered behaviors assuming unit dispersions. The additive model has 5-fold LCV score 0.88578. In comparison, the model of Table 16.11 based on only parent and family types has 5-fold LCV score 0.84992 with distinct PD 4.05% (i.e., greater than the cutoff of 0.40%). Consequently, family management type provides for a distinct improvement. The LCV score for the additive model of Table 16.12 has distinct PD 3.00% compared to the moderation model with 5-fold LCV score 0.91322. Consequently, a distinct moderation effect is identified for the means. The adaptive additive model requires 0.2 min of clock time while the adaptive moderation model requires 2.0 min for a total of 2.2 min.

For the moderation model of Table 16.12, the estimated probability of a high level of intensity of the child's conduct-disordered behaviors is 0.10 for parents in family focused or somewhat family focused families with both parents participating and for parents in somewhat condition focused families, which decreases to 0.03 for mothers in family focused or somewhat family focused families without participating fathers and increases to 0.30 for parents in condition focused families. The estimated correlation is 0.47.

16.4.3 Models Based on Parent, Family, and Family Management Types and on Family Functioning

This section provides a comparison of adaptive additive and moderation models for means in parent, family, and family management types together with family functioning assuming unit dispersions. Parent, family, and family management type are represented by the same indicator variables as in Sect. 16.4.2.

Table 16.13 provides a comparison of adaptively generated additive and moderation models based on parent, family, and family management types together with family functioning for means of the high level of intensity of conduct-disordered behaviors assuming unit dispersions. The adaptive additive model has 5-fold LCV score 0.91785 while the adaptive moderation model has 5-fold LCV score 1.24185. In comparison, the associated models of Table 16.12 based on only parent, family,

Table 16.13 Adaptively generated unit dispersion models based on parent, family, and family management types and on family functioning for means of a high level of intensity of conduct-disordered behaviors for the partnered parents data[a]

Model type	5-fold LCV score	Mean transforms[b]	Clock time (min)
Additive	0.91785	$\text{famfunct}^{-0.64}$, Cfocus	1.2
Moderation	1.24185	$(\text{father}\cdot\text{famfunct}^{5}\cdot\text{Ffocus})^{3.59}$, $\text{famfunct}^{-0.601}$, $(\text{momonly}\cdot\text{F\_SFfocus}\cdot\text{famfunct}^{0.7})^{0.8}$, $(\text{SFfocus}\cdot\text{father}\cdot\text{famfunct}^{b})^{-3.41}$	250.3

[a]Computed using extended linear mixed modeling, exchangeable correlations, and measurement-wise deletion

[b]The transform 1 represents an intercept; otherwise, the intercept is zero. The variable father is the indicator for the parent being a father. The variable momonly is the indicator for a family with only the mother participating. Ffocus, SFfocus, F_SFfocus, and Cfocus are indicators for the family being family focused, being somewhat family focused, being family focused or somewhat family focused, and being condition focused, respectively. The variable famfunct represents general family functioning

and family management types have 5-fold LCV scores 0.88578 and 0.91322 with distinct PDs 3.49% and 26.46%. Consequently, family functioning provides for a distinct improvement in both cases. The LCV score for the additive model of Table 16.13 has distinct PD 26.09% compared to the LCV score for moderation model of Table 16.13. Consequently, a distinct moderation effect is identified. The adaptive additive model requires 1.2 min of clock time while the adaptive moderation model requires 250.3 min for a total of 251.5 min or about 4.2 h, almost all of which is needed to generate the moderation model.

The moderation model of Table 16.13 has estimated exchangeable correlation 0.44. Figure 16.10 provides plots of estimated probabilities (or means) of a high level of intensity of conduct-disordered behaviors as a function of family functioning for parent type and family management type combinations based on the moderation

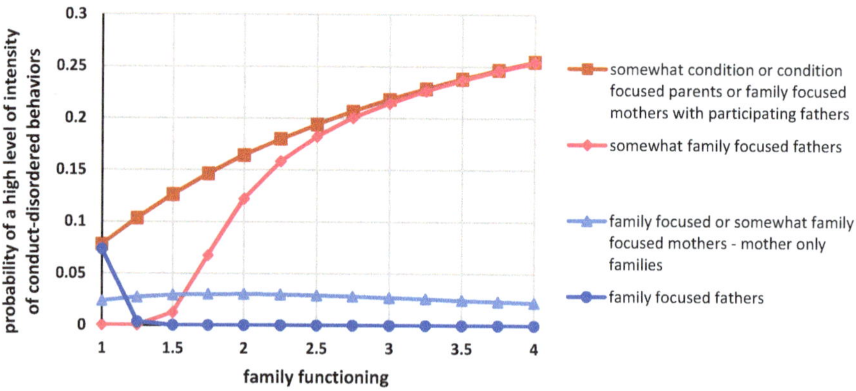

Fig. 16.10 Estimated probability of a high level of intensity of conduct-disordered behaviors in terms of family functioning by combinations of parent type and family management type

model. For fathers in family focused families (37 or 7.9% of the parents), the probability decreases from 0.07 at the lowest (best) value of 1 for family functioning very quickly to essentially 0. For mothers in family focused or somewhat family focused families with only the mother participating (110 or 23.4% of the parents), the probability is relatively constant at 0.02–0.03 for all values of family functioning. Otherwise, the probability increases with family functioning to 0.25 at the highest (worst) value of 4 for family functioning, from essentially 0 for fathers in somewhat family focused families (51 or 10.8% of the parents) and more quickly and from 0.08 for other parents, that is, fathers and mothers in somewhat conditioned and conditioned focused families and mothers in family focused families with both parents participating (273 or 58.0% of the parents).

Standardized residuals of the moderation model range from −2.58 to −0.01 for parents with a high observed level of intensity of conduct-disordered behaviors and from 1.14 to 6.22 for other parents with 10 of these larger than 3.00. The fact that the signs for the standardized residuals are determined by the associated dichotomous outcome values suggests that standardized residuals can sometimes be of limited value for dichotomous outcome variables.

16.4.4 Clock Times for Analyses

Clock times for the analyses of Sect. 16.4 include 1.7 min for the models of Table 16.11, 2.2 min for the models of Table 16.12, and 251.5 min for the models of Table 16.13. Consequently, analyses of a high level of intensity of conduct-disordered behaviors for the partnered parents data require 255.4 min or about 4.3 h altogether.

16.5 Analysis Summary

16.5.1 Analyses of the Single Mothers Data

A summary of the results of analyses of the single mothers data is provided broken down into two categories of results.

1. Models for means and variances in type of scale

The preferable model for the single mothers data has EC correlations with LCV scores based on $k = 10$ folds. All models are generated using linear regression and LMM. The data are analyzed in about 1.7 h of clock time.

Mean difficulty is least problematic (i.e., lowest in value), mean impact is intermediate, and mean effort is most problematic (i.e., highest in value). Difficulty and effort have the same variability that is greater than the variability for impact.

2. Models for means and variances in type of scale and family functioning

Type of scale has a moderation effect on the impact of family functioning on means and variances for scales. Under this model, estimated means are plotted in Fig. 16.1, estimated standard deviations in Fig. 16.2, and standardized residuals in Fig. 16.3.

16.5.2 Analyses of the Intensity of Conduct-Disordered Behaviors

A summary of the results of analyses of the intensity of conduct-disordered behaviors is provided broken down into three categories of results.

1. Models for means and variances in parent and family types

The preferable model for the intensity of conduct-disordered behaviors has EC correlations with LCV scores based on $k = 5$ folds. All models are generated using linear regression and LMM. The data are analyzed in about 2.3 h of clock time.

Means and variances for the intensity of conduct-disordered behaviors are constant in parent and family types.

2. Models based on parent, family, and family management types

Mean intensity of the child's conduct-disordered behaviors is most problematic (i.e., highest in value) for parents in somewhat conditioned or conditioned focused families, intermediate for fathers in somewhat family focused families, and least problematic (i.e., lowest in value) for parents in family focused families and mothers in somewhat family focused families. Variability is lower for parents in family focused, somewhat family focused, and somewhat condition focused families than for parents in condition focused families.

3. Models for means and variances in parent, family, and family management types

Parent, family, and family management types distinctly moderate the effect of family functioning on means and variances for intensity of conduct-disordered behaviors. Under this model, estimated means are plotted in Fig. 16.4, estimated standard deviations in Fig. 16.5, and standardized residuals in Fig. 16.6.

16.5.3 Analyses of the Number of Problematic Conduct-Disordered Behaviors

A summary of the results of analyses of the number of problematic conduct-disordered behaviors is provided broken down into three categories of results.

1. Models for means and dispersions in parent and family types

The preferable model for the number of conduct-disordered behaviors has EC correlations with LCV scores based on $k = 5$ folds. All models are generated using Poisson regression and ELMM. The data are analyzed in about 2.6 h of clock time.

Means and dispersions for the number of conduct-disordered behaviors are constant in parent and family types.

2. Models based on parent, family, and family management types

Mean number of the child's conduct-disordered behaviors is less problematic (i.e., lower in value) for parents in the family focused or somewhat family focused families than for parents in the somewhat condition focused or condition focused families. Dispersions are largest for parents in family or somewhat family focused families with participating fathers and in condition focused families, intermediate for parents in somewhat condition focused families, and lowest for mothers in family focused or somewhat family focused families without participating fathers. The extended variance model is preferable to the associated direct variance model.

3. Models for means and variances in parent, family, and family management types.

Parent, family, and family management types distinctly moderate the effect of family functioning on means and dispersions for number of conduct-disordered behaviors. Under this model, estimated means are plotted in Fig. 16.7, estimated dispersions in Fig. 16.8, and standardized residuals in Fig. 16.9.

16.5.4 Analyses of a High Level of Intensity of Conduct-Disordered Behaviors

A summary of the results of analyses of a high level of intensity of conduct-disordered behaviors is provided broken down into three categories of results.

1. Models for means and dispersions in parent and family types

The preferable model for a high level of intensity of conduct-disordered behaviors has EC correlations with LCV scores based on $k = 5$ folds. All models are generated using logistic regression and ELMM. The data are analyzed in about 4.3 h of clock time.

Means (i.e., probabilities) for a high level of intensity of conduct-disordered behaviors are constant in parent and family types. Unit dispersions are appropriate and so assumed in subsequent models. Consequently, variability is thus entirely determined by the variance function $V(\mu) = \mu \cdot (1 - \mu)$.

2. Models based on parent, family, and family management types

The probability of a high level of intensity of the child's conduct-disordered behaviors is largest for parents in conditioned focused families, intermediate for parents in family focused and somewhat family focused families with both parents participating and for parents in somewhat condition focused families, and smallest for mothers in family focused or somewhat family focused families without participating fathers.

3. Models for means and variances in parent, family, and family management types

Parent, family, and family management types distinctly moderate the effect of family functioning on probabilities of a high level of intensity of conduct-disordered behaviors. Under this model, estimated means are plotted in Fig. 16.10.

References

Epstein, N. B., Baldwin, L. M., & Bishop, D. S. (1983). The McMaster family assessment device. *Journal of Marital & Family Therapy, 9*, 171–180.

Eyberg, S. M., & Pincus, D. (1999). *Eyberg child behavior inventory and Sutter-Eyberg student behavior inventory-revised: Professional manual*. Psychological.

Eyberg, S., & Ross, A. W. (1978). Assessment of child behavior problems: The validation of a new inventory. *Journal of Clinical Child Psychology, 7*, 113–116.

Knafl, K., Deatrick, J. A., Gallo, A., Dixon, J. K., Grey, M., Knafl, G. J., & O'Malley, J. P. (2011). Assessment of the psychometric properties of the family management measure. *Journal of Pediatric Psychology, 36*, 494–505. https://doi.org/10.1093/jpepsy/jsp034

Knafl, K. A., Deatrick, J. A., Knafl, G. J., Gallo, A. M., Grey, M., & Dixon, J. (2013). Patterns of family management of childhood chronic conditions and their relationship to child and family functioning. *Journal of Pediatric Nursing, 38*, 523–535.

Index

G. J. Knafl, *Modeling Correlated Outcomes Using Extensions of Generalized Estimating Equations and Linear Mixed Modeling*,
https://doi.org/10.1007/978-3-031-41988-1

FSC
www.fsc.org
MIX
Papier | Fördert gute Waldnutzung
FSC® C083411

Kolibri 360 GmbH
Ferdinand-Jühlke-Straße 7
99095 Erfurt, Deutschland
produktsicherheit@kolibri360.de